TRAUMA:
CORE KNOWLEDGE IN
ORTHOPAEDICS

Other Volumes in the Core Knowledge in Orthopaedics Series

Spine

Hand, Elbow, and Shoulder

Sports Medicine

Trauma

Foot and Ankle

Pediatric Orthopaedics

Adult Reconstruction & Arthroplasty

TRAUMA:
CORE KNOWLEDGE
IN ORTHOPAEDICS

ROY SANDERS, MD

Chief, Department of Orthopaedics,
Tampa General Hospital, Tampa, FL;
Director, Orthopaedic Trauma Services,
Florida Orthopaedic Institute, Tampa, FL

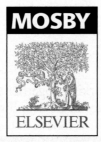

MOSBY

ELSEVIER

1600 John F. Kennedy Blvd.
Ste 1800
Philadelphia, PA 19103-2899

TRAUMA: CORE KNOWLEDGE IN ORTHOPAEDICS   ISBN: 978-0-323-03424-1

Notice

Knowledge and best practice in this field are constantly changing. As new research and experience broaden our knowledge, changes in practice, treatment, and drug therapy may become necessary or appropriate. Readers are advised to check the most current information provided (i) on procedures featured or (ii) by the manufacturer of each product to be administered to verify the recommended dose or formula, the method and duration of administration, and contraindications. It is the responsibility of the practitioner, relying on their own experience and knowledge of the patient, to make diagnoses, to determine dosages and the best treatment for each individual patient, and to take all appropriate safety precautions. To the fullest extent of the law, neither the Publisher nor the Editor assumes any liability for any injury and/or damage to persons or property arising out or related to any use of the material contained in this book.

The Publisher

Library of Congress Cataloging-in-Publication Data

Trauma : core knowledge in orthopaedics / [edited by] Roy W. Sanders. – 1st ed.
    p. ; cm. – (Core Knowledge in orthopaedics series)
  Includes bibliographical references and index.
  ISBN 978-0-323-03424-1
    1. Orthopedics. 2. Wounds and injuries–Surgery. 3. Fractures–Surgery. I. Sanders, Roy W.
II. Series.
  [DNLM: 1. Fractures, Bone–surgery. 2. Bone and Bones–injuries. 3. Orthopedics–methods.
WE 180 T777 2007]

RD731.T73 2007
617.4′7–dc22   2007003813

Acquisitions Editor: Emily Christie
Developmental Editor: Pamela Hetherington
Project Manager: Bryan Hayward
Design Direction: Steven Stave

Printed in China
Last digit is the print number: 9 8 7 6 5 4 3 2 1

Contributors

JEFFREY ANGLEN, MD, FACS
Professor and Chairman, Department of Orthopaedics, Indiana University, Indianapolis, IN

MICHAEL T. ARCHDEACON, MD, MSE
Associate Professor, University of Cincinnati, Cincinnati, OH; Director, Division of Musculoskeletal Traumatology, Associate Professor, University Hospital, Cincinnati, OH

BRIAN BADMAN, MD
Orthopaedic Surgeon, Department of Orthopaedic Surgery, Hendricks Regional Health, Danville, IN

CARLO BELLABARBA, MD
Associate Professor, Harborview Medical Center, University of Washington School of Medicine, Seattle, WA

BRETT R. BOLHOFNER, MD
Director of Orthopaedic Trauma, Bayfront Medical Center, St. Petersburg, FL

JOSEPH BORRELLI, JR., MD
Professor and Chairman, Department of Orthopaedic Surgery, University of Texas–Southwestern Medical Center, Dallas, TX

MICHAEL P. CLARE, MD
Director of Fellowship Education, Foot and Ankle Fellowship, Division of Foot and Ankle Surgery, Florida Orthopaedic Institute, Tampa, FL

CORY A. COLLINGE, MD
Staff Physician, John Peter Smith Orthopaedic Residency Program, Fort Worth, TX; Director of Orthopaedic Trauma, Harris Methodist Hospital, Fort Worth, TX

THOMAS G. DIPASQUALE, DO
Affiliate Assistant Professor, Department of Orthopaedic Surgery, College of Medicine, University of South Florida, Tampa, FL; Clinical Associate Professor, Orthopaedics, Michigan State University, East Lansing, MI; Associate Director of Orthopaedic Trauma Service, Tampa General Hospital, Tampa, FL

A. SAMUEL FLEMISTER, JR., MD
Associate Professor of Orthopaedics, Department of Orthopaedic Surgery, University of Rochester School of Medicine, Rochester, NY

SETH I. GASSER, MD
Co-Director, Sports Medicine Department, Florida Orthopaedic Institute, Medical Director, Florida Orthopaedic Institute Surgery Center, Tampa, FL

GEORGE J. HAIDUKEWYCH, MD
Orthopaedic Traumatologist, Florida Orthopaedic Institute, Tampa, FL

KEITH HEIER, MD
Chief, Department of Orthopaedics, Presbyterian Hospital of Plano, Plano, TX

DOLFI HERSCOVICI, JR., DO
Clinical Associate Professor, Orthopaedic Traumatologist, University of South Florida, Tampa, FL; Attending, Orthopaedic Trauma, Tampa General Hospital, Florida Orthopaedic Institute, Tampa, FL

ALFRED V. HESS, MD
Clinical Associate Professor, University of South Florida College of Medicine, Department of Surgery, Division of Plastic Surgery; Director, Division of Hand Surgery, Florida Orthopaedic Institute, Tampa, FL

ANTHONY F. INFANTE, JR., DO
Clinical Faculty Orthopedics, MSU School of Osteopathic Medicine, Michigan State University, East Lansing, MI; Orthopedic Trauma Faculty, Tampa General Hospital, Tampa, FL; AO Teaching Faculty, AO North America; Vice Chief of Staff, South Bay Hospital, Sun City Center, FL

ERIC M. LINDVALL, DO
Assistant Clinical Professor, University of California–San Francisco, Fresno Medical Education Program, Fresno, CA; Orthopaedic Traumatologist, Community Regional Medical Center–Fresno, Fresno, CA

FRANK A. LIPORACE, MD
Assistant Professor, Department of Orthopaedics–University of Medicine and Dentistry of New Jersey-New Jersey Medical School, Newark, NJ

MARK A. MIGHELL, MD
Instructor of Surgery, Uniformed Services, University of the Health Sciences, F. Edward Hebert School of Medicine, Bethesda, MD; Co-Director, Division of Shoulder and Elbow Surgery, Florida Orthopaedic Institute, Tampa, FL

WILLIAM M. RICCI, MD
Associate Professor, Orthopaedic Surgery; Chief, Orthopaedic Trauma; Director, Clinical Operations, Washington University Orthopaedics, St. Louis, MO; Attending Orthopaedic Surgeon, Barnes-Jewish Hospital, St. Louis, MO

H. CLAUDE SAGI, MD
Clinical Assistant Professor of Orthopaedics, University of South Florida; Director of Research, Orthopaedic Trauma Service, Florida Orthopaedic Institute, Tampa General Hospital, Tampa, FL

ROY SANDERS, MD
Chief, Department of Orthopaedics, Tampa General Hospital, Tampa, FL; Director, Orthopaedic Trauma Services, Florida Orthopaedic Institute, Tampa, FL

JULIA M. SCADUTO, ARNP
Florida Orthopaedic Institute, Tampa General Hospital, Tampa, FL

STEVEN SIEGAL, MD
Fellow, Division of Shoulder and Elbow Surgery, Florida Orthopaedic Institute, Tampa, FL

MICHAEL SIRKIN, MD
Chief, Orthopaedic Trauma Service, North Jersey Orthopaedic Institute; Assistant Professor, University of Medicine and Dentistry of New Jersey-New Jersey Medical School, Newark, NJ

STEVEN D. STEINLAUF, MD
Orthopaedic Surgeon, Orthopaedic Associates of South Broward; Chief of Orthopaedics, Memorial Regional Hospital; Foot and Ankle Surgeon, Cleveland Clinic, Weston, FL

NAZEEM VIRANI, MD
Research Fellow, Florida Orthopaedic Institute Research Foundation, Tampa, FL

KEITH WATSON, MD
Tarrant County Clinical Instructor, John Peter Smith Orthopaedic Surgery Residency Program, Fort Worth, TX; Harris Methodist Hospital, Fort Worth, TX

JEFF D. YACH, MD, FRCSC
Assistant Professor of Orthopaedic Surgery, Queen's University at Kingston, Kingston, Ontario, Canada; Orthopaedic Trauma Service Chief, Kingston General Hospital, Kingston, Ontario, Canada; Chief, Orthopaedic Trauma Service, Kingston General Hospital, Kingston, Ontario, Canada

Contents

Foreword

During the past 25 years Orthopaedic Trauma has evolved into a mature subspecialty, complete with national and international societies and journals dedicated to the discipline. Throughout this period, the Orthopaedic Trauma Service (OTS) at Tampa General Hospital (www.ots1.com) has been in the forefront of this development. Started in the 1980s by Drs. Phillip Spiegel and Jeffrey Mast, the emphasis on teaching, training, innovating, and publishing concepts and surgical skills has been an ongoing process. Additionally, since 1985, the OTS in Tampa has trained more than 50 orthopaedic trauma fellows who, in many cases, have gone on to become Chiefs of Orthopaedic Trauma Services. These graduates are now running academic trauma services and training and teaching their own residents and fellows. This program has also been honored by having three of its members become Presidents of the Orthopaedic Trauma Association (Drs. David Helfet, Roy Sanders, and Jeff Anglen), and two members are now Orthopaedic Department Chairmen (Drs. Jeff Anglen [Indianapolis] and Joseph Borrelli [Dallas]). Last, the faculty/graduates of the program have produced well over 200 publications, several of which have become classics in Orthopaedic Trauma.

To have a complete textbook exclusively written by graduates of the program in Tampa is both humbling and unique. This book's goal is to present their knowledge, experience, and understanding of Orthopaedic Trauma in a format that is useful for their students—residents and fellows alike. I thank each and every author, and feel proud to have been associated with them during their education, training, and subsequent careers.

I would also like to especially acknowledge and thank those individuals who have helped make this happen in Tampa over the years. David Helfet, who was instrumental in bringing me to Tampa. Thomas DiPasquale and Dolfi Herscovici, my partners through the "rough" years, who helped build a world-class orthopaedic trauma unit through their team spirit and hard work. The staff of the OTS, especially Dawne Phillip, our tireless coordinator who always managed to defuse multiple crises. Phillip Spiegel, our former Chairman, who afforded me an opportunity to grow academically as a teacher and surgeon starting from when I was a green attending just out of fellowship. His genuine interest in the advancement of our subspecialty is not lost on anyone who had the privilege to work with him. Most important, I would like to thank my wife, Melanie, for her unending support, without which none of this would have been possible.

Roy Sanders, MD
Orthopaedic Trauma Services
Tampa, Florida
June 2007

1

Compartment Syndromes and Open Fractures

Michael Sirkin, MD

Open Fractures

Grading

- The most commonly used open fracture classification grading system was described by Gustilo and Anderson.[1] It still remains the most widely used scheme despite its moderate to poor interobserver (60% agreement) reliability.[2–4]
- The initial grade is assigned at the time of injury during the emergency debridement. Final grading is done in the operating room (OR) after debridement and wound closure, even if this occurs several days or debridements later.[3–5] It is not infrequent that a fracture initially graded as III-A is reassessed as a III-B, because flap coverage becomes necessary. The soft tissue condition and status is the most important determinant of fracture grade.

Type I

- Type I open fractures are those that have skin wounds, are less than 1 cm in length, and are usually from an inside-out injury with the sharp spike of bone creating the wound. There is minimal muscle contusion, and the fracture pattern is typically simple transverse or oblique. The infection rates in these fractures are similar to those seen in closed fractures.

Type II

- In type II fractures, the open wound measures between 1 and 10 cm. There should be only minimal periosteal stripping and minimal contamination. There may also be a minimal to moderate crushing component. Fracture patterns are typically short transverse or oblique with little comminution.

Type III

- In type III fractures, there is significant crushing and injury to the soft tissues. Wounds are greater than 10 cm in length with wide periosteal stripping and contamination. Fracture patterns may be more complex, with noticeable comminution.
  - Not all fractures with wounds less than 10 cm are classified as grade II. When there is severe soft tissue injury or contamination, they should be correctly classified as grade III. All open segmental fractures should be considered grade III.
  - Since 1984, the classification of type III fractures has been further divided[6] based on the vascular status and whether a flap will be required for wound coverage.

III-A

- The III-A open fracture has adequate bone coverage and a traumatic wound that will be not need flap coverage.

III-B

- Flap coverage changes the designation of an open grade III fracture from A to B. These fractures typically have more soft tissue crush and tissue or bone loss. They are frequently highly contaminated.
  - Coverage options may include rotational flaps, such as the gastrocnemius or soleus flap in the leg. Free-tissue transfer may use muscle flaps, such as the rectus dorsi, latissimus dorsi, or fasciocutaneous flaps.

III-C

- The III-C fractures are open fractures that have vascular injury and require repair of the vessel. Muscle ischemia may result from the vascular injury.

- Farm injuries are also considered to be III-C injuries as a result of the level of contamination.
- Both farm injuries and injuries with significant ischemia carry greater risk of anaerobic infection. As a result, antibiotic prophylaxis should target these types of bacteria.
- These fractures have reportedly had high amputation rates and in some series as high as 50%.[6,7]

Initial Evaluation and Treatment

- Open fractures are frequently caused by high-speed or high-energy injuries, such as motor vehicle accidents, falls from heights, or pedestrians struck by automobiles. Whenever fractures result from these mechanisms, care must be taken to avoid missing associated injuries that may threaten life or limb. Care should integrate a general trauma or surgical service. In most instances, these patients should be admitted to the trauma service for the first 24 hours to avoid missing any other nonorthopaedic injuries.
- Initial evaluation should include a complete history when possible. The mechanism, location, and timing of the injury all may play a role in treatment and should be investigated. Any patient comorbidities should be identified, especially those that play a role in the patient's ability to heal or prevent infection (such as diabetes or human immunodeficiency virus [HIV] status). Smoking, alcoholism, homelessness, job status, and workers' compensation all affect outcome and should be carefully considered, especially in those patients with severe high-grade open injuries.[8-12]
- In addition to close inspection of the injured extremity, a careful neurologic and vascular examination is performed, which may include the ankle brachial index, especially for any extremity that may have compromised circulation, decreased pulses, or injuries with high index of injury (such as knee dislocation or medial tibial plateau fractures). A complete musculoskeletal examination should be done to avoid missing other injuries, especially in the foot, hand, and spine. Any area of the body that is tender should be imaged, as should any bruised area in the unconscious or intubated patient. Reevaluation with secondary and tertiary surveys are necessary in the patient with multiple injuries to avoid missing injuries.[13-15] The most frequently missed injuries[16] who are in the most severely injured patients.[17] These measures will decrease, but not eliminate, missed injuries.
- Initially all wounds should be evaluated in the emergency department (ED) and covered with a sterile dressing. Dressings should remain in place until the patient is in the OR. Avoid multiple reevaluations of the traumatic wound. If the initial dressing is placed by a junior caregiver, the tendency to reevaluate by someone more senior should be avoided.

- The injured extremity should be immobilized with a well-padded splint over the sterile dressing. Exploration, irrigation, and debridement should not be routinely performed while the patient is in the ED. Cultures of traumatic wounds are not routinely performed in the ED. Although up to 80%[1,18,19] of these cultures will be positive, leading to the current recommendations for prophylactic antibiotics, late infections usually involve different organisms.[20,21]
- Antibiotic prophylaxis should be given as early as possible to decrease the risk of infection.[1,18]
- Tetanus immunization status must be assessed, and prophylaxis should be administered as follows:
  - If more than 5 years since last booster, patients need tetanus vaccine (Td).
  - If more than 10 years since last booster, patients need tetanus vaccine (Td) and human tetanus immunoglobulin (HTIG).
  - If more than 5 years and a wound prone to tetanus, patients should also receive HTIG.

Antibiotics

- Almost all open fractures are contaminated at the time of presentation to the hospital. The most common organism is coagulase-positive *Staphylococcus*. In higher energy injuries or those with more contaminated wounds, gram-negative bacilli may be present. Anaerobes may exist in ischemic wounds or those resulting from farm injuries.[18,19] Antibiotic selection should take these trends into account to prevent infection from these organisms.[22]
- In low-grade (I and II) open fractures, antibiotics should be directed at gram-positive and gram-negative coverage. A first-generation cephalosporin, such as cefazolin, should be used. A 2-g loading dose is given, followed by 1 g every 8 hours. Ciprofloxacin has been shown to be effective in these low-grade open fractures. It is initially given in a dosage of 400 mg intravenously every 12 hours, followed by 500 mg orally every 12 hours after surgical debridement.[23]
- For the higher grade fractures (III-A and III-B), the treating physician must also worry about gram-negative coverage. An aminoglycoside (gentamycin or tobramycin) must be added to help prevent infections.[6] Gentamycin, given once daily, has been shown to be an effective and safe dosing regimen.[24] This method of dosing has the benefit of being potentially safer and more effective. The effectiveness of gentamycin in killing bacteria is related to the highest peak value attained, whereas the associated nephrotoxicity is related to sustained trough levels. By dosing at the higher dose once daily, both parameters are optimized.
- For grade III-C fractures (dysvascular limbs and farm injuries), the presence of anaerobes is more likely. In addition to a cefazolin and gentamycin, aqueous penicillin G 4 million units every 4 hours, must be added.

- The duration of antibiotic therapy was historically 7 to 10 days.[1] Most likely this was recommended to simulate the duration of wound healing. Although definitive work is not available, current recommendations for uncomplicated, grade I or II fractures is 24 to 48 hours after wound closure. For grade III fractures, this should be extended to 48 to 72 hours after definitive wound closure.[18,25,]

Operative Debridement

- The timing of debridem ent is somewhat controversial. Although no study has shown that there is an adverse outcome with delayed debridement of open fractures, no study has ever looked at delaying surgery as part of the treatment protocol. Several studies show no difference in the infection rates when the treatment of open fractures in less than 6 hours versus more than 6 hours (but usually within the first 24 hours).[26–31] The conclusion of these studies is that early debridement is recommended, but more evidence is needed on this subject. In cases in which patient or institutional factors delay surgery, no adverse results have been reported. One study showed that when debridement was delayed greater than 5 hours, there was an increase in the infection rate.[32] Even though there is considerable debate on this topic, the standard of care is to treat open fractures as emergencies with immediate debridement.
- All necrotic or severely contaminated tissue must be removed. To perform an effective debridement, it is necessary to enlarge the traumatic wound. Adequate exposure is necessary to asses all muscle and bone. If there are two separate traumatic wounds, it is advantageous to "connect the dots." This allows for a complete assessment of the zone of injury. If not done, there is a chance of missing necrotic tissue or contaminants that must be removed to prevent infection.
- A thorough debridement should begin from the outside and work in toward the bone. Begin with the skin edges, then the fascia and muscle, and finally clean and debride the bone.
- Fascia underlying the cutaneous tissues is usually expendable and can be removed if devitalized or contaminated. Contrary to a commonly held belief, open fractures do not decompress fascial compartments, and if excessive swelling is noted beneath the fascia, then prophylactic fasciotomy may be warranted.
- The viability of the muscle is assessed by its contractility, consistency, color, and the capacity to bleed (the 4 Cs). All nonviable muscle and foreign material should be removed.
- Assessment of the bone begins in most cases with inspection of the bone ends. At times, the fracture is delivered through the wound for better inspection. This allows the surgeon to look for gross contamination within the intramedullary canal or behind the bone ends. Although full inspection is needed, care should be taken to try to minimize the amount of additional periosteal stripping that is done. Excessive periosteal stripping will lead to avascular bone, which inhibits the ability to heal the fracture.

Irrigation of Wound

- The main purpose of irrigation is to decrease the bacterial counts that are present in the wound to a level that the human body (with the aid of antibiotics) can eliminate. A failure to adequately debride or decrease the bacterial counts may lead to an infection.[19] Common amounts of irrigation fluid currently used are three 3-L bags, but at times more may be necessary. Newer devices to assist with debridement and irrigation are currently under investigation and show some promise.[33]

Additives

- The addition of additive to the irrigation solution has been questioned. Antibiotics, such as bacitracin and polymyxin, added to the irrigant have marginal benefit and may increase the wound complication rate when compared to other additives like castile soap.[34] The overall importance of these additives is most likely as a detergent to wash away the contamination.

Delivery Method

- Wound irrigation can be performed in a number of different ways. Gravity feed with arthroscopy tubing, low-pressure irrigation (bulb syringe), and high-pressure irrigation are typical methods employed. All deliver high volumes of liquid and serve to decrease the bacterial counts of the wounds. High-pressure irrigation is the most efficacious at removing dirt, debris, and bacteria, (especially after a delay of 3 hours or more) but may damage bone.[35] In the early phase, fracture healing may be delayed, but as fracture healing progresses, there are no ill effects.[36,37] In addition, multiple irrigations may impede fracture healing.[38] Current recommendations are to use high-pressure pulse lavage in fractures with significant contamination, because fracture healing will only be delayed in the earlier phases. In cases in which fracture healing will be delayed and there is minimal contamination, a bulb syringe will be equally effective.[37,39] Fear of driving particulate debris deeper into wounds with high pressure lavage have not been substantiated.[39]

Stabilization

- Fracture stabilization is needed in most, if not all, open fractures. It serves to limit further soft-tissue injury and allows healing of the bone and soft tissues. Pain is decreased and mobility increased when open fractures have been stabilized. In addition, fracture fixation allows for optimal wound and nursing care.

- Initially, internal fixation was thought to be contraindicted in open fractures. It was theorized that treatment should only be with external fixation.[1] With the routine use of antibiotics, care in soft-tissue handling, and better understanding of the injury, internal fixation can be performed safely when applied for the right indications.
- Stabilization methods can be thought of as those that are soft-tissue friendly, and those that are not. In general, plaster splints and casts along with plates are not thought to preserve soft tissue, whereas intramedullary nails and external fixation are considered to be soft-tissue sparing.
  - Although plaster or fiberglass splints are mandatory to immobilize an open fracture after initial evaluation, they should not be used for definitive care in open-fracture management. They do not easily allow for soft-tissue management and do not adequately stabilize the bone to obtain the necessary goals.
  - Plate fixation for most open fractures should be avoided on the day of admission. Although late plate fixation is safe, especially for articular injures, such as the tibial plateau or pilon, it must be avoided early. In general, the use of plates requires added soft-tissue dissection, stripping, and devitalization of bony fragments, all which will increase the infection rate. For open articular injuries, a period of external fixation is warranted, and for diaphyseal fractures, other better methods, such as intramedullary nails, are available.
    Fractures of the forearm,[40–42] humerus,[43,44] and ankle can be treated with plates in most cases without additional damage to the soft tissue and without any increase in the infection rates.
  - Intramedullary nailing has become the mainstay of treatment for open diaphyseal fractures of the lower extremity. This treatment has low infection, malunion, and nonunion rates. Patients regain function quickly, and in most cases, intermedullary devices are superior to plates or external fixation for these injuries.[45–48]
  - External fixation is a useful tool, not only in severe articular fractures, but also in diaphyseal fractures. There are several indications for external fixation of the diaphysis, including:

    Extremely dirty wounds in which intramedullary nailing would preclude a second look behind the bone or when there is dirt in the intramedullary canal. If there is extensive muscle damage behind the bone external fixation will be helpful. In these cases, at the time of second debridement, the fixator can be loosened and the intramedullary canal can be reexamined and further cleaned or debrided. During any of these subsequent surgeries, exchange nailing can be performed as definitive treatment.[49,50]
    Patients with multiple orthopaedic injuries who have open fractures and are too sick to undergo definitive

treatment can have external fixation performed safely and effectively.
Concomitant injuries around joints with diaphyseal fractures may make intramedullary nailing difficult, and therefore the role of external fixation may become more important, whether as a temporizing measure or as definitive treatment.

Postoperative Wound Management

Primary Closure

- Primary wound closure in open fractures can be performed if debridement has been done by an experienced trauma surgeon with removal of all necrotic tissue and contaminants. If there is any concern regarding the potential for more necrotic tissue or having not removed all debris, then primary closure is unwise.
- If at any time in the early postoperative period, there are any signs of inappropriate wound healing, such as persistent drainage, cellulitis, or purulence, then the patient should return to the OR without delay.

Secondary Closure

- Secondary wound closure may be a safer more effective measure when dealing with wounds that have persistent contamination or when there is a question of necrotic tissue forming after the initial debridement, as in fractures with a significant crush component. Delayed closure may also be beneficial for that surgeon who lacks the experience or expertise in complicated traumatic wound debridement.
- There are number of methods available to deal with the traumatic wound between debridements and before definitive wound closure.
  - Loose reapproximation of the skin edges to serve as a biologic dressing. Care must be taken not to place tension on the skin edges, because this may increase the risk of skin necrosis. Retraction of the skin ends may increase the rate of free-tissue transfer for wound management. Some have advocated the use of rubber bands in preventing retraction of the skin edges.

Antibiotic Beads

- The antibiotic bead pouch has been shown to decrease the infection rates of open fractures when used between debridements. Vancomycin and gentamycin or tobramycin are mixed with polymethyl methacrylate (PMMA) and allowed to dry on either suture, such as prolene, or steel wire. Once hardened, the beads are placed into the wound, after which if possible, the skin can be closed or an Ioban® (3M corp.) drape can be used to cover the wound. With time, the antibiotic leaches out of the PMMA and into the blood from the open fracture. This hematoma with its high concentration of antibiotic will keep bacterial counts down. In addition, it will keep the tissue from desiccating.

- Final wound closure can be performed with or without beads. For those fractures that will not require bone grafting, beads are routinely not placed. If bone graft is planned because of bone loss, then antibiotics beads may be used as a spacer, as described by Mescale. It is important to pressure the membrane that forms around these beads, because it has been found to contain osteoprogenitor cells.

Vacuum-Assisted Wound Closure

- Vacuum-assisted closure (VAC) is effective in the management of open-fracture wounds. Its use has been associated with a low incidence of infection and a reduction of the use of muscle flaps to gain wound coverage. It promotes the formation of granulation tissue, which may only require skin grafting. When soft-tissue coverage is still needed, VAC may decrease the size of the flap that is needed. For example, a rectus or a fasciocutaneous flap may be used instead of a latissimus flap.[51,52]

Open Wound

- Leaving the wound completely open for a period of time is the best method when there are areas of extensive crush and contamination that may persist in the wound for unusual reasons. This prevents the occurrence of gas gangrene and allows drainage of any offending agents that may be locked into the wound.

Soft-Tissue Coverage

- Different flaps are available for soft-tissue coverage in open fractures. The size of the area to be covered and type of tissue needed will ultimately determine which flap is used.
- Whether a rotational flap or a free tissue transfer is needed depends on the status of the remaining tissue, the size of the defect, and the training of the surgeon. The classic teaching of the proximal tibia being covered by the gastrocnemius, the middle tibia being covered by the soleus, and the distal tibia needing a free flap has been challenged by the lower extremity assessment project (LEAP) study, suggesting free flaps perform better in all cases of open fractures of the tibia.[53] Nevertheless, rotational flaps are used quite often in many trauma centers.
- Timing of wound closure and soft-tissue transfer should be early. Although some authors recommend immediate flap coverage,[54-56] most surgeons wait until the traumatic wound is felt to be clean and free of necrotic tissue. Several studies have shown that the early flap does better with a lower infection rate,[56,57] although this is not always possible.[58] A good rule of thumb is the earlier the better. After 5 to 10 days, flaps are associated with a much higher incidence of infection,[59] although there is some evidence that the use of the VAC changes this time frame.[60]

- There has been a trend over the last several years for surgeons to use fewer free flaps and more delayed closures and skin grafts. This is mostly a result of better soft-tissue management techniques and the use of the VAC.[52]

Compartment Syndrome

- Compartment syndrome is a condition characterized by raised pressure within a closed space that if left untreated will cause muscle and cell death and may lead to loss of limb.
- Compartment syndrome occurs in open and closed fractures. Almost all fracture types have been associated with compartment syndrome.[61]
- The most common location for compartment syndrome to occur is in the anterior and deep posterior compartment of the leg and the volar compartment of the forearm.[62] Other common areas are the other compartments of the leg, forearm, and thigh.[63]
- The most common associated risk factor for compartment syndrome is a fracture, with the tibia being the most common site. Young men are more likely to have compartment syndrome associated with a fracture. The second most common association was a soft-tissue injury and a bleeding disorder or anticoagulants use.[62]

Causes

Pathophysiology of Compartment Syndrome

- Normal tissue pressure should be between 0 to 4 mm Hg. Tissue perfusion is based on the difference between diastolic pressure and tissue pressure. It is this pressure gradient that allows the tissues to be perfused by allowing flow down the pressure gradient. When tissue pressure equals or exceeds the diastolic pressure, there can be no effective perfusion of the tissues.
- Ischemia fewer than 4 hours is typically reversible. After 4 to 6 hours, the outcome is uncertain, and greater than 8 hours irreversible damage has occurred.[64]
- Compartment syndrome can result from tight dressings or casts. Circular casts that are initially put on with room may become tight as limb swelling from injury occurs. Dressings initially dry that become soaked with blood may also become tight as the blood dries. Other outside constrictors may include burns, which cause a tightening of the skin with an inability to expand. Muscle damage also occurs with burns, which increases the internal pressure.
- Increased volume in a compartment may be caused by hemorrhage into the compartment, which will increase

the pressure. Typical causes of bleeding include fractures, vascular, or soft-tissue injuries.

- Other increases in volume within a compartment may occur from swelling of muscle secondary to injury or trauma. This muscle injury may be associated with fracture but not in all cases. Burns, snake bites,[65] crush injuries, or gunshot wounds may cause enough damage to precipitate a compartment syndrome without fracture.[66]
- In addition to hemorrhagic causes of increased pressure, arterial injuries can cause compartment syndrome after revascularization. Ischemia causes damage to the basement cell membranes, which will allow leakage of fluid. With restoration of blood flow, edema occurs with a resultant increase in the compartment pressure.

Diagnosis

Subjective Evaluation

- The clinical signs of compartment syndrome have been classically described as the five *P*'s: pain, pallor, paralysis, pulselessness, and paresthesia. These are unreliable in establishing the diagnosis, and these signs are more consistent with an established compartment syndrome in which ischemic injury has already occurred. In a majority of these latter cases, it is already too late for effective treatment and release.
- Palpable pulses are usually present unless an arterial injury occurs. In the absence of an arterial injury, it would be necessary for the compartment pressure to exceed systolic blood pressure to stop the blood flow.
- Sensory changes and paralysis occur after at least 1 hour of ischemia.
- Of these clinical signs, the earliest and most important symptom is pain. Specifically, pain out of proportion to the injury and pain with passive stretch of the involved compartment are common. Disproportionate pain may be difficult to identify but can be used in addition to pain with passive stretch. Another somewhat reliable tool to aid in establishing if the pain is appropriate or not is elevation of the extremity. If the pain is from swelling, elevation of the limb should decrease the pain, whereas if the pain is a result of a compartment syndrome, the pain should increase.

Usefulness of Clinical Signs

- Not having clinical findings is associated with a good negative predictive value. In other words, in the absence of clinical signs, there is little chance the patient has a compartment syndrome.
- Be aware that this assumes a normal sensory examination. It has been shown that patients with altered sensorium, whether induced by drugs, head trauma, alcohol, or the presence of an underlying disease, like schizophrenia, may have their symptoms masked.[67]
- In addition, when patients have positive clinical findings, these findings have a poor sensitivity, and therefore other measures are frequently needed to confirm the diagnosis, such as compartment pressure measurements.

Objective Evaluation

- These are necessary because of the poor sensitivity of clinical findings and the need for a cooperative, awake, sober patient who has no head trauma or other cause of altered sensorium. A more objective measure is measurement of compartment pressures.
- There are several ways to determine compartment pressures, but all of the currently available methods consist of placing a needle into the involved compartment and measuring the corresponding pressure.
  - The needle infusion technique was first described by Whitesides and others[68] and was the earliest description for a simple way to measure compartment pressures with standard hospital items. Although it really took two people, all that was required was intravenous (IV) tubing, a manometer, and three-way stopcock. However, even this became a timely procedure when needed quickly and often.
  - A handheld device made by Stryker® (Kalamazoo, MI) became available to try to make compartment pressure measurement easier and more ubiquitous throughout the hospital. This device is self-contained with use of a disposable kit that includes the needle and transducer.
  - In addition to these methods, an arterial line can be used to measure intracompartmental pressure. This method is primarily used where arterial lines and monitors are frequently used, as in an OR and the intensive care unit (ICU).
- The accuracy of these three have been compared.[69] The most accurate of these appears to be the arterial manometer with use of a slit catheter. The Stryker® monitor is accurate as well, with the Whitesides technique lacking the accuracy that is needed for patient care. Side-port needles or slit catheters are more accurate than straight needles, which tend to overestimate the pressure.
- McQueen has recommended continuous monitoring to minimize the delay in diagnosis of compartment syndrome and subsequent decompression. Those patients with less delay in decompression had no long-term sequelae.[70] Continuous monitoring might not be possible in all situations or settings but when available should be considered.
- Noninvasive techniques being examined that may have promise in the future include ultrasound (US)[71] and near-infrared.[72]
- Heckman[73] has shown that the pressure within the compartment is not uniform. The area closest to the fracture or injured area shows the highest pressure, and measurement should occur within 5 cm of this area. In addition, if clinical suspicion is high and pressure values fail to demonstrate

compartment syndrome, repeat measurement is warranted in zones just proximal or distal to determine the highest pressure. Both anterior and deep posterior compartments and any other compartment that has clinical signs should be measured.

- Hargens and others[74] demonstrated that intracompartmental pressure above 30 mm Hg will cause significant muscle necrosis. Whitesides and others[75] showed that compartment syndrome was more dependent on the relation of the compartment pressure and the diastolic blood pressure. Others have also shown that the pressure difference between compartment pressure and diastolic pressure to be the most important factor. The smaller the pressure differential is, the more damage that will occur to the tissues.
- Current recommendations suggest a compartment syndrome is present when clinical signs are present and the compartment pressure is within 20 to 30 mm Hg of the diastolic pressure.[64,76-78]

Treatment

- Treatment for acute compartment syndrome involves decreasing the pressure within the compartment to allow reperfusion of the tissues.
- The pressure can be relieved by removal of constricting bandages or casts if external constrictors are the cause and if significant muscle damage has not already occurred. If done early, these impending compartment syndromes can be reversed by simply removing the dressing causing the pressure.
- If the elevated internal compartment pressure is the cause of the compartment syndrome, then release of the skin and fascia must occur to reestablish tissue perfusion. Releasing the fascia will decrease compartment pressure and increase the pressure differential with diastolic pressure, allowing tissue perfusion and oxygenation to return.
  - There must be an adequate release of the skin and the underlying fascia. The skin causes a significant impedance to pressure reduction if not adequately released.[79]
- Early decompression has been shown to be effective in decreasing the long-term sequelae[70,80] and in reducing the indemnity risk.[81]
- Patients with compartment syndrome of the tibia should be treated with prompt decompression followed by stable internal fixation.[82] There is some evidence to support the fact that compartment syndrome may increase the time to healing in tibia fractures.[83]

Forearm

- There are three compartments in the forearm: the superficial flexor, the deep flexor, and the extensor compartments.

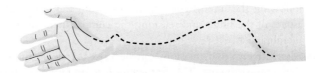

Figure 1–1: Typically the superficial and deep flexor compartments can be released through a single incision. This approach has been described by Henry and uses a skin incision that begins proximal to the antecubital fossa and extends to the palm across the carpal tunnel. (Redrawn from Browner, et al: *Skeletal trauma*, ed 3, Philadelphia, 2002, W.B. Saunders, Fig. 12–20.)

Compartment release of the forearm begins with release of the volar flexor compartments.

- Typically the superficial and deep flexor compartments can be released through a single incision. This approach uses a skin incision that begins proximal to the antecubital fossa and extends to the palm across the carpal tunnel.[75] The skin incisions begins medial to the biceps tendon and crosses the elbow crease. It is carried down the radial side of the forearm along the medial border of the brachioradialis and continues across the palm along the ulnar crease (Figure 1–1).
- The fascia over the superficial compartment is readily identified and released. It is important to release the fascia over each of the deep compartment flexors to adequately decompress the volar forearm.
- After full release of the flexors, the pressure in the extensor compartment should be remeasured and if elevated, released though a dorsal Thompson approach. A straight incision from the lateral condyle to the midline of the wrist is used, and the interval between the extensor carpi brevis and extensor digitorum communis is identified and a fasciotomy is performed.

Leg

- The leg contains four compartments: the superficial and deep posterior, the anterior, and the lateral compartments.
- In most circumstances associated with trauma to the leg, all four compartments must be released. Limited fasciotomy is almost never indicated.
- These compartments can be released by using either a single incision centered over the fibula[84] or through the more classic two-incision fasciotomy.
- When performing a single-incision fasciotomy, an incision is made that extends from the fibula head to the ankle following the fibula. The intermuscular septum between the anterior and lateral compartments is identified, and the fascia is incised approximately 1 cm anterior and 1 cm posterior to the septum. The superficial posterior compartment is readily identified posterior to the lateral compartment and is released. The lateral compartment is retracted anteriorly, and the superficial posterior compartment is retracted laterally to reach the deep posterior compartment. The deep posterior compartment is reached by

following the interosseous membrane from the posterior aspect of the fibula and releasing the compartment of this membrane.

- Alternatively, two incisions can be used to release these four compartments. The first incision is lateral and centered between the anterior and lateral compartments. These two compartments can easily be released after identification of the septum separating them. The second incision is made 1 to 2 cm posterior to posteromedial border of the distal third of the tibia. The fascia overlying the gastrocnemius soleus complex is incised, and the deep compartment is exposed in the distal third of the leg. To fully release the deep compartment, the soleus bridge must be detached from the back of the tibia. This allows exposure of the fascia covering flexor digitorum and the deep posterior compartment. After incising this, the fasciotomy is complete.

Thigh

- There are three compartments of the thigh: the anterior, posterior, and adductor compartments. Typically it is only necessary to release the anterior and posterior compartments. After release of these two compartments, the adductor compartment pressure typically will no longer be elevated or require release.
- Compartment pressure measurements will confirm which compartments are involved and should be performed after release of the anterior and lateral compartments.
- To release the anterior and posterior compartments, a single lateral incision is used. The iliotibial band is split, and the fascia overlying the vastus lateralis is incised over its length. The intermuscular septum can then be divided thereby releasing the posterior compartment.

Aftercare

- There are several methods available for aftercare of fasciotomy wounds. A sterile dressing with xeroform or similar covering can be used until swelling has decreased allowing delayed primary closure or split-thickness skin grafting. VAC dressings have been gaining popularity to decrease the time necessary to obtain wound closure.[85] Another technique uses vessel loops as a means to help prevent retraction of the skin ends and by sequential tightening gain wound closure.[86]

Annotated References

1. Gustilo RB, Anderson JT: Prevention of infection in the treatment of one thousand and twenty-five open fractures of long bones: retrospective and prospective analyses, *J Bone Joint Surg Am* 58:453-458, 1976.

Classic Article: 673 open long-bone fractures treated from 1955 to 1968. Infection rate was 12% from 1955 to 1960 and 5% from 1961 to 1968. In a prospective study from 1969 to 1973, 352 patients were managed by a protocol consisting of irrigation and debridement and antibiotics for 3 days postoperatively. In grade I and II fractures, the infection rate was 2.5%, and grade III fractures were 9%

2. Brumback RJ, Jones AL: Interobserver agreement in the classification of open fractures of the tibia: the results of a survey of two hundred and forty-five orthopaedic surgeons. *J Bone Joint Surg Am* 76:1162-1166, 1994.

This study tested the reliability of the Gustilo and Anderson open-fracture classification. The level of agreement for the classification of each fracture was determined according to the largest percentage of observers who chose a single classification type. The average agreement among the observers for all 12 fractures was 60%. The overall agreement for each fracture ranged from 42% to 94%. The respondents were divided into groups based on their level of experience. The more the experience the surgeon had, the more the agreement there was.

3. Faraj AA: The reliability of the pre-operative classification of open tibial fractures in children a proposal for a new classification, *Acta Orthop Belg* 68:49-55, 2002.

4. Horn BD, Rettig ME: Interobserver reliability in the Gustilo and Anderson classification of open fractures, *J Orthop Trauma* 7:357-360, 1993.

This study tries to assess the interobserver reliability of the Gustilo and Anderson classification. Agreement was determined by kappa analysis, which demonstrated only moderate agreement. This seems to indicate that, although useful, the Gustilo and Anderson open-fracture classification system does have limitations; studies and treatment recommendations based on it should be interpreted with caution.

5. Gustilo RB, Anderson JT: JSBS classics. Prevention of infection in the treatment of one thousand and twenty-five open fractures of long bones: retrospective and prospective analyses, *J Bone Joint Surg Am* 84-A:682, 2002.

6. Gustilo RB, Mendoza RM, Williams DN: Problems in the management of type III (severe) open fractures: a new classification of type III open fractures, *J Trauma* 24:742-746, 1984.

This study looks at 87 type III open fractures and creates a new classification system in these injuries with massive soft-tissue injuries. The authors felt the current designation of type III was too inclusive. They created three sub types: Type III-A—Adequate soft-tissue coverage of a fractured bone despite extensive soft-tissue laceration or flaps or high-energy trauma irrespective of the size of the wound. Type III-B—Extensive soft-tissue injury loss with periosteal stripping and bone exposure. This is usually associated with massive contamination. Type III-C—Open fracture associated with arterial injury requiring repair. Wound sepsis in the three subtypes were: type III-A, 4%; III-B, 52%; and III-C, 42%; whereas amputation rates were, respectively, 0%, 16%, and 42%. The bacterial pathogens in infected open fractures have changed dramatically over the years. In the present series 1976 to 1979), 77% of infections were a result of gram-negative bacteria, compared with 24% previously (1961 to 1975). A change of antibiotic therapy from a first-generation cephalosporin alone to a combination of a cephalosporin and an aminoglycoside or a third-generation cephalosporin, is currently indicated in type III open fractures.

7. Gustilo RB, Gruninger RP, Davis T: Classification of type III (severe) open fractures relative to treatment and results, *Orthopedics* 10:1781-1788, 1987.

8. MacKenzie EJ, Bosse MJ, Kellam JF, et al: Early predictors of long-term work disability after major limb trauma, *J Trauma* 61:688-694, 2006.

9. Mackenzie EJ, Bosse MJ: Factors influencing outcome following limb-threatening lower limb trauma: lessons learned from the Lower Extremity Assessment Project (LEAP), *J Am Acad Orthop Surg* 14:S205-S210, 2006.

The lower extremity assessment project (LEAP) is a multicenter study of severe lower extremity trauma in the U.S. civilian population. At 2- and 7-year follow-ups, the LEAP study found no difference in functional outcome between patients who underwent either limb salvage surgery or amputation. However, outcomes on average were poor for both groups. This study and others provide evidence of wide-ranging variations in outcome following major limb trauma, with a substantial proportion of patients experiencing long-term disability. In addition, outcomes often are more affected by the patient's economic, social, and personal resources than by the initial treatment of the injury, specifically, amputation or reconstruction and level of amputation. A conceptual framework for examining outcomes after injury may be used to identify opportunities for interventions that would improve outcomes. Because of essential differences between the civilian and military populations, the findings of the LEAP study may correlate only roughly with combat casualty outcomes.

10. MacKenzie EJ, Bosse MJ, Kellam JF, et al: Characterization of patients with high-energy lower extremity trauma, *J Orthop Trauma* 14:455-466, 2000.

This prospective study of 601 patients reports the demographic, socioeconomic, behavioral, social, and vocational characteristics of patients enrolled in a study to examine outcomes after high-energy lower extremity trauma (HELET) and to compare them with the general population; to determine whether characteristics of patients undergoing limb salvage versus amputation after HELET are significantly different from each other. Patients were followed up for 24 months post-injury. Characteristics of patients undergoing limb salvage versus amputation are also compared. Most patients were male (77%), white (72%), and between the ages of 20 and 45 years (71%). Seventy percent graduated from high school (compared with 86% nationally; $p<0.05$). One fourth lived in households with incomes below the federal poverty line, compared with 16% nationally ($p<0.05$). The percentage with no health insurance (38%) was also higher than in the general population (20%; $p<0.05$). The percentage of heavy drinkers was over two times higher than reported nationally ($p<0.01$). Study patients were slightly more neurotic and extroverted and less open to new experiences. When patient characteristics were compared for those undergoing amputation versus limb salvage, no significant differences were found among any of the variables ($p>0.05$). In conclusion, LEAP patients differ in important ways from the general population. However, the decision to amputate verus reconstruct does not appear to be significantly influenced by patient characteristics.

11. Castillo RC, Bosse MJ, MacKenzie EJ, et al: Impact of smoking on fracture healing and risk of complications in limb-threatening open tibia fractures, *J Orthop Trauma* 19:151-157, 2005.

This study looked at the role of smoking in complications in patients with open tibia fractures. After adjusting for covariates, current and previous smokers were 37% ($p = 0.01$) and 32% ($p = 0.04$) less likely to achieve union than nonsmokers, respectively. Current smokers were more than twice as likely to develop an infection ($p = 0.05$) and 3.7 times as likely to develop osteomyelitis ($p = 0.01$). Previous smokers were 2.8 times as likely to develop osteomyelitis ($p = 0.07$) but were at no greater risk for other types of infection. Conclusion: Smoking places the patient at risk for increased time to union and complications. Previous smoking history also appears to increase the risk of osteomyelitis and increased time to union. The results highlight the need for orthopaedic surgeons to encourage their patients to enter a smoking cessation programs.

12. MacKenzie EJ, Bosse MJ, Kellam JF, et al: Factors influencing the decision to amputate or reconstruct after high-energy lower extremity trauma, *J Trauma* 52:641-649, 2002.

Factors thought to influence the decision for limb salvage include injury severity, physiologic reserve of the patient, and characteristics of the patient and his or her support system. Data collected at enrollment relevant to the decision-making process included injury characteristics and its treatment and the nature and severity of other injuries. Logistic regression and stepwise modeling were used to determine the effect of each covariate on the variable salvage/amputation. Of 527 patients included in the analysis, 408 left the hospital with a salvaged limb. Of the 119 amputations performed, 55 were immediate and 64 were delayed. The multivariate analysis confirmed the bivariate analysis: All injury characteristics remained significant predictors of limb status with the exception of bone loss, and soft-tissue injury and absence of plantar sensation were the most important factors in accounting for model validity. Soft-tissue injury severity has the greatest impact on decision making regarding limb salvage versus amputation.

13. Buduhan G, McRitchie DI: Missed injuries in patients with multiple trauma, *J Trauma* 49:600-605, 2000.

This is a retrospective review to identify the incidence, contributing factors, and clinical outcomes of missed injuries. Forty-six of 567 patients (8.1%) had missed injuries. Patients with missed injuries had higher mean injury severity scores (ISSs) and longer stays in the hospital and intensive care unit (ICU) compared with patients without missed injuries ($p<0.05$). Patients with missed injuries were more likely to have lower Glasgow Coma Scale (GCS) scores and to have required pharmacologic paralysis ($p<0.05$). Of the factors contributing to missed injuries, 56.3% were potentially avoidable, and 43.8% were unavoidable. Patients with missed injuries tend to be more severely injured with initial neurologic compromise. The majority of missed injuries are potentially avoidable with repeat clinical assessments and a high index of suspicion.

14. Janjua KJ, Sugrue M, Deane SA: Prospective evaluation of early missed injuries and the role of tertiary trauma survey, *J Trauma* 44:1000-1006, 1998. discussion 1006–1007.

This study prospectively evaluated the prevalence, clinical significance, and contributing factors to early missed injuries and the role of tertiary survey in minimizing frequency of missed injuries in admitted trauma patients. Tertiary survey was conducted within 24 hours. Of 206 patients, 134 (65%) had 309 missed injuries composing 39% of all 798 injuries seen. Tertiary trauma survey detected 56% of early missed injuries and 90% of clinically significant missed injuries within 24 hours. Secondary trauma survey is not a definitive assessment and should be supplemented by tertiary trauma survey.

15. Howard J, Sundararajan R, Thomas SG, et al: Reducing missed injuries at a level II trauma center, *J Trauma Nurs* 13:89-95, 2006.

16. Rizoli SB, Boulanger BR, McLellan BA, et al: Injuries missed during initial assessment of blunt trauma patients, *Accid Anal Prev* 26:681-686, 1994.

17. Kalemoglu M, Demirbas S, Akin ML, et al: Missed injuries in military patients with major trauma: original study, *Mil Med* 171:598-602, 2006.

18. Gustilo RB: Use of antimicrobials in the management of open fractures, *Arch Surg* 114:805-808, 1979.
The role of antibiotic therapy in open fractures is secondary to adequate debridement, irrigation, and definitive wound care. Experimental and clinical studies indicate that parenteral administration of appropriate antibiotics within 3 hours after injury helps to prevent wound sepsis. Initial wound cultures of 158 open-fracture wounds revealed bacterial growth in 70.3%. Eighty-six were gram-positive, 57 were gram-negative, and 32 yielded mixed bacterial growth. Sensitivity studies of these organisms suggest that cephalothin sodium is the most effective antibiotic for prophylaxis. In a prospective study from 1969 to 1975, treatment of 520 patients was as follows: debridement, copious irrigation, and primary closure for types I and II fractures and secondary closure for type III fractures. No primary internal fixation was done except in vascular injuries. Cultures were taken of all wounds and antibiotics were given before surgery and for 3 days postoperatively. In type III open fractures, severe soft-tissue injury, and segmental or traumatic amputation, the infection rate was 9%, compared to a 44% infection rate in the retrospective study from 1955 to 1968.

19. Robinson D, On E, Hadas N, et al: Microbiologic flora contaminating open fractures: its significance in the choice of primary antibiotic agents and the likelihood of deep wound infection, *J Orthop Trauma* 3:283-286, 1989.
This is a prospective study of the contaminating microbial flora in 89 open fractures. Wound cultures were positive in 83% of all fractures, and a total of 84 strains of bacteria were isolated. In 39.3% of cultures, various species of aerobic gram-negative rods (most commonly *Pseudomonas aeruginosa*) were retrieved, followed by *Staphylococcus epidermidis* (34.5%) and *Staphylococcus aureus* (26.1%). We conclude that (a) most open fractures are already contaminated on the patient's arrival at the ED in many cases by potentially pathogenic staphylococci and gram-negative organisms; (b) contaminating organisms are community acquired and, as such, are sensitive to most routine antibiotics; and (c) persistence of the same organisms in a repeat culture taken 1 day after debridement signifies technical failure of debridement and a subsequent high risk of infection. Therefore achieving adequate wound asepsis immediately following debridement is of the utmost importance.

20. Sanders R, Swiontkowski MF, Nunley JA II, et al: The management of fractures with soft-tissue disruptions, *Instr Course Lect* 43:559-570, 1994.

21. Valenziano CP, Chattar-Cora D, O'Neill A, et al: Efficacy of primary wound cultures in long bone open extremity fractures: are they of any value? *Arch Orthop Trauma Surg* 122:259-261, 2002.
This prospective study examined whether primary wound cultures predict which wounds will become infected and whether bacterial growth on primary wound cultures correlates with bacteria cultured from infected wounds. Before any interventions were performed, initial aerobic and anaerobic cultures of the wounds of 117 consecutive open extremity fractures grades I to III were obtained. The results of these cultures were correlated with the development of a wound infection, and if an infection occurred, the organism grown from the infected wound was compared with any organism grown from the primary wound cultures. Of the initial cultures, 76% (89 of 117) did not demonstrate any growth, while the other 24% (28 of 117) only grew skin flora. There were only seven (6%) wound infections, and 71% (5 of 7) initially did not grow any organisms. Of the isolates that grew from the initial cultures, none were the organisms that eventually led to wound infections. The use of primary wound cultures in open extremity injuries has no value in the management of patients suffering long-bone open extremity fractures.

22. Gustilo RB: Current concepts in the management of open fractures. *Instr Course Lect* 36:359-366, 1987.

23. Patzakis MJ, Bains RS, Lee J, et al: Prospective, randomized, double-blind study comparing single-agent antibiotic therapy, ciprofloxacin, to combination antibiotic therapy in open fracture wounds, *J Orthop Trauma* 14:529-533, 2000.
The purpose of this prospective, double-blind, randomized, clinical trial was to compare the efficacy of a single agent, ciprofloxacin, with that of combination antibiotic therapy consisting of cefamandole and gentamicin in all types of open-fracture wounds. One hundred sixty-three consecutive patients with 171 open fractures were enrolled over a 20-month period. The infection rates in type I, II, and III fractures were calculated for the two treatment groups. The infection rate for types I and II open fractures in the ciprofloxacin group was 5.8% and 6% for the cefamandole/gentamicin group ($p = 1$). The infection rate for type III open fractures for the ciprofloxacin group was 31% (8 of 26) versus 7.7% (2 of 26) for the cefamandole/gentamicin group ($p = 0.079$). There were no statistically significant differences in infection rate between the group treated with ciprofloxacin and the one treated with cefamandole/gentamicin for types I and II open-fracture wounds. However, there appeared to be a high failure rate for the ciprofloxacin type III open-fracture group, with patients being 5.33 times more likely to become infected than those in the combination therapy group. Although this difference was not statistically significant, possibly because of the small sample size, there was a definite trend toward statistical significance. Single-agent antibiotic therapy with ciprofloxacin is effective in treatment of types I and II open-fracture wounds but cannot be recommend ciprofloxacin alone for type III wounds.

24. Sorger JI, Kirk PG, Ruhnke CJ, et al Once daily, high dose versus divided, low dose gentamicin for open fractures, *Clin Orthop Relat Res* 1999: 197–204.

This prospective, randomized study was performed on 75 Gustilo grades II and III open fractures to determine the efficacy of once daily, high-dose aminoglycoside therapy compared with more conventional dosing in reducing the infection rate when used in conjunction with an aggressive operative treatment protocol. Patients in group I received gentamicin 5 mg/kg divided into twice daily doses, and patients in group II received gentamicin 6 mg/kg given once daily. All patients were monitored for renal toxicity and observed for radiographic and clinical signs of infection until fracture union. The results of the study revealed no statistically significant difference between once daily, high-dose versus divided, low-dose gentamicin in infection rates. Thus, daily dosing of gentamicin was found to be safe, effective, and cost efficient in the treatment of open fractures when combined with a cephalosporin and aggressive operative debridement and stabilization.

25. Dellinger EP, Caplan ES, Weaver LD, et al: Duration of preventive antibiotic administration for open extremity fractures, *Arch Surg* 123:333-339, 1988.

This is a double-blind prospective trial of 248 patients with open fractures that either received 1 or 5 days of cefonicid sodium therapy or 5 days of cefamandole nafate therapy as part of the initial treatment. Rates of fracture-associated infections in the three groups were 10 (13%) of 79, 10 (12%) of 85, and 11 (13%) of 84, respectively. The 95% confidence limit for the difference in infection rates between the 1-day group and the combined 5-day groups was 0% to 8.3%. The actual difference was 0.2%. A brief course of antibiotic administration is not inferior to a prolonged course of antibiotics for prevention of postoperative fracture-site infections.

26. Noumi T, Yokoyama K, Ohtsuka H, et al: Intramedullary nailing for open fractures of the femoral shaft: evaluation of contributing factors on deep infection and nonunion using multivariate analysis, *Injury* 36:1085-1093, 2005.

27. DeLong WG Jr, Born CT, Wei SY, et al: Aggressive treatment of 119 open fracture wounds, *J Trauma* 46:1049-1054, 1999.

The purpose of this study was to determine whether immediate primary closure of open-fractures wounds can be performed without increasing the incidence of infections and delayed unions or nonunions. Of the 127 patients with open fractures, 90 patients (119 open fractures) were initially treated within 24 hours of injury, had fractures proximal to the carpus or tarsals, and were followed-up until fracture union. All patients underwent emergent wound irrigation and debridement. The method of fracture immobilization and timing of wound closure were left to the discretion of the attending orthopaedic surgeon. Immediate primary closure was used in 22 of 25 grade I open fractures (88%), 37 of 43 grade II fractures (86%), 24 of 32 grade IIIA fractures (75%), 4 of 12 grade IIIB fractures (33%), and 0 of 7 grade IIIC fractures (0%). Eight fractures (7%) were complicated by a deep wound infection or osteomyelitis, and 19 fractures (16%) developed a delayed union or nonunion. Statistical analysis revealed no significant difference in delayed union or nonunion and infection rates between immediate and delayed closures. Immediate primary closure of open-fracture wounds after a thorough debridement by an experienced fracture surgeon appears to cause no significant increase in infections or delayed union or nonunions. In addition, early closure may decrease the requirement for subsequent debridement and soft-tissue procedures, thereby minimizing surgical morbidity, shortening hospital stays, and reducing costs.

28. Khatod M, Botte MJ, Hoyt DB, et al: Outcomes in open tibia fractures: relationship between delay in treatment and infection, *J Trauma* 55:949-954, 2003.

The purpose of this study was to evaluate the infectious outcome of open tibia fractures relative to the time from injury to operative irrigation and debridement. One hundred seventy-eight patients with 191 consecutive fractures were retrospectively reviewed. Of these, 103 patients with 106 fractures were available for this study, with an average follow-up of 10.23 months. Results revealed 21.7% type I fractures, 43.4% type II fractures, 16.0% type III-A fractures, 11.3% type III-B fractures, and 7.5% type III-C fractures. Of all fracture types, 22.6% became infected, and 5.7% went on to have osteomyelitis. The average time to treatment was not significantly different in infected versus noninfected fractures across fracture types. No infection occurred when the time to surgery was within 2 hours; however, no significant increase in infection was discovered with respect to patients treated after 6 hours compared with those treated within 6 hours. The results support the Gustilo grading system of open fractures as a significant prognostic indicator for infectious complication. We continue to support the emergent treatment of open tibia fractures.

29. Harley BJ, Beaupre LA, Jones CA, et al: The effect of time to definitive treatment on the rate of nonunion and infection in open fractures, *J Orthop Trauma* 16:484-490, 2002.

This retrospective study tried to determine the association between time to definitive surgical management and the rates of nonunion and infection in open fractures resulting from blunt trauma. A total 215 fractures were available for review at a minimum of 12 months post-injury. The occurrence of deep infections or nonunions after fracture treatment was evaluated. The mean time to definitive treatment was 8 hours and 25 minutes (range 1 hour 35 minutes to 30 hours 40 minutes). Forty patients went on to nonunion, and 20 developed a deep infection. In the final multivariate regression model, time was not a significant factor in predicting either nonunion or infection ($p > 0.05$). The strongest determinants for nonunion were found to be presence of infection and grade of injury ($p < 0.05$). The strongest predictors for the development of a deep infection were fracture grade and a lower extremity fracture ($p < 0.05$). The risk of developing an adverse outcome was not increased by aggressive debridement or lavage and definitive fixation up to 13 hours from the time of injury, when early prophylactic antibiotic administration and open-fracture first aid were instituted.

30. Spencer J, Smith A, Woods D: The effect of time delay on infection in open long-bone fractures: a 5-year prospective audit from a district general hospital, *Ann R Coll Surg Engl* 86:108-112, 2004.

31. Pollak AN: Timing of debridement of open fractures, *J Am Acad Orthop Surg* 14:S48-S51, 2006.

Review article looking at multiple studies suggesting time is not an independent predictor of wound infection.

32. Kindsfater K, Jonassen EA: Osteomyelitis in grade II and III open tibia fractures with late debridement, *J Orthop Trauma* 9:121-127, 1995.

The purpose of this study was to compare the incidence of infection in grade II and III open tibia fractures with respect to early and late debridement. Forty-seven fractures (25 grade II and 22 grade III) in 46 patients were evaluated. In all grade II and III fractures, one of 15 fractures (7%) debrided in less than or equal to 5 hours became infected. Twelve of 32 fractures (38%) debrided greater than 5 hours after injury became infected ($p < 0.03$). Overt manifestations of infection did not appear until an average of 4.8 months from the time of injury, and the infecting organisms correlated with the initial cultures in only 25% of the cases. Negative postdebridement cultures did not preclude subsequent infection. The injury severity score (ISS) did not appear to correlate with increased risk of subsequent osteomyelitis. In this study, time to debridement was associated with increased risk of infection if more than 5 hours after debridement.

33. Granick M, Boykin J, Gamelli R, et al: Toward a common language: surgical wound bed preparation and debridement, *Wound Repair Regen 14 Suppl* 1:S1-S10, 2006.

34. Anglen JO: Comparison of soap and antibiotic solutions for irrigation of lower-limb open fracture wounds: a prospective, randomized study, *J Bone Joint Surg Am* 87:1415-1422, 2005.

This study was performed to compare the efficacy of those two solutions in the treatment of open fractures in humans. Adult patients with an open fracture of the lower extremity were prospectively randomized to receive irrigation with either a bacitracin solution or a nonsterile castile soap solution. The patients were followed clinically to assess for the development of infection, healing of the soft-tissue wound and union of the fracture. Between 1995 and 2002, 400 patients with a total of 458 open fractures of the lower extremity were entered into the study. One hundred ninety-two patients were assigned to the bacitracin group (B), and 208 were assigned to the castile soap group (C). The mean duration of follow-up was 500 days. An infection developed at 35 (18%) of the 199 fracture sites in group B and at 26 (13%) of the 199 fracture sites in group C. This difference was not significant ($p = 0.2$). Bone healing was delayed for 49 (25%) of the 199 group B fractures and 46 (23%) of the 199 group C fractures ($p = 0.72$). Wound-healing problems occurred in association with 19 group B fractures (9.5%) and 8 group C fractures (4%). This difference was significant ($p = 0.03$). Irrigation of open-fracture wounds with antibiotic solution offers no advantages over the use of a nonsterile soap solution, and it may increase the risk of wound-healing problems.

35. Bhandari M, Schemitsch EH, Adili A, et al: High and low pressure pulsatile lavage of contaminated tibial fractures: an in vitro study of bacterial adherence and bone damage, *J Orthop Trauma* 13:526-533, 1999.

This study was designed to examine the effect of pulsatile irrigation on microscopic bone architecture and its time-dependent efficacy in removing adherent slime-producing bacteria from cortical bone. High-pressure pulsatile lavage (HPPL) resulted in significantly greater macroscopic damage than was seen with low pressure pulsatile lavage (LPPL) or in controls (ANOVA, $p < 0.001$). Histomorphometry revealed that HPPL was associated with significantly larger and more numerous fissures or defects in the cortical bone when compared with low-pressure irrigation ($p < 0.001$). However, high- and low-pressure lavage were associated with similar degrees of periosteal separation from the cortical bone surface ($p = 0.87$). Both high- and low-pressure lavage were effective in removing adherent bacteria from bone at 3-hours' irrigation delay, but only high-pressure lavage removed adherent bacteria from bone at 6-hours delay. In this in vitro study, LPPL compared to HPPL led to less structural damage and was equally effective in removing bacteria within 3-hours' debridement delay; however, the efficacy of LPPL at 6-hours' debridement delay is questionable. This finding may have clinical significance in the development of infection following open tibial fractures.

36. Adili A, Bhandari M, Schemitsch EH: The biomechanical effect of high-pressure irrigation on diaphyseal fracture healing in vivo, *J Orthop Trauma* 16:413-417, 2002.

This study was done to evaluate the effect of both high-pressure pulsatile lavage (HPPL) and bulb syringe (BS) irrigation on the biomechanical parameters of fracture healing using an in vivo open noncontaminated diaphyseal femoral fracture model in rats. The 37% lower peak bending force and 32% lower stiffness in the HPPL group after 3 weeks of fracture healing were not present in the femora tested at 6 weeks. The findings of this study suggest that selective use of high-pressure irrigation in the management of open fractures appears warranted. In situations in which HPPL may be deleterious to bone healing, alternative strategies that optimize bacterial removal from soft tissues, while preserving bone architecture will need to be investigated.

37. Dirschl DR, Duff GP, Dahners LE, et al: High pressure pulsatile lavage irrigation of intraarticular fractures: effects on fracture healing, *J Orthop Trauma* 12:460-463, 1998.

This study was done to evaluate the effects of pulsatile lavage and bulb syringe (BS) irrigation on fracture healing in vivo. The control group (C) underwent osteotomy of the medial femoral condyle, stabilization, and closure. The BS and pulsatile lavage groups underwent the same procedure as group C, with the addition of irrigation with 1 L of normal saline via a bulb syringe (B) or a pulsatile lavage system (P). Union was determined by examination of microradiographs under light microscopy and the viability of bone along the fracture site was determined. Twenty percent of the osteotomies in groups C and B did not unite, compared with 30% in group P ($p > 0.5$). Pulsatile lavage irrigation of fresh intraarticular fractures in rabbits has a detrimental effect on early new bone formation; this effect, however, is no longer apparent 2 weeks following irrigation. Although this study evaluated the effects of pulsatile lavage irrigation in noncontaminated fractures without extensive soft-tissue injury, the detrimental effects observed on early new bone formation may translate to an increased risk of nonunion in the setting of a contaminated open fracture with extensive soft-tissue injury. Based on the results of this investigation, the selective use of pulsatile lavage irrigation appears warranted. In the absence of gross wound contamination, irrigation with a bulb syringe appears less likely to impair fracture healing than does pulsatile lavage irrigation.

38. Park SH, Silva M, Bahk WJ, et al: Effect of repeated irrigation and debridement on fracture healing in an animal model, *J Orthop Res* 20:1197-1204, 2002.

This study looked at effect of repetitive washouts on a rabbit osteotomy model. The osteotomy sites in the study groups underwent repeat irrigation and debridement on either the third day (group II), the fourth day (group III), or consecutively on the first and second days (group IV) after the index procedure. In group I (control), all osteotomies healed radiographically before the tenth week. In group II, 5 of 6 osteotomies healed radiographically before the tenth week. In Group III, only 2 of 5 osteotomies healed before the tenth week. In group IV, none of the osteotomies had healed by the fifteenth week. Compared to the control group at the tenth week, the average bone mineral content at the osteotomy site, and the area of high mineral density callus ($>$or $= 890$ mg/cm^3) were significantly lower in groups III (63%, $p = 0.002$ and 95%, $p = 0.05$, respectively) and intravenously (99%, $p < 0.001$ and 100%, $p = 0.05$, respectively). The results of this study suggest that repeated irrigation and debridement, associated with persistent rigid immobilization, may contribute to the development of delayed unions or atrophic nonunions.

39. Lee EW, Dirschl DR, Duff G, et al: High-pressure pulsatile lavage irrigation of fresh intraarticular fractures: effectiveness at removing particulate matter from bone, *J Orthop Trauma* 16:162-165, 2002.

This study was done to determine the effectiveness of high-pressure pulsatile lavage (HPPL) versus bulb syringe (BS) irrigation in removing particulate matter from metaphyseal cancellous bone. Particulate debris was placed into osteotomy sites and then irrigated using either HPPL or BS irrigation. A representative coronal section from each specimen was then prepared for histologic evaluation using 400× light microscopy. The number and distribution of graphite particles—present as small (less than 20 μm), medium (20 to 50 μm), and large (greater than 50 μm) aggregates—were then recorded. Results: The mean maximum perpendicular distance of graphite aggregates of all sizes from the osteotomy site was measured. Separate analyses controlling for aggregate size of the specimens also revealed no significant differences between HPPL and BS irrigation. HPPL and BS irrigation appear equally effective in removing particulate matter from metaphyseal cancellous bone in an intraarticular fracture model. Furthermore, HPPL does not appear to drive particulate matter farther into metaphyseal cancellous bone than BS irrigation.

40. Anderson LD, Sisk D, Tooms RE, et al: Compression-plate fixation in acute diaphyseal fractures of the radius and ulna, *J Bone Joint Surg Am* 57:287-287, 1975.

This article looks at 244 patients (216 were closed and 28 were open) with 330 fractures of the radius and ulna treated with open reduction internal fixation (ORIF). Union rate for the radius was 97.9% and for the ulna 96.3%. Compression plating was a successful method of treatment for both open and closed fractures.

41. Moed BR, Kellam JF, Foster RJ, et al: Immediate internal fixation of open fractures of the diaphysis of the forearm, *J Bone Joint Surg Am* 68:1008-1017, 1986.

Between 1975 and 1983, 57 patients with an open diaphyseal fracture of the forearm were treated with immediate internal plate fixation. The injuries were classified on the basis of the extent of soft-tissue injury as defined by Gustilo and Anderson and consisted of 20 type I injuries, 19 type II injuries, and 11 type III injuries. The complications included deep infection in two patients and nonunion in six. The functional results were excellent or good in 85% of the series. This study demonstrates that immediate stable plate fixation is a beneficial method of treatment of open fractures of the forearm. The results are related to the severity of the initial soft-tissue injury and the surgical technique. Autogenous cancellous bone-grafting at the time of closure of the wound in comminuted fractures in which interfragmental compression cannot be obtained is recommended.

42. Hadden WA, Reschauer R, Seggl W: Results of AO plate fixation of forearm shaft fractures in adults, *Injury* 15:44-52, 1983.

43. Dabezies EJ, Banta CJ II, Murphy CP, et al: Plate fixation of the humeral shaft for acute fractures, with and without radial nerve injuries, *J Orthop Trauma* 6:10-13, 1992.

44. Hee HT, Low BY, See HF: Surgical results of open reduction and plating of humeral shaft fractures, *Ann Acad Med Singapore* 27:772-775, 1998.

45. Tigani D, Sabetta E, Specchia L, et al: A comparison between delayed and immediate intramedullary nailing in the treatment of comminuted and open fractures (grade 1) of the tibia, *Ital J Orthop Traumatol* 15:25-31, 1989.

46. Ruedi T: Intramedullary nailing with interlocking, *Arch Orthop Trauma Surg* 109:317-320, 1990.

47. Piccioni L, Guanche CA: Clinical experience with unreamed locked nails for open tibial fractures, *Orthop Rev* 21:1213-1219, 1992.

48. Rand N, Mosheiff R, Liebergall M: The role of intramedullary nailing in modern treatment of open fractures of the tibia and femur, *Mil Med* 159:709-713, 1994.

49. Maurer DJ, Merkow RL, Gustilo RB: Infection after intramedullary nailing of severe open tibial fractures initially treated with external fixation, *J Bone Joint Surg Am* 71:835-838, 1989.

The study looked at 24 patients who had a severe open fracture of the tibia that was initially treated by external fixation and subsequently by reamed intramedullary nailing. The external fixation had been maintained for an average of 52 days (range, 7 to 230 days). The mean interval between removal of the external fixator and intramedullary nailing was 65 days (range, 3 to 360 days). In 5 of the 7 patients who had had an infection at one or more of the pin sites, an infection later developed around the intramedullary nail. In comparison, only 1 of the 17 patients who had not had a pin-site infection had an infection later around the nail ($p = 0.003$). An analysis of other variables, including the duration of external fixation, wound coverage, other injuries, and the type of fracture, showed that none was a predictor of infection either at the pin sites or around the intramedullary nail. This study concludes that a pin-site infection that develops during external fixation is a contraindication to the subsequent use of reamed intramedullary nailing in patients who have a fracture of the tibia.

50. Tornetta P III, DeMarco C: Intramedullary nailing after external fixation of the tibia, *Bull Hosp Jt Dis* 54:5-13, 1995.

51. Herscovici DJ, Sanders RW, Scaduto JM, et al: Vacuum-assisted wound closure (VAC therapy) for the management of

patients with high-energy soft tissue injuries, *J Orthop Trauma* 17:683-688, 2003.

This study was done to evaluate the results of a vacuum-assisted closure (VAC) device in patients presenting with open high-energy soft-tissue injuries. There were 21 patients, with 21 high-energy soft-tissue wounds (6 tibial, 10 ankle, and 5 with wounds of the forearm, elbow, femur, pelvis, and a below-knee stump) treated with a VAC device. Infected wounds had dressings changed every 48 hours, whereas all others had dressings changed every 72 to 96 hours. The duration of VAC use, final wound closure outcome, costs versus standard dressing changes or free flaps, and a list of all complications were recorded. All patients were followed for 6 months post-coverage. Patients averaged 4.1 sponge changes, 77% performed at bedside, with the device used an average of 19.3 days. Twelve wounds (57%) required either no further treatment or a split-thickness skin graft, and nine (43%) required a free tissue transfer. The VAC appears to be a viable adjunct for the treatment of open high-energy injuries. This device does not replace the need for formal debridement of necrotic tissue, but it may avoid the need for a free-tissue transfer in some patients with large traumatic wounds.

52. Parrett BM, Matros E, Pribaz JJ, et al: Lower extremity trauma: trends in the management of soft-tissue reconstruction of open tibia-fibula fractures, *Plast Reconstr Surg* 117:1315-1322; discussion 1323–1314, 2006.

53. Pollak AN, McCarthy ML, Burgess AR: Short-term wound complications after application of flaps for coverage of traumatic soft-tissue defects about the tibia. The Lower Extremity Assessment Project (LEAP) Study Group, *J Bone Joint Surg Am* 82:1681-1691, 2000.

This was part of the lower extremity assessment project (LEAP) study. The treatment data consisted of the type of flap, the timing of the flap coverage, and the type of fixation. Eighty-eight limbs were treated with a rotational flap, and 107 limbs were treated with a free flap. Second, the injury severity score (ISS) was significantly higher ($p = 0.001$) in the rotational flap group (mean, 14 points) than in the free-flap group (mean, 11 points), suggesting that patients in the former group had sustained more substantial total body trauma. Of the limbs that sustained an ASIF/OTA type-C osseous injury, those that were treated with a rotational flap were 4.3 times more likely to have a wound complication requiring operative intervention than were those treated with a free flap.

54. Hertel R, Lambert SM, Muller S, et al: On the timing of soft-tissue reconstruction for open fractures of the lower leg, *Arch Orthop Trauma Surg* 119:7-12, 1999.

The purpose of this study was to determine the most adequate timing in the management of soft-tissue injuries in open fractures. Twenty-nine consecutive open fractures of the tibia, including 24 grade III-B and 5 grade III-C fractures, were treated using a protocol of immediate debridement, early definitive skeletal stabilization, and early soft-tissue reconstruction. Fifteen lower legs were reconstructed after a mean delay of 4.4 days (range 1 to 9 days), whereas 14 lower legs were reconstructed immediately, that is, as an emergency procedure on the day of admission. Both groups were comparable. In the delayed reconstruction group the time to full, unprotected weight-bearing ($p = 0.0021$),

the time to definitive union ($p = 0.0049$), the number of reoperations ($p = 0.0001$), and the infection rate ($p = 0.0374$) were significantly higher. The data suggest that immediate reconstruction is the timing of choice for soft-tissue coverage.

55. Cole JD, Ansel LJ, Schwartzberg R: A sequential protocol for management of severe open tibial fractures, *Clin Orthop Relat Res* 84–103, 1995.

In this study 50 consecutive open fractures of the tibia, including 22 grade III-B and 4 grade III-C, were treated using a protocol of debridement, immediate wound coverage, and intramedullary nailing. Fasciocutaneous flaps were used extensively to cover areas of exposed bone. The severity of the soft-tissue injury dictated the timing of definitive fixation. Ninety-eight percent of the fractures united <6 months postoperatively. There was one infection (2%), two malunions (4%), and one case of partial flap necrosis. Locking screws broke in one patient (2%); the fracture united with <5 mm of shortening. Immediate postdebridement wound coverage and intramedullary nailing after reconstruction of the soft-tissue envelope facilitate fracture healing in these complex open injuries. Intramedullary nailing can be performed safely to include all grades of open tibial fractures from the proximal to distal metaphysis.

56. Gopal S, Majumder S, Batchelor AG, et al: Fix and flap: the radical orthopaedic and plastic treatment of severe open fractures of the tibia, *J Bone Joint Surg Br* 82:959-966, 2000.

This is a retrospective review of the case notes of 84 consecutive patients who had suffered a severe (Gustilo III-B or III-C) open fracture of the tibia after blunt trauma between 1990 and 1998. All had been treated by a radical protocol which included early soft-tissue cover with a muscle flap by a combined orthopaedic and plastic surgery service. The ideal management in this study is a radical debridement of the wound outside the zone of injury, skeletal stabilization and early soft-tissue cover with a vascularized muscle flap. Debridement and stabilization of the fracture were invariably performed immediately. In 33 cases the soft-tissue reconstruction was also completed in a single stage, whereas in a another 30, it was achieved within 72 hours. In the remaining 21, there was a delay beyond 72 hours, often for critical reasons unrelated to the limb injury. Overall, there was a rate of superficial infection of the skin graft of 6%, of deep infection at the site of the fracture of 9.5%, and of serious pin-track infection of 37% in the external fixator group. The treatment of these severe injuries by an aggressive combined orthopaedic and plastic surgical approach provides good results; immediate internal fixation, and healthy soft-tissue cover with a muscle flap is safe. Indeed, delay in cover (>72 hours) was associated with most of the problems.

57. Fischer MD, Gustilo RB, Varecka TF: The timing of flap coverage, bone-grafting, and intramedullary nailing in patients who have a fracture of the tibial shaft with extensive soft-tissue injury, *J Bone Joint Surg Am* 73:1316-1322, 1991.

This article reviews 43 patients who had a type III-B open fracture of the tibial shaft were reviewed to determine the effect of treatment of the soft-tissue injury on the rate of major complications. An infection developed in 2 of 11 patients who had early muscle-flap coverage compared with 10 of 13 who had been managed by open care of the wound and 9 of 13 who had later flap coverage. Patients who had had bone-grafting after complete reepithelialization of the wound, regardless of the method of closure, had a lower rate of early infection (0 of 16 compared with 4 of 15) and an earlier average time to union (54 compared with 63 weeks) than those in whom the wound was not completely closed or was draining at the time of bone grafting. Delayed intramedullary nailing with reaming was associated with a high rate of infection (9 of 19 patients), regardless of the condition of the soft tissue at the time of nailing. In my opinion, adequate debridement and early assessment of the soft-tissue defect are necessary so that appropriate soft-tissue coverage can be provided within the first 1 to 2 weeks. When the soft-tissue portion of the injury is addressed promptly and definitively and then allowed to heal completely, secondary osseous reconstruction may proceed with fewer complications.

58. Hong SW, Seah CS, Kuek LB, et al: Soft tissue cover in compound and complicated tibial fractures using microvascular flaps, *Ann Acad Med Singapore* 27:182-187, 1998.

59. Breugem CC, Strackee SD: Is there evidence-based guidance for timing of soft tissue coverage of grade III B tibia fractures? *Int J Low Extrem Wounds* 5:261-270, 2006.

60. Steiert AE, Partenheimer A, Schreiber T, et al: [The V.A.C. system (vacuum assisted closure) as bridging between primary osteosynthesis in conjunction with functional reconstructed of soft tissue—open fractures type 2 and type 3]. *Zentralbl Chir* 129 Suppl 1:S98-S100, 2004.

61. Joseph J, Giannoudis PV, Hinsche A, et al: Compartment syndrome following isolated ankle fracture, *Int Orthop* 24:173-175, 2000.

62. McQueen MM, Gaston P, Court-Brown CM: Acute compartment syndrome: who is at risk? *J Bone Joint Surg Br* 82:200-203, 2000.
This article analyzed associated factors in 164 patients with acute compartment syndrome who were treated over an 8-year period. In 69%, there was an associated fracture, about half of which were of the tibial shaft. Most patients were men, usually under 35 years of age. Acute compartment syndrome of the forearm, with associated fracture of the distal end of the radius, was again seen most commonly in young men. Injury to soft tissues, without fracture, was the second most common cause of the syndrome and one tenth of the patients had a bleeding disorder or were taking anticoagulant drugs. Young patients, especially men, were at risk of acute compartment syndrome after injury.

63. Heidepriem RW, Frey SE, Robinson D, et al: Thigh compartment syndrome: diagnosis and surgical treatment, *Vascular* 12:271-272, 2004.

64. Whitesides TE, Heckman MM: Acute compartment syndrome: update on diagnosis and treatment, *J Am Acad Orthop Surg* 4:209-218, 1996.
This is a review article on compartment syndrome. Because unusual pain may be the only symptom of an impending problem, a high index of suspicion, accurate evaluation, and prophylactic treatment will allow the physician to intervene in a timely manner and prevent irreversible damage. Muscles tolerate 4 hours of ischemia well, but by 6 hours the result is uncertain; after 8 hours, the damage is irreversible. Ischemic injury begins when tissue pressure is 10 to 20 mm Hg below diastolic pressure. Therefore, fasciotomy generally should be done when tissue pressure rises past 20 mm Hg below diastolic pressure.

65. Hardy DL Sr, Zamudio KR: Compartment syndrome, fasciotomy, and neuropathy after a rattlesnake envenomation: aspects of monitoring and diagnosis, *Wilderness Environ Med* 17:36-40, 2006.

66. Hope MJ, McQueen MM: Acute compartment syndrome in the absence of fracture, *J Orthop Trauma* 18:220-224, 2004.

67. Murthy BV, Narayan B, Nayagam S: Reduced perception of pain in schizophrenia: its relevance to the clinical diagnosis of compartment syndrome, *Injury* 35:1192-1193, 2004.
This article points out the need to have a high index of suspicion with patients that have an altered sensorium especially in the schizophrenic patients. Classic symptoms cannot be trusted.

68. Whitesides TE Jr, Haney TC, Harada H, et al: A simple method for tissue pressure determination, *Arch Surg* 110:1311-1313, 1975.
The classic article describes the technique for measuring intracompartment pressure with hospital devices.

69. Boody AR, Wongworawat MD: Accuracy in the measurement of compartment pressures: a comparison of three commonly used devices, *J Bone Joint Surg Am* 87:2415-2422, 2005.
This study evaluates the accuracy of the Stryker Intracompartmental Pressure Monitor System, an arterial line manometer, and the Whitesides apparatus. Most methods demonstrated excellent correlation ($R^2 > 0.95$) between calculated and measured pressures. The arterial line manometer with the slit catheter showed the best correlation ($R^2 = 0.9978$), and the Whitesides apparatus with the side-port needle showed the worst ($R^2 = 0.9115$). Furthermore, the Stryker system with the side-port needle demonstrated the least constant bias (+0.06 kPa). Straight needles tended to overestimate pressure. Two of the three needle configurations involving the Whitesides apparatus overestimated pressure. The data for the Whitesides methods had the highest standard errors, showing clinically unacceptable scatter. Side-port needles and slit catheters are more accurate than straight needles are. The arterial line manometer is the most accurate device. The Stryker device is also accurate. The Whitesides manometer apparatus lacks the precision needed for clinical use.

70. McQueen MM, Christie J, Court-Brown CM: Acute compartment syndrome in tibial diaphyseal fractures, *J Bone Joint Surg Br* 78:95-98, 1996.
This articles reviews 25 patients with tibial diaphyseal fractures, which had been complicated by an acute compartment syndrome. Thirteen had undergone continuous monitoring of the compartment pressure, and the other 12 had not. The average delay from injury to fasciotomy in the monitored group was 16 hours and in the nonmonitored group 32 hours ($p < 0.05$). Of the 12 surviving patients in the monitored group, none had any sequelae of acute compartment syndrome at final review at an average of 10.5 months. Of the 11 surviving patients in the nonmonitored group, 10 had definite sequelae with muscle weakness and contractures ($p < 0.01$). There was also a significant delay in tibial union in the nonmonitored group ($p < 0.05$). The authors felt that, when equipment is available, all patients with tibial fractures should have continuous

compartment monitoring to minimize the incidence of acute compartment syndrome.

71. Lynch JE, Heyman JS, Hargens AR: Ultrasonic device for the noninvasive diagnosis of compartment syndrome, *Physiol Meas* 25:N1-N9, 2004.

72. Gentilello LM, Sanzone A, Wang L, et al: Near-infrared spectroscopy versus compartment pressure for the diagnosis of lower extremity compartmental syndrome using electromyography-determined measurements of neuromuscular function, *J Trauma* 51:1-8, 2001. discussion 8–9

73. Heckman MM, Whitesides TE Jr, Grewe SR, et al: Compartment pressure in association with closed tibial fractures: the relationship between tissue pressure, compartment, and the distance from the site of the fracture. *J Bone Joint Surg Am* 76:1285-1292, 1994.
This article looks the relationship between compartment pressure and the distance at which the pressure was measured from the site of the fracture. Tissue pressure was measured in all four compartments of the leg at the level of the fracture and at 5-cm increments proximal and distal to the fracture. The peak pressure was usually found at the level of the fracture and was always located within 5 cm of the fracture. The highest pressures were recorded in the anterior and the deep posterior compartments in 20 patients. The measured pressure decreased steadily when sampled at increasing distances proximal and distal to the site of the highest recorded pressure. Decreases of 20 mm Hg (2.67 kilopascals) 5 cm adjacent to the site of the peak pressure were common. Failure to measure tissue pressure within a few centimeters of the zone of peak pressure may result in a serious underestimation of the maximum compartment pressure. These results suggest that measurements should be performed in both the anterior and the deep posterior compartments at the level of the fracture and at locations proximal and distal to the zone of the fracture to determine reliably the location of the highest tissue pressure in a lower extremity when a compartment syndrome is suspected clinically.

74. Hargens AR, Schmidt DA, Evans KL, et al: Quantitation of skeletal-muscle necrosis in a model compartment syndrome, *J Bone Joint Surg Am* 63:631-636, 1981.
In this article skeletal-muscle necrosis was evaluated in previously pressurized canine compartments. Intracompartmental necrosis was quantitated in the anterolateral muscle compartment of each dog by uptake of 99 mTc stannous pyrophosphate using the contralateral anterolateral compartment as an internal control. Muscle necrosis was assessed in compartments 48 hours after pressurization to levels of 10 to 120 mm Hg for 8 hours in 27 dogs. In another dog, neither anterolateral compartment was pressurized so that both compartments acted as control muscle. The results in these experiments identify a threshold pressure level (30 mm Hg) and duration (8 hours) at which significant muscle necrosis occurs at normal blood pressure. These findings suggest significant muscle necrosis associated with an impending compartment syndrome occurs at a threshold intracompartmental pressure of 30 mm of Hg of mercury after 8 hours. Because time variables are often unknown in suspected compartment syndromes, fasciotomy is recommended when intracompartmental pressure exceeds 30 mm Hg in a patient with normal blood pressure.

75. Whitesides TE, Haney TC, Morimoto K, et al: Tissue pressure measurements as a determinant for the need of fasciotomy, *Clin Orthop Relat Res* 1975: 43–51.
This is an experimental and clinical technique of measuring tissue pressures within closed compartments demonstrates a normal tissue pressure is approximately 0 mm Hg and increased markedly in compartmental syndromes. There is inadequate perfusion and relative ischemia when the tissue pressure within a closed compartment rises to within 10 to 30 mm Hg of the patient's diastolic blood pressure. Fasciotomy is usually indicated, therefore, when the tissue pressure rises to 40 to 45 mm Hg in a patient with a diastolic blood pressure of 70 mm Hg and any of the signs or symptoms of a compartmental syndrome. There is no effective tissue perfusion within a closed compartment when the tissue pressure equals or exceeds the patient's diastolic blood pressure. A fasciotomy is definitely indicated in this circumstance, although distal pulses may be present.

76. Heckman MM, Whitesides TE Jr, Grewe SR, et al: Histologic determination of the ischemic threshold of muscle in the canine compartment syndrome model, *J Orthop Trauma* 7:199-210, 1993.
This article tries to define the critical tissue pressure at which irreversible muscle damage occurs. A standard plasma infusion compartment syndrome model was created in a canine model. Four dogs were in each of four experimental groups with compartment pressure maintained as follows: (a) 30 mm Hg with support of diastolic blood pressure to a level > 50 mm Hg; (b) 20 mm Hg less than diastolic pressure; (c) 10 mm Hg less than diastolic blood pressure; (d) a level equal to the animal's diastolic blood pressure. All animals were sacrificed 14 days after the procedure. Histology revealed the following: (a) tissues pressurized to 30 mm Hg in a normotensive dog demonstrated no significant abnormalities; (b) tissues pressurized to 20 mm Hg less than diastolic revealed occasional cells undergoing regeneration but no evidence of infarction or fibrosis; (c) tissues pressurized to 10 mm Hg less than diastolic showed scattered small areas of infarction and fibrosis; and (d) tissues pressurized to diastolic blood pressure demonstrated more widespread infarction and scarring. The ischemic threshold of muscle, beyond which irreversible tissue damage occurs, is directly related to the difference in compartment and perfusion pressure. These findings document this pressure to be 10 mm Hg less than diastolic blood pressure or within 30 mm Hg of mean arterial pressure. This data refutes the use of absolute tissue pressure values as a guide to the necessity of fasciotomy. To abort an impending compartment syndrome and avoid irreversible tissue injury and their sequelae, fasciotomy should be done if tissue pressure reaches within 10 to 20 mm Hg of diastolic pressure.

77. McQueen MM, Court-Brown CM: Compartment monitoring in tibial fractures: the pressure threshold for decompression, *J Bone Joint Surg Br* 78:99-104, 1996.
This study is a prospective study of 116 patients with tibial diaphyseal fractures who had continuous monitoring of anterior compartment pressure for 24 hours. Three patients had acute compartment syndrome (2.6%). In the first 12 hours of monitoring, 53 patients

had absolute pressures over 30 mm Hg and 30 had pressures over 40 mm Hg, with four higher than 50 mm Hg. Only one patient had a differential pressure (diastolic minus compartment pressure) of less than 30 mm Hg; he had a fasciotomy. In the second 12-hour period 28 patients had absolute pressures over 30 mm Hg and 7 over 40 mm Hg. Only two had differential pressures of less than 30 mm Hg; they had fasciotomies. None of the 116 patients had any sequelae of the compartment syndrome at their latest review at least 6 months after injury. A threshold for decompression of 30 mm Hg would have indicated that 50 patients (43%) would have required fasciotomy and at a 40 mm Hg threshold 27 (23%) would have been considered for an unnecessary fasciotomy. The use of a differential pressure of 30 mm Hg as a threshold for fasciotomy led to no missed cases of acute compartment syndrome and decompression should be performed if the differential pressure level drops to under 30 mm Hg.

78. Ozkayin N, Aktuglu K: Absolute compartment pressure versus differential pressure for the diagnosis of compartment syndrome in tibial fractures, *Int Orthop* 29:396-401, 2005.

79. Cohen MS, Garfin SR, Hargens AR, et al: Acute compartment syndrome: effect of dermotomy on fascial decompression in the leg, *J Bone Joint Surg Br* 73:287-290, 1991.

This study investigated the skin envelope as a potential contributing factor. Wide fascial releases were performed through limited 8-cm incisions in eight cases of posttraumatic lower extremity compartment syndrome. In 9 of 29 compartments, the pressure remained greater than 30 mm Hg. Lengthening the skin incisions to an average of 16-cm decreased intracompartmental pressures significantly. This study documents the skin envelope as a contributing factor in acute compartment syndromes of the leg.

80. Middleton C: Compartment syndrome: the importance of early diagnosis, *Nurs Times* 99:30-32, 2003.

81. Bhattacharyya T, Vrahas MS: The medical-legal aspects of compartment syndrome, *J Bone Joint Surg Am* 86-A:864-868, 2004.

This study looks at factors of a successful defense in malpractice claims related to compartment syndrome. Nineteen closed claims, involving 16 patients and encompassing a total liability of $3.8 million, were found in the data for malpractice claims closed between 1980 and 2003. Ten claims were resolved in favor of the physician. The average time to closure was 5.5 years. All three claims that went to trial resulted in a verdict for the physician. Evidence of poor physician-patient communication was found in six cases, all of which resulted in an indemnity payment ($p < 0.01$). Increasing time from the onset of symptoms to the fasciotomy was linearly associated with an increased indemnity payment ($p < 0.05$). A fasciotomy performed within 8 hours after the first presentation of symptoms was uniformly associated with a successful defense. While malpractice claims involving compartment syndrome were uncommon, they resulted in a high rate and amount of indemnity payments. Early fasciotomy not only improves patient outcome but is also associated with decreased indemnity risk.

82. Gershuni DH, Mubarak SJ, Yaru NC, et al: Fracture of the tibia complicated by acute compartment syndrome, *Clin Orthop Relat Res* 1987: 221-227.

This is a consecutive series of 32 patients with tibia fractures complicated by compartment syndrome was treated with fasciotomy. One group was also treated with closed reduction of the fracture and cast immobilization and compared with a comparable group treated with internal fixation without case immobilization after fasciotomy. The anatomic and functional results in the internal fixation group were better than those treated with fasciotomy and cast immobilization. All fractures were united by 20 weeks. Complications in both groups were similar, although one deep infection, which was resolved with appropriate treatment, occurred in the group treated with internal fixation. Six open tibia fractures were treated with external skeletal fixation after fasciotomy; the results were less satisfactory, but the initial injuries were also more severe in this group. Patients with closed tibial fractures complicated by compartment syndromes should be treated expeditiously with fasciotomy, followed by stable internal fixation.

83. Court-Brown C, McQueen M: Compartment syndrome delays tibial union, *Acta Orthop Scand* 58:249-252, 1987.

84. Matsen FA III, Winquist RA, Krugmire RB Jr: Diagnosis and management of compartmental syndromes, *J Bone Joint Surg Am* 62:286-291, 1980.

85. Yang CC, Chang DS, Webb LX: Vacuum-assisted closure for fasciotomy wounds following compartment syndrome of the leg, *J Surg Orthop Adv* 15:19-23, 2006.

This study evaluated the efficacy of vacuum-assisted closure (VAC) for treatment of fasciotomy wounds for traumatic compartment syndrome. The records of 34 patients were reviewed who had compartment syndrome of the leg requiring the standard two-incision release of all four compartments and received the application of VAC therapy until the time of definitive wound closure or coverage. A matched series of 34 consecutive patients were also studied and served as a control group. The main parameter of interest was the time to "definitive closure" (delayed primary closure with sutures or skin graft coverage) of the wounds. Of the 68 wounds in 34 patients managed with VAC, the average time to definitive closure for both the lateral and the medial wounds was 6.7 days. For the 70 wounds in the 34 control patients, the average time to definitive closure was 16.1 days. This difference in time to wound closure between the VAC group and the non-VAC group was statistically significant ($p < 0.05$). Experimental work has shown VAC wound management to be effective in hastening the resolution of wound edema, enhancing local blood flow, promoting granulation tissue, and thwarting bacterial colonization. These factors may account for its utility in the management of fasciotomy wounds in the setting of compartment syndrome of the leg.

86. Asgari MM, Spinelli HM: The vessel loop shoelace technique for closure of fasciotomy wounds, *Ann Plast Surg* 44:225-229, 2000.

CHAPTER 2

Polytrauma Considerations

Jeff D. Yach, MD, FRCSC

- Polytrauma presents distinct challenges in diagnosis and management, requiring a well-organized multidisciplinary team approach in which injuries are identified and treated in order of priority.
- Musculoskeletal injuries are common in polytrauma, and ideally, an orthopaedic surgeon should be a member of the trauma team.
- Treatment priorities in the patient with multiple injuries may necessitate different orthopaedic management strategies as compared to isolated fractures.
- Frequently, temporizing or damage control measures will be necessary in the initial management of the unstable patient with multiple injuries.
- This chapter will outline treatment guidelines for initial assessment, resuscitation, and the principles of orthopaedic management in polytrauma, but it should be emphasized that algorithms and protocols are designed to serve as guidelines and are not a substitute for clinical judgment.

Initial Diagnosis, Management, and Resuscitation: The Primary Survey

- Polytrauma patients commonly sustain injuries that are an imminent threat to life.
- A systematic approach to assessment and management of patients in which injuries that are the greatest threat to life are identified and treated first can be invaluable in prioritizing care, particularly in centers in which patients who have sustained multiple injuries are infrequently encountered.
- The American College of Surgeons has devised an approach to injured patients known as Advanced Trauma Life Support (ATLS), which has become the standard of care for initial management of trauma victims worldwide.[1]
- Resuscitation of the patient begins in the prehospital phase.

- Depending on the skill and training of the emergency services personnel, the patient's airway is secured, spinal precautions are initiated, and intravenous (IV) access is obtained to administer an infusion of crystalloid fluid.
- Debate exists regarding the merits of more aggressive on-scene measures versus immediate transport to a trauma center.
- When possible, a trauma team should be activated either in the prehospital phase or during the initial assessment.
- Ideally, a trauma team consists of a trauma specialist acting as trauma team leader, an orthopaedic surgeon, general surgeon, neurosurgeon, thoracic surgeon, physician skilled in airway management, such as an anesthesiologist, radiologist, nurses, and radiology technicians.[2]
- If emergent operative intervention is anticipated, the OR personnel should be notified.
- The following sections outline the initial sequence of assessment and resuscitation, although it should be noted that some interventions can be performed concurrently in the trauma team setting.
- If a significant abnormality is encountered during the primary survey, treatment is initiated before moving on to the next step.

Airway Assessment and Management

- Establishing a secure airway is the first priority in the patient with multiple injuries to protect against aspiration and obstruction and allow ventilation.
- Patients who are unable to protect their airway from potential aspiration or impending obstruction should undergo immediate endotracheal intubation to establish a definitive airway.
- During assessment and management of the patient's airway, care must be taken to avoid excessive cervical spine (c-spine) movement as a result of the potential presence of an unstable c-spine fracture.

- The patient should initially be managed with spinal precautions including a rigid cervical collar, rigid spine board, and log-rolling.
- A quick and easy way to assess the need for immediate intubation is to speak to the patient and if the patient can speak, the airway is patent, at least for the moment.
- Physical signs of impending airway compromise include stridor, hoarseness, intercostal indrawing, and nasal flaring.
- The oropharynx is assessed next and should be cleared of debris, such as blood, teeth, and vomit, using suction.
- The patient vomiting on a spinal immobilization board should be log-rolled to prevent aspiration.
- The face and neck should be examined for open wounds, enlarging hematomas, or fractures that may cause airway compromise.
- Initial airway management maneuvers include a manual chin lift or jaw thrust (with appropriate c-spine precautions) to help relieve obstruction.
- In obtunded patients, an oral airway can be placed to prevent obstruction by soft tissues in the oropharynx, but the awake patient will usually not tolerate an oral airway, and a nasopharyngeal airway may be favored (provided there is no contraindication to placement, such as a suspected basal skull fracture).
- A definitive airway, when indicated, usually consists of either orotracheal or nasotracheal intubation.
- If airway obstruction prevents successful intubation, emergency cricothyroidotomy or tracheostomy must be performed.
- Patients with decreased levels of consciousness may need to be intubated for airway protection and as a guideline, a Glasgow Coma Scale (GCS) score of 8 or less is generally considered an indication for intubation.
- Patients with inhalation injuries are at high risk of developing airway obstruction resulting from laryngeal edema.
- Signs of inhalation injuries include burns to the oropharynx, singed nasal hairs, and carbonaceous sputum, and ideally, these patients should be intubated before signs of airway obstruction develop.
- Efforts should be made to avoid maneuvers and pharmacologic agents that cause raised intracranial pressures (ICPs) in the patient with head injuries, and rapid sequence induction (RSI) is generally the preferred method.
- If endotracheal intubation is indicated but cannot be achieved, a surgical airway must be performed.

Breathing

- Once a patent airway has been established, the next step is to ensure adequate ventilation and oxygenation.
- Great efforts should be made to avoid even transient hypoxia and hypoventilation because these can have profound impact on the prognosis of patients with severe injuries.
- Supplemental oxygen and an oxygen saturation monitor should be used in all trauma patients.

- The patient should be exposed and inspected for tracheal deviation, jugular venous distension, open thoracic wounds, subcutaneous emphysema, intercostal indrawing, and asymmetric chest movements.
- The chest should be auscultated bilaterally to assess air entry.
- Percussion resonance can be used to help identify intrathoracic injuries, although its use in the noisy trauma room may be limited.
- Severe injuries that are most likely to cause immediate ventilatory compromise include tension pneumothorax, open pneumothorax, massive hemothorax, and large flail chest.
- A tension pneumothorax is characterized by ipsilateral decreased breath sounds and hyperresonance, tracheal deviation to the opposite side, and jugular venous distension (Figure 2–1).
- A tension pneumothorax is treated by immediate decompression with a large-bore angiocatheter placed in the second interspace in the midclavicular line followed by tube thoracostomy.

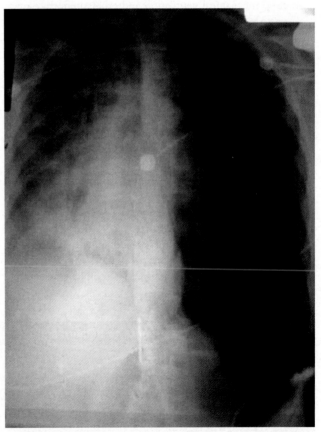

Figure 2–1: **Left-sided tension pneumothorax secondary to blunt chest trauma that was initially undetected. Note the deviation of the heart, mediastinum, and trachea to the right and depression of the left hemidiaphragm. Treatment consisted of needle decompression followed by tube thoracostomy.**

- An open pneumothorax (also known as a sucking chest wound), as the name implies, can usually be immediately identified by inspection.
- If the size of the defect is larger than approximately two-thirds the diameter of the trachea, air will preferentially enter the thoracic cavity via the chest wound.
- Treatment consists of an occlusive dressing over the wound, taped on three sides to create a one-way valve (allowing air to escape but not enter via the chest wall).
- A massive hemothorax is characterized by dullness to percussion and decreased breath sounds and may be the source of impaired ventilation and hypovolemic shock.
- Management of these problems consists of placement of a large-caliber thoracostomy tube.
- Multiple chest tubes may need to be placed and connected to a water-sealed collection device with suction drainage, noting the amount of initial drainage and the rate of ongoing bleeding.
- A flail segment is defined as the fracture of two or more ribs in two or more places; large flail segments can result in paradoxical chest movement, which impairs ventilation.
- Flail chest injuries may also have underlying pulmonary contusions, pneumothoraces, and hemothoraces and may require mechanical ventilation and other supportive measures to ensure optimal ventilation.

Circulation

- The next priority in the management of the patient with multiple injuries is the recognition and treatment of shock.
- Shock is considered to be the inadequate perfusion and oxygenation of the tissues and in the trauma setting, may be subdivided into hemorrhagic and nonhemorrhagic.
- In trauma, hemorrhagic or hypovolemic shock is the most commonly encountered; however, one must also consider nonhemorrhagic causes, such as cardiogenic and neurogenic shock.
- As the patient is being assessed, members of the trauma team are assigned to establish IV access, usually with two large-bore peripheral IV lines and to apply blood pressure and cardiac monitors.
- A sterile pressure dressing should be applied to actively bleeding wounds.

- Hypovolemic shock is identifiable via the effects on the cardiovascular system and by signs of decreased end-organ perfusion, but it must be remembered that these responses can have great variability depending patient factors, such as fitness, medical comorbidities, medications, and age (Table 2–1).
- The initial response to blood loss is an increase in heart rate until decompensation occurs, at which point, hypotension will occur.
- Hypotension is a relatively late finding and may not be identifiable until as much as 2 L of blood have been lost.
- Signs of impaired end-organ perfusion include altered mentation, cold, mottled skin, and decreased urine output.
- Fluid resuscitation is the initial treatment of hemorrhagic shock until a bleeding source can be identified and controlled and usually begins with a 2-L bolus of warmed crystalloid.
- Under most circumstances, the initial choice for fluid resuscitation is crystalloid, because it replenishes both the intravascular and interstitial compartments.[3]
- The general rule for crystalloid replacement of blood loss is 3:1.
- Progression to blood transfusion is considered if homeostasis cannot be achieved with the crystalloid fluid bolus.
- More recent work has examined the role of permissive hypotension in penetrating trauma and the role of hypertonic saline as an initial resuscitation fluid.
- Sources of life-threatening blood loss to consider are the thoracic and abdominal cavities, pelvis, femora, and open wounds.
- Blood loss in the chest may be attributable to intercostal artery or major vessel injury and may be noted by physical examination findings and on chest X-ray (CXR).
- A hemothorax is treated with tube thoracostomy and greater than 1500 ml of initial blood loss or continued blood loss of greater than 200 ml/hr over 4 hours are generally considered indications for operative intervention.
- Traumatic aortic disruption usually results in immediate death; however, some patients may survive and make it to hospital where prompt recognition and intervention is required to ensure continued survival.
- The diagnosis is usually suspected by a widened mediastinum on CXR (Figure 2–2) and is usually confirmed by

CLASS	BLOOD LOSS (% TOTAL BLOOD VOLUME)	BLOOD LOSS VOLUME (ml)*	PHYSIOLOGIC RESPONSE
I	0–15	0–750	None (amount consistent with blood donation)
II	15–30	750–1500	Tachycardia (>100), normal blood pressure, decreased pulse pressure, tachypnea, anxiety, mildly decreased urine output (20–30 ml/hr)
II	30–40	1500–2000	Tachycardia (>120), hypotension, decreased pulse pressure, tachypnea, confusion, decreased urine output (5–15 ml/hr)
IV	>40	>2000	Tachycardia (>140), marked hypotension, tachypnea, obtundation, anuria

Table 2–1: Physiologic Response to Hemorrhage by Volume

*Assume 70-kg ideal body weight male.

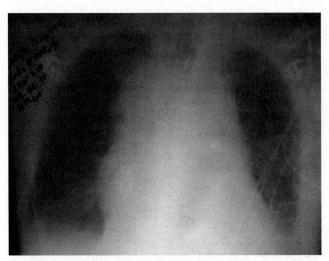

Figure 2–2: **Blunt chest trauma resulting in aortic injury and resultant widened mediastinum on chest X-ray.**

angiography or helical contrast computed tomography (CT).

- Blood loss in the abdomen can be difficult to identify, particularly in the patient who is unresponsive or impaired.
- Signs of peritoneal irritation generally warrant exploratory laparotomy; however, pelvis and rib fractures and abdominal wall contusions can cause muscular spasm that mimic peritoneal irritation.
- Adjunct diagnostic tests, such as focused abdominal sonography of trauma (FAST), diagnostic peritoneal lavage (DPL), and CT, may be required.
- The choice of investigation is dependent on a number of factors, the most important of which is the stability of the patient.
- Management of suspected intraabdominal hemorrhage usually consists of exploratory laparotomy.
- Other abdominal injuries requiring urgent laparotomy can be detected when assessing the abdomen for occult blood loss.
- Patients with generalized peritonitis should be taken to the OR for exploratory laparotomy because a perforated hollow viscus is the most likely etiology.
- The pelvis may be examined for stability by applying an anteroposterior force to each anterior superior iliac spine followed by lateral compression over the iliac wings.
- It is important to avoid repetitive manipulation of the unstable pelvis, which may exacerbate bleeding and patient discomfort.
- Blood loss from unstable pelvis fractures can be diagnosed by the identification of shock together with a pelvis injury pattern consistent with disruption of pelvic vessels (this will be discussed in greater detail later in the chapter).
- A management dilemma may arise when the patient has suspected bleeding from more than one site, such as a pelvis fracture and abdominal visceral injury.

- A team approach with close collaboration between the orthopaedic and general surgeons is critical in this setting to ensure optimal patient care.
- Nonhemorrhagic shock, such as pericardial tamponade, myocardial contusion, and neurogenic shock, may also occur.
- Pericardial tamponade results in insufficient preload to maintain cardiac output (CO) resulting from increased pressure from a hemopericardium.
- Pericardial tamponade diagnosis is described classically by Beck's triad, consisting of muffled heart sounds, hypotension, and elevated venous pressure.
- Initial treatment consists of needle pericardiocentesis; however, a definitive open procedure may ultimately be required.
- Blunt cardiac injury may also be the source of cardiogenic shock secondary to impaired contractility.
- Spinal cord injuries may also cause, or at least exacerbate, shock as a result of a loss of sympathetic tone with resultant peripheral vasodilation and hypotension.

Disability

- Pupillary responses and GCS are assessed quickly to identify head injury requiring urgent operative intervention and the need for intubation.
- The patient is also examined for movement of the extremities either spontaneously or to stimuli.
- A more detailed neurologic examination should be performed; however, depending on the patient's stability, this may be deferred to the secondary survey (Box 2–1).

Environment/Exposure

- It is important to ensure the patient is fully exposed to allow a rapid head-to-toe examination.
- This is an appropriate time to log-roll a patient on a spine board, perform a rectal examination, and remove the board.
- Once the patient has been fully exposed, efforts should be made to warm the patient with blankets or an external warmer to avoid hypothermia.

Investigations

- Trauma patients should initially have oxygen saturation, cardiac and blood pressure monitors applied, and in some cases, more invasive monitoring, such as a central or arterial line may be indicated.
- Standard trauma panel blood work and a sample for type and cross-matching, and when applicable, arterial blood gas (ABG) are sent to the laboratory for testing.
- Initial X-rays usually include a lateral c-spine, anteroposterior (AP) chest, and AP pelvis.
- In most patients, a baseline electrocardiogram (ECG) is obtained.
- Additional radiographs and other investigations are directed by the findings of the primary and secondary survey, in conjunction with the patient's status.

Box 2–1	Secondary Survey

History

- Complete history including events leading up to, and including the injury, comorbid conditions likely to influence management, such as coronary artery disease (CAD) or bleeding disorders, medications and allergies, and previous operative history.
- If a life-threatening injury necessitates an immediate trip to the OR, history can be limited to an AMPLE history, consisting of allergies, medications, past medical history, last meal, and events surrounding the injury.

Examination

- Complete head-to-toe physical examination identifies additional injuries that may not be immediately life-threatening.

Head and Neck

- Reevaluate pupils and level of consciousness.
- Inspect for signs of fractures or open wounds.
- Examine eyes for evidence of intraocular injury, foreign bodies, and visual acuity.
- Examine ears and nose for bleeding or signs of cerebrospinal fluid (CSF) leakage, which may indicate a basal skull fracture.
- Do a maxillofacial examination to look for fractures or tenderness and inspection of the oropharynx to look for bleeding, inhalational injury, or loose teeth.
- Complete a cranial nerve examination.
- Determine if trachea is midline and inspect for neck swelling, subcutaneous emphysema, or expanding hematoma.
- Auscultate and palpate of the carotid arteries.
- The cervical collar can be opened with in-line stabilization to facilitate this portion of the examination and palpating for tenderness, which may indicate cervical spine fracture or ligamentous injury.

Chest

- The chest is reevaluated for signs of tenderness or deformity and auscultated for air entry and heart sounds.
- Interventions, such as tube thoracostomy or pericardiocentesis, can be completed as indicated.

Abdomen

- Inspect the abdomen for external signs of injury, such as open wounds or bruising.
- Palpate for tenderness, guarding, and rebound.
- Abdominal examination in the neurologically impaired patient may be equivocal.
- Diagnostic peritoneal lavage (DPL), focused abdominal sonography of trauma (FAST), or computed tomography (CT) may be employed, depending on clinical judgment and the stability of the patient.

Pelvis

- Avoid repeat manipulation of the unstable pelvis and consider application of temporary stabilization if indicated.
- Examine genitalia and perineum for evidence of bleeding and open wounds, including vaginal examination in females.
- Rectal examination for tone and bleeding and in males, the location of the prostate (a high-riding prostate may indicate a urethral injury).

Musculoskeletal/Neurologic

- Axial and appendicular skeleton are assessed for tenderness, deformity, instability, and open wounds.
- A thorough neurovascular examination of all four extremities should be performed and documented.
- Radiographs of suspected fractures or dislocations are obtained, and deformities are provisionally reduced and splinted.
- Open wounds are covered with a sterile dressing, and tetanus immunization and antibiotics are administered as indicated.

- Under many circumstances, a CT scan will be useful; however, it is rarely appropriate in the patient who is critically unstable.

Reevaluation and Response to Resuscitation

- At this point, the patient's response to initial resuscitation is assessed, and the primary survey is quickly repeated to look for any change in status.

- If the patient is located in a peripheral center, consideration should be given to the timing and appropriateness of transfer to a trauma center.
- If the patient's status permits, a more detailed secondary survey is completed in conjunction with treatment adjuncts and investigations as indicated.
- A urinary catheter is placed as long as there is no sign of urethral disruption, such as blood at the urethral meatus or a high-riding prostate.

- If a urethral or bladder injury is suspected, this can be evaluated with a retrograde cystourethrogram.
- A nasogastric tube is also placed to decompress the stomach, but care should be taken to ensure there is no evidence of basal skull fracture before insertion.
- It is also important to understand the significance and sequelae of the patient's injury pattern in an attempt to avoid or minimize secondary complications (Box 2–2).
- Various scoring systems have been proposed in an attempt to guide prognosis and management and for research purposes (Box 2–3).

Orthopaedic Management in the Patient with Multiple Injuries

- As outlined in the previous section, a team approach is important to providing organized, efficient, and comprehensive management of the patient with multiple injuries.
- As a result of the high incidence of musculoskeletal injuries in the patient with multiple injuries, the orthopaedic surgeon is often a vital member of the trauma team.
- It is important for the orthopaedic surgeon to not only recognize the extent and severity of injuries but also the immediate and long-term sequelae of those injuries.

- The goal of the trauma team is to identify and treat injuries based on priority.
- The initial management focuses on the preservation of life and limb.
- Orthopaedic management strategies will vary depending on the patient's status and may range from temporizing or damage control measures in the unstable patient to more definitive treatment in the stable patient to maximize long-term outcome and function.
- The general consensus based on the literature favors early stabilization of musculoskeletal injuries to improve outcome, mobility, and pain control.[4]
- Many of the popularly cited studies on the subject are retrospective in nature and involve relatively small numbers of patients.
- Conclusions drawn from historical comparisons may also be limited because there have been many advances in critical care, which may also be responsible for improved outcomes.
- A management plan must be individualized to the patient and be coordinated with other team members.
- The following sections review some of the orthopaedic considerations in the patient with multiple injuries.

Limb Ischemia

- Ischemia is a time-sensitive injury requiring emergent measures for limb preservation.

Box 2–2	**Postresuscitation Considerations**

- A considerable proportion of victims of polytrauma that survive their initial injuries will go on to prolonged intensive care unit (ICU) and hospital stays.
- Therapeutic measures during the initial resuscitation of these patients can influence their hospital course and ultimate prognosis.
- Hypovolemic shock results in tissue hypoxia and lactic acidosis, local tissue damage, and release of inflammatory mediators.
- These inflammatory mediators, with or without superimposed infection, contribute to the systemic inflammatory response.
- The systemic inflammatory cascade may lead to multiple organ dysfunction, and this can be the cause of many late deaths in polytrauma patients.
- Hypothermia can result in uncontrollable coagulation disorders, and therefore initial preventative measures are crucial (warming blankets, warmed IV fluids).
- Coagulopathy may also arise in association with massive blood loss and fluid resuscitation and may delay all but the most crucial lifesaving procedures until it can be corrected.
- Initially patients in hypovolemic shock undergo a period of increasing oxygen debt and lactic acidosis.
- After the patient has been resuscitated and bleeding stopped, this is followed by a hypermetabolic period with increased caloric requirements and a generalized catabolic state.
- Early enteral feeding is essential to protect gut mucosal integrity and prevent infection, and tight glycemic control is important.
- Many trauma patients develop the systemic inflammatory response syndrome (SIRS) and still others develop adult respiratory distress syndrome (ARDS) or sepsis with multiple organ dysfunction.
- These syndromes can be difficult to manage once they have developed, and therefore there has been considerable focus on prevention during the initial resuscitation phase.
- Treatment of these disorders consists largely of support of the failing systems with mechanical ventilation, vasopressors, and dialysis with a search for and treatment of underlying causes of infection.
- In ventilated patients, prophylaxis against pneumonia by keeping the head of the bed elevated is indicated.
- Prophylaxis against stress ulceration of the gastric mucosa using a histamine$_2$ blocker and deep venous thrombosis prophylaxis should be considered.
- Adequate cerebral perfusion pressure must be maintained in patients with head injuries by avoiding hypotension and raised intracranial pressure.

Box 2–3 Scoring Trauma Injuries

- Several different scoring systems for assessing the severity of injury in polytrauma exist and are listed here.
- These systems have evolved in an attempt to refine prognosis and triage decisions and for resource allocation and outcomes research.

Glasgow Coma Scale

- The Glasgow Coma Scale (GCS) is a simple scoring system and is used in patients with closed head injuries and evaluates eye opening (1 to 4), best motor response (1 to 6), and verbal response (1 to 5) for a score out of 15.
- General guidelines recommend that patients with GCS < 13 should be transferred to a trauma center, and patients with GCS of 8 or less have a severe head injury and should be intubated for airway protection.

Revised Trauma Score

- The revised trauma score (RTS) system is widely used for triage decisions.
- Patients receive a score of 0 to 4 for each of GCS, systolic blood pressure, and respiratory rate and patients with a combined score < 11 should be taken to a trauma center.

Abbreviated Injury Scale

- The abbreviated injury scale (AIS) was initially devised for blunt trauma but updated to include penetrating trauma, this system assigns a score of 0 to 6 based on each anatomic region of the body, in which 0 indicates no injury and 6 represents a nonsurvivable or fatal injury. (Examples include 1 for a minor injury, such as an abrasion, 2 for an undisplaced pelvic fracture, 3 for a displaced long-bone fracture, 4 for a displaced pelvic fracture, 5 for multiple open fractures, and 6 for a fatal injury.)
- This system is most useful in polytrauma when used to create an injury severity score.

Injury Severity Score

- The injury severity score (ISS) system utilizes the AIS and takes the highest score from the three most severely injured anatomic regions and sums their squares, for a score of 0 to 75.
- A patient with a score of 6 for any one region is given an ISS of 75.
- The ISS correlates well with mortality, but it is limited in that other physiologic indicators of survival, such as age and comorbidities, are not considered, and it may underestimate the severity of injury for patients with multiple injuries that include closed head injury.

Trauma and Injury Severity Score

- The trauma and injury severity score (TRISS) system combines the anatomic and physiologic elements of ISS and RTS to produce a better predictive model of survival after trauma but is generally too cumbersome for clinical use.
- This scoring system is primarily a research and quality control tool.
- TRISS estimates probability of survival by the formula $P = 1/(1 + e^b)$ in which $b = b0 + b1(RTS) + b2(ISS) + b3$, and values for b0 to b3 depend on whether the trauma is blunt or penetrating and on patient age.

- Based on early animal studies and clinical experience, the threshold for salvage appears to be between 6 and 8 hours of warm ischemia time.
- Initial resuscitation focuses on the support of the patient's systemic hemodynamics.
- As always, a careful neurovascular examination of the extremities is important but is sometimes limited in cases, such as the patient who is unconscious or impaired.
- Limb ischemia can still occur in the patient who is normotensive and may be related to compartment syndrome or distortion or disruption of vessels in association with fractures and dislocations.
- Open sites of active bleeding should be controlled with direct pressure as part of the initial resuscitation phase.
- Deformed extremities should be realigned and splinted, which may help to correct the distortion of vessels and restore circulation.

- A high index of suspicion is important in the patient who is unresponsive to avoid missed injuries, such as evolving compartment syndrome.
- Compartment syndrome can develop from direct injury and indirect sources, such as reperfusion after a period of ischemia, which is particularly prevalent if the ischemic period has been greater than 4 hours.
- As intracompartment pressure increases, it can exceed capillary perfusion pressure and lead to ischemic necrosis of muscles and nerves within the compartment.
- Physical findings associated with compartment syndrome include tenseness on palpation, increasing pain, pain on passive stretch of muscles, paraesthesia, and impaired motor function (late compartment syndrome).
- It should be noted that the arterial pulse is not obliterated, and the presence of a distal pulse does not rule out compartment syndrome.

- Compartment pressures can also be measured using specialized monitors or an arterial line.
- There is no consensus as to an absolute pressure, which is diagnostic of compartment syndrome because perfusion also depends on the differential with the diastolic blood pressure.
- A general guideline is that compartment pressures within 30 mm Hg of the diastolic pressure represent a significant likelihood of compartment syndrome.[5]
- Fasciotomy is indicated for compartment syndrome and should be considered prophylactically in the at-risk patient, such as following revascularization of an ischemic limb or the patient who is unresponsive with a high energy tibia fracture.
- In the situation of an ischemic limb requiring surgical revascularization, it is important to coordinate with the vascular surgeon regarding the timing, sequence, and method of treatment of associated musculoskeletal injuries.
- Time permitting, it may be advantageous to stabilize associated fractures, at least on a provisional basis, before undertaking vascular repair to restore stability, length, and alignment.
- If ischemia time does not permit this approach, temporary vascular shunts can be used to allow limb realignment and stabilization before definitive vascular reconstruction.
- Limb position and length must be carefully considered, particularly if the vascular repair is performed first because it may be feasible to perform a primary vascular repair with the limb in a shortened or deformed position. This may be jeopardized if the subsequent fracture repair restores the anatomy to normal.

Pelvic Fractures

- Unstable pelvic fractures can be associated with life-threatening blood loss.
- In addition to examination for stability and initial radiographs, it is important to examine for open wounds, genitourinary, gastrointestinal (GI), and neurovascular injuries.
- Pelvic fractures can be classified by the degree and pattern of instability.
- Tile[6] described a classification system that distinguished stable from unstable pelvic fractures.
- The unstable pattern was further differentiated into rotationally or vertically unstable.
- Young and others[7] further expanded on the patterns to refine prognosis and guide treatment.
- The pattern of injury (AP compression, lateral compression, or vertical shear) can help to predict associated injuries.
- AP compression or open-book injuries may result in tearing of vessels and an increased intrapelvic volume that may allow a significant amount of blood loss (Figure 2–3).
- Open-book pelvic injuries may be temporarily stabilized with devices, such as a pelvic binder, sheet, bean bag, or C-clamp, which may help to control hemorrhage by

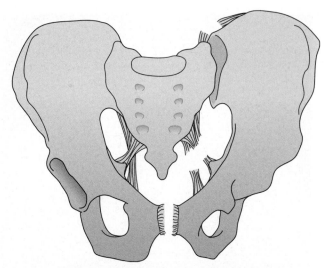

Figure 2–3: Illustration showing anteroposterior compression injury with symphysis and left sacroiliac joint disruption with resultant widening and increased intrapelvic volume.

decreasing the intrapelvic volume and tamponade bleeding (Figure 2–4).
- Ideally, the emergent measures should still permit access to the patient and other potential sources of blood loss.
- It may be difficult to determine if a patient with a pelvic fracture also has a significant intraabdominal injury.
- If DPL is undertaken, it should generally be performed above the umbilicus in a patient with an associated pelvic fracture to avoid entering an extraperitoneal hematoma.
- There is some debate as to the role of angiography and embolization versus surgical stabilization for the patient with an unstable pelvic fracture and ongoing blood loss.
- Some authors have reported good results using embolization as the first-line treatment; however, others suggest that only 15% of cases have an minor arterial source of bleeding that is amenable to embolization.[8]
- Bleeding from the extensive sacropelvic venous plexus is not amenable to embolization.
- In most centers, surgical stabilization in the OR is a more reliable management technique, and it offers the advantage of concomitant treatment of other injuries.
- If the patient is persistently hypotensive, he or she may be taken to the angiography suite for attempted embolization.
- Surgical stabilization often involves the application of an anterior external fixator (Figure 2–5) or a posterior ring resuscitation clamp under fluoroscopic guidance.
- Ideally, these should be applied so as to permit access to the abdomen in case a laparotomy is required.
- In patients requiring both a laparotomy and pelvic stabilization, it is important to have close communication among team members and realistic estimates of operative time and blood loss when formulating a treatment plan.
- Immediate definitive surgical stabilization (plate osteosynthesis, percutaneous screws) may also have a role in

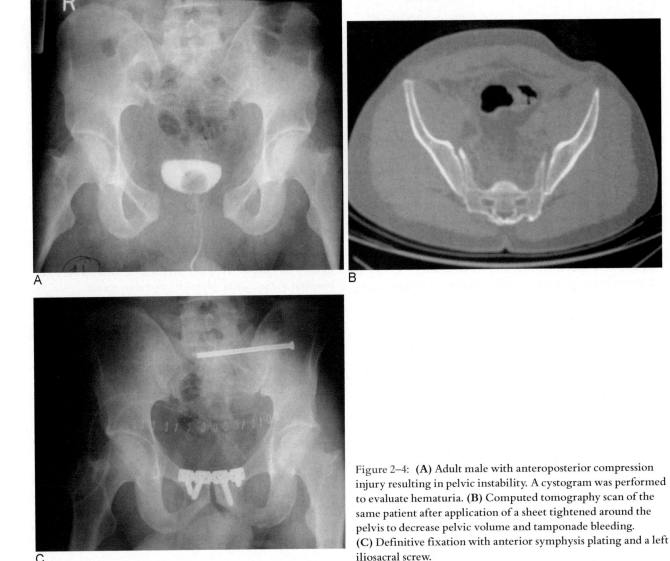

Figure 2–4: **(A)** Adult male with anteroposterior compression injury resulting in pelvic instability. A cystogram was performed to evaluate hematuria. **(B)** Computed tomography scan of the same patient after application of a sheet tightened around the pelvis to decrease pelvic volume and tamponade bleeding. **(C)** Definitive fixation with anterior symphysis plating and a left iliosacral screw.

selected cases (depending on surgeon expertise), but disadvantages include decompression of the pelvic hematoma with increased blood loss and increased operative time.

Open Fractures

- Open fractures are time-sensitive injuries as a result of the risk of infection; however, the exact time threshold and indications for surgical debridement are debatable.[9]
- Most surgeons would agree that wounds with significant soft-tissue injury or contamination require urgent surgical debridement.
- Initial management of the wound includes coverage with a sterile dressing, and the administration of wound appropriate antibiotic coverage and tetanus prophylaxis.[10]

- If the patient's status permits, irrigation and debridement should be performed in the OR in conjunction with some form of fracture stabilization (provisional or definitive) as indicated (Figure 2–6).
- Irrigation and debridement can potentially be performed concurrently with other procedures by a second surgical team.

Long-Bone Fractures

- Long-bone fractures can be associated with significant blood loss and secondary pulmonary dysfunction resulting from adult respiratory distress syndrome (ARDS) and fat embolism syndrome (FES).

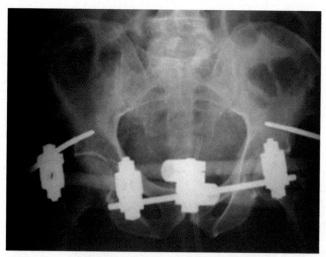

Figure 2–5: Application of a two-pin anterior external fixator for a patient with hemodynamic instability following an anteroposterior compression injury. The frame is adjusted to allow access to the abdomen to address concomitant injuries.

- Femur fractures are usually the most significant of the long-bone fractures.
- Controversy surrounds many aspects of femoral fracture treatment in the patient with multiple injuries, including the timing of fixation and implications of concomitant head or pulmonary injuries.
- Under most circumstances, the procedure of choice for the treatment of a femoral diaphyseal fracture is a reamed, locked intramedullary nail.[11]
- In the unstable patient with multiple injuries, temporary external fixation is an option to provide initial stability.
- The advantage of external fixation is that it can usually be applied quickly with minimal blood loss.
- External fixation generally does not provide a definitive solution as a result of the risk of malunion, nonunion, and pin-tract infection.
- External fixation is usually converted to an intramedullary nail within the first week to avoid disseminating a pin-tract infection to create a pan-diaphyseal osteomyelitis, although the exact window for safe conversion is not known.
- Plate osteosynthesis is also an option in selected patients, if, for example, patient position or concomitant injuries make nailing suboptimal.
- The timing of femoral fracture stabilization has been the subject of much debate.
- Numerous retrospective studies support the early (within 24 hours) stabilization of femoral fractures in the patient with multiple injuries, citing improved outcome and decreased incidence of ARDS,[12] but many authors have challenged this premise.
- Most studies are limited by heterogeneity within the study population and the lack of control as to the cause for surgical delay.

- In many cases, increased surgical delay is secondary to the patient's physiologic status, and therefore there is a bias for the more severely injured and unstable patients to experience a longer surgical delay.
- Bone and others[13] performed a prospective randomized study comparing patients with multiple injuries with early (<24 hours) versus delayed (>48 hours) fixation of femoral fractures and found a decrease in pulmonary complications, intensive care unit (ICU) requirements, and length of stay, although the delayed group had a significantly higher number of patients with pulmonary injury.
- The combination of femur fracture and pulmonary injury has also been the topic of much debate.
- It has been proposed that marrow emboli incite an inflammatory response in the lungs, which leads to ARDS and FES.
- Some authors have proposed delayed fixation of long-bone fractures in patients with associated pulmonary injuries and avoidance of reamed intramedullary nailing.[14]
- Intramedullary reaming has been shown to produce marrow emboli in animal and clinical studies, although the clinical significance is still unclear.
- Several authors have advocated early stabilization based on improved outcome, whereas others have found that the most significant determinant of outcome is the severity of the chest injury.
- Bosse and others[15] could not find a difference in pulmonary complications or mortality in patients with femoral shaft fractures and pulmonary injury treated with either plate osteosynthesis or reamed intramedullary nailing.
- A number of retrospective studies have also sought to address the issue of femoral fracture fixation in the patient with multiple injuries including a closed head injury.
- Initial management of a traumatic brain injury (TBI) includes support of oxygenation and perfusion while controlling ICP.
- It is unclear whether the timing of fracture stabilization has any effect on ultimate neurologic outcome, and many retrospective studies on the subject use GCS as a measure of outcome, which may not be a specific and precise enough parameter to accurately assess global cognitive function.
- As always, it is important to have close collaboration between the neurosurgeon and the orthopaedic surgeon and carefully weigh the case-specific risks and benefits when formulating a treatment plan.
- Unfortunately, there is no consensus on the timing of fixation of long-bone fractures in the patient with multiple injuries; however, the general trend is to favor early fixation in patients who are stable and delayed fixation in unstable patients whose status can be improved with supportive management (e.g., the patient who is hypothermic and coagulopathic).

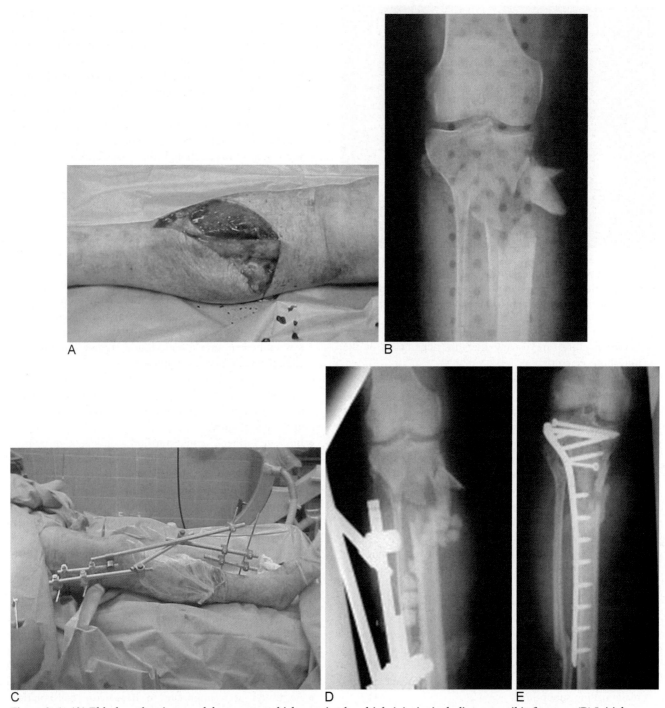

Figure 2–6: **(A)** Elderly pedestrian struck by a motor vehicle sustained multiple injuries including open tibia fracture. **(B)** Initial anteroposterior X-ray. **(C)** and **(D)** Post-debridement, insertion of antibiotic beads, and spanning external fixation. **(E)** Delayed definitive fixation with a locked plate.

Spine Fractures

- The patient with multiple injuries should be considered to have a potential spine injury until proven otherwise.
- Patients are initially managed with spinal precautions including a cervical collar, spine board for transport, and log-rolling.
- Care should be taken to avoid prolonged immobilization on a rigid spine board as a result of the potential for pressure ulceration.
- In the awake, alert, and cooperative patient, significant spinal injury can potentially be excluded by a careful physical examination (+/− radiographs); however, many patients may be cognitively impaired (head injury, intoxication) or suffer from distracting injuries.
- Resulting from the potentially catastrophic neurologic complications with a missed unstable spine fracture, it is generally recommended to err on the side of caution.
- It is also important to maintain a high index of suspicion for multiple, sometimes noncontiguous fractures.
- The use of methylprednisolone was advocated in patients with spinal cord injury (SCI) to improve neurologic outcome,[16] however the conclusions of the landmark study have been questioned.
- Methylprednisolone remains an option for the treatment of early (<8 hours) partial cord injuries.
- The initial IV bolus of 30 mg/kg is administered followed by an infusion of 5.4 mg/kg for 24 hours.
- Relatively few spine fractures require immediate operative intervention.
- The main indication for emergent decompression and stabilization is neurologic deterioration. however there is limited evidence to support improved outcome with early intervention in patients with a partial cord deficit.[17]
- Unstable injuries without progressive neurologic deficit are generally managed on a semiurgent basis to provide stability, prevent further deformity or neurologic deterioration, and to enhance mobility and pain control.

Fractures and Dislocations

- Some musculoskeletal injuries may have time-sensitive associations with long-term sequelae.
- Certain fractures, such as talar neck and femoral neck, have been associated with a high incidence of avascular necrosis (AVN), which can lead to significant long-term disability.
- It has been proposed and there is some limited clinical evidence, that the risk of AVN can be decreased by the prompt reduction and stabilization of these fractures.
- Similarly, hip dislocations have been found to have an AVN rate, which is related to the duration of time from injury to reduction.[18]
- Other dislocations or fracture dislocations may cause pressure and stretch-related injuries to the surrounding soft-tissue envelope and neurovascular structures.

- The orthopaedic surgeon must be aware of the immediate and long-term implications of these injuries and collaborate with the trauma team accordingly to develop a treatment plan.
- In many instances, a quick, closed reduction can be performed during a window of opportunity during the initial management of the patient with multiple injuries without causing significant delay in the treatment of other injuries.

Periarticular Fractures

- High-energy intraarticular and periarticular fractures can be challenging injuries to treat under ideal circumstances.
- There are several reasons why the acute phase of management of the patient with multiple injuries may not be the ideal time to undertake definitive treatment of intraarticular and periarticular fractures.
- High-energy fractures usually have concomitant injuries to the soft tissues, even if the fractures are not open, and early, open reduction and internal fixation may increase the incidence of wound complications.
- Staged treatment protocols for injuries, such as pilon and calcaneal fractures (with delayed definitive fixation), have been reported and demonstrate improved results with respect to wound complications.[19]
- Optimal treatment of complex periarticular injuries sometimes requires further imaging, such as CT scan, to assist in preoperative planning, and in the unstable patient with multiple injuries, these additional investigations may need to be deferred.
- Reconstruction of periarticular fractures can sometimes require several hours and subspecialty expertise, and this may not be appropriate in the initial management of the patient with multiple injuries.
- In most cases, provisional reduction and splinting or spanning external fixation can be safely performed with relatively little time and blood loss.
- Spanning external fixation has the advantage of more rigidly realigning the extremity and still allowing access to the soft tissue for wound care, neurovascular, and compartment pressure monitoring.
- Provisional fixation allows the patient's physiologic status and local soft tissues to stabilize, and subsequent definitive reconstruction can be undertaken in the ensuing weeks by an appropriately rested and prepared surgical team.

The Mangled Extremity

- The patient with severe bone and soft-tissue injury to an extremity (mangled extremity) should still be managed using standard trauma guidelines.
- Life-threatening injuries should be identified and treated before limb-threatening injuries.
- The decision for limb salvage versus amputation must take into consideration the patient factors and physiologic status of the patient with multiple injuries.

- Limb salvage procedures may require soft-tissue reconstructive procedures, such as free flaps, that may be impractical or ill-advised in the unstable patient who is already facing significant physiologic stress and metabolic load (Figure 2–7).
- Various scoring systems have been proposed in an effort to guide the decision of limb salvage versus amputation, including the mangled extremity severity score (MESS).
- The MESS considers age, shock, energy of injury, and ischemia, and scores of 7 or less have been suggested to be compatible with limb salvage.[20]
- Although scoring systems can be helpful, they do not provide a definitive answer for all cases. and the surgeon's clinical judgment is paramount.
- Although it is generally true that amputation can always be performed at a later date, the presence of necrotic or infected tissue can have systemic sequelae, which may further compromise the critically injured patient.

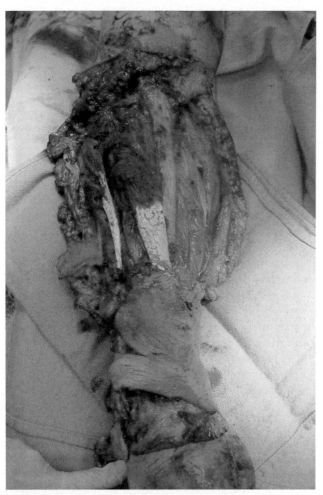

Figure 2–7: Adult woman sustained severe soft-tissue and bone disruption secondary to being struck by a train. Decision to amputate was guided by patient's associated vascular and tibial nerve disruption and hemodynamic instability.

- If limb salvage is proposed, the injured limb may be provisionally stabilized with an external fixator, and open wounds should be debrided of necrotic tissue and gross contamination.
- Staged reconstructive efforts for limb salvage must be re-evaluated at each stage with respect to timing and indication based on the status of the patient.
- It may be helpful to document the recommendations of two or more qualified surgeons when proposing immediate amputation, particularly if the patient is unresponsive or impaired.
- It is also useful to photograph the injured limb for documentation purposes.

Lesser Fractures

- The patient with multiple injuries may also have a variety of less severe fractures that are not immediately life threatening or limb threatening.
- These injuries may nonetheless cause pain, complicate nursing care, and impair mobilization.
- Definitive stabilization of these fractures can often be helpful with short-term mobilization, pain control, and long-term function.
- The decision as to the timing and type of treatment should be based on the status of the patient.
- Timing of definitive fracture care is sometimes complicated by sepsis, multiple organ dysfunction, and other secondary sequelae that may develop while the patient is in the ICU.
- In some cases, it may be simpler and safer to treat a malunion in the future than to proceed with fixation in a compromised patient.

Nerve Injury

- Peripheral nerve deficits may be missed or difficult to initially diagnose in the patient with multiple injuries, and ongoing vigilance and careful examination and documentation are crucial.
- Nerves injuries may be classified by the extent of disruption.
- Neurapraxia refers to a loss of conduction within a segment of a nerve, which is still in continuity, possibly secondary to stretch or contusion, and can generally be expected to recover.
- Axonotmesis occurs when the endoneurial sheath remains intact, but there is axonal disruption.
- Neurotmesis occurs when the nerve is completely disrupted and generally carries the worst prognosis for spontaneous recovery.
- Open injuries have been associated with a higher incidence of neurotmesis.
- Some injuries may be heterogeneous, and it may be initially difficult to ascertain the ultimate zone of injury.

- As a result, definitive reconstructive procedures are often delayed until the patient is more stable, and the extent of the injury is better understood.
- In the meantime, the injured extremity should be otherwise stabilized as needed and splinted in a position of function to help prevent contractures.

Summary

- The patient with multiple injuries presents unique challenges in diagnosis and management.
- A team approach with a trauma team and experienced trauma team leader has been adopted in most centers to facilitate the diagnosis and treatment of injuries in the order of priority.
- The orthopaedic surgeon is usually a vital member of the team as a result of the high frequency of musculoskeletal injuries.
- It is important to recognize the immediate and lasting implications of specific musculoskeletal injuries and collaborate with other members of the trauma team to develop an appropriate treatment plan.

Acknowledgments

The author would like to thank Trevor Bardell, MD, for his help in manuscript preparation and Ann Taite for her original artwork.

Annotated References

1. American College of Surgeons Committee on Trauma: *Advanced Trauma Life Support for doctors: student manual*, ed 7, Chicago: 2004, American College of Surgeons.

This manual is produced to support the ATLS course provided worldwide by the American College of Surgeons. The ATLS approach allows a basic framework for managing trauma patients that is applicable to physicians who manage trauma infrequently or daily, allowing a common understanding of treatment priorities and objectives.

2. Hoyt DB, Coimbra R, Potenza BM: Trauma systems, triage, and transport, In: *Trauma*, ed 5, New York, 2004 McGraw-Hill.

A comprehensive textbook of trauma including prehospital, emergency department, operative, and critical care management of the trauma patient written by world leaders in this field.

3. Finfer S, Bellomo R, Boyce, N, et al: A comparison of albumin and saline for fluid resuscitation in the intensive care unit, *N Engl J Med* 350:2247–2256, 2004.

In this large-blinded, randomized controlled trial from Australia, the investigators found that 4% albumin was as safe as normal saline for fluid resuscitation. Subgroup analysis suggests that saline may be better in trauma patients, with albumin possibly preferable in severe sepsis.

4. Riska EB, von Bondsdorff H, Hakkinen, S, et al: Primary operative fixation of long bone fractures in patients with multiple injuries, *J Trauma* 17:111–121, 1977.

The authors review 47 cases of multiple, long-bone injuries in the polytrauma patient over a 5-year period and conclude that primary internal fixation is preferable to conservative management.

5. McQueen MM, Court-Brown CM: Compartment monitoring in tibial fractures, *J Bone Joint Surg Br* 78:99–104, 1996.

Based on continuous compartment pressure monitoring in their prospective cohort of 116 patients with tibial shaft fracture, the authors recommend assessing the difference between diastolic blood pressure and compartment pressure, with a difference of less than 30 mm Hg as a threshold for consideration of fasciotomy.

6. Tile M: Pelvic ring fractures: should they be fixed? *J Bone Joint Surg Br* 70:1–12, 1988.

In this review article, Tile classifies pelvic disruption according to rotational and vertical stability and relates operative and nonoperative management to this classification system.

7. Young JWR, Burgess AR, Brumbach, AR, et al: Pelvic fractures: value of plain radiography in early assessment and management, *Radiology* 160:445–451, 1986.

Young and others retrospectively reviewed anteroposterior (AP), pelvic inlet, and pelvic outlet radiographs in 142 cases of pelvic fracture and through correlation with clinical assessment, identified four patterns of injury recognizable with plain films.

8. Ben-Menachem Y, Coldwell DM, Young, JWR, et al: Hemorrhage associated with pelvic fractures: causes, diagnosis and emergent management, *AM J Roentgenol* 157:1005–1014, 1991.

In this review article, the authors describe their approach to management of hemorrhage associated with pelvic fractures according to mechanism of injury and anatomic considerations.

9. Olson SA: Open fractures of the tibial shaft, *J Bone Joint Surg Am* 78:1428–1436, 1996.

In this comprehensive review of open tibial shaft fractures, Olson describes and justifies the principles of treatment in the emergency department (ED) and OR, in addition to wound care rehabilitation.

10. Tscherne H, Gotzen L: *Fractures with soft tissue injuries*, Berlin, 1984, Springer-Verlag.

The author reports that covering the open-fracture wound with a sterile dressing immediately and leaving it in place until surgical debridement results in a threefold to fourfold decrease in long-term infection rates, as compared to dressing changes or leaving the fracture open.

11. Winquist RA, Hansen ST, Clawson DK, et al: Closed intramedullary nailing of femoral fractures: a report of five hundred and twenty cases, *J Bone Joint Surg Am* 166:529–539, 1984.

In this large retrospective review, Winquist and others review their experience with predominantly closed intramedullary nailing and find a union rate of greater than 99% and a low complication rate.

12. Johnson, KD, Cadambi, A, Seibert, GB: Incidence of adult respiratory distress syndrome in patients with multiple musculoskeletal injuries: effect of early operative stabilization of fractures, *J Trauma* 25:375, 1985.

A retrospective review of 132 patients with at least two long-bone fractures and an injury severity score of at least 18. The authors found that greater delay in operative stabilization of fractures was related to increased incidence of adult respiratory distress syndrome (ARDS), particularly in the patient with more severe injuries.

13. Bone, LB, Johnson, KD, Weigelt J, et al: Early vs, delayed stabilization of femoral fractures, *J Bone Joint Surg Am* 71:336, 1989.

The authors performed a prospective trial in which 178 patients were randomized to receive early (<24 hours) versus delayed (>48 hours) stabilization of femoral fractures. The early stabilization group was found to have less incidences of adult respiratory distress syndrome (ARDS), fat embolism syndrome (FES), pneumonia with shorter intensive care unit (ICU) and hospital stays.

14. Pape HC, Auf'm'Kolk M, Paffrath, T, et al: Primary intramedullary femur fixation in multiple trauma patients with associated lung contusion—a cause of posttraumatic ARDS. *J Trauma* 34:540–547, 1993.

This retrospective study from Germany assessed 766 victims of multiple trauma over a decade. The authors concluded that multiple trauma patients without pulmonary contusion benefit from early intramedullary stabilization, but that patients with traumatic lung injury may be at even greater risk of adult respiratory distress syndrome (ARDS) with primary stabilization.

15. Bosse MJ, Mackenzie EJ, Riemer, BL, et al: Adult respiratory distress syndrome, pneumonia, and mortality following thoracic injury and a femoral fracture treated either with intramedullary nailing with reaming or with a plate, *J Bone Joint Surg Am* 79: 799–809, 1997.

In comparing the incidence of pulmonary complications between two centers, one using intramedullary nailing with reaming and the other using a plate, the authors found no difference. They conclude that reaming is safe in patients with multiple injuries including thoracic injury in the absence of significant comorbidity.

16. Bracken MB, Shepard MJ, Collins, WF, et al: A randomized, controlled trial of methylprednisolone or naloxone in the treatment of acute spinal-cord injury, *N Engl J Med* 322:1405–1411, 1990.

This multicenter, randomized, blinded, placebo-controlled trial assessed the use of two drugs that had shown promise in animal models for the treatment of spinal cord injuries (SCIs): methylprednisolone and naloxone. At 6-month follow-up, a larger proportion of patients given methylprednisolone within 8 hours of injury had improved motor and sensory function when compared to the naloxone and placebo groups.

17. Aebi M, Mohler J, Zach, GA, et al: Indication, surgical technique, and results of 100 surgically-treated fractures and fracture-dislocations of the cervical spine, *Clin Orthop Rel Res* 203:244–257, 1986.

Based on observations in this retrospective review of 100 patients, the authors concluded that immediate reduction is the most important predictor of better neurological outcomes.

18. Reigstad A: Traumatic dislocation of the hip, *J Trauma* 20: 603–606, 1980.

In his review of 57 cases of traumatic hip dislocation, Reigstad reported posttraumatic osteoarthritis of the hip in 9.1% of patients and avascular necrosis (AVN) of the femoral head in 5.5%. No cases of AVN were found in patients reduced within 5 hours of injury.

19. Sirkin M, Sanders R, DiPasquale, T, et al: A staged protocol for soft tissue management in the treatment of complex pilon fractures, *J Orthop Trauma* 13:78–84, 1999.

The authors reported a staged protocol for the treatment of complex tibia fractures with immediate fixation of the fibula and spanning external fixation of the ankle followed by definitive fixation of the pilon once soft-tissue swelling resolved. The authors found a significantly decreased wound infection rate as compared to historical reports of immediate definitive fixation.

20. Johansen, K, Daines, M, Howey T, et al Objective criteria accurately predict amputation following lower extremity trauma, *J Trauma* 30:568–572, discussion 572–572, 1990.

Johansen and others derived the mangled extremity severity score (MESS) with a retrospective study of 25 patients with mangled lower extremity and then validated the system with a prospective cohort of 26 patients. All patients with MESS>6 required amputation.

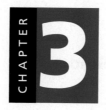
Proximal Humeral Fractures

Mark A. Mighell, MD; Brian Badman, MD; and Nazeem Virani, MD

- Proximal humeral fractures account for 4% to 8% of all fractures and are the third most common type of injury in patients over 65 years of age.[3,5,39]
- The incidence of these fractures has increased in the past decade, likely attributable to the aging population and the associated increase in the incidence of osteoporosis.[6,31,37]
- Despite the relative frequency of these fractures, 80% are minimally displaced and amenable to nonoperative management with good functional outcomes.[26,32,48]
- The treatment of displaced fractures, although controversial, generally involves any number of methods of open reduction and internal fixation (ORIF) or prosthetic replacement as a result of the poor historical outcomes when managed conservatively.[16,18,20,22,29,34,35,41,45,47,48–51,55,59–62,66,68]
- Operative treatment can be quite challenging as a result of the poor bone quality and the naturally deforming forces of the surrounding musculature, which is likely the cause for high failure rates seen with early attempts at osteosynthesis.[2]
- Based on these early failures, many alternative open techniques were proposed with mixed results and no definitive treatment was identified.[16,18,20,22,29,34,35,41,45,47,48–51,55,59–62,66,68]
- Several authors contend that based on the high failure rates with ORIF, the majority of displaced three-part and four-part fractures should be treated by primary prosthetic replacement.[27,43,49,50,62]
- There is a recent trend in the use of locked-plate technology. This can be attributed to the ability to obtain more rigid fixation in compromised bone, thereby eliminating many of the problems associated with standard plating and resulting in improved outcomes.[6,19,21,26,56,60,68,70]

Anatomy

- As initially described by Codman,[13] the proximal humerus can be divided into four anatomic parts based on its epiphyseal lines: the head, the greater tuberosity, the lesser tuberosity, and the proximal shaft (Figure 3–1).
- The average neck–shaft angle is 145 degrees, and the average retroversion of the articular surface, relative to the transepicondylar axis, is 30 degrees[13,17,38,72] (Figure 3–2).
- The greater tuberosity serves as the attachment for three of the four rotator cuff muscles: the supraspinatus, infraspinatus, and teres minor. These muscles serve to abduct and externally rotate the shoulder.
- The lesser tuberosity serves as the attachment for the subscapularis, which internally rotates the shoulder.
- The pectoralis attaches on the lateral edge of the bicipital groove, and the latissimus dorsi attaches on the medial edge.
- With disruption of the anatomy through fractures, the muscles pull on the fragments in a predictable manner, and an understanding of the force vectors can aid in proper treatment of the injury.
- When fractured, the greater tuberosity is displaced superiorly and posteriorly by the outward pull of its attached muscles.
- The lesser tuberosity is pulled medially by the subscapularis.
- The combined forces of the deltoid and pectoralis pull the shaft proximally and medially, respectively, with resultant varus deformity (Figure 3–3).
- Nerve injury must be entertained as a result of the proximity of the brachial plexus. A careful neurologic examination of the upper extremity must be performed.
- Neural injuries may be the result of minor trauma and do not necessarily involve a high-impact injury.
- Nerve injury may occur in up to 67% of patients. Although most of these injuries are transient, an increased incidence of nerve injury is found in displaced fractures (82%) compared to nondisplaced fractures (59%).[4,7]
- The most common nerve injured is the axillary nerve, and the suprascapular nerve is the second most common injured nerve.[4,7]

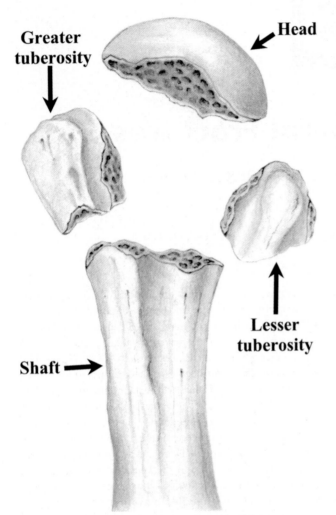

Figure 3–1: Four anatomic parts of the proximal humerus. Codman[13] divided the proximal humerus into four major anatomic parts based on its epiphyseal lines: the head, the greater tuberosity, the lesser tuberosity, and the proximal shaft.

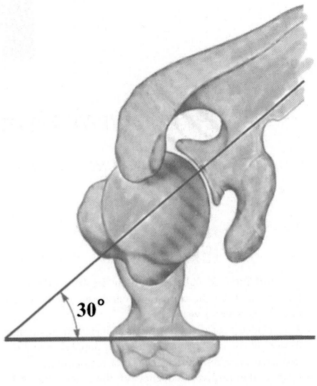

Figure 3–2: Normal position of humeral head. The articular surface of the humeral head is retroverted 30 degrees with respect to the transepicondylar axis. (Modified from Neer CS II: *Shoulder reconstruction*, pp. 143–271. Philadelphia, 1990, W. B. Saunders Company.)

- The major blood supply to the proximal humerus is from the anterior humeral circumflex artery with the majority of the head supplied by the ascending arcuate artery of Laing, located in the lateral portion of the bicipital groove.[27]
- The remaining blood supply is derived from a branch of the posterior humeral circumflex artery and small perforating branches from the overlying rotator cuff.
- Major arterial injury is uncommon in association with proximal humeral fractures.[4,7]
- However, if a major arterial injury is left undiagnosed, the results can be devastating.[4,7]
- Resulting from the proximity of the axillary artery to the brachial plexus, an arteriogram should be performed in any patient with neurologic deficit or absence of pulse in the affected upper extremity.

- In addition to the presence of a brachial plexus injury, age greater than 50 is another factor associated with a major arterial injury.[4] This may be the result of hardening of arteries from atherosclerosis.
- Almost 90% of axillary artery injuries involve the third part of the axillary artery,[4] resulting from the tethering effect of the anterior and posterior circumflex humeral arteries.

Classification

- Although many classification systems have been proposed, the two most popular systems are the Neer classification and the Arbeitsgemeinschaft für Osteosynthesefragen (AO) classification.[36,48]
- The Neer classification, which is the most widely used system, categorizes displaced proximal humerus fractures from two to four parts according to its anatomic segments. Displacement is defined as separation of a fragment by greater than 1 cm or angulation of a fragment greater than 45 degrees. Fracture lines in nondisplaced segments are not included (Figure 3–4).
- The AO classification, a more complex system, is based on the vascular supply of the articular segments. It is

divided into three categories (A, B, C) of increasing severity with each category further split into numerical subgroupings.[36]

- Both classifications have been criticized based on poor interobserver reliability,[58] and debates continue for the development for a more precise system.[5]

Radiographic Analysis

- Accurate imaging is crucial to proper diagnosis and treatment (Box 3–1).
- An initial radiographic assessment should include an anteroposterior (AP) view in the scapular plane, a scapular Y view, and an axillary lateral view.

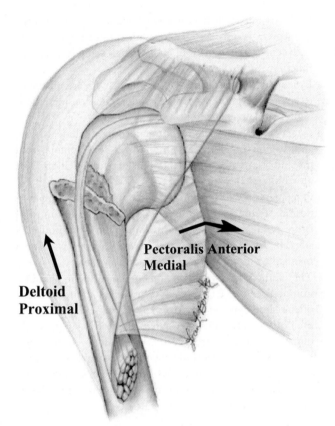

Figure 3–3: Varus deformity seen after two-part fractures. The varus deformity is often the result of the unopposed muscle forces of the deltoid and pectoralis.

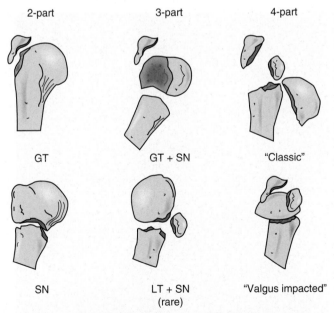

Figure 3–4: Neer's classification system of displaced proximal humerus fractures. The most widely used system used to classify displaced proximal humerus fractures is based on the major anatomic segments of the proximal humerus as defined by Codman.[13] To be considered displaced, the fragment must be displaced at least 1 cm or angulated at least 45 degrees. Note that fractures do not observe segmental description in all cases.[58] GT, greater tuberosity; LT, lesser tuberosity; SN, surgical neck.

Box 3–1	**Considerations when Radiographically Assessing Proximal Humerus Fractures***		

- The classification system is "head-centered," with displacement of the other fragments related to the position of the humeral head.
- Fracture lines may be difficult to see because of osteopenia, obesity, nondisplacement, or overlapping fractures. Note that a fracture may be indicated by a change in metaphyseal bone texture or a double-convex contour.
- In some cases, displacement can be borderline; consider the fragment displaced if there is >1 cm of separation or an angulation that exceeds the normal anatomic angle in a given projection by 45 degrees. When in doubt, obtain additional imaging studies.
- The fracture does not observe segmental description in all cases; for example, half of the lesser tuberosity or greater tuberosity may remain with the head fragment.
- The relationship between the shaft and the remaining fragments may change with arm movement between radiographs. This is most dramatic in the axillary view: If taken with the arm in extension, it may create a high degree of apex anterior angulation. Consider what may happen with fragment position once arm extension is eliminated; use the 40-degree posterior oblique and the scapular lateral (Y) view to judge humeral head-shaft alignment.
- Head-shaft comminution may be difficult to differentiate from a tuberosity fracture.
- Humeral head-shaft shortening is usually not considered displacement.
- Consider head-splitting or impaction only if >20% of the articular surface is affected. If there is impaction or splitting, the fracture should be classified as such and not according to the number of parts.
- When there is a dislocation with an intact head-shaft relationship and a tuberosity fracture, a postreduction radiograph is needed before classifying displacement.

*Modified from Shrader MW, Sánchez-Sotelo J, Sperling JW, et al: Understanding proximal humerus fractures: image analysis, classification, and treatment, *J Shoulder Elbow Surg* 14:497–505, 2005.

- The axillary view is critical and should be obtained at all times because it is important in assessing the extent of tuberosity displacement, determining if a posterior dislocation is present (Figure 3–5), and assessing the integrity of the glenoid. This view can easily be obtained by gently abducting the arm, or if the patient is in too much pain, a Velpeau view can also be obtained.
- In tolerant patients, internal and external views can also be helpful.
- Computed tomography (CT) with 2-mm cuts and three-dimensional (3D) reconstructions, although not necessary in all cases, may be helpful in more complex articular fractures to better assess the fracture type and the extent of fracture displacement.
- Magnetic resonance imaging (MRI) is generally not helpful but can assist in the diagnosis of avascular necrosis (AVN) in the more chronic situation.

Nonoperative Management

- Of the number of proximal humeral fractures, 80% are minimally displaced and amenable to conservative management with good to excellent results.[26,32,48]
- Although debatable in younger patients, Court-Brown and McQueen[15] demonstrated that nonoperative management

for varus-impacted fractures with angulation greater than 40 degrees is also acceptable, with no correlation found between final angulation and overall shoulder pain or function.
- Patients with significant comorbidities, who are unable to tolerate a surgical procedure, should be considered for conservative management.
- General nonoperative recommendations include a sling and swathe or shoulder immobilizer for comfort with the initiation of gentle pendulum activities within 7 to 10 days after the injury.
- Overaggressive early motion can compromise the fracture position resulting from the pull of the rotator cuff musculature, which may end in a malunion. If early motion is advised, routine imaging at 2-week intervals is recommended to monitor for potential displacement.
- The authors' preferred treatment includes a shoulder immobilizer for 4 to 6 weeks with rigid immobilization of the shoulder and emphasis on elbow and wrist range of motion only. Shoulder range of motion is generally initiated at the fourth week, with passive motion and active-assisted motion only for the next 6 weeks or until radiographic union is achieved. Rotator cuff strengthening is usually started at 3 months or with radiographic confirmation of union.

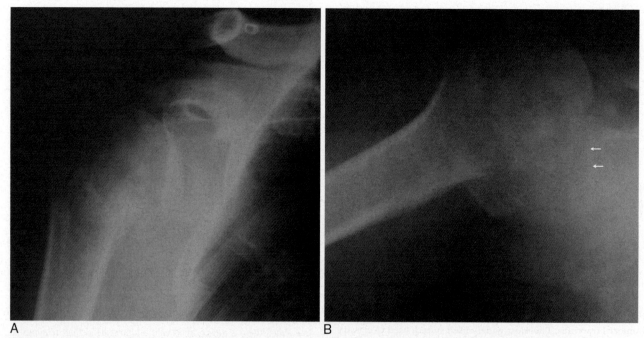

A   B

Figure 3–5: Preoperative radiograph of a patient with a posterior dislocation in addition to a proximal humerus fracture. **A,** Note that the posterior dislocation is not apparent on the anteroposterior radiograph, and the diagnosis may be missed if other views are not obtained. **B,** The preoperative axillary view clearly demonstrates the posterior dislocation that was not evident on the anteroposterior radiograph. Arrows are pointing to the glenoid.

General Surgical Considerations

- Surgical intervention is generally recommended for most displaced Neer two-part, three-part, and four-part fractures as a result of the high complication rates noted with conservative management of these difficult injuries.[12,49,59]
- The two main approaches for operative intervention include either ORIF or prosthetic replacement.
- Although several ORIF techniques have been described, including percutaneous fixation, various methods of tension-band fixation, standard plate and screw fixation, and intramedullary fixation using various techniques, the published outcomes have been mixed, with no definite treatment identified. Several of the described techniques are also associated with a relatively high complication rate, including hardware failure, hardware pain, and injury to adjacent neurovascular structures.[16,18,20,22,29,34,35,41,45,47,48–51,54,55,59–62,66,68]
- Recent interest has been sparked with the advent of locked plating, based on its early success in multiple European series and the avoidance of many of the complications associated with the previous techniques, such as hardware failure or hardware pain.[6,21,53]
- Several recent biomechanical studies confirm improved fixation with the use of a locked plate, as compared to other fixation techniques.[19,25,57,65,67]
- Unlike standard plating, which compresses the screws to the bone, the locked plate functions more like a lever beam. Biomechanical studies have shown that in the locked group the linear range until failure was extended by 64%.[57]
- Despite the improvements in torsional strength with locked plates compared to blade plates,[65] basic orthopaedic principles must be adhered to and cortical contact must be achieved. Therefore, in cases in which a comminuted humeral metadiaphyseal segment exists, it may be beneficial to shorten the humerus by impacting the shaft into the humeral head.
- In elderly patients with osteoporotic bone, the tuberosities are thinned down to a shell or wafer of bone. The most reliable way to achieve an anatomic reduction in these patients is to use heavy sutures passed through the tendon/bone interface of the rotator cuff and secured to the suture islets of the locked plate. This is necessary to balance the forces of the rotator cuff.
- Anatomic studies show that the strongest bone is located in the posterior-medial portion of the humeral head.[30]
- Despite recent advances in internal fixation, several authors still contend that acute hemiarthroplasty should be the treatment of choice for most three-part and four-part fractures in elderly patients.[28,43,49,50,62]
- Hemiarthroplasty for fracture shows predictable improvements in terms of pain relief, but functional improvements are not as predictable.[8,28]
- We believe that with new locked-plate fixation many of the previous fractures treated with hemiarthroplasty are now amenable to internal fixation, even in the elderly population.

Surgical Technique for Locked Plating

- A more detailed description of the surgical technique can be found in the Journal of the American Academy of Orthopaedic Surgeons.[2]

Anesthesia

- An interscalene block is recommended to minimize postoperative pain.
- The endotracheal tube should be positioned on the opposite side of the surgical field to prevent inadvertent dislodgement during surgery.

Positioning

- Adequate fluoroscopic imaging is crucial to the procedure, and appropriate time should be taken to position the patient and the C-arm fluoroscopy unit.
- Most operating tables are equipped with a radiolucent footplate. The table is rotated 180 degrees so that the patient's head is sitting at the foot of the table over the radiolucent portion (Figure 3–6).
- Once on the table, the patient's head and torso are elevated approximately 30 degrees, with the head supported on a jelly doughnut and taped into place.
- The table is then turned 90 degrees relative to the anesthesiologist to allow the C-arm to be positioned parallel to the patient at the head of the bed. This allows for an unobstructed view of the shoulder and avoids interference with the anesthesiologist.
- The C-arm can be rotated over the top so that a direct AP view is obtained. Once adequate imaging is confirmed,

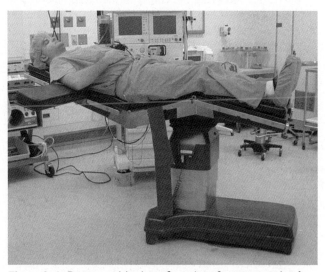

Figure 3–6: **Proper positioning of a patient for open proximal humerus fracture surgery. The patient's head and torso are elevated approximately 30 degrees. Note rotation of the table 180 degrees, so that the patient's head is placed at the foot of the table over the radiolucent portion.**

the C-arm can be pulled straight back so as to not interfere with prepping. If adequate imaging is not obtained, the patient and C-arm should be repositioned before sterile prepping.

Approach

- A standard deltopectoral approach is used.
- A Mayo stand is used and can help support the arm in slight abduction, avoiding the need for an extra assistant and minimizing the tension on the deltoid.
- The cephalic vein is taken medially with the pectoralis muscle to avoid inadvertent injury during retraction of the deltoid.
- Gelpi retractors may be placed superficially, allowing for the development of the subdeltoid space.
- The Browne deltoid retractor (made by Innomed Inc., Savannah, Georgia) is placed next and is essential in aiding proper exposure.
- The clavipectoral fascia should be released, and the subcoracoid space should be developed. Up to 25% of the lateral portion of the conjoined tendon can be released off the coracoid tip to facilitate exposure. We do not recommend placing a self-retaining retractor beneath the conjoined tendon to avoid the risk of musculocutaneous nerve neuropraxia.
- The biceps tendon is now identified deep to the pectoralis tendon and can easily be palpated as it rolls under the pectoralis insertion on the humeral shaft. Hematoma can often obscure the obvious landmarks, so using this as a reference can be helpful. Occasionally, the bicep tendon may be interposed in the fracture fragments and may require mobilization.
- After identifying the bicep tendon, the rotator interval is opened by following the course of the bicep tendon as it enters the glenohumeral joint to its superior attachment on the glenoid. The bicep tendon can be preserved or cut. In cases in which the biceps tendon is injured or entrapped in the fracture site, we believe that this tendon will never function normally. Therefore, to avoid a source of postoperative pain, we perform a subpectoral tenodesis.
- We do not routinely release the pectoralis tendon, but up to 20% of its upper border can be cut to facilitate exposure.

Fracture Preparation

- The fracture hematoma is debrided, and the tuberosities are mobilized if they are separate fragments. A heavy composite suture is placed around the bone/tendon interface of each tuberosity.
- If a tuberosity remains attached to the head segment, then a Krackow stitch is placed in the substance of the attached tendon.
- We routinely place two sutures in the subscapularis and at least two in the supraspinatus and infraspinatus. These stitches serve as traction sutures to assist with the overall

reduction of the fracture and help to counter the deforming forces of the rotator cuff.
- To expose the proximal shaft, extend the arm.
- The clot and hematoma is then removed from within the medullary canal.
- The first step to reconstruction requires anatomic reduction of the head segment.
- A Key or a Cobb elevator is used to elevate the head. This reduction may be held by either placing a Kirschner wire (K-wire) through the head segment into the glenoid or pinning the head segment to the shaft. The provisional K-wire should then be bent to avoid obstructing application of the locked plate.
- Fluoroscopy is used to confirm adequate reduction of the head, and if unacceptable, the K-wire is removed and the reduction is repeated until alignment is deemed satisfactory by the surgeon.
- Once the head is anatomically reduced, the tuberosities beneath the head fragment should also be reduced using the traction sutures previously placed in the cuff.
- In fractures with extensive comminution in which a large metaphyseal void is encountered after reduction of the tuberosities, we advise the use of a structural allograft in the form of a tricortical iliac crest graft or fibular cortical strut. This can be placed intramedullary within the proximal canal and will serve to support the head fragment in situations in which a metaphyseal void is present. A structural graft can prevent subsequent collapse of the head postoperatively. For small voids, corticocancellous bone graft is recommended.
- The shaft is then reduced to the proximal segment, and the head is provisionally pinned to the shaft to maintain the overall reduction. If a greater tuberosity segment is present, it can also be pinned by passing a K-wire from the posterolateral edge of the acromion with capture of the tuberosity and fixation into the shaft. Fluoroscopy is once again used to confirm acceptable reduction.

Plate Application

- The fracture must be anatomically reduced before application of the locked plate.
- Although many different locking plates are available, the following design features are particularly important:
  - A low profile to reduce the risk of overhead impingement on the acromion.
  - Divergent proximal locking screw options to reduce the risk of pullout and improve head fixation.
  - The presence of multiple suture eyelets on the plate that allow for passage of the locking sutures within the rotator cuff after the plate is secured to the bone.
- General manufacturer recommendations include positioning the plate just lateral to the bicipital groove, typically between 1 and 3 cm distal to the top of the humeral head based on the plate type. Most plates offer a gliding hole

for shaft fixation, and this should be drilled first at its center to allow minor adjustments in plate height after viewing with fluoroscopy. This screw should also be nonlocking to allow for proper reduction and compression of the plate to the shaft. Shaft screws typically measure 28 mm in length.

- Once the plate height is acceptable, most plates allow for a central K-wire to be passed through the plate and into the head. We most frequently use the Hand Innovations S3 (DePuy Orthopaedics, Warsaw, Indiana, USA) plate, and when placed appropriately, the K-wire should pass through the center of the humeral head on the AP image (Figure 3–7).
- Proximal head screws are then sequentially placed in a standard fashion after drilling the outer cortex and measuring the appropriate length. We prefer to hand tap all head screws to avoid inadvertent articular penetration of the thin cortical shell because we feel it provides better tactile feedback than when tapping with power.

- With the Hand Innovations system, screws and pegs are both offered for the head fragment. In general, screws are only used when treating an anatomic neck fracture in which additional purchase into the head fragment is critical for stable fixation. In all other circumstances, smooth pegs are preferred because if the head does collapse and the screws subsequently penetrate the joint, we believe a smooth peg would inherently cause less destruction to the joint than a sharp screw tip. The smooth peg also presents a greater surface area for support of the strong subchondral bone of the head segment.
- Once all head screws are placed, the shaft screws are drilled; at least three shaft screws are used.
- Illustrative cases are presented in Figures 3–8 and 3–9.

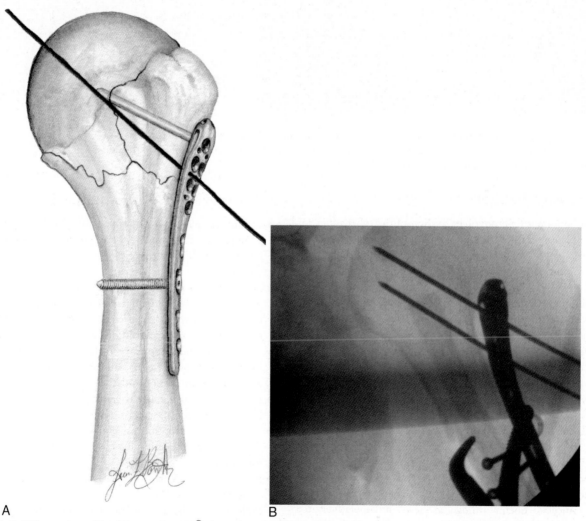

A   B

Figure 3–7: When using a Hand Innovations S3® plate, the centering K-wire should bisect the humeral head. **A,** Diagram showing K-wire passing through the center of the humeral head. **B,** Before placing multiple divergent locked screws in the humeral head, plate position is intraoperatively confirmed by fluoroscopy. Note that an intramedullary allograft strut was used in this patient.

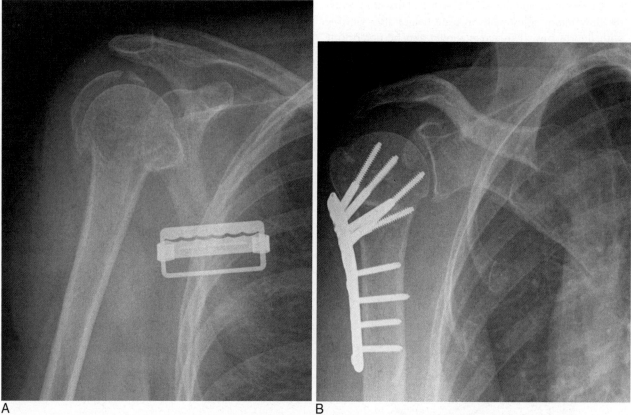

A   B

Figure 3–8: Illustrative case: three-part fracture in a 62-year-old woman treated with locked plating.
A, Preoperative anteroposterior image demonstrating a deformed head. **B,** Postoperative image of the same patient with a locked proximal humeral plate used to fix the fracture.

Tuberosity Fixation

- An important tenet involves fixation of the tuberosities to the plate. Similar to the principles involved with hemiarthroplasty for fracture, the deforming forces of the rotator cuff must be neutralized to avoid subsequent displacement and failure. The pull of the cuff is counterbalanced by using heavy sutures in the rotator cuff and tying them to the plate via suture eyelets at the plate's proximal end. Plates that require the sutures to be passed before plate application to the shaft should be avoided because this is extremely time consuming and could force the surgeon to skip this crucial step.

- Typically one to two sutures are placed through the subscapularis, and two to three sutures are passed into the substance of the supraspinatus and infraspinatus for a total of at least three to five locking sutures tied to the plate (Figure 3–10).

- Once fixation is secure, the arm is rotated to ensure fracture stability and final fluoroscopic imaging is obtained. It is critical to obtain orthogonal views intraoperatively to ensure all screws are the appropriate lengths and that none are intraarticular.

- The rotator interval is closed with a No. 2 Ethibond or FiberWire, and the wound is closed in a standard fashion.

Postoperative Management

- Patients are placed in a shoulder immobilizer and typically admitted postoperatively for a period of 24 hours for intravenous (IV) antibiotics and 1 to 2 days for pain control.

- For stable two-part fractures, the immobilizer is discontinued at 2 weeks, allowing gentle pendulum and passive motion and active-assisted range of motion with the contralateral extremity, focusing on forward flexion.

- Three-part and four-part fractures are usually rigidly immobilized for 4 weeks with an emphasis on wrist and elbow range of motion only.

- Formal physical therapy is generally not initiated until at least 4 weeks for all fracture types.

- Active range of motion usually begins at 8 weeks or with the first radiograph showing evidence of callous formation.

- Strengthening is started in the last phase of formal therapy, typically at 12 weeks.

- Follow-up radiographs are obtained at the initial postoperative visit and then at 6 weeks, 3 months, 6 months, and annually thereafter for a period of at least 2 years.

- It is important to monitor for the late development of AVN.

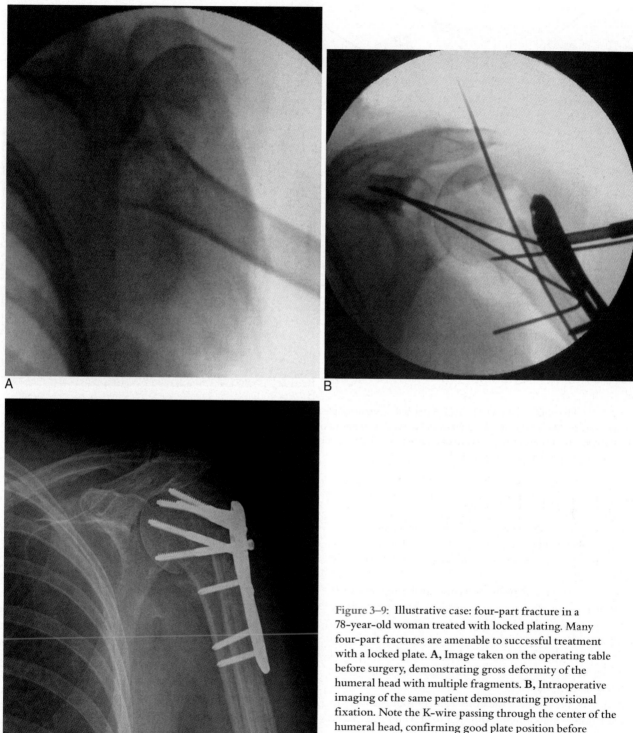

Figure 3–9: Illustrative case: four-part fracture in a 78-year-old woman treated with locked plating. Many four-part fractures are amenable to successful treatment with a locked plate. **A,** Image taken on the operating table before surgery, demonstrating gross deformity of the humeral head with multiple fragments. **B,** Intraoperative imaging of the same patient demonstrating provisional fixation. Note the K-wire passing through the center of the humeral head, confirming good plate position before placement of multiple head screws. **C,** Postoperative anteroposterior image of the same patient demonstrating good fixation with a locked proximal humerus plate. Note that an intramedullary allograft strut was used in this patient.

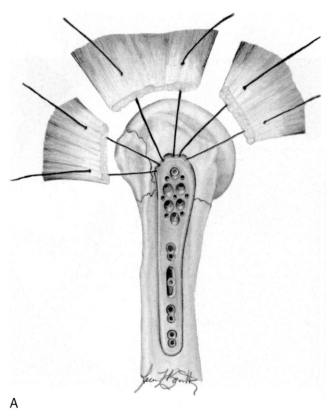

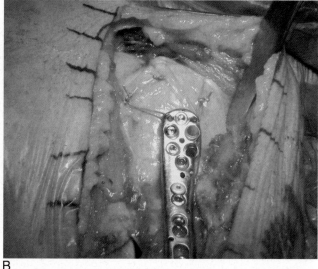

A   B

Figure 3–10: **The pull of the rotator cuff is balanced using multiple heavy sutures. A,** Heavy sutures are passed through suture islets in the proximal plate and tied to the tendons of the subscapularis, supraspinatus, and infraspinatus. **B,** Intraoperative picture of an attempt to balance rotator cuff forces using multiple heavy sutures tied via suture islets to the rotator cuff muscles.

Pearls: Locked Plates

- Confirm that adequate orthogonal fluoroscopic images can be obtained before prepping. This will hasten the case and avoid much unnecessary frustration intraoperatively (Box 3–2).
- Avoid excessive soft-tissue dissection in the region of the bicipital groove to prevent injury to the arcuate artery and to preserve the blood supply to the head segment.
- Minimize handling of the tuberosities. It is preferable to manipulate the bone fragments by traction stitches placed in the substance of the rotator cuff or passed around their bone/tendon interface.
- Anatomic reduction of the head segment is the first key to reduction. To accomplish this, the rotator interval can be opened to allow for direct visualization of the glenohumeral relationship.
- In difficult fracture patterns, the head segment can be pinned into the glenoid vault and used as a keystone for reconstruction of the tuberosities.
- Impaction of the cancellous bone of the proximal humerus often requires a structural graft to support the humeral head and tuberosities. This can help prevent postoperative collapse of the head into the bony void.
- The fracture must be reduced before application of the locked plate.
- Cortical contact must be achieved between the shaft and proximal segment. It is often necessary to impact the shaft segment into the head in cases with significant metadiaphyseal comminution.
- We feel that locked plates with multiple divergent head screws improve fixation when compared to locked plates with limited head screws or convergent screws that act similar to a blade plate.
- In osteoporotic bone, special attention should be made to place head screws or pegs into the strong subchondral bone of the posteromedial head segment.[30]
- The surgeon should attempt to place the maximum number of screws into the proximal bone.

Box 3–2	**Basic Principles of Locked Plating for Proximal Humerus Fractures**

- Cortical contact
- Anatomic reduction of tuberosities
- Counterbalance the deforming forces of the rotator cuff

- Locked plates do not allow for capture of small greater tuberosity fragments, and it is imperative to use heavy sutures or wires to minimize the possibility of tuberosity failure.
- Heavy sutures placed through the cuff and tied to the plate can effectively counterbalance the deforming forces of the rotator cuff.
- Avoid aggressive postoperative range of motion, especially in the three-part and four-part fractures to allow for adequate healing and to potentially minimize failures.

Surgical Technique for Hemiarthroplasty

Indications

- Hemiarthroplasty is typically reserved for comminuted four-part fractures in patients older than 60, anatomic neck fractures in patients older than 40, all head-splitting fractures, and fracture-dislocations.[14]
- The results of internal fixation for four-part fracture-dislocations have been extremely poor.[16] Therefore we now recommend arthroplasty for all four-part fracture-dislocations.

Important Design Features when Selecting an Implant

- Modularity of head and distal stem[46] (Figure 3–11).
- Version guides to allow for predictable placement of the implant in 20 to 40 degrees of retroversion.
- The proximal body of the implant should be small and serve as a scaffold to reconstruct the tuberosities.
- Centralizer or centering sleeve to prevent placing the prosthesis in varus or valgus. A larger diameter distal stem will also prevent malpositioning of the prosthesis. Avoid selection of an implant based on shaft canal diameter because it will often result in an oversized proximal body and an inability to reduce the tuberosities.
- Implants with design features that allow for passage of cerclage sutures.

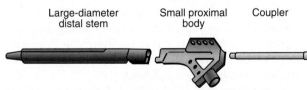

Large-diameter distal stem   Small proximal body   Coupler

Figure 3–11: **Modular hemiarthroplasty stem. The modularity of the fracture stem shown allows a surgeon to couple a small proximal body (for better tuberosity fixation) with a variable diameter distal stem. In elderly patients, whose intramedullary canal diameter often exceeds 10 mm, a larger diameter distal stem is more appropriate. (Reprinted with permission from Encore Medical Corporation [Austin, TX].)**

- Filleted holes that reduce the possibility of suture breakage.
- Implants with roughened proximal body surfaces or irregularity of the proximal body to facilitate stability and ingrowth.[40]

Anesthesia and Positioning

- Anesthesia and position are the same as described earlier in "Surgical Technique for Locked Plating" except that the patient is typically seated in a full beach chair position.
- The C-arm is a useful tool to evaluate tuberosity position relative to the modular head of the prosthetic device.

Approach

- Deltopectoral approach—the cephalic vein should be taken medially to minimize injury during retractor placement and preparation of the humeral canal.
- Develop the spaces—it is important to palpate the axillary nerve in the subcoracoid space so that it can be protected throughout the procedure. We do not routinely dissect out the nerve during the exposure.
- Develop the subdeltoid and subacromial spaces.
- The Browne deltoid retractor is placed next and is essential in aiding proper exposure.
- The arm may be placed onto a well-padded Mayo stand for support during the procedure.

Mobilization of the Tuberosities

- Identify the lesser tuberosity, and place a traction stitch at the tendon/bone interface.
- Enter the joint through the lateral fracture line. In most cases, the greater tuberosity is fractured off just posterior to the bicipital groove. The fracture line may be entered with an osteotome and the cuff split to the supraglenoid tubercle to allow for mobilization of the greater tuberosity. We recommend that the cuff split be co-linear with the fracture line.
- Remove the head segment, and measure the height and diameter with calipers.
- The cancellous bone from the head segment is harvested and morselized for later use as a bone graft.
- Mobilization of the greater tuberosity is then performed. Abduct and internally rotate the arm on a well-padded Mayo stand. Place a traction stitch in the supraspinatus to assist in delivering the fragment into the surgical field. Heavy sutures placed at the tendon/bone interface should be used to manipulate the greater tuberosity to avoid the fragmentation that often occurs from excessive handling of the bone.

Placement of Prosthesis

- Prepare the humeral canal with hand reamers. In elderly patients, the canal diameter often exceeds 10 mm.

- Place drill holes in the humeral canal for placement of heavy sutures that can be used to obtain vertical fixation. We typically place at least two sutures in the bicipital groove because this is where the strongest bone is located. This prevents cutout of the sutures through the bone.
- In most fractures, a portion of the medial calcar remains intact.
- A practical way to determine height is to seat the prosthesis so that the inferior portion of the trial head is flush with any remaining medial calcar (Figure 3–12).
- Alignment or version guides can be used to dial in the appropriate amount of retroversion of the humeral prosthesis. In most cases, 20 to 30 degrees of retroversion is appropriate for reconstruction of the tuberosities.

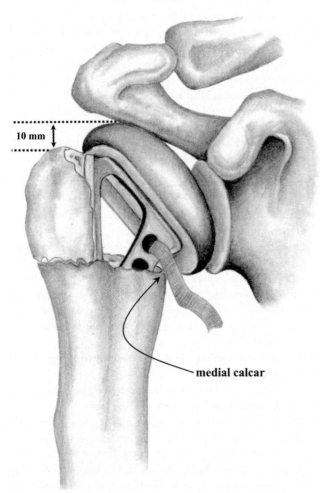

Figure 3–12: **Proper placement of the hemiarthroplasty, so that the inferior portion of the head lies on the medial calcar of the remaining humerus, allows a surgeon to accurately gauge the correct height for the prosthesis. The superior aspect of the greater tuberosity should be 10 mm below the top of the articular surface of the humeral head. Having a head-to-tuberosity distance that is too great is one of the pitfalls of hemiarthroplasty for fracture.**

- In addition to external jigs to determine version, aligning the anterior fin of the stem with the biceps groove will help place the prosthesis in the appropriate amount of retroversion in most prosthetic designs that have at least two fins.
- When selecting the final prosthesis, keep in mind that the proximal body of the prosthesis should serve as a scaffold for reconstruction. The body size should be minimized so that the tuberosities can be reduced to the prosthesis. If necessary, bone graft taken from the head can be used to fill metaphyseal voids. The key to good function requires union of the tuberosities.
- Perform a trial reduction of the tuberosities on the prosthetic body.
- Trial head sizes of varying heights and diameters.
- The glenoid vault and native head segment can be helpful in determining the appropriate diameter for the prosthetic head.
- Place several heavy sutures in the holes previously drilled in the humeral shaft before inserting the final prosthesis.
- Place a cement restrictor in the humeral canal and introduce cement in a doughy state. Remove all excess cement.
- Place one or two cerclage sutures through the medial holes in the prosthesis, and insert the final prosthesis into the humeral canal. We commonly use either two No. 3 cottony Dacrons or two Fibertape sutures (Arthrex, Naples, Florida).
- The prosthesis is fixed distally with cement, and the proximal centimeter of the humeral canal is packed with bone graft harvested from the fractured head segment.
- The cement is allowed to cure.
- The selected modular head segment is then impacted.

Reconstruction of Tuberosities

- The cerclage sutures are placed around the tuberosities at the tendon/bone junction (Figure 3–13A).
- Horizontal fixation is then achieved by placing the heavy sutures from the greater tuberosity through the holes in the anterior fin. These sutures may be tied or passed through the subscapularis to capture the lesser tuberosity (Figure 3–13B).
- When assessing the fracture reduction, the greater tuberosity should be positioned approximately 10 mm from the top of the articular surface of the humeral head (see Figure 3–12). The C-arm may be brought in to confirm that the greater tuberosity is positioned approximately 10 mm beneath the humeral head.
- Horizontal fixation is completed before securing the tuberosities to the shaft.
- The shaft sutures are then placed around the tuberosities in a figure-of-eight fashion for vertical fixation and to complete the reconstruction.
- The arm should be abducted 45 degrees before tying the shaft sutures to the tuberosities. If the sutures are tied with

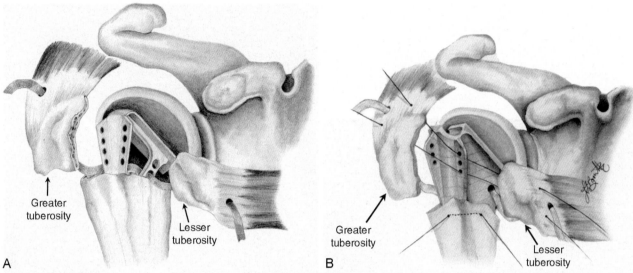

Figure 3–13: Achieving anatomic position of the tuberosities in hemiarthroplasty requires use of a sufficiently small proximal stem combined with cerclage and heavy sutures. **A,** First, cerclage sutures are fed through holes in the medial stem and passed through the tendon-bone junctions of the rotator cuff muscles attached to the greater and lesser tuberosity. **B,** Next, horizontal fixation is achieved by placing heavy sutures from the greater tuberosity through the holes in the anterior fin. These sutures may then be passed through the subscapularis to capture the lesser tuberosity.

the arm at the side, any elevation of the arm will result in loosening of the vertical sutures.
- See illustrative case in Figure 3–14.

Pearls: Hemiarthroplasty

- Minimize handling of the tuberosities to avoid fragmentation (Box 3–3).
- The tuberosities should be mobilized via the heavy sutures placed at the tendon/bone interface.
- Never debulk the tuberosities. If it is difficult to reduce the tuberosities to the prosthetic body, then select a smaller body size.
- In the treatment of fractures, the prosthesis should always be cemented as there is no other consistent way to hold and maintain the prosthesis at the correct height and version.[9]
- The biceps groove is S-shaped, with the groove being more anterior at the level of the surgical neck. If used as a landmark to determine version, it will lead to increased retroversion by 10 to 20 degrees with respect to the retroversion determined by using the transepicondylar axis of the elbow as a guide.[10]
- Excessive retroversion of the prosthesis will lead to limited internal rotation and contribute to increased traction forces on the greater tuberosity repair.
- The prosthesis should be in contact with the medial calcar whenever a portion of the calcar remains.
- Maximal tuberosity stability is provided by one or two heavy cerclage sutures that circumferentially go around the tuberosities and prosthesis. This is most effective when the prosthesis has an irregular geometry.[23,24]

- In the horizontal plane, the greater tuberosity should abut the anterior fin of the prosthesis in a three-fin design or should overhang the lateral fin if only one fin exists.
- The greater tuberosity should be 10 mm beneath the superior aspect of the articular surface of the prosthetic head.[42,44]
- The superior aspect of the humeral articular surface should be 5.5 ± 0.5 cm proximal to the superior border of the pectoralis major tendon. This is a useful relationship in determining whether proper humeral length is restored.[48]

Pitfalls: Hemiarthroplasty

- Technical errors that can result in an increased head-to-tuberosity distance include humeral lengthening by cementing the prosthesis proud, using a head segment that is too thick, and overreducing the greater tuberosity.[23]
- Prosthetic malposition can contribute to poor reduction of the tuberosities. If the prosthesis is excessively retroverted, then all subsequent steps will be compromised. The position of the tuberosities relative to the prosthesis may appear to be acceptable; however, in reality, they are poorly rotated.[70]
- Abnormal bone junction stress may result in early tuberosity failure.
- A prosthesis cemented proud alters the ability to reconstruct the tuberosities accurately.
- Overreduction is required to obtain apposition of the tuberosity with the shaft. This will result in a decreased joint volume. The clinical consequence will be the theoretic possibility of poor function resulting from increased

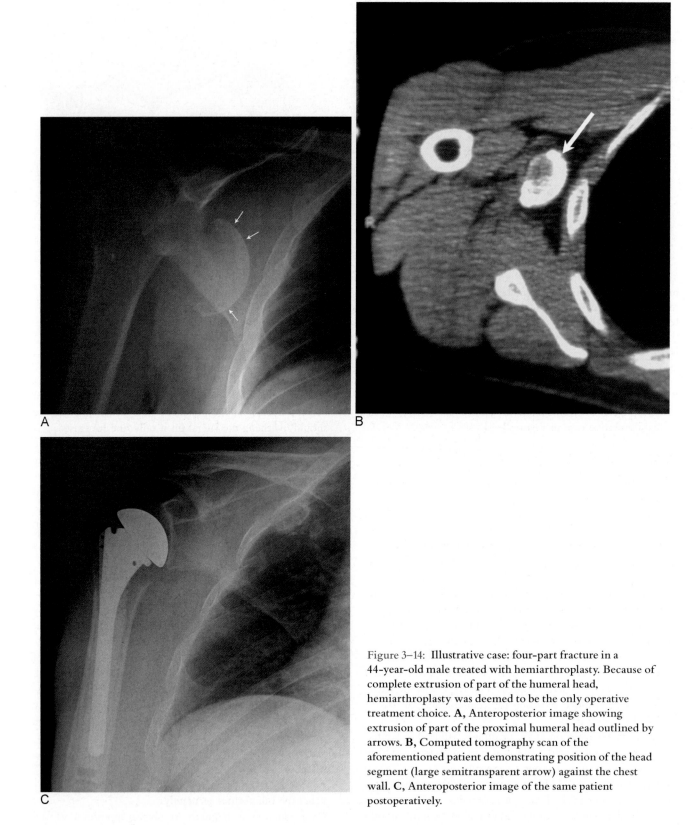

Figure 3–14: Illustrative case: four-part fracture in a 44-year-old male treated with hemiarthroplasty. Because of complete extrusion of part of the humeral head, hemiarthroplasty was deemed to be the only operative treatment choice. **A,** Anteroposterior image showing extrusion of part of the proximal humeral head outlined by arrows. **B,** Computed tomography scan of the aforementioned patient demonstrating position of the head segment (large semitransparent arrow) against the chest wall. **C,** Anteroposterior image of the same patient postoperatively.

Box 3–3	Key Points of Surgical Technique for Hemiarthroplasty

- Height
- Version
- Stable anatomic reduction of the tuberosities

tension within the rotator cuff. This can be avoided by decreasing the thickness of the head segment to balance the joint volume.

- It is essential to secure the prosthesis at the proper height and version to avoid later alterations in tuberosity reduction and fixation.[34]

Common Complications
Avascular Necrosis

- Incidence is most likely related to the complexity of the fractures treated and degree of displacement of the fracture fragments.[26]
- Four-part fractures have the highest incidence of AVN, with rates between 41% and 59%.[41,59]
- The primary blood supply to the head is derived from the ascending branches of the anterior circumflex artery.[27]
- Recent literature has shown that there exists a watershed area on the lateral cortex of the humerus that may be the ideal location for plate application.
- Valgus-impacted four-part fractures have a lower incidence of AVN. This may be the result of preservation of the medial capsular vessels, which may not be disrupted in this injury pattern.[11,35]
- Anatomically reduced fractures of the proximal humerus that go on to AVN may be functionally satisfactory and not require any further surgical intervention.[26,68]

Nonunion

- The risk of nonunion may be broken down into three broad categories related to the fracture pattern, host factors, and surgical technique.
- Fractures that are severely displaced and have significant comminution are at a greater risk for nonunion.[7,56]
- Limited motion of the glenohumeral joint before injury as a result of arthritis, previous trauma, or capsular contracture may also increase the risk for nonunion. In this setting, it is imperative to avoid early aggressive physiotherapy.[7]
- Interposition of the biceps or other soft tissues may also lead to the development of a nonunion.
- Patient factors that contribute to nonunion include obesity, alcoholism, nicotine use, and medical problems, such as diabetes and osteoporosis. These problems often cannot

be corrected but should be addressed with the patient before revision surgery.[63]

- Poor surgical technique may also result in nonunion, and surgical dissection should be performed with an emphasis on limited periosteal stripping and preservation of the remaining vascular supply to the humeral head.
- Cortical contact between the proximal segment and shaft should be achieved, and we recommend impaction of the shaft into the proximal segment to accomplish this in cases of metadiaphyseal comminution.
- The fracture should be anatomically reduced before plate application. If a locked plate is applied to an inadequately reduced fracture, then the fracture will remain poorly reduced or even locked in distraction.[2]
- For patients who develop a nonunion after surgical treatment, always consider deep infection as a possible etiology for nonunion.
- The clinical presentation of patients with radiographic evidence of nonunion is varied. Some patients present with relatively few complaints, whereas others have severe disabling pain and loss of motion.
- Surgical indications include significant pain, loss of function, and deformity.[7]
- The preferred surgical treatment is ORIF.
- Ring and others[52] reported on the use of a blade plate and bone graft and achieved union in 92% of cases with 80% good-to-excellent results.
- Fracture union can be expected with fixed angle devices and bone grafting, but clinical outcomes are inferior as a result of preoperative soft-tissue contracture and capsulitis form prolonged disuse and immobility.
- Structural bone graft may be used in the form of an intramedullary dowel placed in the shaft and left slightly proud to fill the metaphyseal void and allow for impaction of the proximal segment.
  1. Autograft struts have been employed with success but are related to fairly high donor site morbidity.[64]
  2. Allograft struts have also been used with predictable results, and this avoids all donor site morbidity.[3,69]
  3. Structural graft may also be beneficial in cases of severe comminution and osteoporosis. Cortical contact should be achieved in all cases in which a structural graft is used as an intercalary strut or dowel.

Treatment of Nonunion with a Locked Plate

- Expect altered surgical field with significant scar tissue (Figure 3–15).
- Obtain cultures to rule out deep infection in cases of failed internal fixation.
- Minimize bone loss while removing previous hardware.
- Mobilize the fracture fragments, and remove all interposed and fibrous tissue.
- Open the medullary canal of the humeral shaft to facilitate blood flow.

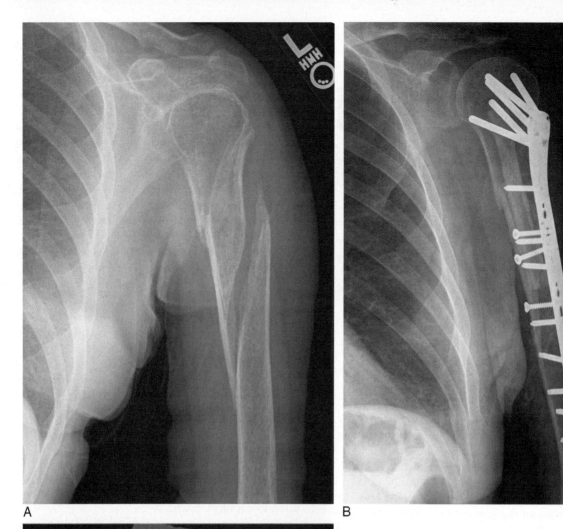

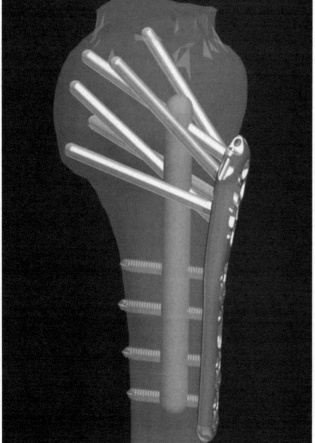

Figure 3–15: Illustrative case: proximal humerus nonunion with failed hardware in a 57-year-old woman treated with locked plating and a fibular strut allograft. **A,** Preoperative X-ray demonstrating a proximal humerus nonunion. The patient sustained a fracture 5 months before this X-ray and was treated conservatively with a brace and a bone stimulator. **B,** Postoperative anteroposterior radiograph of the same patient after a locked plate with a fibular strut allograft. Note the oblique nature of the shaft fracture allowed multiple lag screws to be placed for fracture fixation. **C,** Computer-generated image demonstrating the use of a fibular strut allograft in conjunction with a locked plate. (Reprinted with permission from Hand Innovations [Miami, FL].)

- Structural graft can be placed into the canal to support the humeral head and improve screw purchase (see Figure 3–15C).[3]
- Anatomically reduce and compress the nonunion site.
- In fracture patterns with obliquity, fixation should be performed with lag screws. In this situation, the plate is used as a neutralization device.
- Heavy sutures placed in the tendons of the rotator cuff should be secured to the plate to counterbalance deforming muscular forces.

Treatment of Nonunion with Humeral Head Replacement

- Indication for humeral head prosthesis[1,7] (Figure 3–16).
  - Articular damage.
  - Inadequate bone in the humeral head to hold the fixation.
- Surgical exposure similar to the one described previously.
- Technical points include use of the hand burr. Do not broach the proximal humerus because the bone is often avascular and sclerotic and can easily be fractured.
- As a result of distorted anatomy, it is often prudent to use the smallest prosthetic body possible. This serves to

prevent inadvertent cortical penetration with the hand reamers and may decrease the need to perform a greater tuberosity osteotomy.
- Do not osteotomize the greater tuberosity unless absolutely necessary. Patients with greater tuberosity osteotomies have worse clinical outcomes.[40]
- We recommend a cemented prosthesis because bone ingrowth may not occur in situations with significant sclerosis and areas of avascular bone.
- Obtain intraoperative images to ensure that the canal is not perforated before placement of bone cement to prevent extrusion.

Tuberosity Failure after Hemiarthroplasty for Fracture

- Detachment and migration of the tuberosities is the most common complication after hemiarthroplasty for fractures.[14]
- Poor reduction of the greater tuberosity was by far the most common complication in our series of patients. Overreduction of the greater tuberosity leads to poor outcomes and superior migration of the prosthesis.[44]

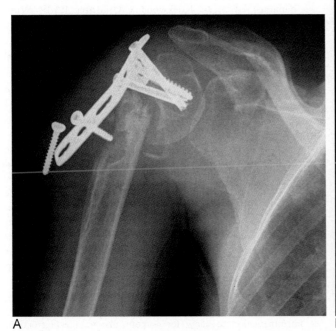
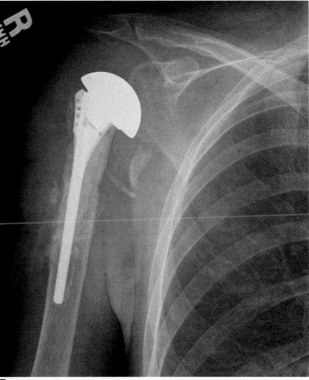

A   B

Figure 3–16: Illustrative case: Proximal humerus nonunion with failed hardware in a 46-year-old woman treated with hemiarthroplasty. This nonunion was not amenable to locked plating, because the head segment had significant cavitary defects and not enough bone to hold fixation. **A,** Preoperative anteroposterior radiograph shows nonunion and failed hardware with extensive damage to the humeral head. **B,** Postoperative anteroposterior radiograph of the same patient after hemiarthroplasty. Significant bone loss is noted.

Conclusions

- Proper diagnosis includes obtaining AP, scapular lateral, and axillary views. CT may be helpful to better assess the fracture type and the extent of fracture displacement.
- Eighty percent of proximal humeral fractures are minimally displaced and amenable to nonoperative management.
- Operative management is recommended for most displaced Neer two-part, three-part, and four-part fractures.
- Anatomic reconstruction using locked plating should be performed whenever possible to allow for the best functional outcomes.
- Key tenets of locked plating include anatomic reduction of the tuberosities, ensuring cortical contact, and counterbalancing the deforming forces of the rotator cuff using heavy sutures.
- Hemiarthroplasty should be reserved for comminuted four-part fractures in patients older than 60, anatomic neck fractures in patients older than 40, all head-splitting fractures, and most fracture-dislocations.
- Key tenets of hemiarthroplasty for fracture include stable reconstruction of the tuberosities and ensuring correct height and version.
- Key complications of operative management of proximal humerus fractures include nonunion, AVN, and tuberosity failure after hemiarthroplasty.
- Nonunions requiring operative management should be treated in most cases with locked plating, using a fibular strut allograft. Hemiarthroplasty should be used when there is articular damage or inadequate bone in the humeral head to hold fixation.

Annotated References

1. Antuña SA, Sperling JW, Sánchez-Sotolo J, et al: Shoulder arthroplasty for proximal humeral nonunions, *J Shoulder Elbow Surg* 11:114-121, 2002.

The authors concluded that shoulder arthroplasty may be beneficial in patients who have significant functional impairment from a nonunion of the humeral surgical neck with failed internal fixation, severe osteoporosis, cavitation of the humeral head, or secondary osteoarthritis.

2. Badman BL, Mighell M: Fixed-angle locked plating of two, three, and four part proximal humerus fractures, *J Am Acad Orthop Surg* in press.

The authors present their surgical technique for internal fixation of two-part, three-part, and four-part proximal humerus fractures. They contend that a reproducible surgical technique using locked plating, suture fixation of the tuberosities, and use of structural allograft in cases with large metaphyseal voids are the main components to a good surgical outcome.

3. Badman BL, Mighell MA, Drake GN: Proximal humeral nonunions: surgical technique with fibular strut allograft and fixed-angle locked plating, *Tech Shoulder Elbow Surg* 7:95-100, 2006.

This article presents a safe and reliable method for treatment of nonunions of the proximal humerus using an inlay fibular strut allograft, compression through the nonunion site with heavy suture, and secure fixation with a fixed-angle locked plate. The authors comment on their positive early results with a radiographic healing rate of 100% in eight surgical neck nonunions.

4. Barei DP, Taitsman LA, Nork SE: Fractures about the shoulder, In Trumble TE, Budof JE,, Cornwall R (eds.), *Hand, elbow and shoulder: core knowledge in orthopaedics*. Philadelphia, 2006, Mosby, Inc.

5. Bigliani LU, Flatow EL, Pollock RG: Fractures of the proximal humerus, In Rockwood CA, Green DP, Bucholz RW, et al (eds.), *Rockwood and Green's fractures in adults*. ed 4, Philadelphia, 1996, Lippincott-Raven Publishers.

6. Björkenheim JM, Pajarinen J, Savolainen V: Internal fixation of proximal humeral fractures with a locking compression plate: a retrospective evaluation of 72 patients followed for a minimum of 1 year, *Acta Orthop Scand* 75:741-745, 2004.

The authors retrospectively reviewed the complications and functional outcomes after a minimum follow-up of 1 year in 72 patients treated with a variable angle Proksimal Humerus Internt Låse System (PHILOS) locking plate. Two fractures failed to unite, and three patients developed avascular necrosis (AVN) of the humeral head. In addition, two implant failures were observed. According to the Constant score, the functional outcome was acceptable, even in elderly patients. The authors conclude that the PHILOS method appears to be safe and can be recommended for the treatment of proximal humerall fractures in patients with poor bone quality.

7. Blaine TA, Bigliani LU, Levine WN: Fractures of the proximal humerus, ed 3, In Rockwood CA, Master FAIII, Wirth MA, et al (eds.), The Shoulder, ed 3, vol 1. Philadelphia, 2004, Saunders.

A comprehensive discussion of proximal humerus fractures and nonunions.

8. Boileau PS, Krishnan G, Tinsi L, et al: Tuberosity malposition and migration: reasons for poor outcomes after hemiarthroplasty for displaced fractures of the proximal humerus, *J Shoulder Elbow Surg* 11:401-412, 2002.

The purpose of this prospective multicenter study was to evaluate the results after hemiarthroplasty for displaced proximal humeral fractures. Subjectively, 44% of patients were very satisfied, 14% were satisfied, and 42% were unsatisfied. Postoperative active elevation averaged 101%. Final tuberosity malposition occurred in 50% of patients and correlated with an unsatisfactory result. Factors associated with failure of tuberosity osteosynthesis included: poor initial position of the prosthesis (specifically, excessive height or retroversion), poor position of the greater tuberosity, and women over the age of 75 (likely with osteopenic bone). The authors concluded that techniques to improve tuberosity osteosynthesis, including modifications to current prosthetic design and instrumentation to allow for a more anatomic reconstruction, should lead to more predictable and satisfactory results.

9. Boileau P, Walch G, Krishnan S: Tuberosity osteosynthesis and hemiarthroplasty for four-part fractures of the proximal humerus, *Tech Shoulder Elbow Surg* 1:96-109, 2000.

10. Boileau P, Walch G: The three-dimensional geometry of the proximal humerus: implications for surgical technique and prosthetic design, *J Bone Joint Surg Br* 79:857-865, 1997.

The three-dimensional geometry of the proximal humerus was studied on human cadaver specimens. Findings demonstrated that the geometry of the proximal humerus is extremely variable. The authors evaluated the effectiveness of the bicipital groove as a means of determining retroversion of the prosthesis. If the biceps groove is used as a landmark at the level of the shaft, the fracture prosthesis was found to be retroverted an additional 10 degrees with respect to the transepicondylar axis. Variations in the geometry of the humerus may not be accommodated by the designs of most contemporary human proximal humerus fracture systems.

11. Brooks CH, Revell WJ, Heatly FW: Vascularity of the humeral head after proximal humeral fractures: an anatomical cadaver study, *J Bone Joint Surg Br* 75:132-136, 1993.

12. Clifford PC: Fractures of the neck of the humerus: a review of the late results, *Injury* 12:91-95, 1980.

13. Codman EA: *The shoulder*, Boston, 1934, Thomas Todd.

14. Compito CA, Self EB, Bigliani LU: Arthroplasty and acute shoulder trauma: reasons for success and failure, *Clin Orthop Relat Res* 307:27-36, 1994.

Fractures that require prosthetic replacement as the definitive treatment include four-part fractures and fracture-dislocations, head-split fractures with >40% articular surface involvement, and selected three-part fractures. Of 70 cases treated with prosthetic replacement that were retrospectively reviewed by the authors, results were excellent in 31, satisfactory in 22, and unsatisfactory in 17.

15. Court-Brown CM, McQueen MM: The impacted varus (A2.2) proximal humeral fracture: prediction of outcome and results of nonoperative treatment in 99 patients, *Acta Orthop Scand* 75:736-740, 2004.

The authors prospectively reviewed 99 varus impacted fractures of the proximal humerus. After nonoperative management, the outcome was good, regardless of the degree of varus, 1 year after fracture. Physiotherapy did not improve outcome.

16. Darder A, Darder A Jr, Sanchis V, et al: Four-part displaced proximal humeral fractures: operative treatment using Kirschner wires and a tension band, *J Orthop Trauma* 7:497-505, 1993.

Thirty-five patients with four-part displaced proximal humeral fractures and fracture-dislocations were retrospectively reviewed. All cases of fracture-dislocations corresponded with unsatisfactory and poor results. Prosthetic replacement should be considered as the primary treatment in cases of four-part fracture-dislocations.

17. Dempster WT: Mechanisms of shoulder movement, *Arch Phys Med Rehabil* 46:49-70, 1965.

18. DePalma AF, Cautilli RA: Fractures of the upper end of the humerus, *Clin Orthop* 20:73-93, 1961.

19. Edwards SL, Wilson NA, Zhang L, et al: Two-part surgical neck fractures of the proximal humerus: a biomechanical evaluation of two fixation techniques, *J Bone Joint Surg Am* 88:2258-2263, 2006.

The locked compression proximal humeral plate demonstrated superior biomechanical characteristics compared with the proximal humeral nail when tested cyclically in both cantilevered varus bending and torsion. The rate of early failure of the proximal humeral nail could reflect the high moment transmitted to the locking proximal screw-bone interface in this implant.

20. Esser RD: Treatment of three- and four-part fractures of the proximal humerus with a modified cloverleaf plate, *J Orthop Trauma* 8:15-22, 1994.

The modified cloverleaf plate proved to be a good method of fixation of three-part and four-part fractures. In this series of younger patients (average age 55), midterm follow-up revealed no avascular necrosis (AVN).

21. Fankhauser F, Boldin C, Schippinger G, et al: A new locking plate for unstable fractures of the proximal humerus, *Clin Orthop Relat Res* 430:176-181, 2005.

Data from this prospective study of 28 patients with 29 proximal humeral fractures revealed that using the locking proximal humerus plate is a reliable treatment method for complex proximal humerus fractures.

22. Flatow EL, Cuomo F, Maday MG, et al: Open reduction and internal fixation of two- and three-part displaced surgical neck fractures of the proximal humerus, *J Shoulder Elbow Surg* 1:287-295, 1992.

23. Frankle MA, Mighell MA: Techniques and principles of tuberosity fixation for proximal humeral fractures treated with hemiarthroplasty, *J Shoulder Elbow Surg* 13:239-247, 2004.

A review of literature on outcomes and complications of shoulder hemiarthroplasty is presented. This article also reviewed the pertinent anatomic landmarks that help achieve a proper reduction of the tuberosities and defined the biomechanical and clinical consequences of malunion and nonunion. The importance of achieving a stable, anatomic tuberosity fixation is underscored. This requires a reproducible technique, a reliable instrumentation system, and a fracture prosthesis that can optimize tuberosity reconstruction.

24. Frankle MA, Ondrovic LE, Markee BA, et al: Stability of tuberosity reattachment in proximal humeral hemiarthroplasty, *J Shoulder Elbow Surg* 11:413-420, 2002.

This study compares different tuberosity reconstruction methods for four-part humeral fractures. The use of a circumferential medial cerclage during hemiarthroplasty for four-part humeral fractures decreased interfragmentary motion and strain, maximized fracture stability, and facilitated postoperative rehabilitation.

25. Fulkerson E, Egol KA, Kubiak EN, et al: Fixation of diaphyseal fractures with a segmental defect: a biomechanical comparison of locked and conventional plating techniques, *J Trauma* 60:830-835, 2006.

These results support the use of locked-plating techniques for comminuted diaphyseal fractures in osteoporotic bone.

26. Gerber C, Werner CL, Vienne P: Internal fixation of complex fractures of the proximal humerus, *J Bone Joint Surg* 86:848-855, 2004.

Thirty-four consecutive articular fractures of the proximal humerus in 33 patients with good bone quality were treated by open reduction and internal fixation. Anatomic or nearly anatomic reduction was achieved in 30 patients at a mean follow-up of 63 months. Complete or partial avascular necrosis (AVN) occurred in 12 cases (35%). Two patients who developed AVN subsequently underwent arthroplasty. The other 10 patients with AVN were functionally satisfactory. If AVN ensues, the clinical result may remain satisfactory with Constant scores comparable to hemiarthroplasty for fractures.

27. Gerber C, Schneeberger AG, Vinh TS: The arterial vascularization of the humeral head: an anatomical study, *J Bone Joint Surg Am* 72:1486-1494, 1990.

This study reaffirmed that the main arterial supply of the humeral head is the anterolateral ascending branch of the anterior circumflex artery. That vessel ran parallel to the lateral aspect of the tendon of the long head of the biceps and entered the humeral head where the proximal end of the intertubercular groove met the greater tuberosity. When the intraosseous (terminal) part of the anterolateral branch, the so-called arcuate artery, had been perfused, almost the entire epiphysis was radiopaque. Injury to this artery may cause avascular necrosis (AVN) even in the absence of displacement of the head.

28. Goldman RT, Koval KJ, Cuomo F, et al: Functional outcome after humeral head replacement for acute three- and four-part proximal humeral fractures, *J Shoulder Elbow Surg* 4:81-86, 1995.

This study indicates that hemiarthroplasty for acute three-part and four-part fractures generally can be expected to result in pain-free shoulders. However, recovery of function and range of motion are much less predictable.

29. Hawkins RJ, Bell RH, Gurr K: The three-part fracture of the proximal part of the humerus: operative treatment, *J Bone Joint Surg Am* 68:1410-1414, 1986.

The authors recommend operative treatment for the healthy, active individual who has a three-part fracture of the proximal part of the humerus. They found that the best results with these difficult fractures are obtained using tension-band wiring.

30. Hepp P, Lill H, Bail H, et al: Where should implants be anchored in the humeral head? *Clin Orthop Relat Res* 415:139-147, 2003.

The medial and posterior aspects of the proximal humeral head were found to be the areas of highest bone strength.

31. Hertel R: Fractures of the proximal humerus in osteoporotic bone, *Osteoporosis Int* 16:S65-S72, 2005.

Selection of a balanced osteosynthesis, adapted to osteoporotic bone, is mandatory.

32. Iannotti JP, Ramsey ML, Williams GR, et al: Nonprosthetic management of proximal humeral fractures, *J Bone Joint Surg* 85:1578-1593, 2003.

33. Iannotti JP, Williams GR: Total shoulder arthroplasty: factors influencing prosthetic design, *Orthop Clin North Am* 29:377-391, 1998.

Prosthetic designs should attempt to facilitate the surgical correction of the pathology encountered, with the goal of reproducing normal anatomy.

34. Jaberg H, Warner JJ, Jakob RP: Percutaneous stabilization of unstable fractures of the humerus, *J Bone Joint Surg Am* 74:508-515, 1992.

Forty-eight of 54 patients who had closed reduction and percutaneous pinning of an unstable fracture of the proximal end of the humerus were available for retrospective clinical and roentgenographic follow-up at an average of 3 years. Four patients had loss of fixation and had repeat fixation with percutaneous pinning after a second closed reduction. Only one of them had a poor result because of malunion. Four patients had a superficial pin-track infection and loosening of pins, one patient had a deep infection, and two had a nonunion. Complete avascular necrosis (AVN) with collapse of the humeral head developed in only two patients. However, eight patients had localized AVN with transient cyst formation and sclerosis in the humeral head that resolved over 1 to 2 years. The authors concluded that closed reduction and percutaneous pinning is a technically demanding procedure, but it may offer results that are comparable with previously described operative methods for the treatment of unstable fractures of the proximal end of the humerus.

35. Jakob RP, Miniaci A, Anson PS, et al: Four-part valgus impacted fractures of the proximal humerus, *J Bone Joint Surg Br* 73:295-298, 1991.

There is a specific type of displaced four-part fracture of the proximal humerus that consists of valgus impaction of the head fragment. This deserves special consideration because the rate of avascular necrosis (AVN) is lower than that of other displaced four-part fractures. Using either closed reduction or limited, open reduction and minimal internal fixation, 74% satisfactory results can be achieved in this injury.

36. Jakob RP, Kristiansen T, Mayo K, et al: Classification and aspects of treatment of fractures of the proximal humerus. In Bateman JE, Welsh RP editors: *Surgery of the shoulder,* Philadelphia, 1984, BC Decker.

37. Kannus P, Palvanen M, Niemi S, et al: Osteoporotic fractures of the proximal humerus in elderly Finnish persons: sharp increase in 1970–1998 and alarming projections for the new millennium, *Acta Orthop Scand* 71:465-470, 2000.

38. Keene JS, Huizenga RE, Engber WD, et al: Proximal humeral fractures: a correction of residual deformity with long-term function, *Orthopedics* 6:173-178, 1983.

39. Koukakis A, Apostolou CD, Taneja T, et al: Fixation of proximal humerus fractures using the PHILOS plate, *Clin Orthop* 442:115-120, 2006.

40. Kralinger F, Schwaiger R, Wambacher M, et al: Outcome after primary hemiarthroplasty for fracture of the head of the humerus: a retrospective multicentre study of 167 patients, *J Bone Joint Surg Br* 86:217-219, 2004.

The authors examined 167 patients who had a hemiarthroplasty for three-part and four-part fractures and fracture-dislocations of the head of the humerus in a multicenter study involving 12 Austrian hospitals. All patients were followed for more than 1 year. Anatomical healing of the tuberosity significantly influenced the outcome as measured by the Constant score and subjective patient satisfaction. With regard to pain, the outcome was generally satisfactory, but only 41.9% of patients were able to flex the shoulder above 90 degrees. The age of the patient and the type of prosthesis significantly influenced the healing of the tuberosity, but bone grafting did not. Achievement of healing of the tuberosity was inferior in institutions at which fewer than 15 hemiarthroplasties had been performed.

41. Kristiansen B, Christensen SW: Plate fixation of proximal humeral fractures. *Acta Orthop Scand* 57:320-323, 1986.

42. Loebenberg MI, Jones DA, Zuckerman JD: The effect of greater tuberosity placement on active range of motion after hemiarthroplasty for acute fractures of the proximal humerus, *Bull Hosp Jt Dis* 62:90-93, 2005.

43. Mansat P, Guity MR, Bellumore Y, et al: Shoulder arthroplasty for late sequelae of proximal humeral fractures, *J Shoulder Elbow Surg* 13:305-312, 2004.

Twenty-eight patients with sequelae of proximal humeral fractures were treated with shoulder arthroplasty and were reviewed with a mean follow-up of 47 months. The prognosis was influenced positively by the integrity of the rotator cuff at surgery, whereas the need for greater tuberosity osteotomy worsened the final result.

44. Mighell MA, Kolm GP, Collinge CA, et al: Outcomes of hemiarthroplasty for fractures of the proximal humerus, *J Shoulder Elbow Surg* 12:569-577, 2003.

Outcomes of 80 shoulders treated with hemiarthroplasty were reviewed. At follow-up, 93% of patients were pain free and satisfied with their results. The mean American Shoulder and Elbow Surgeons score was 76.6, the mean Simple Shoulder Test score was 7.5, forward flexion was 128 degrees, external rotation was 43 degrees, and internal rotation was to L2. The authors recommend placement of the greater tuberosity 10 mm below the superior aspect of the prosthetic humeral head.

45. Mouradian WH: Displaced proximal humeral fractures: seven years' experience with a modified Zickel supracondylar device, *Clin Orthop* 212:209-218, 1986.

46. Murachovsky J, Ikemoto RY, Nascimento LG, et al: Pectoralis major tendon reference (PMT): a new method for accurate restoration of humeral length with hemiarthroplasty for fracture, *J Shoulder Elbow Surg* 15:675-678, 2006.

The authors dissected 20 cadavers (40 shoulders), and the distance between the upper border of the pectoralis major tendon insertion on the humerus and the top of the humeral head was measured (PMT). The PMT averaged 5.6 ± 0.5 cm. In only 4 of 40 shoulders did this distance exceed 6 cm, and there was no correlation between the size of the patient and this measurement. The PMT is a useful landmark that will aid in accurate restoration of humeral length when reconstructing complex proximal humeral fractures in which landmarks are otherwise lost because of fracture comminution.

47. Naranja RJ Jr, Iannotti JP: Displaced three- and four-part proximal humerus fractures: evaluation and management, *J Am Acad Orthop Surg* 8:373-382, 2000.

The authors note that vertical fixation alone with Rush rods in patients with poor bone quality and in those with four-part fractures is no longer considered adequate and should not be used.

48. Neer CS: Displaced proximal humeral fractures: Part I. Classification and evaluation, *J Bone Joint Surg Am* 52:1077-1089, 1970.

49. Neer CS: Displaced proximal humeral fractures: Part II. Treatment of three part and four part fracture displacement, *J Bone Joint Surg Am* 52:1090-1103, 1970.

50. Norris TR, Green A, McGuigan FX: Late prosthetic shoulder arthroplasty for displaced proximal humerus fractures, *J Shoulder Elbow Surg* 4:271-280, 1995.

Late surgery for failed early treatment is technically difficult, and the results are inferior to those reported for acute humeral head replacement. These findings should be considered when treatment is selected for acute three-part and four-part proximal humerus fractures. Nonetheless, late arthroplasty is a satisfactory reconstructive option when primary treatment of proximal humerus fractures fails.

51. Paavolainen P, Björkenheim JM, Slatis P, et al: Operative treatment of severe proximal humeral fractures, *Acta Orthop Scand* 54:374-379, 1983.

Results after the operative treatment of 41 severe proximal fractures of the humerus were retrospectively reviewed. The most common technical error was excessively high positioning of the AO plate and persistent varus deformation of the head of the humerus.

52. Ring D, Mckee MD, Perey BH, et al: The use of a blade plate and autogenous cancellous bone graft in the treatment of ununited fractures of the proximal humerus, *J Shoulder Elbow Surg* 10:501-507, 2001.

Stable internal fixation is essential to obtain healing of an ununited fracture of the proximal humerus. Standard plate and screw fixation may be inadequate to secure a small, osteopenic proximal fragment. The authors used blade plates and autogenous, cancellous bone graft to repair ununited fractures of the proximal humerus in 25 patients with a mean age of 61 years. Healing was documented in 23 of 25 patients (92%). Objective and subjective instruments documented substantial functional improvement in patients with healed fractures. The results were classified as good or excellent in 20 of 25 patients, and few complications were encountered. Blade-plate fixation facilitates successful treatment of ununited fractures of the proximal humerus.

53. Rose PS, Adams CR, Torchia ME, et al: Locking plate fixation for proximal humeral fractures: initial results with a new implant, *J Shoulder Elbow Surg* 16:202-207, 2007.

Sixteen patients treated with a Synthes LCP locking proximal humerus plate were reviewed retrospectively. Patients were followed until union or revision with a mean of 12 months' follow-up. The authors did not comment on use of heavy suture or cerclage wires to counterbalance the forces of the rotator cuff. In those cases with comminution, it was not clear if the head was impacted into the shaft. Twelve of 16 patients healed without complications. There were four nonunions; all occurred in patients with three-part fractures with metadiaphyseal comminution, three of whom were heavy smokers. These fractures remain challenging despite the availability of locked-plating systems.

54. Rowles DJ, McGrory JE: Percutaneous pinning of the proximal part of the humerus: an analtomic study, *J Bone Joint Surg Am* 83-A:1695-1699, 2001.

55. Savoie FH, Geissler WB, Vander Griend RA: Open reduction and internal fixation of three-part fractures of the proximal humerus, *Orthopedics* 12:65-70, 1989.

Eleven patients with 12 three-part fractures of the proximal humerus were treated by open reduction and internal fixation using AO/ASIF buttress plating. All of the fractures healed. There were no failures of fixation. Nine of these patients returned for a follow up of more than 2 years and had a satisfactory rating using Neer's shoulder rating system.

56. Scheck M: Surgical treatment of nonunions of the surgical neck of the humerus, *Clin Orthop* 167:255-259, 1982.

End-to-end alignment of the fragments usually does not provide good bone contact or stability for fractures of the surgical neck of the humerus, because cavitation of the head fragment and comminution constitute bone stock deficiency. Painful and disabling nonunions of the surgical neck of the humerus in five patients were repaired by impaling one fragment into the other, usually the shaft into the head. A corticocancellous iliac graft bridged the nonunion by extending from the interior of the head to the shaft, where it was fixed by screws. Rush rods were used for internal fixation. All five patients obtained union without evidence of avascular necrosis (AVN) during the period of observation (12 to 39 months), had good pain relief, and regained satisfactory function.

57. Seide K, Triebe J, Faschingbauer M, et al: Locked vs. unlocked plate osteosynthesis of the proximal humerus: a biomechanical study, *Clin Biomech* in press.

Locked plates (internal fixators) have been found to be an optimal method for fixation in proximal humeral fractures. In a biomechanical cadaver study, the difference between locked and nonlocked osteosynthesis was investigated. Paired humeri were harvested and bone density was measured. Locked internal fixators were mounted on one specimen. Identical plate-screw systems without a locking mechanism were applied to the contralateral specimen for comparison. Linear range until failure was extended in the locked group by 64% (92 N versus 56 N), which was statistically significant.

58. Shrader MW, Sánchez-Sotelo J, Sperling JW, et al: Understanding proximal humerus fractures: image analysis, classification, and treatment, *J Shoulder Elbow Surg* 14:497-505, 2005.

Proximal humerus fractures are difficult to define because of their extreme variability and potential for complexity. The authors designed a study to evaluate further why this is true. Radiographs of 113 proximal humeral fractures were assessed by three knowledgeable observers. Ten learning points enhanced the ability to interpret images at the second review and provided more consistent fracture classification with statistically significant improvements. The problem was understanding the images of complex fractures not the classification system. To enhance consistency in understanding these fractures, imaging of complex fractures must be enhanced.

59. Stableforth PG: Four-part fractures of the neck of the humerus, *J Bone Joint Surg Br* 66:104-108, 1984.

Four-part fractures of the upper end of the humerus are uncommon injuries, and there is still dispute about the best form of management. A retrospective study of 32 patients with these injuries showed that nonoperative management is frequently followed by persistent pain, stiffness, and dysfunction of the shoulder. A prospective study of 49 patients with this injury presenting at the Bristol Royal Infirmary showed that reconstruction of the upper end of the humerus with insertion of a Neer prosthesis will usually restore comfort and function. Whichever regimen is employed, disability is prolonged and dedicated physiotherapy is essential in their management.

60. Sturzenegger M, Fornaro E, Jakob RP: Results of surgical treatment of multifragmented fractures of the humeral head, *Arch Orthop Trauma* 100:249-259, 1982.

61. Szyszkowitz R, Seggl W, Schleifer P, et al: Proximal humeral fractures: management techniques and expected results, *Clin Orthop Relat Res* 292:13-25, 1993.

62. Tanner MW, Cofield RH: Prosthetic arthroplasty for fractures and fracture-dislocations of the proximal humerus, *Clin Orthop Relat Res* 179:116-128, 1983.

63. Volgas DA, Stannard JP, Alonso JE: Nonunions of the humerus, *Clin Orthop Relat Res* 419:46-50, 2004.

Humerus fractures comprise 5% to 8% of all fractures. Nonunions are uncommon, but when they occur, they present a challenge to the orthopaedic surgeon and often are debilitating to patients. There are risk factors that may predispose patients to nonunion. Many methods of treating these nonunions have been described with varying degrees of success. The literature concerning the treatment of proximal, midshaft, and distal humeral nonunions were reviewed, and the authors' treatment protocol based on the literature was described.

64. Walch G, Badet R, Nové-Josserand L, et al: Nonunions of the surgical neck of the humerus: surgical treatment with an intramedullary bone peg, internal fixation, and cancellous bone grafting, *J Shoulder Elbow Surg* 5:161-168, 1996.

Twenty patients with pseudoarthrosis of the upper humerus underwent surgery with the intramedullary bone peg technique. A 6- to 10-cm corticocancellous autogenous bone graft (11 iliac crest, 6 anterior tibial crest, 3 middle-third of the fibula) was pegged into the humerus and bridged the pseudoarthrosis. Stability of the fracture site was obtained by plate osteosynthesis. As a result of the large size of the graft, there were several reports of donor site morbidity. The rate of union was 96%, underlining the importance of an intramedullary bone graft in association with peripheral osteosynthesis in the treatment of pseudoarthrosis of the surgical neck of the humerus.

65. Weinstein DM, Bratton DR, Ciccone WJ, et al: Locking plates improve torsional resistance in the stabilization of three-part proximal humeral fractures, *J Shoulder Elbow Surg* 15:239-243, 2006.

This study quantified the torsional resistance provided by locking plates and angled blade plates used to stabilize proximal humeral fractures. Three-part proximal humeral fractures were created in six pairs of cadaveric humeri. One specimen of each pair was reconstructed with a proximal humeral locking plate, whereas the other specimen was reconstructed with an angled blade plate. An external rotation torque, varying from 0 to 5 Newton Meters (N-m), was applied to the humeral head until the head rotated 30 degrees or 10,000 loading cycles were applied. The mean initial torsional stiffness was significantly larger for the locking plates (0.99 N-m/degree) than for the blade plates (0.59 N-m/degree). For each pair, the maximum rotation was larger for the blade plate than for the locking plate. For this in vitro model of a reconstructed three-part proximal humeral fracture, the locking plate provided better torsional fatigue resistance and stiffness than the blade plate.

66. Weseley MS, Barenfeld PA, Eisenstein AL: Rush pin intramedullary fixation for fractures of the proximal humerus, *J Orthop Trauma* 17:29-37, 1977.

67. Wheeler DL, Colville MR: Biomechanical comparison of intramedullary and percutaneous pin fixation for proximal humeral fracture fixation, *J Orthop Trauma* 11:363-367, 1997.

68. Wijgman AJ, Roolker W, Patt TW, et al: Open reduction and internal fixation of three and four-part fractures of the proximal part of the humerus, *J Bone Joint Surg Am* 84-A:1919-1925, 2002.
The authors assessed the intermediate and long-term results for 60 patients with a three-part or four-part fracture of the proximal part of the humerus who had undergone open reduction and internal fixation with cerclage wires or a T-plate. The Constant score and a visual analog score for pain were calculated, and radiographs of the proximal part of the humerus were evaluated. After an average of 10 years of follow-up, 52 patients (87%) had good or excellent results. Twenty-two patients (37%) had development of avascular necrosis (AVN) of the humeral head, and 17 of these 22 (77%) patients had a good or excellent Constant score. The surgical option discusses above should be considered even for patients with fracture-dislocation patterns that are associated with a high risk for AVN of the humeral head, because this complication did not preclude a good result.

69. Wright TW: Treatment of humeral diaphyseal nonunions in patients with severely compromised bone, *J South Orthop Assoc* 6:1-7, 1997.
Twenty-eight patients were treated for humeral shaft nonunions. Host factors associated with humeral nonunion included a high rate of significant medical problems and significant local tissue trauma from the initiating injury. Comminuted fractures and fractures that were either long oblique or spiral in configuration were also heavily represented in this series. Midshaft was the most common anatomic location ($n = 17$). In patients with severely compromised bone from osteoporosis or multiple fixation attempts, a reconstruction using an intramedullary fibular graft and dynamic compression plate with screws, obtaining four cortices of fixation (quadricortical) was used. This construction was also augmented with iliac crest bone graft. In this difficult subgroup of patients, the authors' technique of intramedullary quadricortical fixation yielded an 89% union rate (17 of 19). Patients with humeral union were satisfied and had functional range of motion of the shoulder and elbow.

Further Reading

70. Frankle MA, Greenwald DP, Markee BA, et al: Biomechanical effects of malposition of tuberosity fragments on the humeral prosthetic reconstruction for four-part proximal humerus fractures, *J Shoulder Elbow Surg* 10:321-326, 2001.
Nonanatomic tuberosity reconstruction led to significant impairment in external rotation kinematics and an eightfold increase in torque requirements ($p = 0.001$). In contrast, anatomic reconstruction produced results indistinguishable from normal shoulder controls. This study underscores the importance of rotational alignment of tuberosities during reconstruction. Failure to properly position tuberosity fragments in the horizontal plane may result in insurmountable postoperative motion restriction.

71. Moeckel BH, Dines DM, Warren RF, et al: Modular hemiarthroplasty for fractures of the proximal part of the humerus, *J Bone Joint Surg Am* 74:884-889, 1992.
This article discusses the importance of modularity in humeral prosthetic design as a way to accommodate to the variable anatomy of the proximal humerus. This was the first article to recognize a specific fracture stem to maximize proximal humeral reconstruction.

72. Neer CS II: *Shoulder reconstruction*, Philadelphia, 1990, WB Saunders Company.
Chapter 3 is a comprehensive review of glenohumeral arthroplasty.

CHAPTER 4

Fractures of the Scapula

Dolfi Herscovici, Jr., DO, and Julia M. Scaduto, ARNP

- The scapula is important for normal function of the arm. It acts as a bony bridge linking the upper extremity to the axial skeleton. As the scapula rotates, it allows the arm and shoulder to function smoothly. Any fracture, soft-tissue scaring, or damage to the muscle or nerve will decrease the motion of the scapular, ultimately affecting the function of the shoulder.
- First described in 1805, these fractures have become recognized entities in trauma patients. They are uncommon injuries representing only 0.4% to 1% of all fractures and 3% to 5% of all shoulder girdle injuries.
- Reasons for this low occurrence include its mobility on the thoracic wall, the protection offered by the rib cage, and the thick covering of the posterior soft tissues. This protection requires that a significant force be generated to create a fracture. High-energy mechanisms produce almost 90% of these fractures, usually resulting from either motor vehicle or motorcycle accidents or falls from significant heights. In addition, fractures can also occur with forceful muscle contractions associated with seizures, electrical injuries, or electroconvulsive therapy.
- The significant trauma necessary to produce these fractures results in 80% to 95% of the patients with associated injuries.[1] In addition to other injuries of the shoulder girdle, concomitant injuries can also include 24% of patients with skull fractures, a 27% to 54% incidence of rib fractures, a 5% to 12% prevalence of brachial plexus injuries, vascular injuries seen in 2% to 10% of patients, and 50% to 62% of patients with intrathoracic injuries.
- The anatomic distribution of fractures consist of 50% involving the body or spine, 25% with fractures of the neck, 10% involving the glenoid fossa and fractures of the acromion, spine, or the coracoid process, each contributing to the remainder of cases.[2]

Examination and Diagnosis

- The diagnosis of a scapular fracture is most often made as an incidental finding on routine chest X-rays (CXRs).
- The reason for this is that these fractures often present in conjunction with multiple, life-threatening or limb-threatening injuries, resulting in attention being directed toward those other injuries, which produces a delay in the diagnosis and treatment of scapular fractures (Figure 4–1).
- Historically, patients often complain of shoulder pain and hold the arm in adduction to avoid any movement of the shoulder. Local tenderness may exist, but the normal findings of edema and ecchymosis may be masked or less than expected, especially if associated chest injuries are present.

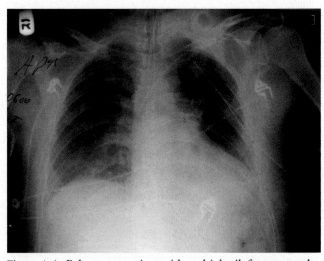

Figure 4–1: Polytrauma patient with multiple rib fractures and pneumothorax (chest tube). Left scapular neck fracture was identified on serial chest X-rays.

- As a result the potential for associated injuries, it is important to examine and document the neurovascular status of the upper extremity during the initial physical examination of the patient.
- In the absence of a clavicle or humerus fracture, any passive motion eliciting pain about the shoulder in a polytrauma patient should be suspicious for a scapular fracture.
- When the radiographic evaluation for fractures of the scapula is performed, there may be some difficulty viewing the scapula because of the superimposition of the thorax. Therefore, multiple views should be taken.
- The initial workup should consist of plain radiographs. An anteroposterior (AP) view will allow visualization of the body, neck, and acromion. The y-view allows the body, spine, acromion, and coracoid process to be visualized, whereas an axillary view is helpful for viewing the acromion, glenoid rim, and position of the glenohumeral joint. Other initial plain films can include the cephalic tilt or Stryker notch view, which is useful in evaluating fractures of the coracoid. (Figure 4–2, *A-C*)
- One should be cautious when attempting to identify fractures in the presence of skeletal anomalies. The four most common scapular abnormalities are epiphyseal lines, seen at the coracoid process or the inferior angle, the presence of an os acromiale, identified by its rounded borders when it is located even with or above the posterior edge of the acromion and the fact that 60% are bilateral, dysplasia of the scapular neck, which can be associated with acromiale or humeral head abnormalities, and a scapular foramina, which often appear benign and well circumscribed.
- A computed tomography (CT) scan is useful when evaluating glenoid fossa fractures, comminuted fractures of the body and neck, or for its ability to provide a three-dimensional (3D) reconstruction, which can be used to evaluate the shoulder girdle complex.
- The use of magnetic resonance imaging (MRI) or radioisotope studies have not been found helpful for the management of acute scapular fractures but may be useful in identifying associated soft-tissue injuries, nonunions, or infections of the scapula.

Classification and Treatment

- Although it is certainly possible to describe every fracture of the scapula as a separate anatomic entity, the areas of primary concern are the acromion, coracoid, body, neck and the glenoid fossa.

Acromial Fractures

- These fractures usually occur as a result of a direct blow, from a superior dislocation of the humeral head, or as a result of repetitive stress, as seen in athletes, or produced iatrogenically after aggressive arthroscopic subacromial decompression.

- They are usually seen lateral to the acromioclavicular (AC) joint or at the base, near the spine of the scapula and need to be distinguished from an os acromiale. (Figure 4–3)
- Nondisplaced fractures respond well to symptomatic care. This includes a sling for the first 2 to 3 weeks followed rehabilitation consisting of passive exercises and active-assisted exercises for the second 3 weeks. At 6 weeks, the patient can be advanced to progressive-resistive exercises.
- Displaced fractures, especially those near the base of the spine or those resulting in a decrease in the subacromial space may require an open-reduction technique. Using a posterior approach to the scapula, either screw and plates or some kind of a tension-band fixation technique is recommended.
- The use of an acromionectomy is not recommended unless it is a small and insignificant fragment.

Coracoid Fractures

- Of all scapular fractures, 2% to 5% consist of coracoid fractures.[2] These occur as a result of a direct blow, in association with AC separations, or by severe contractions of the muscles attached to it.
- The coracoid is important for the integrity of the superior shoulder suspensory complex (SSSC)[3] because some fractures will produce instability between the clavicle and scapula during shoulder motion.
- Although different authors have suggested classifications based on small patient series,[4] there are essentially two types of coracoid fractures, unstable and stable patterns, depending on whether or not the SSSC is involved.
- In an unstable pattern, the fracture occurs at the base and extends to include the upper border of the glenoid. These are essentially intraarticular fossa fractures that also produce instability of the SSSC. To avoid joint incongruity of the fossa and to stabilize the SSSC, surgical stabilization of these fractures is recommended.
- Surgical management of an unstable pattern consists of an anterior open-reduction technique using lag screws or lag screw and plate techniques. These can be placed anteriorly through the tip into the remaining process, superiorly from the clavicle into the coracoid or through a posterior approach, when the fragment is large and involves the superior margin of the glenoid fossa.
- Stable patterns are all other coracoid fractures (Figure 4–4). These can be managed nonoperatively provided the patient does not have glenohumeral instability, obstruction to reducing an anterior shoulder dislocation, or instability of the SSSC occurring with the coracoid fracture and with either an associated clavicle or acromion fracture.

Body Fractures

- Fractures of the body, including those of the scapula spine and avulsion injuries through the main body, are the most

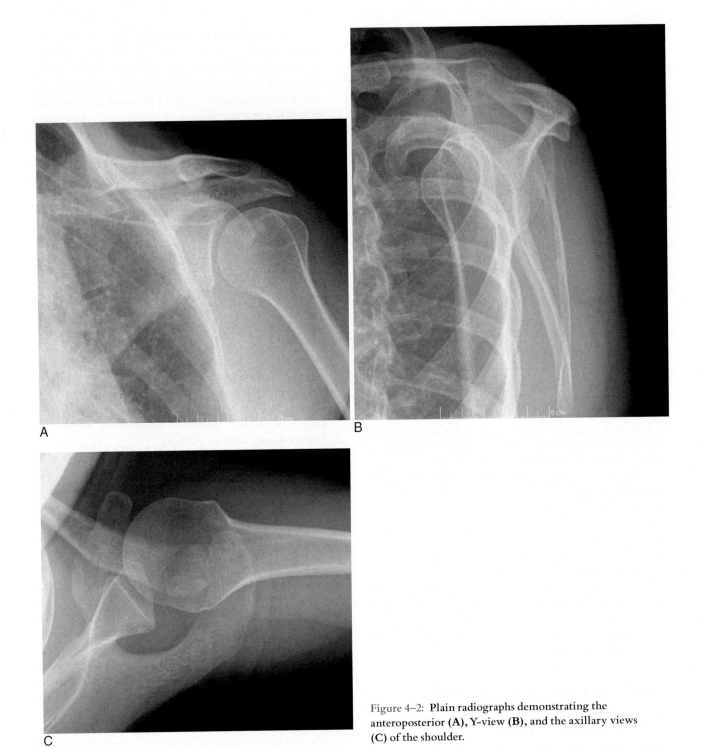

Figure 4–2: **Plain radiographs demonstrating the anteroposterior (A), Y-view (B), and the axillary views (C) of the shoulder.**

common fractures of the scapula. They have the highest incidence of associated injuries and often present as displaced or comminuted patterns.

- With the protection offered by the rib cage and the thick covering of the posterior soft tissues, a substantial force is needed to produce a fracture. This occurs either from direct blows or sudden contraction of opposing muscles, seen with seizures or electroconvulsive therapy (Figure 4–5).

- Patients often have pain about the shoulder or the back and may complain about decreased or painful shoulder motion especially if a bony spike impinges or penetrates an adjacent muscle.

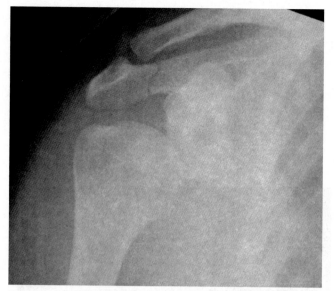

Figure 4–3: Radiograph demonstrating a fracture at the base of the acromion.

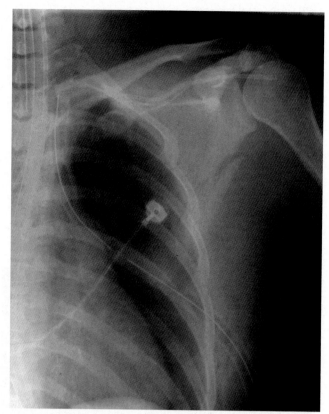

Figure 4–5: Fracture of the body that occurred after being struck in the back during an assault. Radiograph demonstrates a stable pattern and symptomatic care is indicated.

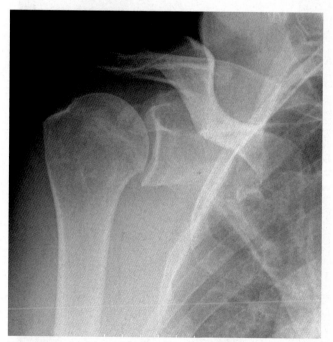

Figure 4–4: Avulsion of the tip of the coracoid process. Fracture pattern is stable and can be treated conservatively.

produces extensive scarring, resulting in a decrease in scapular motion.

- In long-term evaluation of body fractures, however, Nordqvist and Petersson[5] reported that not all body fractures had good outcomes. In patients with greater than 10 mm of displacement only 3 of 7 had good results, whereas 29 of 34 patients with less than 10 mm of displacement had good results.

- If surgery is contemplated, a posterior approach applying fixation is along the medial and lateral borders of the scapula and near the base of the scapular spine is recommended. Smaller-sized implants should be used, and care should be taken to avoid prominence of the screws anteriorly.

Neck Fractures

- A scapular neck fracture is the second most common fracture of the scapula and is produced as a result of a direct blow to the anterior shoulder, a fall onto an outstretched arm, impacting the humeral head against the glenoid, or a force applied to the superior aspect of the shoulder.

- A scapular neck fracture is recognized on plain films as beginning on the lateral border of the scapula, inferior to the glenoid fossa, and exiting along the superior border, medial to the coracoid process. On the basis of plain

- The most common method of treatment is nonoperative care. This method uses a sling worn for 1 to 2 weeks during which time pendulum exercises are instituted. Active exercises and active-assisted exercises are then gradually introduced depending on the comfort levels of the patient.

- Normal bony anatomy of the body is not required to obtain good outcomes because scapulothoracic irritation does not restrict shoulder function unless the fracture films, fractures have been divided into type I (nondisplaced) patterns or type II (displaced) patterns, empirically defined as translation 1 cm or greater or angulation in the coronal or sagittal plane 40 or greater degrees. (Figure 4–6 *A*)

● Based on 3D CT scans however, three different patterns for this injury exists. The first pattern results in the fracture extending across the entire scapula exiting on the medial border, effectively dividing the scapula in half.

The second pattern is the one most commonly recognized as a neck fracture, exiting along the superior border. The third pattern begins similar to the first pattern but turns and exits at the inferior margin of the scapula. (see Figure 4–6 *B-E*)

● Over the last 10 to 15 years, no injury pattern of the scapula has produced more controversy concerning its management than this area of the scapula. The debate is whether or not all of these fractures are benign injuries

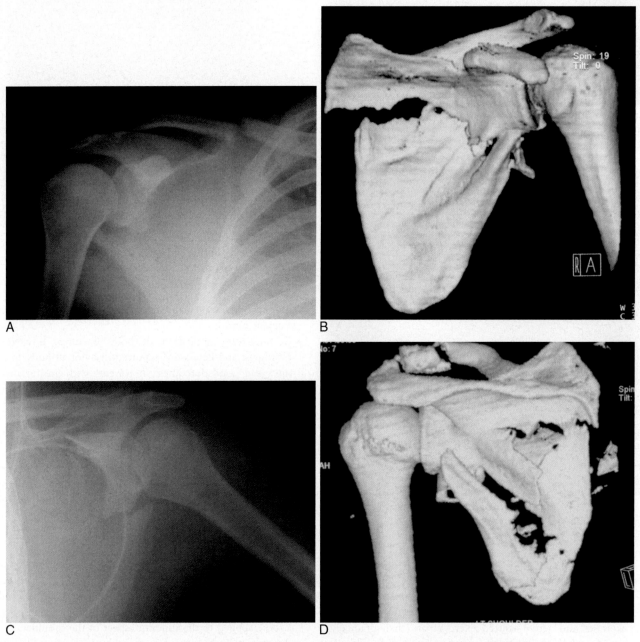

Figure 4–6: An anteroposterior radiograph (**A**) demonstrating a right scapular neck fracture. A three-dimensional computed tomography (CT) scan viewed posterior of the same patient demonstrates that this fracture has a transverse pattern exiting at the medial border (**B**). This patient also has a left scapular neck fracture (**C**), but CT scan shows fracture exiting inferiorly (**D**).

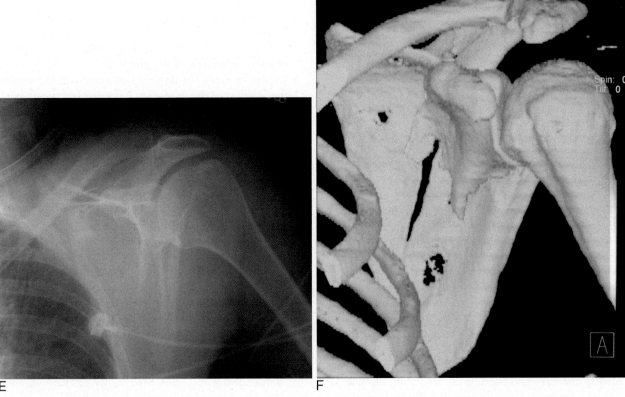

Figure 4–6, cont'd: **Third patient has traditional neck pattern exiting through the superior border (E, F).**

that can be treated using conservative care or whether certain patterns have poor outcomes unless they are managed surgically.

- For some surgeons, the problem is in determining how much displacement or angulation is acceptable before the outcome is affected. In an attempt to quantify displacement some authors have discussed using of the glenopolar angle (GPA)[6] as a method to evaluate fractures, with angles greater than 20 to 30 degrees as indications to fix these fractures.

- In addition, debate has also developed regarding the management of a "floating shoulder" injury (ipsilateral neck and clavicle fracture as defined by Herscovici and others)[7] especially as it relates to the SSSC. The concern is that a neck fracture that produces instability to the SSSC will eventually produce adverse healing and compromise function to the shoulder girdle.[3]

- When reviewing results of injuries to the scapula, studies have demonstrated that that the pain associated with a scapular fracture improves at a mean of 2.7 months and that almost 70% to 80% of fractures involving the body or neck of the scapula, especially those healing with moderate or pronounced deformities, especially with large GPAs, result in only slight or moderate disabilities.[6,8]

- One reason for good outcomes of these nonoperatively treated fractures may be explained through biomechanical

studies, which have demonstrated that even patterns suggesting a potential injury to the SSSC, tend to be inherently stable and may not require surgical intervention, if they present with intact AC and coracoacromial ligaments.[9]

- In addition, recent clinical studies have also demonstrated that although surgically treated neck fractures may have improved motion compared to those treated nonoperatively, overall, those treated with open reduction techniques tended to have a marked decrease in strength of the shoulder versus those that had been treated nonoperatively.[10]

- Although this injury can have significant displacement, the actual motion obtained in the upper extremity is primarily the result of the shoulder complex of the glenohumeral and scapulothoracic joints. This complex has greater motion than almost any other joint in the body and is principally the result of the synergistic effects of these two joints, whose primary function is to produce elevation of the arm. This function will be retained despite this neck fracture because the ability to elevate the arm above 90 degrees horizontal (abduction) will be preserved and has even been demonstrated in patients who have undergone a fusion of the glenohumeral joint.

- If surgical management is contemplated, then the use of a posterior surgical approach to the scapula with rigid fixation of the neck fracture, using plate and screw fixation, is recommended.

Glenoid Fossa and Rim Fractures

- Fractures of the glenoid fossa constitute 10% of scapular fractures, but of these, only 10% of fractures are significantly displaced and should be considered for surgical management.
- Fractures of the rim (Figure 4–7) are located along the periphery of the fossa and occur when the humeral head strikes the glenoid. These are true fractures but are often grouped together with avulsion injuries that occur with dislocations of the shoulder.
- Along with plain X-rays, the radiographic workup of these injuries should also include a two-dimensional (2D) CT scan and a 3D reconstructive CT scan to determine displacement and joint incongruity.
- Ideberg,[11] based on 300 cases, classified glenoid fractures (Figure 4–8) into five different types: type I, fractures of the glenoid rim, subdivided into IA-anterior and IB-posterior; type II, transverse or oblique fractures of the lower half of the fossa, which may present with inferior subluxation of the humeral head; type III, fractures involving the upper-third of the glenoid (Figure 4–9, A-C),which exits superiorly and includes the coracoid process and may also fracture the acromion, clavicle, or produce an AC separation; type IV, fractures extending horizontally through the glenoid to the medial (vertebral) border of the scapula; and type V, which combines the type II and type IV patterns. In addition, a type VI

pattern with severe comminution of the articular surface[12] has also been added to the original description.
- The management of these injuries is dependent on the amount of articular displacement, any associated injuries when first treated, the medical stability of the patient, and the experience of the physician.
- Closed reduction of displaced fractures will not improve the position of the fragments, but some late improvement can occur, which may be the result of molding of the glenoid and the surrounding tissues by the muscle forces acting across the joint.
- If surgery is indicated, there are two approaches for the surgical management: an anterior deltopectoral approach with release of the subscapularis, used for anterior rim fractures; and a posterior approach, using either a vertical incision, to enter the teres minor-infraspinatus interval, or an extensile incision (Judet approach), which begins on the posterior acromion and extends along the spine toward the medial border of the scapula and ends at the inferior angle. This latter approach will elevate the posterior deltoid and the infraspinatus muscle exposing the acromion, spine, glenoid, and all of the infraspinatus fossa. (Figure 4–10, A-G)
- When operatively managing these fractures, rigid fixation using cannulated screws and buttress-plate fixation is recommended. The long-term results of operative intervention are sparse[13] but have shown an 82% excellent-to-good results with operative intervention.

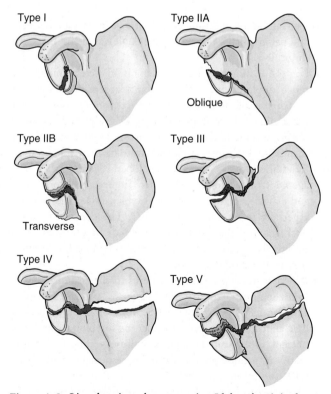

Figure 4–8: Line drawings demonstrating Ideberg's original classification of fractures of the glenoid fossa.

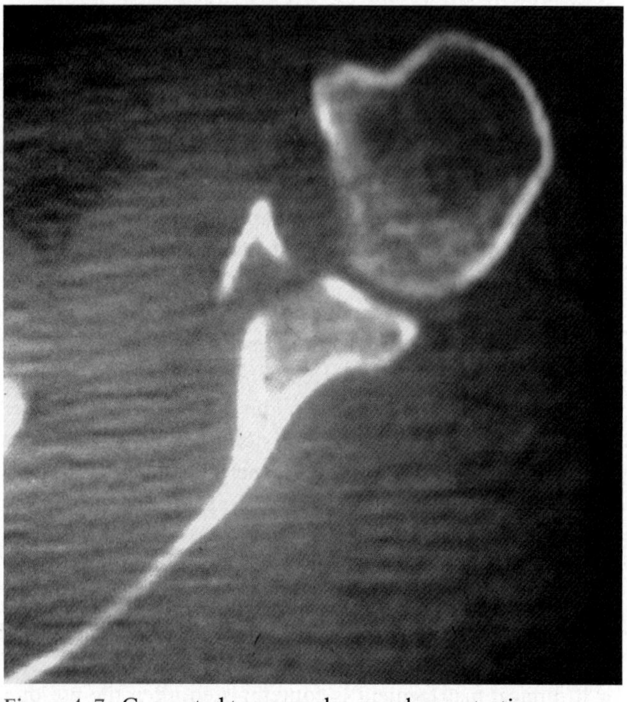

Figure 4–7: Computed tomography scan demonstrating a displaced fracture of the anterior rim of the glenoid fossa.

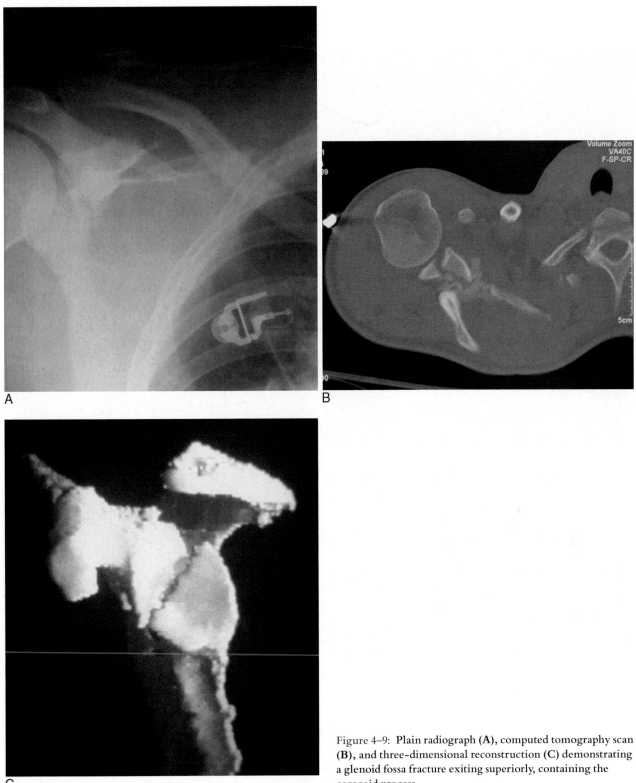

A

B

C

Figure 4–9: Plain radiograph **(A)**, computed tomography scan **(B)**, and three-dimensional reconstruction **(C)** demonstrating a glenoid fossa fracture exiting superiorly, containing the coracoid process.

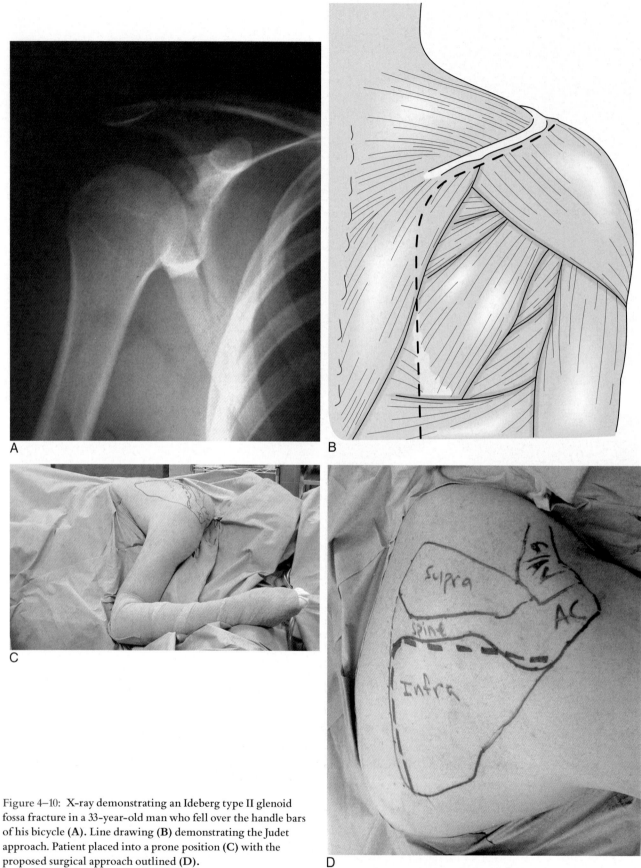

Figure 4–10: X-ray demonstrating an Ideberg type II glenoid fossa fracture in a 33-year-old man who fell over the handle bars of his bicycle (**A**). Line drawing (**B**) demonstrating the Judet approach. Patient placed into a prone position (**C**) with the proposed surgical approach outlined (**D**).

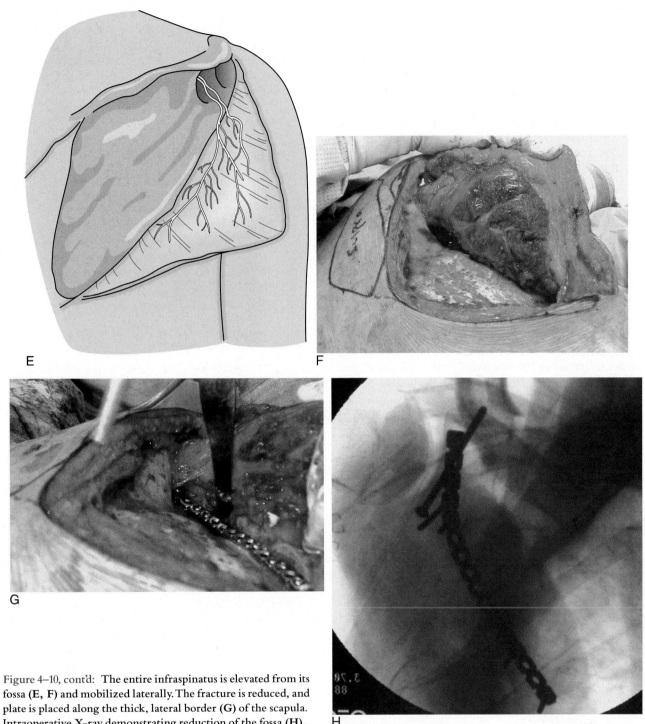

Figure 4–10, cont'd: The entire infraspinatus is elevated from its fossa (**E, F**) and mobilized laterally. The fracture is reduced, and plate is placed along the thick, lateral border (**G**) of the scapula. Intraoperative X-ray demonstrating reduction of the fossa (**H**).

Scapulothoracic Dislocations

Intrathoracic Dislocations of the Scapula

- This is an extremely rare injury caused by direct blunt trauma to the posterior chest wall producing entrapment of the inferior angle of the scapula between third and fourth ribs or the fourth and fifth intercostal space.[14]
- Early recognition may allow a stable reduction to be achieved using hyperabduction of the arm and manually manipulating the scapula into its correct position.
- If discovered late, an open reduction along with the release and reattachment of contracted soft tissues will be needed.

Scapulothoracic Dissociation

- This is a high-energy injury producing a closed, lateral displacement of the scapula, which may be associated with fractures of the ribs, clavicle, scapula, and proximal humerus and disruptions of the glenohumeral, AC, or sternoclavicular (SC) joints.[15]
- Associated soft-tissue injuries include partial or complete tears of scapular or chest muscles; vascular disruptions, most frequently of the subclavian artery; and incomplete (neuropraxia) or complete avulsions of the brachial plexus.
- As a result of the associated bony and soft-tissue pathology associated with this injury, it has often been described as a "closed, forequarter amputation."
- Massive swelling over the shoulder girdle and a pulseless and flail upper extremity are common on physical examination of the patient.

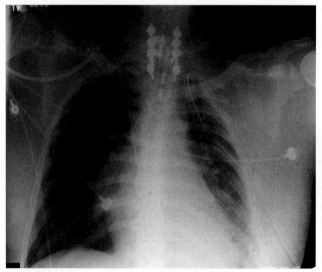

Figure 4–11: Anteroposterior chest X-ray demonstrating a patient with a left-sided scapulothoracic dissociation. Note the rib fractures, prominence of the medial border of the scapula (compared to the right side), and the widened acromioclavicular joint. This patient also presented with a flail left arm, decreased pulses (tear of the axillary artery requiring surgery), cervical spine injuries, and a diaphyseal humeral fracture.

- The diagnosis is made with a nonrotated CXR, which demonstrates a significant lateral displacement of the scapula as measured from the medial border to the spine (Figure 4–11).
- The mortality rate for this injury is high and after successful resuscitation an above-elbow amputation with or without a shoulder arthrodesis should be considered.

Annotated References

1. Thompson DA, Flynn TC, Miller PW, et al: The significance of scapular fractures, *J Trauma* 25:974-977, 1985.
Retrospective review demonstrating scapula fractures occurring in 2.9% of patients with blunt trauma. This article also discusses the high volume of associated injuries seen when patients present with scapular injuries.

2. Ada JR, Miller ME: Scapular fractures: analysis of 113 cases, *Clin Orthop* 269:174-180, 1991.
A study of 113 patients with a variety of scapular fractures followed for a minimum of 15 months. Authors propose a classification of scapula fractures and demonstrate that majority of fractures can be treated nonoperatively.

3. Goss TP: Double disruptions of the superior shoulder suspensory complex, *J Orthop Trauma* 7:99-106, 1993.
Initial description explaining the concept of the superior shoulder suspensory complex as a bony/soft-tissue ring made up of the glenoid, coracoid, distal clavicle, and the coracoclavicular (CC) and acromioclavicular (AC) ligaments designed to maintain a normal relationship between the scapula/upper extremity and the axial skeleton.

4. Eyres KS, Brooks A, Stanley D: Fractures of the coracoid process, *J Bone Joint Surg Br* 77:425-428, 1995.
A review of 12 patients in which the authors present a classification of these fractures and discuss their recommendations for the conservative and surgical management of these injuries.

5. Nordqvist A, Pettersson C: Fracture of the body, neck or spine of the scapula: a long-term follow-up study, *Clin Orthop* 283:139-144, 1992.
This is a retrospective review of 68 patients examined at an average of 14 years after their injury, who were treated conservatively for fractures of the body, neck, or spine. Although 48% had a radiographic deformity, the residual disability to the shoulder was only slight or moderate.

6. Pace AM, Stuart R, Brownlow H: Outcome of glenoid neck fractures, *J Shoulder Elbow Surg* 14:585-590, 2005.
This study evaluated nine patients treated conservatively with neck fractures, followed for an average of 57.3 months. Using radiographs to evaluate the glenopolar angle and glenoid version demonstrated that regardless of X-ray findings 90% of patients achieved good or excellent levels.

7. Herscovici DJr, Fiennes AG TW, Allgower M, et al: The floating shoulder: ipsilateral clavicle and scapular neck fractures, *J Bone Joint Surg Br* 74:362-364, 1992.
Retrospective evaluation of nine patients who sustained ipsilateral midshaft clavicle and scapular neck fractures followed for an

average of 48.5 months. The study showed that the operative fixation of the clavicle prevented anteromedial displacement of the scapular neck, had no complications, and resulted in good outcomes.

8. Lindholm A, Leven H: Prognosis in fractures of the body and neck of the scapula: a follow-up study, *Acta Chir Scand* 140:33-36, 1974.

A review of 19 patients with 20 fractures treated nonoperatively. Normal motion was found in all patients and pain resolved at a mean of 2.7 months.

9. Williams GRJr, Naranja J, Klimliewicz J, et al: The floating shoulder: a biomechanical basis for classification and management, *J Bone Joint Surg Am* 83:1182-1187, 2001.

Twelve fresh-frozen human cadavers underwent ipsilateral clavicle scapular neck fractures, coracoacromial ligament disruption, and acromioclavicular (AC) capsular disruption. The authors found instability of the shoulder girdle occurred with fractures of the clavicle and scapula if there were also disruptions of the associated soft tissues. However, making the diagnosis of these associated soft-tissue problems may be difficult.

10. Egol KA, Connor PM, Karunakar MA, et al: The floating shoulder: clinical and functional results, *J Bone Joint Surg Am* 83:1188-1194, 2001.

Retrospective review of 19 patients, 12 nonoperative and 7 operative (fixation of clavicle and glenoid), found that operatively treated patients had greater amounts of forward flexion, but there was no significant differences between both groups regarding three functional outcome measures.

11. Ideberg R: Fractures of the scapula involving the glenoid fossa, In Bateman JE, Welsh RP editors: *Surgery of the shoulder*, Philadelphia, 1984, BC Decker.

Original description and classification of glenoid fossa fractures proposed by Ideberg after reviewing the trauma registry of 25 hospitals in Sweden.

12. Goss TP: Fractures of the glenoid cavity, *J Bone Joint Surg Am* 74:299-305, 1992.

This is a review summarizing the evaluation, treatment, and rehabilitation of fractures of the glenoid cavity.

13. Mayo KA, Bernirschke SK, Mast JW: Displaced fractures of the glenoid fossa: results of open reduction and internal fixation, *Clin Orthop* 347:122-130, 1998.

Evaluation of 27 patients from two trauma centers assessed at a mean of 43 months who had undergone an open reduction internal fixation of displaced glenoid fossa fractures. Functional ratings demonstrated 82% excellent and good outcomes with low rates of complications regardless of the operative approach.

14. Nettrour LF, Krufty LE, Mueller RE, et al: Locked scapula: intrathoracic dislocation of the inferior angle, *J Bone Joint Surg Am* 54:413-416, 1972.

A case report describing the pathology and treatment of a rare injury involving an intrathoracic dislocation of the scapula.

15. Oreck SL, Burgess A, Levine AM: Traumatic lateral displacement of the scapula: a radiographic sign of neurovascular disruption, *J Bone Joint Surg Am* 66:758-763, 1984.

Original description of scapulothoracic dissociation discussing the physical findings, associated pathology, and the radiographic criteria used to make the diagnosis.

Clavicle Fractures

Cory A. Collinge, MD, and Keith Watson, MD

- Fractures of the clavicle account for 5% to 10% of all fractures and almost half of all shoulder girdle injuries.
- Historically, clavicle fractures have been treated mostly nonoperatively, with an expectation for a return to painless, reliable function.
- Management has typically included using either a shoulder sling or a figure-of-eight brace. Although the majority of these fractures healed, they healed with variable amounts of deformity.
- Recent studies, however, have identified several particular injury patterns that are at significant risk for problems with respect to bony union or compromised function.
- Recent literature on clavicular injuries indicates that non-operative treatment remains the best treatment for most clavicle fractures; however, recommendations regarding the optimal method of treatment have changed for certain clavicular injuries.

Mechanism of Injury

- Clavicle fractures occur from medium to high-energy trauma.
- These injuries may result from a blow to the point of the shoulder, which often occurs when a person is thrown from a motorcycle or strikes the ground in athletics, or a lateral blow to the shoulder and chest wall, such as that which occurs when a person is T-boned in a motor vehicle crash.
- Concomitant injury is common in these settings and can include chest injury and rib fractures, ipsilateral scapula fracture or other upper extremity trauma, and head or neck injuries.

Anatomy and Function

- The clavicle's pertinent surrounding anatomy is illustrated in Figure 5–1.

- The clavicle is an S-shaped bone when viewed from above and straight when viewed from the front.
- The medial clavicle articulates with the sternum at the sternoclavicular (SC) joint where stability is provided mostly by the strong costoclavicular ligaments and the capsule of the SC joint.
- Laterally, the distal clavicle and the acromion meet to form the acromioclavicular (AC) joint.
- The primary stabilizers of the AC joint are the AC ligament, which overlies the AC joint and the stronger coracoclavicular (CC) ligaments. The CC ligaments, the conoid (medial) and the trapezoid (lateral), attach the coracoid process to the inferior surface of the distal clavicle and provide most of the vertical stability of the AC joint.
- The clavicle is quite mobile, and its motion, primarily through the SC joint, allows for rotation, elevation, extension, and flexion of the shoulder as the scapula moves over the chest wall.
- Muscle groups attached to the clavicle perform complex interconnected motions including: the sternocleidomastoid and pectorals (medially) and the trapezius and deltoid (laterally).
- Other important structures in proximity to the clavicle are at risk for injury in conjunction with a clavicle fracture or its treatment (see Figure 5–1).
- The subclavian artery and vein lie posterior and inferior to the middle portion of the clavicle. Additionally, the brachial plexus also passes behind the clavicle and is intertwined around the subclavian vessels. Fortunately, the small but well-placed subclavius muscle lies between the clavicle, and these neurovascular structures and may prevent more frequent damage to these structures.
- The great vessels travel just posterior to the medial extent of the clavicle and the SC joint. Finally, the first rib, the pleura, and apices of the lungs lie beneath the medial clavicle and may be injured in high-energy situations.

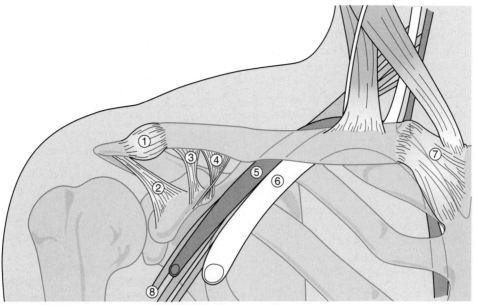

Figure 5–1: The clavicle and its local anatomy are diagrammed. (1) Acromioclavicular ligament; (2) coracoacromial ligament; (3) coracoclavicular ligament (trapezoid); (4) coracoclavicular ligament (conoid); (5) subclavian artery; (6) subclavian vein; (7) anterior sternoclavicular ligament; and (8) brachial plexus.

- The clavicle and the scapula function as struts to suspend the shoulder and upper extremity from the upper thorax.
- Goss[1] described the superior shoulder suspensory complex (SSSC) as a mechanical ring of bony and soft tissues (made up of the glenoid, coracoid process, CC ligaments, distal clavicle, AC joint, and the acromion) at the end of two bony struts (the clavicle and scapula).
- Traumatic injury to one component of the SSSC is common and does not compromise the overall integrity of the complex; therefore, the consequences of these injuries tend to be minor.
- Traumatic disruptions of the complex in two places (double disruptions of the SSSC) can create a potentially unstable anatomical situation that may include long-term problems with healing and functional consequences.

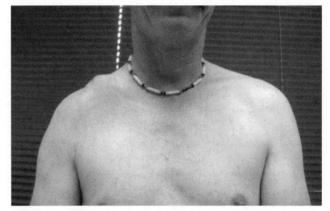

Figure 5–2: Clinical picture of patient with displaced right clavicle fracture.

Physical Examination

Local Examination

- Because the clavicle lies in a largely subcutaneous position, swelling and deformity after fracture is usually obvious (Figure 5–2).
- Tenderness of most clavicle fractures is apparent with simple palpation at the fracture site, and instability is seen in displaced fractures.
- Open fractures of the clavicle are not common but do occur because the bone is subcutaneous. Any skin abrasions or other wounds in proximity to the fracture site must be examined carefully to determine if the fracture is an open injury.

- On occasion, a fracture spike will incarcerate in the skin. This tenting of the skin can cause pressure necrosis and result in an open injury.
- An open fracture and this impending open fracture represent indications for early surgical treatment.
- Some clavicle fractures, especially those occurring with a displaced scapular neck fracture ("floating shoulder" injuries), will lead to a droop of the affected shoulder.
- If the patient is ambulatory, examination of the standing patient with his or her arms hanging down and shoulders exposed will clearly demonstrate this deformity. This cosmetic droop will not be corrected without operative intervention (see Figure 5–2).

Distant Examination

- The affected limb should be assessed carefully for other signs of trauma. A complete neurovascular examination of the involved extremity must be performed and documented.
- Although a variety of neurologic injuries may occur with clavicle injury, the medial cord of the brachial plexus is in closest proximity and, thus, is commonly injured; medial cord injury is manifest distally as "ulnar nerve" findings.
- Pulses are assessed and compared to the contralateral side.
- Katras and others[2] reported four patients with ipsilateral clavicle fracture and subclavian artery injury. The authors noted that findings on clinical examination after subclavian artery occlusion may be subtle because collateral flow in the upper extremity is generally good.
- A comparison of blood pressures taken using each arm can be helpful in identifying occult injury.
- As noted, clavicle fractures occur typically as a result of medium-energy or high-energy trauma; therefore, the Advanced Trauma Life Support (ATLS) protocols for evaluation and treatment should be followed until other injuries have been definitively ruled out.
- Areas of particular interest with clavicle fracture include the chest, where rib fractures or pulmonary injury are common, and head and neck, where significant injury may also occur.

Radiographic Examination

- The initial diagnosis is often made from an anteroposterior (AP) chest X-ray (CXR), which is a good screening study.
- Specific views of the clavicle include AP and 30- to 40-degree cephalic tilt views (Figure 5–3). Both should include the SC joint medially and the AC joint laterally.
- Views of the clavicle aimed at 45 degrees cephalic and at 45 degrees caudal (Quesana views) may better demonstrate fracture displacement compared to other views.
- AP CXR or a view of both clavicles on a single long film may be useful for measuring the amount of fracture shortening by comparing the lengths of the clavicle between the injured and normal sides.

- AP radiograph, which is centered at the AC joint with a 10-degree cephalic tilt (Zanca view), provides excellent visualization of the AC joint and far distal fractures.
- Radiographic evaluation of medial clavicle fractures and SC dislocations may be best seen on computed tomography (CT) or an AP radiograph with cephalic tilt of 40 to 45 degrees (serendipity view).

Classification Systems

- The most commonly used classification system for fractures of the clavicle is that of Allman[3] (Box 5–1).
- Group I fractures, fractures that occur at the middle third, account for 72% to 80% of all clavicle fractures.
- Group II, fractures occurring at the lateral clavicle, make up 10% to 30% of clavicle fractures.

Box 5–1	Combined Allman and Neer Classification Systems for Clavicle Fractures

Group I—Fracture of middle third
Group II—Fracture of the distal third

- Type I—Minimally displaced or interligamentous
- Type II—Displaced as a result of fracture medial to the coracoclavicular ligaments
- Type II-A—Both the conoid and trapezoid remain attached to distal fragment
- Type II-B—Either the conoid is torn or both the conoid and trapezoid are torn
- Type III—Fractures involving articular surface
- Type IV—Ligaments intact to the periosteum with displacement of the proximal fragment
- Type V—Comminuted

Group III—Fracture of the proximal third

- Type I—Minimal displacement
- Type II—Displaced
- Type III—Intraarticular
- Type IV—Epiphyseal separation (observed in young patients)
- Type V—Comminuted

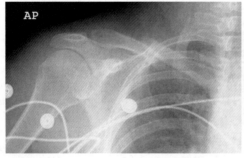 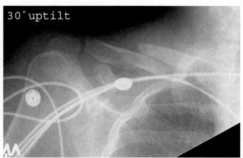

Figure 5–3: Anteroposterior and 30-degree cranial tilt views of a middle-third clavicle fracture. As in this case, the "uptilted" view may best demonstrate the fracture morphology.

- Group III, fractures of the medial clavicle, are quite rare (<5%).
- Group II fractures (distal third) have been subsequently subclassified by Neer[4] into three types based on the location of the clavicle fracture in relation to the CC ligaments (see Box 5–1, Figure 5–4).
- In type I distal clavicle injuries, the CC ligaments are intact and the fracture is usually nondisplaced or minimally displaced.
- Type II distal clavicle fractures are at the level of the CC ligaments and are further subdivided into II-A and II-B fractures.
- In type II-A fractures, both the conoid and trapezoid ligaments remain intact and the fracture is medial to the ligaments.
- Type II-B fractures involve a disruption of the conoid ligament, with the trapezoid ligament remaining intact and attached to the distal fracture fragment.
- Type II-B injuries tend to have significant displacement of the fracture fragments because of the loss of the downward restraint on the medial fragment from the CC ligaments.

- Type III injuries are distal to the CC ligaments and involve the AC joint. These are usually nondisplaced or minimally displaced.

Treatment Options
Medial-Third Fractures

- Recommended management of medial clavicle fractures is typically nonoperative, and results have remained consistently good.
- Significant displacement and healing problems are rare in fractures of the medial clavicle as a result of the extensive soft-tissue attachments.
- If significant displacement does occur with a medial fracture, further imaging studies, such as an AP radiograph with 40- to 45-degree cephalic tilt or CT scan, are warranted.
- The medial clavicle's physis is among the last to fuse in the body; thus, patients from late adolescence into their early 20s may have physeal fractures in this area.

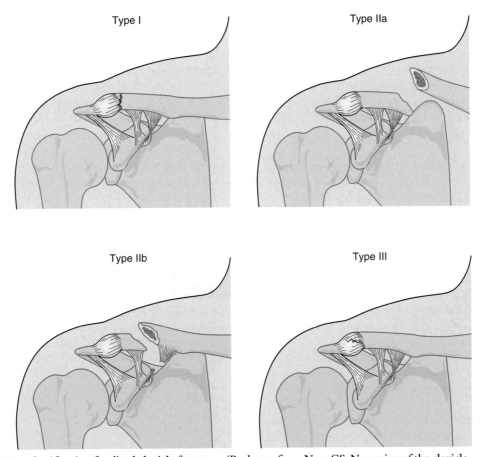

Figure 5–4: **The Neer classification for distal clavicle fractures. (Redrawn from Neer CS: Nonunion of the clavicle,** *JAMA* 172:1002-1011, 1960.)

Middle-Third Fractures

- The majority of clavicle fractures involve the middle third and heal well with nonoperative treatment.
- Nordqvist and others[5] demonstrated that 82% of patients with clavicle fractures were asymptomatic with full return of function an average of 17 years after nonoperative treatment.
- Nondisplaced or minimally displaced clavicle fractures heal well with nonoperative management.
- The typical middle-third clavicle fracture, however, is displaced, with flexion of the major medial fragment and inferior displacement of the major lateral fragment. Simple fractures are usually oblique, with more complex patterns demonstrating a similar pattern with a butterfly fragment or comminution.
- Maintaining any meaningful closed reduction of a clavicle fracture with simple manipulation alone is nearly impossible; therefore, acute reduction maneuvers should be avoided.
- Many displaced middle-third clavicle fractures can be successfully treated nonoperatively as well.
- Displaced fractures heal with varying degrees of cosmetic deformity, often causing a noticeable bump at the fracture site.
- If the goal of surgery is cosmesis, operative repair is indicated rarely, if ever, as the surgical scar will likely be cosmetically displeasing for the patient as well. In the vast majority of cases, trading a bump for a scar is not worth the risks of surgical treatment.
- Nonoperative treatment is managed in two ways, using bracing that provides (1) simple support of the extremity, such as with a sling or sling and swath, or (2) reduction and immobilization, typically with a figure-of-eight brace.
- Many physicians continue to use figure-of-eight bracing with the rationale that it improves reduction and allows for better results than simple immobilization.
- However, Andersen and others[6] demonstrated that functional and cosmetic results were identical between the two methods, and less patient discomfort was noted with treatment using only a sling. In both cases, the alignment of the healed fractures was unchanged from the initial fracture displacement in both treatment groups.
- No difference in the speed of recovery has been demonstrated between those treated with a sling or those treated with figure-of-eight bracing.
- During the period of immobilization, the patient performs pendulum and Codman's exercises to maintain shoulder motion and active range of motion of the elbow, wrist, and hand.
- By 6 weeks, pain is usually well controlled, and limitations involving activities of daily living and use of the sling may be discontinued at 3 weeks as pain allows.

- Clinical healing has usually occurred by 6 to 8 weeks, and radiographic union follows shortly thereafter. A return of full function can usually be expected by 12 weeks.

Surgical Indications

- Although the majority of middle-third clavicle fractures heal well with nonoperative treatment, operative treatment has been recommended under certain circumstances.
- Common indications for the surgical treatment of acute midshaft clavicle fractures (Box 5–2) include: open fracture and impending open fracture, progressive neurologic deficit, and limited mobility as a result of the clavicle fracture in polytrauma patients.
- *Painful* nonunion is also a common indication for operative treatment.
- Additional recommendations for surgery include floating shoulder injuries and shortening of the clavicle expected to result in nonunion or affect function (e.g., shortening >2 cm). These will be discussed further.
- The potential functional significance of displaced ipsilateral fractures of the clavicle and scapular neck (floating shoulder injury) because a double disruption of the SSSC has been mentioned.[1] In this situation, surgical treatment of the clavicle alone has been recommended by several authors.
- Restoration of the superior-anterior bony strut, in theory, restores the clavicular anatomy directly and indirectly improves the scapular anatomy, transforming the injury to a single disruption of the SSSC. Good-to-excellent outcomes have been shown using this treatment approach.[7,8]
- Some evidence suggests that only floating shoulder injuries with significant displacement of the glenoid may be the strongest indications for operative repair.
- One study demonstrated satisfactory results in patients with floating shoulders having mild displacement treated nonoperatively.[9]

Box 5–2 | **Common Indications for the Surgical Treatment of Clavicle Fractures**

- Open fracture and impending open fracture
- Ipsilateral displaced fractures of the clavicle and scapular neck fracture or "floating shoulder" injury
- Shortening of the clavicle expected to result in nonunion or affect function (e.g., shortening > 2 cm)
- Progressive neurologic deficit
- Polytrauma patients in whom mobility is limited as a result the clavicle fracture
- Painful nonunion
- Most displaced type II distal clavicle fractures

- In a nonrandomized, retrospective study of 35 patients with floating shoulder injuries treated operatively and nonoperatively, one study reported similar functional results at 35 months.[10] A subset of six patients with significant caudal displacement of the glenoid experienced dismal results after nonoperative treatment.

- In an effort to decide if the floating shoulder injury pattern required operative stabilization, a biomechanical cadaver sectioning study was performed to determine the osseous and ligamentous contributions to the stability of experimentally created scapular neck fractures.[11] They determined that ipsilateral fractures of the scapular neck and the clavicular shaft do not produce a true floating shoulder, without additional disruption of the coracoacromial and AC ligaments. These and other unstable combined injury patterns are likely to be accompanied by substantial medial displacement of the glenoid fragment.

- It seems reasonable to recommend surgical treatment (e.g., open reduction and internal fixation [ORIF] clavicle) only for those floating shoulders in which there is significant medial or caudle displacement of the scapula fracture or other indications for operative intervention are present, such as in seen in Box 5–2.

- A large series of patients with clavicle fractures treated nonoperatively was reviewed, and the incidence of nonunion was 4.5% of the diaphyseal fractures and 11.5% of the lateral-end fractures.[12] Following a diaphyseal fracture, the risk of nonunion was significantly increased by displacement of the fracture, comminution, advancing age, and female gender. Although most surgeons with substantial experience in treating clavicle fractures believe that the amount of fracture displacement is important in the decision to proceed with surgery, questions remain as to the relative influence of these other factors on that decision.

- Another report found a high rate (15%) of nonunion and a relatively high proportion of unsatisfactory results in fractures in which initial shortening of the fracture was greater than 2 cm.[13] The authors recommended surgical treatment of these injuries.

- Similarly, a study reviewed 39 nonunions of middle-third clavicle fractures initially treated nonoperatively and found a correlation between initial fracture shortening of greater than 2 cm and nonunion.[14] The major complaint for all of these nonunions was pain, and all patients had complete or near-complete resolution of their symptoms after successful operative treatment.

- Finally, a study evaluated the functional results of 15 patients undergoing corrective osteotomy for shortened, malunited clavicular fractures with chronic pain, weakness, neurologic symptoms, and dissatisfaction with the appearance of the shoulder.[15] Postoperatively, primary union was achieved in 14 of 15 patients, clavicular length was predictably restored, and functional results were dramatically improved.

- Other studies have attempted to identify risk factors associated with a compromised outcome of clavicular fractures.[16] The strongest radiographic predictors for sequelae were lack of bony contact (displacement), with comminuted fractures having transverse fragments, and older patients. The effects of these findings on most surgeon's decision making remain unclear to date.

Methods of Operative Treatment

- No consensus as to the best method of operative treatment for these injuries has been reached; most common recommendations have included plating using 3.5-mm plates and small fragment screws, intramedullary fixation, and even external fixation.

- As with most conditions for which numerous treatment options are advocated, established methods for the operative treatment of acute midshaft clavicle fractures and clavicular nonunions have had varying results, and complications are not uncommon and in some series, as high as 75%.

- Complications frequently reported include painful implant prominence, nonunion, and implant breakage or migration.

- More than a few catastrophic complications, such as major neurovascular injury and pneumothorax, have been reported as well.

- Many surgeons now use a technique of anterior-inferior plating for the treatment of those middle-third fractures and painful nonunions of the clavicle that require surgical treatment.[7] The technique is reviewed in this chapter (Figures 5–5 and 5–6). This treatment method results in early healing, few complications, and a return of good-to-excellent function in the majority of patients.

- The rationale for using this technique is to apply modern plating methods, including the use of stiff plates, lag

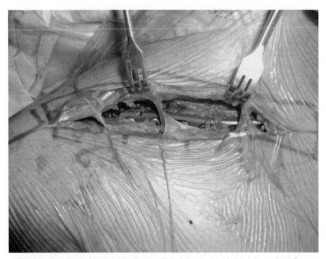

Figure 5–5: "Biologically friendly" fixation of the clavicle after anterior-inferior plating using a 3.5-mm plate.

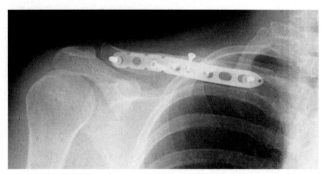

Figure 5–6: **Corresponding postoperative radiograph demonstrating middle-third clavicle fracture after open reduction and anterior-inferior plating.**

screws, and respect for the local biology to achieve stable internal fixation and early healing.

- Furthermore, by placing the implants on the anterior-inferior border of the clavicle, several theoretical benefits may be achieved.
  1. Screws are directed in a posterior-superior direction. Thus, instrumentation and screws are directed safely away from the dangerous infraclavicular anatomy.
  2. Placement in this orientation also allows screws to take advantage of the widest axis of the flattened ends of the clavicle; therefore, longer screws may be placed, resulting in increased fixation strength.
  3. Finally, by applying the plate to the anterior-inferior border of the clavicle, difficulties with implant prominence may be minimized.
- Plating of the anterior-inferior surface of the clavicle does not appear to have a negative effect on mechanical stability.[17,18]

Plating Methods

- Fracture biology is maintained, and the only dissection allowed is that absolutely necessary for a quality reduction and plate application (see Figure 5–5).
- Most fractures are oblique in orientation and should, if possible, be fixed with one or more lag screws, either through or outside the plate (see Figure 5–6).
- A 3.5-mm reconstruction or a dynamic compression plate is recommended because they are sturdy and allow for oblique screw placement (see Figure 5–6).
- For acute fractures, typically, an eight-hole plate fits well and allows the appropriate screws to be placed. To match the normal anatomy of the clavicle, the plate must be bent into an "S" shape when viewed on edge and without bend when viewed with the screw holes in plain view.
- Clavicular nonunions are measured and compared to the normal side. When significant shortening has occurred, a structural iliac crest autograft is used in conjunction with the plating.
- More details for anterior-inferior plating methods are described in Box 5–3.

| Box 5–3 | **Technique for Anterior-Inferior Plating of Middle-Third Clavicle Fractures** |

- Preoperative planning is performed for all cases (see Fig. 5-1).
- Clavicular nonunions are measured and compared to the normal side; when needed, a structural iliac crest bone graft is used in conjunction with the plating.
- The patient is positioned in the supine position with a large bump placed between the scapulae and the spine, allowing the injured shoulder girdle to fall posteriorly and exposing the length of the clavicle.
- The upper chest, sternal notch, and a portion of neck are included in the surgical field. The entire upper extremity is draped free to allow manipulation, if needed.
- The skin incision is centered over the fracture and follows a line connecting the sternal notch to the anterior edge of the acromion (see Fig. 5-5).
- The lateral platysma is released, and the supraclavicular nerves identified on the anterior aspect of the clavicle and spared.
- The clavipectoral fascia is then incised along its attachment to the anterior clavicle and carefully elevated in an inferior direction.
- Dissection is first performed along the flexed medial fragment to protect the vital infraclavicular structures.
- Minimal soft-tissue dissection is performed at the fracture site in the case of acute fracture to maintain "good fracture biology."
- In nonunion cases, the fracture ends are drilled to open up the intramedullary canal.
- Reduction is performed and held with small bone holding clamps. (A minidistractor is sometimes useful tool in holding the bone ends from overlapping.)
- A 3.5-mm dynamic compression plate or a 3.5-mm reconstruction plate is contoured for application to the anterior-inferior edge of the clavicle (see Fig. 5-5). Typically, an eight-hole plate fits well when contoured into a S-shape as viewed on edge and without bend when viewed with the screw holes in plain view.
- Lag screws can be placed either through or outside the plate in the majority of cases, because most of these fractures had an oblique fracture or a sizable butterfly fragment.
- Screws are aimed posteriorly and superiorly (see Fig. 5-6).
- Cancellous or tricortical autologous iliac crest bone graft are added in patients treated for clavicular nonunion.
- The clavipectoral fascia is closed over the implants, and the skin closed in multiple layers.

Intramedullary Fixation

- Proponents of intramedullary fixation of clavicle fractures have demonstrated successful clinical results with this method of treatment.
- Critics of this method, however, point out that many of the clavicle fractures requiring surgery may be treated poorly with intramedullary devices. For example, in comminuted or long-oblique fractures intramedullary devices provide little control of the clavicular length.
- A similar surgical approach for open reduction is performed as described for plating.

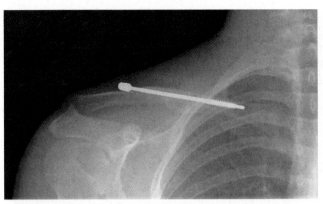

Figure 5–7: **Postoperative radiograph demonstrating middle-third clavicle fracture after open reduction using an intramedullary device.**

- This includes an open approach to the fracture site and preservation of the bone's soft-tissue attachments.
- A Steinman pin, cannulated screw, or specialty clavicle screw is then placed in a retrograde fashion past the fracture site (Figure 5–7).
- It is recommended that implants be threaded in the proximal fragment to prevent migration because catastrophic complications have been seen due to medial migration of implants into the thorax and mediastinum. If a smooth pin is used, bend the distal tip to prevent migration after crossing the fracture site.
- As with plating, grafting with cancellous autograft is indicated in cases of nonunion.

Complications of Surgical Treatment

- Most series reporting results of operative treatment for acute midshaft fractures of the clavicle describe nonunion rates of 3% to 13%, whereas those treating established nonunions report recurring nonunion rates 0% to 15% after surgery.
- Historically, high rates of operative treatment failures appear to have resulted, at least in part, from inadequate internal fixation.
- The need for implant removal is inherent to intramedullary fixation of clavicle nonunions; in recent studies, the removal of 85% to 93% of intramedullary implants was required as a result of painful implant prominence.[19,20]
- Several catastrophic complications, such as major neurovascular and mediastinal injury, have been reported. Most of these have resulted from the medial migration of pins or portions of intramedullary implants. The routine use of smooth pins for intramedullary fixation of these fractures should be avoided.
- Superiorly applied plates are subcutaneous, and in many patients 3.5-mm plates placed here may also cause local tenderness, pain, or cosmetic problems.

- In one study, patients with plates applied to the anterior-inferior surface of the clavicle, only 3 of 58 patients (5%) desired implant removal as result of hardware problems and few other patients described any hardware-related symptoms.[7]

Postoperative Rehabilitation

- Postoperatively, patients are placed in a sling for 7 to 10 days for comfort.
- Patients are instructed in gentle range-of-motion exercises and are encouraged to move the arm without pushing, pulling, or heavy lifting.
- Full return of activities is permitted once healing has occurred, usually by 10 to 12 weeks.

Distal-Third Fractures

- As mentioned previously, these injuries account for about 12% to 15% of all clavicle fractures.
- Neer's classification system of distal clavicle fractures is demonstrated in Figure 5–4.
- As type I and III fractures are often nondisplaced or minimally displaced, they are typically treated with nonoperative treatment and progress to early union and a successful clinical result.[21]
- The few far distal fractures (type III), which do not unite and are painful, may be treated with late distal clavicle resection.
- Much controversy, however, remains in the literature regarding the appropriate management of type II fractures of the distal third of the clavicle (Figure 5–8).
- Neer found that although distal-third clavicle fractures are rare, they account for approximately half of all clavicular nonunions.[22] The incidence of nonunion for these injuries is relatively high, ranging from 28% to 30%.
- As many as 80% of distal clavicle nonunions may cause no pain or other symptoms at long-term follow-up.
- Nordqvist and others[21] found that 5 of 23 (22%) patients with displaced type II distal clavicle fractures had residual shoulder dysfunction and pain when treated nonoperatively.
- Recommendations from the majority of shoulder surgeons are to treat most displaced type II distal clavicle fractures surgically.
- A variety of different procedures have been described for this purpose. Problems that must be overcome with surgical treatment of these injuries include maintaining implant purchase in a short distal fragment in which significant deforming forces are present.
- Many techniques of surgical fixation of distal clavicle fractures have been described in the literature. Resulting from the uncommon nature of the injury, however, no large operative series are available to make treatment recommendations.

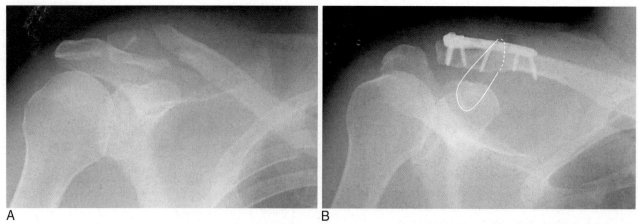

A   B

Figure 5–8: **A,** Radiographs demonstrating a type II fracture of the distal clavicle and its treatment with plate fixation. **B,** A coracoclavicular reconstruction may also performed *(white line)* using Mersilene tape, heavy suture, or other material. These ligatures should be placed in a manner so as not to "saw" through the clavicle.

- Surgical principles, though, include direct visualization and reduction of the fracture fragments.
- Use of plates, Kirschner wires (K-wires), tension banding, CC screws, and CC reconstruction with Dacron or Mersilene tape, or combinations of these have been described (see Figures 5–8 and 5–8).
- Stabilization of the CC interval has been a part of many methods of these surgical reconstructions, with the rationale that placing the medial fragment in an improved position in the superior or inferior plane helps stabilize the fracture repair.
- Reducing the lateral end of the proximal clavicle fragment inferiorly by tethering it to the coracoid, however, also necessarily brings the clavicle anteriorly. Thus, the surgeon must be aware that in some cases this technique may result in a less anatomic repair than originally recognized.
- The surgical treatment of distal clavicle fractures can lead to a variety of complications, and some are unique to this area.
  1. The vast majority of implants require removal after healing has been achieved because they are nearly always symptomatic.
  2. Hook plates may cause erosion of the acromion and AC joint.
  3. Any wires of other implants crossing the AC joint may ultimately break.
  4. Erosion of the clavicle has been seen in some cases wherein techniques such as heavy suture, wire, or tape are used for CC interval reconstruction alone. They may ultimately "saw" through the clavicle, creating secondary injury and symptoms. Some surgeons have applied a thin plate on the superior surface of the clavicle beneath the suture material or placed it through a drill hole in an attempt to prevent these problems.

- After surgery, rehabilitation may be performed in a similar fashion to other operatively treated clavicle fractures (described previously).

Annotated References

1. Goss TP: Double disruptions of the superior shoulder suspensory complex, *J Orthop Trauma* 7:99-106, 1993.
Goss described the "superior shoulder suspensory complex" (SSSC), a bony/soft-tissue structure, important both for its role as an intact unit and for the individual components that make up this unit. Single disruptions in this unit may cause only minor problems, but "double disruptions" of the SSSC frequently create an unstable anatomic situation with potentially adverse long-term healing and functional consequences. This double-disruption principle underlies, unites, and allows one to understand several well-described but difficult-to-treat shoulder injuries that have previously been described in isolation.

2. Katras T, Baltazar U, Rush DS, et al: Subclavian arterial injury associated with blunt trauma, *Vasc Surg* 35:43-50, 2001.

3. Allman FL: Fractures and ligamentous injuries of the clavicle and its articulation, *J Bone Joint Surg Am* 49:774-784, 1976.
This article discusses shoulder injuries and presents the most widely used classification system for clavicular fractures.

4. Neer CS: Fractures of the clavicle, In Rockwood C and Greens D: *Fractures in Adults*, ed 1, Philadelphia, 1984 JB Lippincott.
Classic discussion on clavicle fractures and their treatment.

5. Nordqvist A, Petersson CJ, Redlund-Johnell I: Mid-clavicle fractures in adults: end result study after conservative treatment, *J Orthop Trauma* 12:572-576, 1998.
The authors analyzed the long-term outcome of 225 midclavicle fractures to evaluate the clinical importance of displacement and fracture comminution. At follow-up, 185 (82%) shoulders were asymptomatic, 39 (17%) had moderate pain and were rated as fair, and 1 was rated as poor. There were 7 (4.5%) nonunions in 154 displaced fractures. Forty of 53 (75%)

malunited fractures and 3 of 7 nonunions were clinically rated as good. The authors concluded that few patients with fractures of the midpart of the clavicle require operative treatment.

6. Andersen K, Jensen PO, Lauritzen J: Treatment of clavicular fractures: figure-of-eight bandage versus a simple sling, *Acta Orthop Scand* 58:71-74, 1987.
The authors demonstrated in a prospective, randomized study that functional and cosmetic results were identical between bracing of clavicular fractures with figure-of-eight bracing versus a simple sling. Less patient discomfort was noted with treatment using only a sling. In both cases, the alignment of the healed fractures was unchanged from the initial fracture displacement in both treatment groups.

7. Collinge C, Devinney S, DiPasquale T, et al: Anterior-inferior plate fixation of middle-third fractures and nonunions of the clavicle, *J Orthop Trauma* 20:680-686, 2006.
The authors describe the treatment of 80 consecutive patients treated with open reduction and anterior-inferior plating of acute middle-third fractures and nonunions. Results and outcomes were available in 58 patients; complication rates were low, and a high percentage of good or excellent results were achieved. Problems with implant prominence appeared to be markedly reduced with application of the plate in this manner.

8. Herscovici D Jr, Fiennes AG, Allgower M, et al: The floating shoulder: ipsilateral clavicle and scapular neck fractures, *J Bone Joint Surg Br* 74:362-364, 1992.
A small series of patients treated for ipsilateral midclavicular and scapular-neck fractures advocating internal fixation of the fractured clavicle by a plate and screws. Their rationale for treatment was to restore the mechanical stability of the suspensory structures and to prevent late deformity of the shoulder by directly realigning the clavicle fracture and indirectly reducing of the scapular neck fracture.

9. Edwards SG, Wood GW 3rd, Whittle AP: Factors associated with Short Form-36 outcomes in nonoperative treatment for ipsilateral fractures of the clavicle and scapula, *Orthopedics* 25:733-738, 2002.
The authors demonstrated satisfactory results in patients with floating shoulders with mild displacement of the scapula fracture at average 28-months' follow-up. They concluded that nonoperative treatment of floating shoulder injuries, especially those with less than 5 mm of fracture displacement, can achieve results that are probably equal or superior to those reported after operative treatment without the risk of operative complications.

10. van Noort A, te Slaa RL, Marti RK, et al: The floating shoulder: a multicentre study, *J Bone Joint Surg Br* 83:795-798, 2001.
This is a nonrandomized, retrospective study of 35 patients with floating shoulder injuries treated operatively and nonoperatively. The authors found similar functional results between those patients treated with and without surgery at 35 months. A subset of six patients with significant caudal displacement of the glenoid that were treated nonoperatively experienced dismal results.

11. Williams GR Jr, Naranja J, Klimkiewicz J, et al: The floating shoulder: a biomechanical basis for classification and management, *J Bone Joint Surg Am* 83-A:1182-1187, 2001.
The authors performed a biomechanical cadaver sectioning study to assess whether the "floating shoulder" injury pattern required operative stabilization. They determined that ipsilateral fractures of the scapular neck and the clavicular shaft do not produce a true floating shoulder without additional disruption of the coracoacromial and acromioclavicular ligaments. These and other unstable combined injury patterns are likely to be accompanied by substantial medial displacement of the glenoid fragment.

12. Robinson CM, Court-Brown CM, McQueen MM, et al: Estimating the risk of nonunion following nonoperative treatment of a clavicular fracture, *J Bone Joint Surg Am* 86-A:1359-1365, 2004.
The authors reviewed more than 800 consecutive patients with clavicular fracture treated nonoperatively, including 581 fractures in the middle-third and 263 fractures of the distal clavicle. The incidence of nonunion at 24 weeks after the fracture was 4.5% of the middle-third fractures and 11.5% of the lateral-end fractures. Following a middle-third fracture, the risk of nonunion was significantly increased by advancing age, female gender, displacement of the fracture, and the presence of comminution.

13. Hill JM, McGuire MH, Crosby LA: Closed treatment of displaced middle-third fractures of the clavicle gives poor results, *J Bone Joint Surg Br* 79:537-539, 1997.
The authors evaluated 52 patients treated conservatively for a displaced middle-third fracture of the clavicle at an average of 38 months after injury. Eight of the 52 fractures (15%) had developed nonunion, and 16 patients (31%) reported unsatisfactory results. Initial shortening at the fracture of equal to 20 mm had a highly significant association with nonunion ($p < 0.0001$) and increased risk for an unsatisfactory clinical result. No other patient variable, treatment factor, or fracture characteristic had a significant effect on outcome. The authors recommended open reduction and internal fixation of severely displaced fractures of the middle third of the clavicle in adult patients.

14. Wick M, Muller EJ, Kollig E, et al: Midshaft fractures of the clavicle with a shortening of more than 2 cm predispose to nonunion, *Arch Orthop Trauma Surg* 121:207-211, 2001.
The authors reviewed 39 nonunions of middle-third clavicle fractures initially treated nonoperatively and found a correlation between initial fracture shortening of greater than 2 cm and nonunion. These patients subsequently underwent open reduction and internal fixation with subsequent union of the fracture. The major patient complaint for all of these nonunions was pain, and all patients had complete or near complete resolution of their symptoms after successful operative treatment. Wick and others, however, still recommended a trial of conservative treatment before open reduction and internal fixation of these fractures.

15. McKee MD, Wild LM, Schemitsch EH: Midshaft malunions of the clavicle, *J Bone Joint Surg Am* 85-A:790-797, 2003.
The authors reviewed functional results of 15 patients undergoing corrective osteotomy for malunited clavicular fractures with chronic pain, weakness, neurologic symptoms, and dissatisfaction with the appearance of the shoulder. The mean amount of clavicular shortening found preoperatively was 2.9 cm. Postoperatively, primary union was achieved in 14 of 15 patients,

clavicular length was predictably restored, and functional results were dramatically improved.

16. Nowak J, Rahme H, Holgersson M, et al: Can we predict long-term sequelae after fractures of the clavicle based on initial findings? A prospective study with nine to ten years of follow-up, *J Shoulder Elbow Surg* 13:479-486, 2004.

The authors attempted to identify risk factors associated with a compromised outcome of clavicular fractures. Two-hundred eight patients were followed at 9 to 10 years; 54% had recovered completely, whereas 46% still had sequelae. The strongest radiographic predictor for sequelae was displacement with comminuted fractures with transverse fragments, and older patients also having significantly increased risks for remaining symptoms. In this study, fracture location and shortening did not predict outcome except for cosmetic defects.

17. Ianotti MR, Crosby LA, Stafford P, et al: Effects of plate location and selection on the stability of midshaft clavicle osteotomies: a biomechanical study, *J Shoulder Elbow Surg* 11:457-462, 2002.

18. Harnroongroj T, Vanadurongwan V: Biomechanical aspects of plating osteosynthesis of transverse clavicular fracture with and without inferior cortical defect, *Clin Biomech* 11:290-294, 1996.

Two biomechanical studies comparing osteosynthesis using plates applied superiorly versus anterior-inferiorly. Whereas in certain circumstances one may provide improved stability of one construct over the other, both appeared mechanically acceptable for the vast majority of fracture patterns.

19. Boehme D, Curtis RJ, DeHaan JT, et al: Non-union of fractures of the mid-shaft of the clavicle: treatment with a modified Hagie intramedullary pin and autogenous bone-grafting, *J Bone Joint Surg Am* 73:1219-1226, 1991.

20. Capicotto PN, Heiple KG, Wilbur JH: Midshaft clavicle nonunions treated with intramedullary Steinman pin fixation and onlay bone graft, *J Orthop Trauma* 8:88-93, 1994.

These two studies demonstrated a high percentage of successful clinical results after the intramedullary nailing of middle-third clavicle fracture nonunions. Secondary surgeries were typically necessary to remove implants resulting from tenderness and painful prominence over the implants.

21. Nordqvist A, Petersson C, Redlund-Johnell I: The natural course of lateral clavicle fracture: 15 (11–21) year follow-up of 110 cases, *Acta Orthop Scand* 64:87-91, 1993.

The authors report a large series (110 patients) treated nonoperatively for fractures of the distal clavicle. Follow-up averaged 15 years. Ninety-five patients were asymptomatic. There were only 23 displaced type II fractures. Of these, 28% failed to unite, but 20 of the 23 patients had a good result.

22. Neer CS: Nonunion of the clavicle, *JAMA* 172:1002-1011, 1960.

CHAPTER 6

Fractures of the Humeral Shaft

Anthony F. Infante, Jr., DO, and Eric M. Lindvall, DO

- Fractures of the humeral shaft are common fractures. They are typically treated nonsurgically and have predictable outcomes.[1]
- Surgical treatment for these fractures has evolved over the past 25 years. Operative treatment is commonly performed now compared to the past with predictable outcomes.
- Intramedullary fixation has been improved, both with surgical devices and with techniques.
- Techniques for open reduction and internal fixation (ORIF) have evolved from the early Association for the Study of Osteosynthesis (AO) principles of the 1970s and 1980s to the minimally invasive surgery (MIS) techniques with minimal soft-tissue handling of the 21st century. The implants have developed as well with new screws, new plates, and new devices that allow screws to lock into the plate. Recent literature on plating, nailing, and conservative care has compared all three to show the positives and negatives of each approach.
- With these newer techniques and newer implants, the radial nerve has been shown to be less at risk for iatrogenic injuries.
- Continued research will help future fractures be treated easier and safer. Indications, relative indications, contraindications, and acceptable alignment all continue to evolve with newer techniques and newer implants.

Relevant Anatomy

- The humeral diaphysis starts at the proximal insertion of the pectoralis major and goes to the proximal aspect of the supracondylar ridge of the humerus.[2]
- The location of the fracture in relation to the muscular origin and insertion will determine the angular deformity.[3]
- The pectoralis major and deltoid insertions are the major deforming forces of the humeral shaft fracture.[4] This is important when deciding on a treatment plan for the

patient. The surgeon must realize how nonoperative treatment will control the fracture fragments. If the fracture does not lend itself to nonoperative treatment, a surgical technique must be chosen.

Classification

- The fractures of the humeral shaft do not have a unique classification. They are described by the AO and Orthopaedic Trauma Association (OTA) classification systems using the bone, location, and character of the fracture to classify it. These systems help describe the fracture but have limited usefulness in prognosis, research, and outcome assessments. The AO and OTA classifications have gained acceptance by the orthopaedic community over the past 10 years. The classifications seem difficult to learn at first but with constant use become relatively easy. A wall chart in the operating room (OR) and dictation area is helpful when trying to memorize each fracture.
- Each classification uses an alphanumeric coding system, which is accepted for long bone fractures including the femur and tibia. The system presents the humeral diaphysis as bone 1 and segment 2. The fracture is further defined by the morphologic characteristics. The fracture types are A, B, and C, which stand for simple, wedge, and complex, respectively. The geometry is described next as three different groups, 1, 2, and 3. Types A and B are then divided into subgroups, .1, .2, and .3. The subgroups represent the zones of the fractures .1 (proximal), .2 (middle), and .3 (distal). The type C fractures use the subgroups to define the intermediate fragments. An example would be a distal, comminuted, spiral humeral shaft fracture. Like all of the diaphyseal fractures in the classification system, types A, B, and C represent a spectrum of increasing severity and in theory worsening prognosis.[3]

Clinical and Radiographic Evaluation

- The humeral shaft fracture can occur in many ways. The forces that create the fractures are either direct or indirect (motor vehicle crash, fall, gunshot, stabbings) or direct blow.[1]
- Fractures secondary to extraordinary muscle contraction have also been reported, most frequently caused by torsional forces associated with arm wrestling and throwing a baseball. This sports-related injury typically has a spiral pattern in the middle-third to distal-third of the humerus.[5,6] They can occur when the bone is weakened by a tumor or even in healthy bone as a result of the muscle forces across the humerus.
- The humeral shaft fracture patient will typically have all the signs of a long-bone fracture when seen in the emergency department (ED) or clinic: pain, swelling, deformity, shortening, and abnormal joint motion above and below the fracture segment. This is an easy diagnosis in the awake, alert patient. However this is a challenge in the patient with multiple injuries who is unresponsive.
- A comprehensive examination must be performed initially and then secondary and tertiary examinations can be performed by looking at and palpating all extremities every few days the patient is in the hospital. Pelvic and lower extremity trauma even in responsive patients can cause extreme pain, and the upper extremity fractures can go unnoticed. The examination must include a description of the skin and soft tissues.
- Open fractures are graded using the Gustilo and Anderson classification.[7,8] A complete neurovascular examination must be performed to find associated injuries and to get a baseline examination of the nerves and arteries to make sure they do not deteriorate during the postinjury period. The radial nerve is the nerve most commonly injured, especially in the distal one-third fracture.[9–11]
- Radiographic evaluation must include an anteroposterior (AP) and lateral full length view of the humerus.[2–4] The shoulder and elbow should be evaluated separately to verify that there are no additional fractures, especially in the unresponsive patient. Additional studies are rare, but intraarticular extension may require a computed tomography (CT) scan. Soft-tissue injuries of the elbow ligaments or rotator cuff may require magnetic resonance imaging (MRI).

Treatment

- The question that needs to be answered is: can the fracture be treated with conservative care, does it need open reduction and internal fixation with plates and screws or can it be treated with an intramedullary (IM) nail?

- If conservative care is elected, we start treatment similar to Sarmiento and others[12] with splinting or casting for 7 to 14 days and then convert the treatment to a fracture brace.
- If plating, one must decide which approach would best lend itself to aiding in the plating of the shaft fracture? The four approaches to the humerus; anterior, anterolateral, lateral, or posterior are all considerations.[13,14]
- Once the surgeon decides to nail the fracture as a result of location, fracture pattern, and soft-tissue injury, a decision is made regarding an antegrade or retrograde approach. Lastly, an implant choice must be made regarding standard locking or flexible nails. One should preoperatively plan the surgery with all of these choices and decide which implant to use based on the anatomy and fracture location.
- All things considered, the majority of these fractures can be treated nonoperatively.[12] Over the past 30 years, surgical treatment has been known to increase rates of nonunions, infections, radial nerve palsies, and prolonged disabilities.
- Nonoperative treatment is the initial preferred method for humeral shaft fractures. Operative immobilization is not necessary for healing, and perfect alignment is not essential for an acceptable result. The acceptable result can have a malunited humerus on X-ray. The angles of the humerus that still allow excellent motion of the shoulder and elbow and acceptable appearance of the arm are up to 20 degrees of anterior angulation, 30 degrees of varus, and 1 inch of shortening.[15] Because of this, we can treat these fractures with casts, fracture braces, and nonrigid immobilization techniques while still achieving excellent clinical outcomes. Hanging arm casts, prefabricated functional braces, and coaptation splints have all been associated with excellent results.[12]
- Figures 6–1 through 6–4 demonstrate an example of conservative care. A 26-year-old male sustained a comminuted shaft fracture when involved in a motor vehicle crash. He declined surgery. The risks and benefits of nonoperative care were discussed, and the patient was aware that surgery might become an option if the fracture did not heal. Figures 6–1 and 6–2 demonstrate preoperative X-rays of his comminuted humerus fracture did not heal. Figures 6–3 and 6–4 demonstrate his healing at 4 months. He regained full range of motion of his elbow and shoulder and without restrictions.
- We prefer treatment that is nonoperative, if possible, with initial immobilization in a hanging arm cast or coaptation splint converted to a functional brace in 10 to 14 days. Early motion of the shoulder and elbow begins at the time of brace application. At 6 weeks, when X-rays show acceptable alignment and surgery will not be needed, the patient starts formal therapy, with active and active-assisted motion to increase motion and strength.
- Nonoperative treatment does not work for all humeral shaft fractures. Absolute indications for surgery include

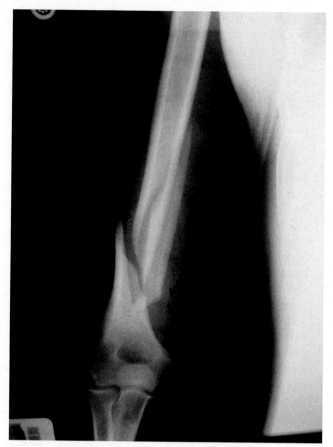

Figure 6–1: **Preoperative anteroposterior X-ray of a comminuted humerus.**

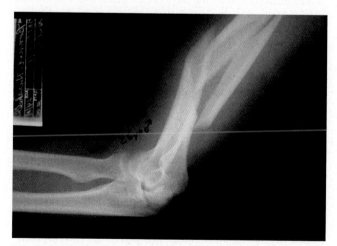

Figure 6–2: **Preoperative lateral X-ray.**

a humeral shaft fracture with a vascular injury and an open humeral shaft fracture. The vascular injury and open wound must go to surgery, but if the fracture is stable, it can still be treated with immobilization techniques. All other indications are relative indications (Box 6-1).

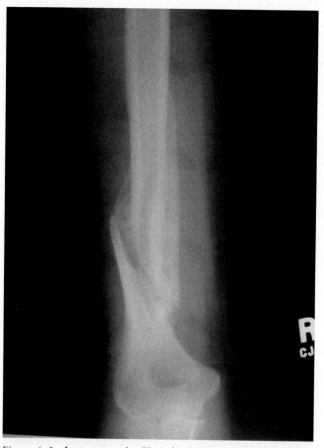

Figure 6–3: **Anteroposterior X-ray healed with fracture brace.**

Surgical Treatment

- If nonoperative treatment fails, a surgical technique is required. There are three options for fixation of humeral shaft fractures: plate and screws, external fixation, and intramedullary fixation.
- Many biomechanical studies have studied the three different techniques for fixation. Unfortunately, these studies use cadaveric bones that are fixed with one of the three techniques but do not have any live muscle function or any bone healing. Therefore all data from these studies must be theorized to the real situation and extrapolated to a human situation. Each technique can be justified by the surgeon who chooses it. Because there is no hard, objective data on one technique versus the other, the choice is really that of the surgeon. One must know the strengths, weaknesses, risks, and benefits of each and pick the appropriate treatment for the individual patient.
- Open humeral shaft fractures require a thorough irrigation and debridement first, followed by treatment of the humeral shaft. The majority of these fractures will be treated with ORIF using a plate and screws. However if multiple debridements will be needed or temporary fixation is required, an external fixator may be chosen. The external

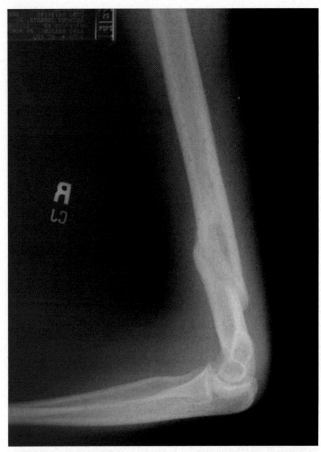

Figure 6–4: Lateral X-ray post–conservative care with fracture brace.

Box 6–1	**Relative Indications for Operative Treatment**

- Failed nonoperative treatment (malalignment or poor patient tolerance)
- Neurologic injury
- Segmental fractures
- Floating elbow
- Bilateral humeral fractures
- Pathologic fractures
- Parkinson's disease
- Polytrauma

fixator can be placed quickly and more easily than plating the humerus. It can also be disassembled to perform a 360-degree irrigation and debridement and reassembled. Plates and screws and intramedullary rods do not have this flexibility. Once the soft tissue and bone is deemed "clean," the bone can then be fixed definitively. Rarely is the external fixator left in place. It is typically converted to a plate or an intramedullary rod. Severe comminution and bone or soft tissue loss may be indications to treat with operative techniques. The gold standard for operative treatment of humeral shaft fractures is compression plating—a broad 4.5 dynamic compression plate if the width of the humerus allows it, and a narrow 4.5 dynamic compression plate if it does not. Before choosing the plate, one must decide the approach to use. Two factors come into play: location of the open wound and which surgical approach would be best for the current fracture. If the surgical wound after debridement lends itself to conversion to an anterolateral or posterior approach, one can use this incision for the ORIF. If, however, the wound is not in an optimal spot, a surgeon should irrigate and debride the wound and then perform a second incision away from the first with a skin bridge. The posterior approach allows a surgeon an exposure from the olecranon fossa with a triceps split to the proximal one third of the humerus. A posterior approach with an olecranon osteotomy allows exposure from the ulnar-humeral joint to the proximal third of the humerus. The anterolateral approach starts as the deltopectoral approach proximally and travels to the elbow laterally. It enables a surgeon to perform fixation from the proximal humerus, including the tuberosities, to the distal humerus, including the epicondyles. It does not lend itself to intra-articular fractures.'

Open Treatment Options for Specific Locations of Fractures

- Proximal third shaft fractures can be treated with an IM nail or with an anterolateral plate. Most of the plates are anatomically designed today to fit the proximal humerus, and they have locking and nonlocking options for the screws.
- Figures 6–5 through 6-8 show a 49-year-old woman with a comminuted humeral shaft fracture that extends to the surgical neck laterally. The patient was treated with ORIF. The surgeon proceeded with a deltopectoral incision so that a plate that was long enough to place screws into the humeral head for proximal fixation could be used. Lag screws were used for fixation of the multiple fragments, and then a neutralization proximal locking plate was placed (Figures 6–7 and 6-8).
- The incision is larger for plating. However, the smaller incision for the nail must include the deltoid and rotator cuff. If one chooses to incise and go through it, our recommendations are to formally open it and carefully repair it. Be careful trying to avoid the rotator cuff. The lateral entry portal for the nail puts a large stress on the area of the head between the articular cartilage and the greater tuberosity. The rigid implants may comminute the proximal humerus by communicating the fracture fragments with the entry portal. This would split off the greater tuberosity and the rotator cuff insertion.

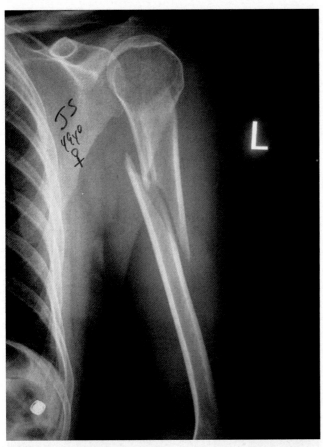

Figure 6–5: Preoperative lateral X-ray of comminuted humerus fracture.

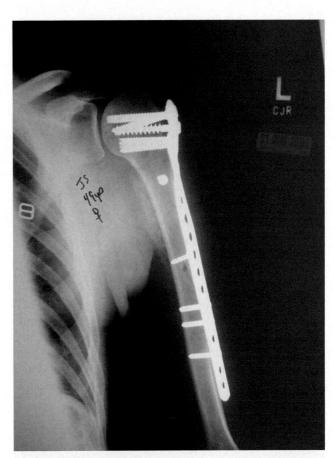

Figure 6–7: Postoperative anteroposterior X-ray treated with open reduction and internal fixation.

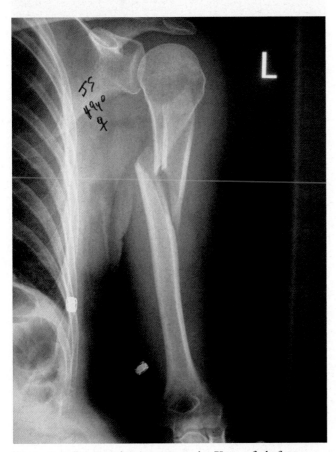

Figure 6–6: Preoperative anteroposterior X-ray of a before comminuted humerus.

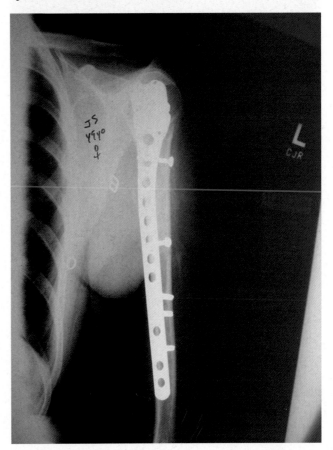

Figure 6–8: Postoperative lateral X-ray treated with open reduction and internal fixation.

- Midshaft fractures can be treated with long IM nails or plating. Either antegrade or retrograde long nails can be used, and they may be either rigid or flexible. The retrograde option allows one to avoid the rotator cuff with a triceps splitting approach at and just above the olecranon fossa. Retrograde flexible nails are an excellent option in this case, allowing a surgeon to avoid undue stress on the anterior cortex and risk comminution that would occur with a rigid nail. A surgeon must have the fracture reduced before reaming and nailing as a result of the risk of injuring the radial nerve. Plating can be performed with a posterior approach or anterolateral approach. Figures 6–9 through 6-12 show an anterolateral plating with a humeral shaft large fragment locking plate. The fracture is reduced and lag screws are placed. The large fragment plate is then placed laterally and used as a neutralization plate. The dissection must include careful handling of the soft tissues near the radial nerve.
- Compression plating with a 4.5 mm. broad plate is the implant of choice if the humerus is wide enough. If not, a 4.5 mm. narrow plate would be the second option.

- Distal-third shaft fractures do not do well with antegrade or retrograde nails. This fracture is too distal and too close to the olecranon fossa, which puts the retrograde insertion point at risk of comminuting the humerus with communication of the fracture. The antegrade nail does not have a large amount of nail distal to the fracture and the locking screws are close to the fracture itself. Plating here with a posterior approach is the treatment of choice. Holstein-Lewis[16] showed care again must be taken to avoid damage to the radial nerve and its posterior interosseous branch. Again a 4.5 broad plate would be the implant of choice. If distal extension occurs into the supracondylar region, double plating with a posterolateral and medial plate is a good option.

Complications

- Although nearly all humerus fractures heal with either closed or open techniques, complications can still occur. These include malunions, nonunions, infection, radial

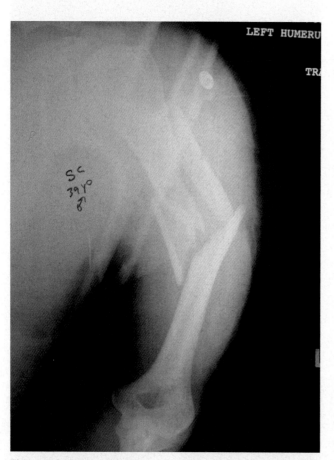

Figure 6–9: **Preoperative anteroposterior X-ray of comminuted humerus.**

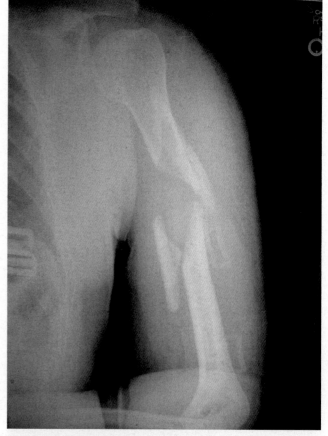

Figure 6–10: **Preoperative lateral X-ray of comminuted humerus.**

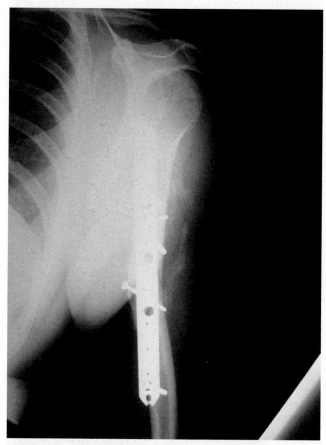

Figure 6–11: Postoperative lateral X-ray of comminuted humerus treated with open reduction and internal fixation.

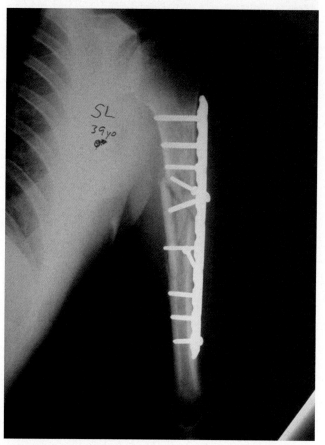

Figure 6–12: Postoperative anteroposterior X-ray treated with open reduction and internal fixation.

nerve palsy, and joint stiffness. Most of these can be avoided with careful planning, excellent surgical technique, and the bone and early range of motion. Once the fracture is stabilized with implants or callus, the shoulder and elbow can be ranged and joint stiffness can be avoided. If a nonunion or malunion is seen and is painful with casting and bracing, the treatment of choice would be compression plating.[17,18] If the primary surgery was an intramedullary rod and it failed, then the nonunion should be stabilized the majority of the time with a compression plating technique and bone grafting.

• Figures 6–13 through 6-17 show a case of a 68-year-old female who was in a motor vehicle crash. She sustained a closed midshaft humerus fracture. She was treated elsewhere with an intramedullary nail. Unfortunately, she was nailed with slight distraction at the fracture site (Figure 6–14). This is one of the main problems with IM nailing of humeral shaft fractures. Because the upper extremity is nonweight bearing. Compression with external devices such as braces or intramedullary nails, are unsuccessful. If this were a tibia or femur, the patient

could bear weight, and the fracture would make callus and heal or the screws would break, the nail would dynamize and then the bone would heal.

We discussed risks and benefits of revision ORIF with compression plating. We also discussed the use of an intercalary fibula graft to help with the poor, osteoporotic bone. Figures 6–16 and 6-17 show the reduced humerus with an intercalary fibula graft for added bone to drill and tap through. This was done through two approaches. First we placed the patient in the beach chair position, removed the nail, and repaired the rotator cuff. We then placed her in the prone position. We performed a posterior approach with a triceps splitting technique. The deep exposure was widened proximal to the nonunion through normal tissue to find the radial nerve. We worked our way distally and gently retracted the radial nerve with its soft-tissue attachments laterally. The nonunion was debrided, and the canals were drilled and reamed. We then placed an intercalary fibula graft and reduced the humerus. We placed a posterior plate and compressed through the plate. Bone morphogenic protein (BMP) graft was then used at the nonunion site.

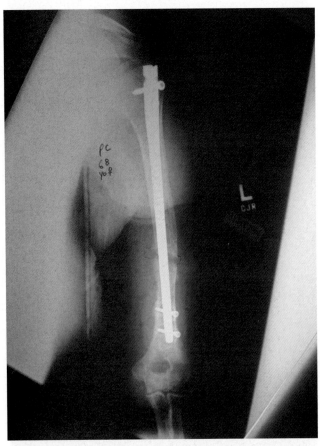

Figure 6–13: Preoperative anteroposterior X-ray of humeral nonunion treated with IM nail.

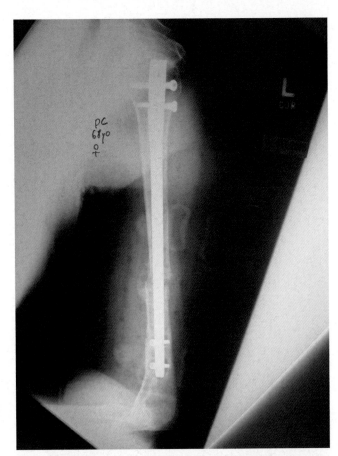

Figure 6–15: Preoperative lateral X-ray of nonunion.

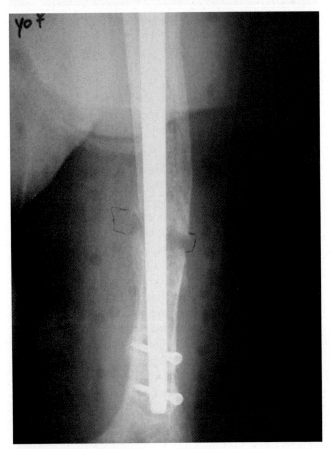

Figure 6–14: Preoperative anteroposterior X-ray of the distraction at nonunion site.

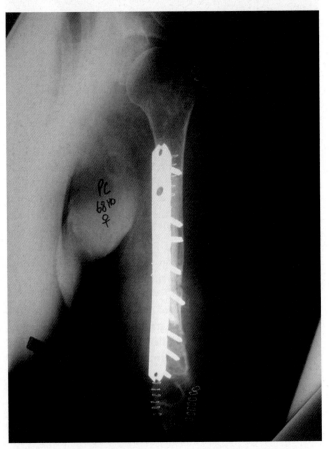

Figure 6–16: Postoperative anteroposterior X-ray of nonunion treated with open reduction and internal fixation, compression, and Intercalary fibula graft.

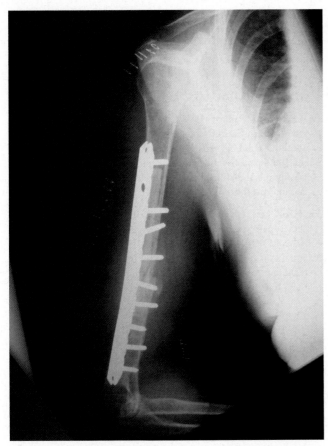

Figure 6–17: **Postoperative lateral X-ray nonunion after open reduction and internal fixation.**

Annotated References

1. Ekholm R, Adami J, Tidermark J, et al: Fractures of the shaft of the humerus: an epidemiological study of 401 fractures, *J Bone Joint Surg Br* 88:1469-1473, 2006.
An interesting study of over 400 patients who sustained humeral shaft fractures and the age at which they occurred.

2. Browner BD, Jupiter JB, Levine AM, et al *Skeletal trauma*, Philadelphia, 2002, WB. Saunders.
An amazing collection of orthopaedic chapters that make up one of the most important books in orthopaedics. A must have in your personal library.

3. Fractures of the humerus: In Baumgaertner M, Tornetta P III editors: *Orthopedic knowledge update: trauma*, ed 3, Rosemont, Ill, 2005, American Academy of Orthopedic Surgeons.
The review book that all residents and fellows should own. Excellent chapter on humeral shaft fractures.

4. Rockwood C Jr, Green DP, Buckholz RW: *Fractures in adults*, ed 6, Philadelphia, 2005, Lippincott.
Fantastic chapter on humeral shaft fractures. Anatomy and treatment options make it excellent reading.

5. DiCicco JD, Mehlman CT, Urse J: Fracture of the shaft of the humerus secondary to muscular violence, *J Orthop Trauma* 7:90-93, 1993.

First paper describing a rotational force so strong on the humerus that the shaft could fracture. A great lead in to Sabick and others' article.

6. Sabick MB, Torry MR, Kim YK, et al: Humeral torque in professional baseball pitchers, *Am J Sports Med* 32:892-898, 2004.
Eleven years after DiCicco and other's article, Hawkins and other's wrote on their experiences with humeral shaft fractures caused by the professional athletes.

7. Gustillo RB, Anderson JT: Prevention of infection in the treatment of one thousand and twenty-five open fractures of long bones: retrospective and prospective analyses, *J Bone Joint Surg Am* 58:453-458, 1976.
The gold standard paper for open fractures. All open fracture papers or presentations quote Gustilo and Anderson.

8. Anderson JT, Gustilo RB: Immediate internal fixation in open fractures, *Orthop Clin North Am* 11:569-578, 1980.
Immediate fixation in open fractures can happen, if in the right place and at the right time, with minimal complications.

9. Shao YC, Harwood P, Grotz MR, et al: Radial nerve palsy associated with fractures of the shaft of the humerus: a systematic review, *J Bone Joint Surg Br* 87:1647-1652, 2005.
The current recommendations for exploring the radial nerve versus watching it over 2 to 3 months after fractures of the humerus.

10. DeFranco MJ, Lawton JN: Radial nerve injuries associated with humeral fractures, *J Hand Surg (Am)* 31:655-663, 2006.
The radial nerve is the most commonly injured nerve associated with humeral shaft fractures. He also teaches the understanding of examples of the humeral fractures and their associated injuries.

11. Ring D, Chin K, Jupiter JB: Radial nerve palsy associated with high-energy humeral shaft fractures, *J Hand Surg Am* 29: 144-147, 2004.
High-energy humeral shaft fractures can lead to injuries to the radial nerve. When and how to explore the injured nerve is discussed.

12. Sarmiento A, Horowitch A, Aboulabia A: Functional bracing for comminuted extra-articular fractures of the distal-third of the humerus, *J Bone Joint Surg Br* 72B:283-287, 1990.
Many descriptions of how to treat these humeral shaft fractures with conservative measures and fracture braces. Fracture bracing will help heal the fracture and help the patient during rehabilitation to obtain good-to-excellent results of shoulder and elbow motion.

13. Zlotolow DA, Catalano LW 3rd, Barron OA, et al: Surgical exposures of the humerus, *J Am Acad Orthop Surg* 14:754-765, 2006.
A must read for upper extremity and trauma surgeons. A synopsis and update for Hoppenfeld's surgical exposure book.

14. Hoppenfeld S, deBoer P: *Surgical exposures in orthopedics: the anatomic approach*, ed 3, Philadelphia, 2003, Lippincott.
The gold standard for surgical exposures. Excellent pictures and descriptions of humeral shaft exposures. The pages make you feel like you are doing the surgery before you get to the operating room.

15. Klenerman L: Fractures of the shaft of the humerus, *J Bone Joint Surg Br* 48B:105-111, 1966.

An early and historic article on humeral shaft fractures. Good reading for a start of knowledge base.

16. Holstein A, Lewis GB: Fractures of the humerus with radial nerve paralysis, *J Bone Joint Surg Am* 45A:1382-1388, 1963.

The classic article on distal humerus fractures and the relationship of the fracture to the radial nerve.

17. Hierholzer C, Sama D, Toro JB, et al: Plate fixation of ununited humeral shaft fractures: effect of type of bone graft on healing, *J Bone Joint Surg Am* 88:1442-1447, 2006.

Current treatment recommendations for nonunions of the humeral shaft. Material looking at the plating and the choice of bone graft to enhance the healing properties of the nonunion.

18. Foster RJ, Dixon GL Jr, Bach AW: Internal fixation of fractures and non-unions of the humeral shaft: Indications and results in a multi-center study, *J Bone Joint Surg Am* 67A: 857-864, 1985.

An early multicenter study on fractures and nonunions of the humeral shaft; educational on indications for surgery and techniques on fixing nonunions.

Further Reading

19. Hall RF Jr, Pankovich AM: Ender nailing of acute fractures of the humerus: a study of closed fixation by intramedullary nails without reaming, *J Bone Joint Surg Am* 69A:558-567, 1987.

A mid-1980s paper by the master technician on placing enders nails to treat humeral shaft fractures. An excellent tool for open reduction and internal fixation (ORIF) to keep in your repertoire.

20. Henly MB, Chapman JR, Claudi BF: Closed retrograde Hack-ethal nail stabilization of humeral shaft fractures, *J Orthop Trauma* 6:18-24, 1992.

An article on nailing of shaft fractures. It is good to learn multiple techniques for open reduction and internal fixation (ORIF) of these fractures.

CHAPTER 7

Fractures of the Distal Humerus

Michael T. Archdeacon, MD, MSE

- Fractures of the distal humerus are common, particularly in children (pediatric supracondylar humerus and lateral condyle fractures) and in patients who are seniors with osteoporotic bone.[1] They occur frequently in high-energy trauma as well.
- The mechanism of injury is typically a fall or high-energy force applied to the extended arm (indirect) or a fall onto the elbow (direct).
- Operative treatment is generally recommended in order to preserve function and decrease postoperative stiffness.
- Fractures occur in common patterns and typically involve the articular surface or the medial or lateral "columns" of the distal humerus.

Functional Anatomy

- The distal humerus is defined as the metadiaphyseal region or the portion of the distal humerus as far proximal as the condyles are wide (Figure 7–1).
- This region is effectively composed of two columns of bone (medial and lateral), which support or "suspend" the trochlea or ulnohumeral articulation (Figure 7–2).
- The elbow is essentially a hinge joint with a single axis of rotation. However this axis of rotation is not perpendicular to the long axis of the limb, but lies in approximately 4 to 8 degrees of valgus with 3 to 9 degrees of external rotation.[2] The exact center of this axis can be visualized on the lateral elbow radiograph with the superimposition of three concentric shadows formed by the trochlear sulcus, the capitellum, and the medial facet of the trochlea.[3] (Figure 7–3).
- The ulnohumeral joint is a constrained joint with the proximal ulna (olecranon) rotating on the fixed axis of the distal humerus (trochlea).
- The flexion/extension arc in normal individuals ranges from 0 degrees (full extension) to approximately 135 degrees (full flexion.)

- The radiocapitellar joint constitutes the remaining articulation of the distal humerus, and this joint is primarily concerned with forearm rotation, with little effect on the elbow flexion extension arc.

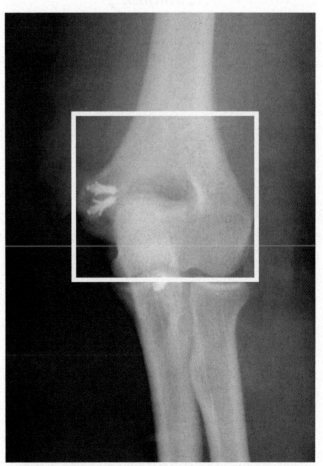

Figure 7–1: Radiographic image of distal humerus demonstrating the supracondylar region.

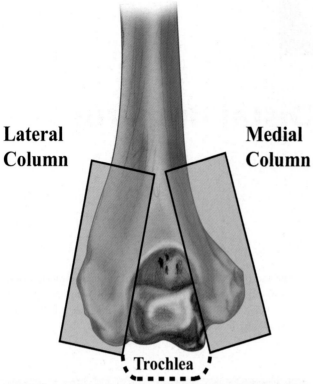

Figure 7–2: The medial and lateral columns of the distal humerus supporting the "suspended" trochlea.

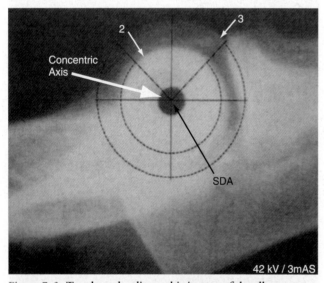

Figure 7–3: True lateral radiographic images of the elbow demonstrating the axis of rotation of the joint. The exact center of this axis can be visualized on the lateral elbow radiograph with the superimposition of three concentric shadows formed by the trochlear sulcus, the capitellum, and the medial facet of the trochlea. (Reproduced from Madey SM, Bottlang M, Steyers CM, et al: *J Orthop Trauma* 14:46, 2000; Figure 8B.)

- The supination/pronation arc ranges from 90 degrees of full supination through 90 degrees of full pronation constituting a 180-degree arc in normal individuals.
- Posteriorly, these bony columns are separated by the olecranon fossa, which accommodates the proximal ulna during full extension (Figure 7–4).
- Anteriorly, the distal humerus consists of the capitellum, the anterior trochlea, and a corresponding coronoid fossa to accommodate the coronoid process during elbow flexion (Figure 7–4).
- The medial column terminates in the medial epicondyle and provides attachment for the anterior and posterior portions of the medial collateral ligament and is the origin for the flexor mass of the forearm.
- The ulnar nerve runs in the cubital tunnel at the inferior portion of the medial column.
- The lateral column terminates in the capitellum anteriorly and the lateral supracondylar ridge and epicondyle laterally. The laterally based structures provide an origin for the extensor mass and a site of attachment for the lateral collateral ligament.

Surgical Anatomy

Vascular Anatomy

- The major arterial vessels in the region of the elbow include the brachial artery and its major tributaries including the radial and ulnar arteries (Figure 7–5).
- The brachial artery enters the cubital fossa region laterally adjacent to the median nerve and superficial to the brachialis muscle. Midway through the cubital fossa it divides into the terminal branches: the radial artery and the ulnar artery.
- The radial artery descends laterally into the forearm beneath the brachioradialis and lies medial to the biceps tendon. The recurrent radial artery ascends toward the supinator muscle and supplies this region with several perforators known as the leash of Henry.
- The ulnar artery branches medially from the brachial artery and dives into the pronator teres muscle before descending into the forearm.
- The major superficial venous branches at the elbow include the cephalic vein on the anteriorlateral aspect of the brachium and the basilic vein coursing anteriormedially along the brachium.

Neurologic Anatomy

- The radial nerve enters the cubital fossa between the brachialis and the brachioradialis and then divides into the posterior interosseous nerve and the superficial radial nerve (see Figure 7–5).
- The ulnar nerve enters the elbow posteriorly along the medial epicondyle and moves anteriorly through the

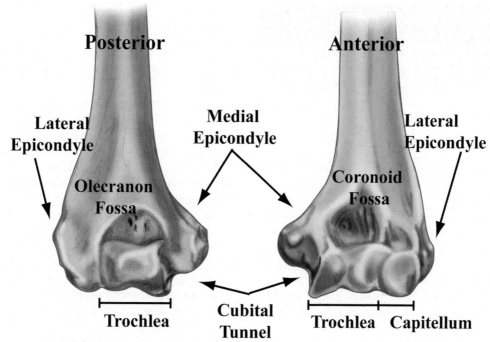

Figure 7–4: Drawings of the distal humerus demonstrating the bony anatomy.

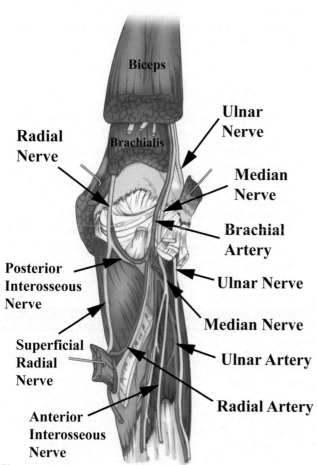

Figure 7–5: **Major neurovascular structures around the elbow.**

cubital tunnel. It then divides the two heads of the flexor carpi ulnaris as it continues into the forearm.

- The median nerve lies deep to the bicipital aponeurosis in the cubital fossa and dives into the interval between the two heads of the pronator teres.

Ligamentous Anatomy

- In terms of the passive elbow stabilizers, the medial collateral ligament complex, which originates from the medial epicondyle, includes the anterior oblique ligament, the posterior oblique ligament, and the transverse ligament.
- The lateral collateral complex includes the radial collateral ligament, the lateral ulnar collateral ligament (LUCL), and the accessory ligament, all arising from the lateral epicondyle.

Muscular Anatomy

- The active elbow stabilizers and the muscular anatomy of the elbow can be divided into the medial group, the lateral group and the posterior group.
- The medial group or common flexors originate from the medial epicondyle and include, from posterior to anterior, the flexor carpi ulnaris (FCU), the palmaris longus, the flexor digitorum superficialis, the flexor carpi radialis, and the pronator teres. All but the FCU (ulnar nerve) are supplied by the median nerve (Table 7–1).
- The lateral muscles originate from the lateral epicondyle and consist of the common extensor origin and the "mobile wad." The common extensors include, from

Table 7–1: Innervation of the Muscles about the Elbow

INNERVATION OF ELBOW MUSCULAR ANATOMY		
RADIAL NERVE	**ULNAR NERVE**	**MEDIAN NERVE**
ECU, EDM, ED, BR, ECRL, ECRB, anconeus, and triceps	FCU	PL, FDS, FCR, and pronator teres

ECRB, extensor carpi radialis brevis; ECRL, extensor carpi radialis longus; ECU, extensor carpi ulnaris; ED, extensor digitorum; EDM, extensor digiti minimi; FCR, flexor carpi radialis; FCU, flexor carpi ulnaris; FDS, flexor digitorum superficialis; PL, palmeris longus.

posterior to anterior, the anconeus, the extensor carpi ulnaris (ECU), the extensor digiti minimi (EDM), and the extensor digitorum (ED). These are supplied by the radial nerve (anconeus) and the posterior interosseous nerve (Table 7–1). The mobile wad consists of the brachioradialis, the extensor carpi radialis longus (ECRL) and the extensor carpi radialis brevis (ECRB), which are all supplied by the radial nerve proper.

- The posterior muscle group includes a portion of the anconeus and the triceps brachii, which are both innervated by the radial nerve.

History, Physical Examination, and Radiographs

- The history is that of a blow or fall onto the limb or an indirect injury secondary to a motor vehicle accident or other high-energy mechanism.
- In patients who are seniors, risks for osteoporosis should be assessed, and a suspicion for pathologic fractures must always be considered, particularly with a history of pain before fracture.
- The physical examination is centered on the injured limb; however, a brief musculoskeletal examination of the other extremities is warranted, especially in the face of high-energy trauma.
- Pain, swelling, deformity, and instability at the elbow are hallmarks, and repeated manipulation of the limb should

be avoided to prevent further pain or neurovascular compromise.

- A careful inspection of the skin is required so as not to miss a subtle open fracture as the distal humerus is essentially a subcutaneous bone posteriorly, medially, and laterally.
- A complete vascular examination is critical, and consists of evaluation of radial and ulnar pulses and an assessment of capillary refill. Although uncommon in distal humerus fractures without vascular compromise, compartment syndrome must always be considered.
- A thorough neurologic examination before manipulation or treatment is paramount from a patient care standpoint and from a medical-legal perspective. This consists of a complete motor examination including components of the median, ulnar, radial, anterior interosseous, and posterior interosseous nerves. A complete sensory examination assessing median, ulnar, and radial nerve sensation must be documented with two-point discrimination utilized in any cases of neurologic deficit (Table 7–2).
- Standard anteroposterior (AP) and lateral radiographs of the elbow are generally sufficient to define the pathology; however, complete views of the entire humerus are necessary. Often, slight traction to the lower arm will improve the quality of the radiograph and further delineate the involvement of the distal humerus fractures (Figure 7–6).

Fracture Classifications

- Fractures can be classified based on a number of parameters, including fracture patterns and anatomic involvement.
- Fracture patterns include transcondylar, lateral condylar, medial condylar, T types, Y types, H types, and λ types based on the fracture configuration in the supracondylar region (Figure 7–7).
- An anatomic classification addresses whether the fracture involves one or both columns, whether the fracture is intraarticular or extraarticular, whether or not the fracture has a simple fracture configuration or is comminuted, and finally based on other associated injuries including

Table 7–2: Neurologic Examination of the Upper Extremity

MOTOR ASSESSMENT				
RADIAL	**ULNAR**	**MEDIAN**	**POSTERIOR INTEROSSEOUS**	**ANTERIOR INTEROSSEOUS**
Thumb extension (EPL)	Finger AB/ADduction	MCP/PIP Flexion	Finger MP extension	DIP flexion (thumb and index)

SENSORY ASSESSMENT		
RADIAL	**ULNAR**	**MEDIAN**
Dorsal radial aspect of hand (thumb, index, and long fingers)	Volar and dorsal ulnar aspect of hand (ulnar ring and small fingers)	Volar radial aspect of hand (thumb, index, long and radial ring)

AB, abduction; DIP, distal interphalangeal; MCP, metacarpal phalangeal; MP, metacarpal phalangeal; PIP, proximal interphalangeal.

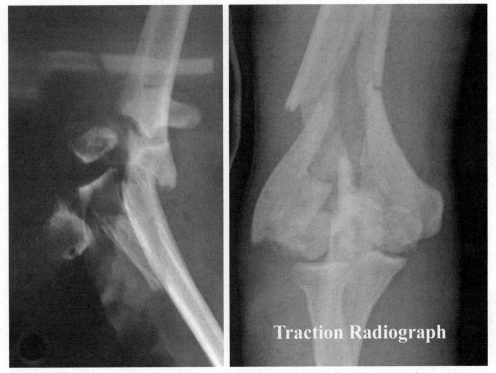

Figure 7–6: Traction radiographs of a complex, comminuted distal humerus fracture demonstrating a better appreciation of the fracture anatomy after traction.

fractures of the olecranon or radial head, elbow dislocation, and other elbow injury (Table 7–3).

Treatment

Goals of Treatment

- The goals of treatment for distal humerus fractures include the soft-tissue injury goals, the bony injury goals, and the functional outcome goals (Box 7–1).

Nonoperative Treatment

- Closed treatment of the majority of these injuries is not advocated for several reasons.
- First, reduction, particularly of intraarticular fractures, is difficult if not impossible to obtain in a closed manner.
- Second, maintaining reduction with cast immobilization is difficult, and residual joint incongruity will result in posttraumatic arthrosis of the elbow.
- Third, elbow stiffness associated with fractures of distal humerus is a major source of disability after any treatment method. This stiffness or joint contracture is only exacerbated with prolonged cast immobilization in closed treatment.
- Thus the vast majority of distal humerus fractures will be managed operatively to obtain as near an anatomic reduction of the articular surface as possible and to allow early elbow range-of-motion exercises to reduce the risk and severity of posttraumatic elbow stiffness.

Preoperative Planning

- Ideally the patient is evaluated, provisionally reduced, splinted, and prepared for surgical intervention on a nonemergent basis. Typically within 24 to 72 hours of injury.
- However provided there is no evidence of vascular compromise or compartment syndrome, the injury can be addressed on a more delayed basis to allow for adequate resuscitation in a patient with multiple injuries or medical clearance in a more senior patient. Reconstruction can be adequately performed up to 1 week after injury.
- General anesthesia is recommended as the procedure can be lengthy and may require the lateral decubitus or prone position. Additionally, muscle relaxation obtained with general anesthesia may be helpful with difficult reductions.
- An olecranon osteotomy will facilitate exposure and reduction of comminuted or complex intraarticular fractures. The surgeon should be prepared for an osteotomy regardless because a fracture that appears simple on plain radiographs often is more complex on exposure.
- Equipment should include a variety of reduction tools and implant or screw configurations for the distal humerus (Box 7–2).

Positioning

- Ideally, the patient is positioned in lateral decubitus on a beanbag with a padded bolster supporting the operative extremity at the elbow. Alternatively, the prone position

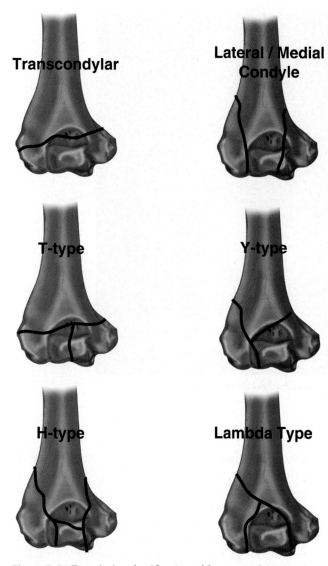

Figure 7–7: **Descriptive classification of fractures of the distal humerus.**

Table 7–3:	Anatomic Fracture Classification of the Distal Humerus
UNICOLUMNAR	

Medial or lateral column
Intraarticular
   Trochlea
   Capitellum
   Extraarticular
   Epicondylar

BICOLUMNAR

Transcondylar
Intracondylar/Intraarticular
   Simple
   T, Y, H, λ types
   Comminuted
   Capitellum shear fractures

ASSOCIATED INJURIES

Olecranon fracture
Radial head fracture/dislocation
Ulnohumeral dislocation
Ligamentous instability

Box 7–1 Goals of Treatment for Fractures of the Distal Humerus

Soft Tissue Injury

Adequate debridement
Wound closure and coverage
Prevention of infection

Bony Injury

Anatomic joint reduction
Restoration of metadiaphyseal bone
Fixation and union of articular block and shaft

Functional Outcome Goals

Stable fixation and union
Mobile elbow joint
Return to activities of daily living and leisure

Box 7–2 Checklist for Operative Treatment of Distal Humerus Fractures

Oscillating saw and osteotomes for olecranon osteotomy
Bone clamps for columnar and intraarticular reduction
Multiple-size Kirschner wires (K-wires) (1.25, 1.6, and 2 mm)
Small fragment 3.5- or 2.7-mm compression plates and
   reconstruction plates
Periarticular elbow plates
Long screws (50 to 90 mm)
Intraarticular screws (variable pitch screws or minifragment screws)
Bioresorbable pins or screws

---

can be used with the affected arm draped over the table edge or an arm table attachment.

- In either case, full access to the upper extremity is necessary, and the arm is draped sterile to the lateral chest wall and flank. A sterile tourniquet can be used on the brachium.
- A minifluoroscopy unit is recommended because it will allow the flexibility needed to obtain both AP and lateral radiographic images in the lateral or prone positions.
- I recommend marking the arm or surgical drapes with a medial or lateral designation before surgery because the injured anatomic landmarks can be confusing with the patient lateral or prone and the hand draped out of view.

Surgical Exposures and Olecranon Osteotomy

- When a simple unicolumnar fracture is being treated, a direct medial or lateral approach is acceptable. However, one must be prepared for a more complex fracture than what is originally anticipated on initial plain radiographs. Thus I advocate the more extensile posterior approach under most circumstances.

- If the direct medial approach is chosen, the incision is centered on the medial epicondyle. The surgical plane lies between the brachialis and triceps proximally and the brachialis and pronator teres distally. Mobilization and possible transposition of the ulnar nerve will be required. Elevation of the triceps with gentle anterior retraction of the ulnar nerve will expose the medial condyle of the humerus.

- If the direct lateral approach is chosen, the incision is centered on the lateral epicondyle and extended distally toward the olecranon. The dissection is between the anconeus and the triceps and allows for exposure of the lateral condyle. Care should be taken not to release more than the posterior third of the extensor mass in order to maintain the integrity of the radial collateral ligament complex.

- In bicolumnar or complex fractures, I recommend a standard posterior approach to the distal humerus. A posterior incision from the midportion of the humerus is extended distally and curves slightly medial around the tip of the olecranon and terminates about 6 to 8 cm distal to the olecranon.

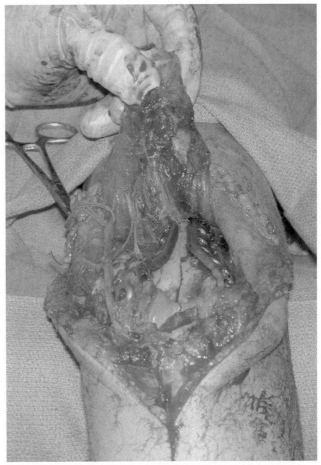

Figure 7–9: **Surgical photograph demonstrating the distal humerus via a standard posterior approach with an olecranon osteotomy.**

- The incision is carried down through subcutaneous tissue to the level of the triceps fascia, developing flaps to expose the distal triceps and intramuscular septum.

- The subcutaneous dissection is continued distally, with care taken to identify and protect the ulnar nerve. If plate fixation is anticipated in the region of the cubital tunnel, the ulnar nerve can be transposed anteriorly at this time.

- An olecranon osteotomy is performed to expose the distal intraarticular portion of the humerus. At a point approximately 2.5 cm from the tip of the olecranon, a single Kirschner wire (K-wire) is passed to the subchondral bone perpendicular to the ulna at the level of the extraarticular portion of the olecranon fossa. The wire then serves as a focal point for a distally oriented chevron osteotomy.

- The osteotomy is performed with an oscillating saw to the level of the subchondral bone. It is then completed with a narrow osteotome. Further dissection along the medial and lateral borders of the triceps allows elevation of the extensor mass at the level of the distal humerus. As the triceps is elevated proximally, the intracondylar or supracondylar portion of the distal humerus is fully exposed (Figures 7–8 and 7–9).

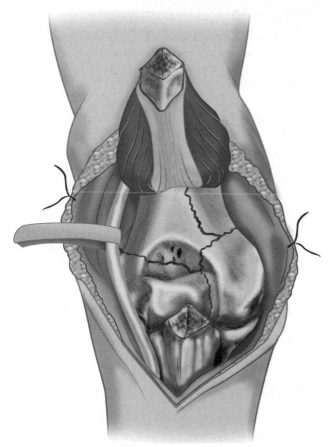

Figure 7–8: **Drawing of the distal humerus via a standard posterior approach with an olecranon osteotomy.**

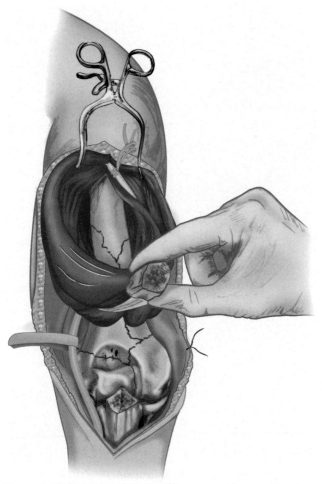

Figure 7–10: Drawing of the distal humerus with a combined posterior approach to the humeral shaft and olecranon osteotomy for distal humeral exposure. This approach is useful for extensive fractures involving the supracondylar regions and the midshaft regions of the humerus.

Combined Triceps Split and Olecranon Osteotomy

- If the fracture pattern is extensive and extends into the humeral shaft, a modification of the standard distal exposure can allow further exposure of the humerus including the proximal and midshaft regions. A standard triceps split exposure is performed concomitantly with the distal exposure.[4]
- Working between the two intervals of the olecranon osteotomy and the posterior triceps split, complete exposure of the shaft and supracondylar or intracondylar humerus can be achieved (Figures 7–10 and 7–11).

Reduction and Provisional Stability

- Reduction is accomplished in one of two manners. One: The articular block is fully reconstructed and then secured

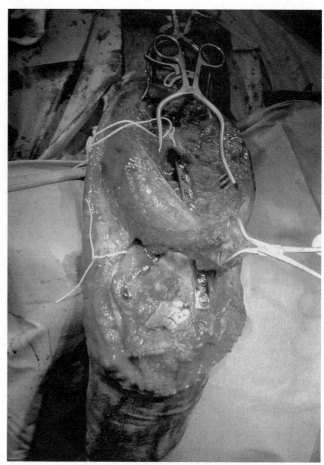

Figure 7–11: Surgical photograph demonstrating the combined posterior approach to the humerus and olecranon osteotomy for the distal humerus.

to the shaft. Two: A stable column is reconstructed and used as a cornerstone for the remaining articular block and opposite column.

- In terms of the intraarticular fractures, fragments are reduced with a combination of small reduction clamps, elevators, and K-wires used as joysticks. Typically, the trochlea can be reconstructed and provisionally stabilized with K-wires, clamps, or small screws (Figure 7–12).
- This is followed by restoration of the trochlea to the capitellum. Frequently, the capitellum or lateral column relationship is easily reduced, and this provides a "base" on which to build the remaining joint.
- As the intraarticular portion is reconstituted, the columns are provisionally reduced. Compression can then be applied across the columns, thus, supporting the reduced articular trochlea (Figures 7–13 and 7-14)

Definitive Fixation

- When provisional reduction is complete, definitive fixation can be applied.

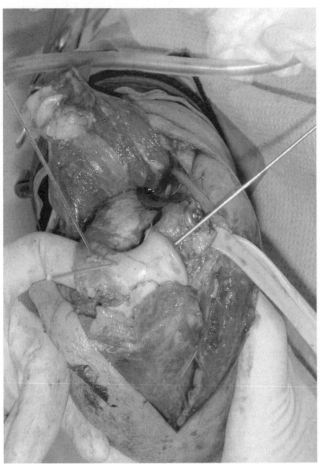

Figure 7–12: Intraoperative photograph demonstrating provisional reconstruction of a comminuted intraarticular supracondylar humerus fracture. The radial column was reconstructed first, followed by reconstruction of the trochlea.

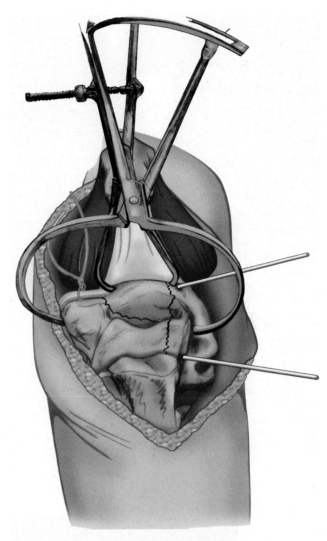

Figure 7–13: Drawing of an intraarticular distal humerus fracture with provisional reduction achieved with clamps and Kirschner wires (K-wires).

Intraarticular Fixation and Resorbable Implants

- The articular reconstruction is stabilized with lag screws, variable pitch intraarticular screws, minifragment screws, and bioabsorbable pins[5] (Figure 7–15).
- Whenever possible, multiple lag screws are used reduce and maintain columnar reconstruction, and all soft-tissue pedicles are left intact to assist in the healing.

Column Fixation

- The reconstruction is completed with compression plating of the shaft to the articular segment.
- Frequently, a 90/90 plating technique with a medial 3.5-mm reconstruction plate and a 3.5-mm dynamic compression plate on the posterior lateral column is used for column stabilization[6] (Figure 7–16).

- Alternatively, recently introduced periarticular distal humerus plates provide precontoured options for both the medial and lateral columns[7] (Figure 7–17). Fixed-angle screws are available in some versions of these implants.

Osteotomy Fixation and Closure

- The olecranon osteotomy is fixated with a tension band wire construct or a 6.5-mm cancellous lag screw augmented with a tension band. Alternatively, a one-third tubular plate can be applied across the osteotomy to obtain stable fixation. Frequently, the olecranon fixation hardware will need to be removed as it is often symptomatic after fracture healing.
- The ulnar nerve is transposed if fixation extends into the cubital tunnel.

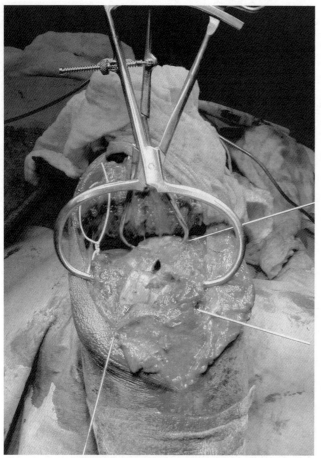

Figure 7–14: **Surgical photograph showing the reduction with clamps and Kirschner wires (K-wires).**

- The triceps split, if used, is approximated with interrupted resorbable suture, and the subcutaneous and skin closure is performed with interrupted sutures or staples.
- The patient is placed in a well-padded posterior mold splint with the arm in 10 to 30 degrees of flexion.
- A complete neurovascular exam must be performed postoperatively to assess for the possibility of iatrogenic neurovascular injury.

Rehabilitation

- The splint is applied for 1 to 5 days to allow wound healing.
- As soon as the wound is sealed, the splint is removed and an active-assisted range-of-motion program is initiated. Activities of daily living are encouraged as soon as the wound is healed (Table 7–4).
- It is paramount to obtain as rigid fixation as possible to advance range-of-motion exercises early in the postoperative course. Posttraumatic elbow stiffness is a major impairment for patients, and all efforts should be made to minimize this potentially adverse outcome.
- All patients with traumatic injury or fractures in the elbow region should be told to expect some loss of terminal extension. This is particularly relevant for fractures that extend into the olecranon fossa. However most patients are able to achieve functional range of motion (30 to 130 degrees.)
- The supination or pronation arc should be exercised early as well. Fractures involving the capitellum will often result in a loss of the supination or pronation arc.

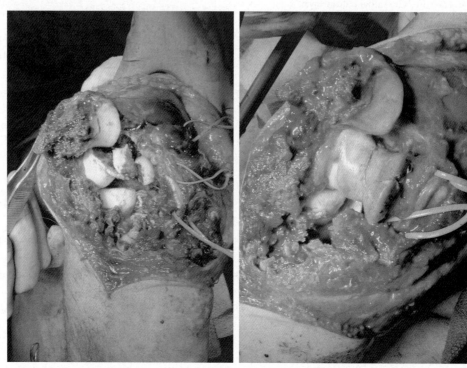

Figure 7–15: Intraoperative photographs demonstrating an extensively comminuted articular surface, and the articular reconstruction using bioresorbable pins for the articular fragments. The blue vessel loops are retracting the ulnar nerve.

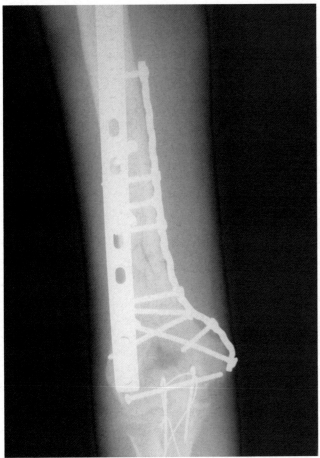

Figure 7–16: Radiograph demonstrating a 90/90 plate configuration. Independent compression lag screws are noted to cross the trochlea region, and a tension-band wire technique was used to repair the olecranon osteotomy.

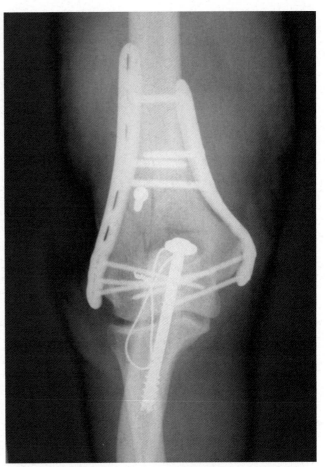

Figure 7–17: Radiograph demonstrating "periarticular" distal humerus "column" plates and screw fixation from each column into the articular segments. An olecranon screw and tension-band technique were used to repair the olecranon osteotomy.

- Active triceps extension is avoided for 6 weeks to allow healing of the olecranon osteotomy, and resistance exercises should be limited until fracture healing is evidenced on plain radiographs, usually about 10 to 14 weeks.
- Active shoulder, wrist, and hand range of motion and passive range of motion should be employed early to prevent stiffness and impairment in the uninjured upper extremity joints.

Special Cases
Capitellum Shear Fractures

- The coronal shear fracture has been described in the literature as an isolated injury or in combination with other distal humerus fracture variants[8] (Figure 7–18). When isolated, it typically occurs with a fall from a standing height, and when combined with other distal humerus fracture components, it often results from high-energy trauma.
- This injury is typically identified on the lateral elbow radiograph with proximal and anterior migration of the fragment. The radiographic finding termed the "double-

Table 7–4:	Rehabilitation Protocols for Fractures of the Distal Humerus	
REHABILITATION	**TIME RANGE**
Posterior splint 20 to 30 degrees of flexion	Immediately postoperatively
Shoulder, wrist, and hand AROM and PROM	Immediately postoperatively
Elbow (flexion/extension and supination/pronation) AAROM	1 to 4 days postoperatively
Light resistance exercises	Early fracture healing ≈ 12 weeks
Progressive resistance exercises and early noncontact sport/exercise motions	Fracture healing ≈ 4 to 7 months

AROM, Active range of motion; AAROM, active-assisted range of motion; PROM, passive range of motion.

arc" sign represents the displaced osteochondral fragment consisting of the capitellum and a portion of the lateral trochlea.[8]
- Fixation can be performed anterior to posterior with intraarticular, buried implants or bioresorbable implants, or fixation can be performed posterior to anterior with small lag screws.

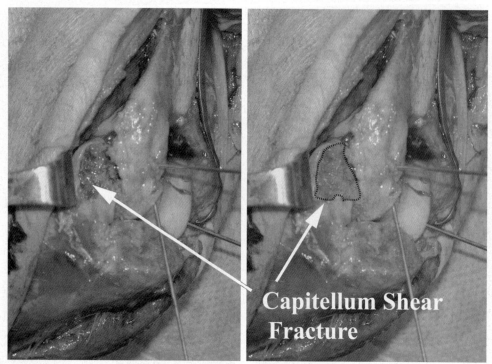

Figure 7–18: **Surgical photograph showing the capitellum shear fracture.**

- Results typically demonstrate satisfactory elbow function with moderate limitation of motion and a low risk of osteonecrosis of the reconstructed capitellum fragment.[8]

Seniors and Osteoporotic Fractures

- Recently published data from Finland demonstrate an increasing incidence in osteoporotic fractures of the distal humerus in women older than 60 years of age.[1] In 1970, 12 of 100,000 women were admitted with this diagnosis, and the number increased to 28 of 100,000 women in 1995.
- The goals and treatment principals for this group of patients may need to be modified compared to those for a younger population with more stable bone. Alternative strategies including locked-plating constructs, prolonged postoperative immobilization, and immediate total elbow arthroplasty (TEA) should be considered in patients who are seniors or osteoporotic.
- It has been hypothesized that a locked-plating constructs would provide superior stability in osteoporotic bone when compared to conventional plating techniques. In a cadaveric biomechanics study comparing plate configuration and locked plating to conventional plating, only the plate configuration (90/90 plate construct) not plate type (locked versus conventional) demonstrated a significant difference in stability.[9]
- Other strategies for improved fixation in osteoporotic bone include triple plating of the distal humerus,[10] autogenous tricortical grafting to replace significant column

loss,[11] and shortening of the metadiaphyseal region to obtain bony contact.[7]
- Even with new-generation locked plating, rigid fixation may not be obtainable; therefore, prolonged cast or brace immobilization at the expense of early motion may be required.[11] Resultant late postoperative elbow stiffness can be addressed on an elective basis with elbow release after soft-tissue and fracture healing.
- In select patients, TEA may be a viable option to preserve elbow function in distal humerus fractures for patients with "unreconstructable" osteoporotic bone or rheumatoid arthritis.[12,13]
- When evaluating the options for reconstruction of these difficult injuries in patients who are seniors with comorbidities, the results of TEA appear superior to open reduction and internal fixation (ORIF).[13] It must be recognized that the majority of good or excellent results for TEA in elderly patients with distal humerus fractures come from a small number of subspecialty trained elbow surgeons. It may not be possible to extrapolate these excellent results to the general orthopaedic community.

Complications
Elbow Stiffness, Heterotopic Ossification, and Posttraumatic Arthritis

- Residual loss of motion at the elbow may be secondary to bony incongruity, hardware impingement, soft-tissue and capsular adhesions, heterotopic bone formation, nonunion, or posttraumatic arthrosis.

- Articular incongruity and posttraumatic arthritis can be addressed with excision of osteophytes, interposition arthroplasty, or TEA. Hardware impingement can be resolved with hardware removal once fracture union has occurred. Capsular adhesions are addressed with open or arthroscopic release. All of these treatments may be used individually or in combination as needed.

- Heterotopic ossification at the elbow after fracture is uncommon in the absence of spinal cord injury or head injury.[14] Other risk factors include open fractures, fracture dislocations, burns, and infection.

- Heterotopic ossification can be treated by prevention with prophylaxis or after its occurrence by resection. Prophylaxis includes oral nonsteroidal antiinflammatories, such as indomethacin, or external beam radiation therapy. Resection of heterotopic bone should be considered in light of clinically significant residual loss of elbow motion. It generally is performed in conjunction with the previous surgical modalities for improving elbow motion after distal humerus fracture.

- Posttraumatic arthropathy after distal humerus fracture occurs frequently but is rarely severely disabling because the elbow is not a weight-bearing joint. Loss of motion is more common, but arthrosis can be treated with osteophyte excision, interposition arthroplasty, or TEA.

Nonunion and Malunion

- Nonunion occurs in 2% to 10% of distal humeral fractures with the majority of intracondylar fractures progressing to union and the majority of nonunions occurring in the supracondylar region.[7,10]

- Techniques to prevent nonunion in the supracondylar region have been described[7] (Box 7-3).

- When nonunion does occur, repair follows the same basic techniques described for primary fixation with the following caveats. Ulnar neurolysis or transposition may be required. Nonunion "take-down" and excision of nonviable bone must be performed to restore motion and allow bony union. Stable fixation must be achieved. Autogenous bone grafting should be used liberally. Finally, occult infection must be considered with deep bone biopsy performed at the time of revision, and staged reconstruction for infected cases.

- Nonunion of the olecranon osteotomy has been reported in 2% to 30% of cases.[15,16] The risk of olecranon osteotomy nonunion can be decreased with careful surgical technique during the osteotomy and repair. First, the osteotomy should be performed at the central sulcus in the region of minimal articular cartilage. Second, the osteotomy must be initiated with a narrow saw or osteotome, and completed by cracking the subchondral bone with a narrow osteotome. Third, if a large compression screw is to be used

---

> **Box 7–3** **Technical Considerations in Fixation of Distal Humerus Fractures to Reduce the Risk of Nonunion or Failure of Fixation**
>
> - Every screw must pass through a plate.
> - Every screw should capture a fragment of the opposite column, which is also fixed to a plate.
> - Every screw should be as long as possible.
> - As many screws as possible should be placed in the distal segments.
> - Every screw should capture as many articular fragments as possible.
> - Plates should achieve compression of both columns at the supracondylar region.
> - Plates must have sufficient fatigue resistance to allow for bony union of the supracondylar region.
> - Diaphyseal bone stock must be restored using autogenous graft as necessary to maintain width and length.

---

for repair, it should be predrilled before the osteotomy. Finally, the repair should be performed with subchondral compression ensuring as much attention to detail as the supracondylar reconstruction.

Ulnar Neuropathy

- Ulnar neuropathy can occur as a result of the initial trauma to the distal elbow or as an iatrogenic injury after surgical treatment. Most incomplete palsies and neuropathic symptoms can be adequately treated with neurolysis and transposition.[16] However, minimizing the risk of ulnar nerve injury with meticulous surgical technique and adequate mobilization at the index procedure cannot be overemphasized.

Summary

- Fractures of the distal humerus including the intracondylar region are common, and fractures in patients who are seniors or osteoporotic will continue to increase in frequency as the prevalence of osteoporosis in society increases.

- The distal humerus is composed of two columns of bone supporting the trochlea.

- A meticulous neurovascular examination of the upper extremity is critical in the face of fractures of the distal humerus because of the nearby brachial, radial, and ulnar vessels and the median, radial, and ulnar nerves.

- High-quality radiographs, including a traction radiograph, are necessary to fully delineate the extent of fracture in the supracondylar or intracondylar region.

- Fractures are classified based on injury patterns or based on anatomic involvement of the columns and articular components.

- Operative treatment is the standard with ORIF. The goals of surgery include soft-tissue management to prevent infection, anatomic articular reconstruction, bicolumnar stabilization with plates, and early motion to reduce posttraumatic elbow stiffness.
- Coronal shear fractures of the capitellum occur as isolated injuries or in combination with other intracondylar fractures.
- Osteoporotic fractures require adjunctive techniques, and TEA should be considered in patients with extreme osteoporosis or rheumatoid arthritis.
- Complications include elbow stiffness, heterotopic bone, arthritis, nonunion, and ulnar neuropathy, with posttraumatic elbow stiffness being the most common.
- Treating physicians should expect predictable good-to-excellent results if attention is provided to anatomic reconstruction, bicolumnar fixation, and early elbow range of motion.[5,7,8,16]

Annotated References

1. Palvanen M, Kannus P, Niemi, S, et al: Secular trends in the osteoporotic fractures of the distal humerus in elderly women, *Eur J Epidemol* 14:159-164, 1998.

A European epidemiology study from Finland that demonstrates an increasing incidence of osteoporotic fractures of the distal humerus in women greater than 60 years of age. Over a 25-year period the incidence in this population has more than doubled from 12 of 100,000 in 1970 to 28 of 100,000 women in 1995.

2. London JT: Kinematics of the elbow, *J Bone Joint Surg Am* 63:529-536, 1981.

This is a descriptive article that details the motion or kinematics of the elbow joint in relation to the anatomic constraints about the elbow.

3. Madey SM, Bottlang M, Steyers, CM, et al: Hinged external fixation of the elbow: optimal axis alignment to minimize motion resistance, *J Orthop Trauma* 14:41-47, 2000.

This article describes the anatomic axis of rotation of the elbow joint and uses the application and function of an articulated elbow fixator to demonstrate the importance of reestablishing this axis of rotation. Additionally, the article describes the radiographic landmarks of the trochlear sulcus, the capitellum, and the medial facet of the trochlea, which are radiographically superimposed to create the axis of rotation of the elbow joint.

4. Archdeacon MT: Combined olecranon osteotomy and posterior triceps splitting approach for complex fractures of the humerus, *J Orthop Trauma* 17:368-373, 2003.

A technique article describing a modification of the standard olecranon osteotomy combined with a triceps splitting approach to the humeral shaft. The approach allows extensive access to the humerus from the proximal-middle third junction distally to the articular block.

5. Ring D, Jupiter JB, Gulotta L: Articular fractures of the distal part of the humerus, *J Bone Joint Surg Am* 85A:232-238, 2003.

A retrospective review of 21 patients with an intraarticular fractures of the distal humerus revealed five common fracture components: (1) capitellum and lateral trochlea; (2) lateral epicondyle; (3) posterior aspect of the lateral column; (4) posterior aspect of the trochlea; and (5) medial epicondyle. Buried intraarticular screws for reconstruction resulted in satisfactory elbow function.

6. Schemitsch EH, Tencer AF, Henley MB: Biomechanical evaluation of methods of internal fixation of the distal humerus, *J Orthop Trauma* 8:468-475, 1994.

A cadaver model was used to examine the relative stability of 10 fixation constructs for a distal humerus fracture model. A 90/90 construct was the most stable in the face of bony contact and a precontoured lateral buttress plate with a medial plate provided the most stability in the absence of bony contact.

7. O'Driscoll SW, Sanchez-Sotelo J, Torchia ME: Management of the smashed distal humerus, *Orthop Clin North Am* 33:19-33, 2002.

This is a comprehensive technique article emphasizing principles of fixation that have improved the author's results and ability to treat difficult distal humerus fractures. The technique addresses screw-and-plate application and encourages the use of periarticular plates for bicolumn stabilization.

8. McKee MD, Jupiter JB, Bamberger HB: Coronal shear fractures of the distal end of the humerus, *J Bone Joint Surg Am* 78A:49-54, 1996.

A retrospective review of six patients with a coronal shear fracture of the distal humerus. The fracture is typically identified on the lateral elbow radiograph with the "double-arc" sign. This represents the displaced osteochondral fragment consisting of the capitellum and a portion of the lateral trochlea. Fixation resulted in satisfactory elbow function with a low risk of osteonecrosis of the capitellum fragment.

9. Korner J, Diederichs G, Arzdorf, M, et al: A biomechanical evaluation of methods of distal humerus fracture fixation using locking compression plates versus conventional reconstruction plates, *J Orthop Trauma* 18:286-293, 2004.

This biomechanics study performed in 40 fresh-frozen human cadavers compared 90/90 plating with dual-dorsal plating using both conventional and locked plating constructs. Primary stiffness in bending and torsion demonstrated that the 90/90 construct was significantly stiffer regardless of the plate type. The authors recommend 90/90 plating in distal humerus fracture fixation and suggest the benefits of a locked plating construct may bear out in diminished bone quality or severe comminution.

10. Ring D, Jupiter JB: Fractures of the distal humerus, *Orthop Clin North Am* 31:103-113, 2000.

An excellent review article from thought leaders in the treatment and management of fractures of the distal humerus.

11. Hausman M, Panozzo A: Treatment of distal humerus fractures in the elderly, *Clin Orthop* 425:55-63, 2004.

A thorough review of the treatment and modifications of typical strategies for distal humerus fractures in the senior patient population.

12. Cobb TK, Morrey BF: Total elbow arthroplasty as primary treatment for distal humerus fractures in elderly patients, *J Bone Joint Surg Am* 79A:826-832, 1997.

This is a retrospective review of 21 distal humerus fractures treated with primary total elbow arthroplasty in elderly patients (mean age 72) with osteoporosis and/or rheumatoid arthritis. At 3.3 years average follow-up, 20 elbows had good or excellent results, with only one revision surgery secondary to acute fracture. The authors conclude total elbow arthroplasty is a reasonable option for elderly distal humerus fractures.

13. Frankle MA, Herscovici D, DiPasquale, TG, et al: A comparison of open reduction and internal fixation and primary total elbow arthroplasty in the treatment of intraarticular distal humerus fractures in women older than age 65, *J Orthop Trauma* 17:473-480, 2003.

In this retrospective cohort study of 24 female patients over age 65, patients were treated with either open reduction and internal fixation (ORIF) or total elbow arthroplasty (TEA). Using the Mayo Elbow Performance score, good or excellent outcomes were achieved in 66% of the ORIF group and in 100% of the TEA group. A poor result in three patients in the ORIF group resulted in conversion to TEA. The authors believe TEA can produce excellent results for distal humerus fractures in women over 65, particularly in patients with comorbidities including osteoporosis, rheumatoid arthritis, and steroid dependence.

14. Garland DE, O'Hollaren RM: Fractures and dislocation about the elbow in the head-injured adult, *Clin Orthop* 168:38-41, 1982.

In a series of 496 patients with spinal cord injury or head injury, elbow heterotopic ossification was noted in 5% of patients without elbow trauma and in 89% of those with elbow trauma.

15. Henley MB, Bone LB, Parker B: Operative management of intra-articular fractures of the distal humerus, *J Orthop Trauma* 1:24-35, 1987.

This article highlights surgical technique and mentions olecranon osteotomy nonunion as a complication of treating these difficult injuries.

16. Jupiter JB: Complex fractures of the distal part of the humerus and associated complications, *Instr Course Lect* 44:187-198, 1995.

A thorough review of complications encountered when treating distal humerus fractures.

CHAPTER 8

Fractures of the Olecranon and Complex Fracture-Dislocations of the Proximal Ulna and Radial Head

Mark A. Mighell, MD, and Steven Siegal, MD

This chapter provides the practicing or resident orthopedic surgeon with a guide for rational preoperative and intraoperative decision making in the treatment of olecranon fractures. Technical points and the pearls and pitfalls of fixation are emphasized.

- The ulna is a superficial osseous structure and is therefore readily susceptible to trauma. It is a common site of fracture for the same reason.
- Fracture patterns exist along a continuum, from simple transverse and oblique patterns to complex transolecranon fracture-dislocations, "terrible triads," and Monteggia equivalents. Because of this variability, understanding the pathoanatomy of individual injury patterns is essential because no single treatment is appropriate for all fracture types.
- Regardless of the complexity of the injury, the primary objective of treatment remains straightforward: definitive stable fixation that allows early progression to motion.

Relevant Anatomy

- The elbow is one of the most congruous joints in the body and is subsequently one of the most inherently stable.[1-4]
- The ulna is particularly susceptible to direct trauma, and essentially, all olecranon fractures are intraarticular.[2] Displaced fractures of the ulnohumeral joint threaten to compromise stability.
- Elbow stability is conferred by the conforming geometry of the articular surfaces and by soft-tissue stabilizers.[2,5]
- The semilunar notch imparts intrinsic stability to the ulnohumeral articulation, and the coronoid and olecranon processes act as buttresses to prevent anterior and posterior displacements.
- The saggital geometry of the semilunar notch is that of an ellipse rather than a semicircle because of the transverse bare area located between the coronoid and olecranon processes (Figure 8–1). This must be appreciated in the reconstruction of the ulnohumeral articulation because direct apposition of the hyaline cartilage surfaces will result in overcompression of this region and consequently an incongruous joint.
- It is apparent that the coronoid and olecranon processes act to prevent trochlear subluxation. Given the resectability of the proximal olecranon, primacy must be given to the coronoid as the most important articular stabilizer of this joint.
- The triceps, the biceps, and the brachialis add to a posteriorly directed force vector with a resultant tendency for the elbow to sublux posteriorly with active contraction (Figure 8–2).
- An anterior buttress is required to prevent posterior joint dislocation. This buttress is composed of the coronoid process of the ulna and the radial head. The greatest threat to ulnohumeral stability occurs when both the coronoid and radial head are fractured.
- Biomechanical studies have demonstrated that at least 50% of the coronoid is necessary to achieve functional stability because the ulnohumeral joint nears extension regardless of the integrity of the other articular elements.
- With an intact radial head, 75% of the coronoid can be removed, and the elbow is still stable to within about 30 degrees of full extension.[6] For this reason and because the radial head serves as a secondary stabilizer to valgus

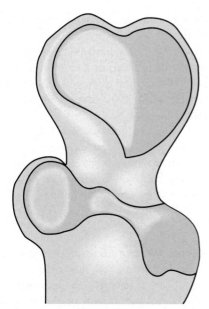

Figure 8–1: The saggital geometry of the semilunar notch is that of an ellipse rather than a bare area because of the transverse bare area located between the coronoid and the olecranon process.

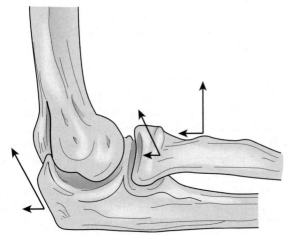

Figure 8–2: Active contraction of the muscles around the elbow results in a posteriorly directed force vector. Those forces may result in the posterior dislocation of the elbow as a result of acute trauma.

stress,[7,8] we recommend radial head reconstruction or replacement for all complex elbow fractures and fracture-dislocations with associated Mason type II and type III fractures. In such cases, the radial head should not be excised.

- The osseous anatomy of the patient is also important when a fixation strategy is developed.
- The olecranon consists of a relatively thin dorsal cortical shell (1- to 2-mm thick) that surrounds a bulbous mass of cancellous bone.[9]
- The dorsal cortex increases in thickness distal to the coronoid process approximately 35 mm from the tip of the olecranon.

- It is essential to gain purchase in this region of the ulna to maximize the rigidity of fixation of the olecranon fracture. It is also desirable to obtain screw purchase in the anterior cortex at the base of the coronoid process. The longitudinal axis of the ulna also must be kept in mind.
- The medullary canal follows a serpentine curve. Baratz and Shanahan have shown that a 6.5-mm screw does not engage the cortex with three-point fixation until it is at least 55 mm from the tip of the olecranon.[9]
- At 65 mm from the tip of the olecranon, it becomes difficult to advance the screw because the diameter of the medullary canal decreases to 5.5 mm. Care must then be taken to hand tap the distal medullary canal, particularly in osteoporotic bone, to avoid distal cortical compromise.

Soft-Tissue Constraints

- Soft-tissue constraints also play an important role in the pathoanatomy of proximal ulna fractures. This is true primarily with increasing fracture complexity, particularly when associated with ulnohumeral or radiocapitellar dislocation patterns.
- The triceps, brachioradialis, and biceps muscles generate the forces that displace the fracture fragments.
- Resisting this tendency to displacement and instability are the medial and lateral expansions of the triceps fascia that blend into the anconeus aponeuroses and common extensor origins.
- Once torn, bony fragments are then free to separate and displace. Negation of these displacing forces is necessary to achieve stable fixation. When plating is indicated, we recommend posterior placement in virtually all settings.
- The elbow is stabilized by both dynamic and static soft-tissue restraints. The primary static restraints are the medial collateral and ulnar lateral collateral ligaments.
- The medial collateral ligament (MCL) is the primary stabilizer to valgus stress, the anterior band being the most critical. The MCL originates from the anteroinferior surface of the medial epicondyle and inserts at a mean of 18 mm distal to the coronoid tip near the sublime tubercle.[10,11]

Classification and Differential Diagnosis

- The ossification center of the olecranon fuses by the age of 14 years.[14]
- Persistent physeal lines and patella cubiti (an accessory ossicle in the triceps tendon) have been reported.[12,13] These structures are usually bilateral; hence, the results of contralateral radiographs may prove informative if the diagnosis is in question.
- In isolation, a small fleck of bone posterosuperior to the tip of the olecranon may indicate a triceps avulsion injury.
- In cases of direct trauma, the olecranon is impacted against the distal humerus; this may result in comminution and

fragment depression. Indirect trauma entails, for example, a fall on an outstretched hand in conjunction with a forceful triceps contraction. This usually results in a transverse or short oblique fracture pattern.

Classification Systems

- Numerous classification systems have been proposed for olecranon fractures. These include the Colton, Arbeitsgemeinschaft für Osteosynthesefragen, Mayo, and Schatzker classification schemes.[14–17]
- However universal fracture descriptors become unwieldy or less than adequate when complex fractures that may include the radial head, coronoid, and soft-tissue restraints are considered.
- Interobserver reliability is also an issue.
- Schatzker's classification of olecranon fractures (Figure 8–3) implies that mechanical considerations are related to the type of internal fixation required.[17] Thus the choice of internal fixation is based on the fracture pattern.
- We present a modified version of Schatzker's classification that provides the surgeon with a treatment-based classification system (Figure 8–4. See Figure 8–5 for Mayo Classification).

Treatment

- The goals of any treatment protocol should be to maximize the restoration of joint stability, power, and range of motion while minimizing morbidity. This can be achieved largely by the stable anatomic reconstruction of the articular surface, which enables progression to early motion.

Nonoperative Treatment

- Mayo type I nondisplaced fractures may be treated nonoperatively with the application of a cast or splint. Some

authors have recommended that these fractures be evaluated under real-time fluoroscopy for stability.[8,18]
- Patients should be treated in neutral rotation, and range of motion should be initiated in 7 to 28 days.
- In general, rehabilitation protocols should avoid elbow flexion greater than 90 degrees to avoid excessive distraction forces.
- A need to splint in full extension is also a relative contraindication to nonoperative treatment. Early reports of this treatment method describe stiffness and a nonfunctional arc of motion that are caused by prolonged immobilization in an extended position.[19]

Surgical Objectives

- The goals of olecranon fracture fixation include the anatomic reconstruction of the articular surface and restoration of joint stability, the prevention of joint stiffness, and the maximization of power with minimal morbidity. To accomplish these goals, we recommend the following systematic approach:
  - Avoid narrowing the greater sigmoid notch.
  - Use pointed reduction forceps to minimize soft tissue stripping.
  - Use a smaller screw or threaded Kirschner wires (K-wires) to assemble fragments when there is significant comminution.
  - If the coronoid is a separate fragment, it must be secured or the construct will fail.
  - The coronoid is often accessed through the fracture defect. When possible, reduce the coronoid to the shaft before attempting the reduction of the olecranon.
  - We prefer lag screw fixation of the coronoid. When this is not possible, FiberWire suture through drill holes is a viable option.
  - Lag screws should be placed perpendicular to the fracture line before plate application when oblique fractures are reconstructed.

Transverse Fractures

- The tension band fixation method is ideally suited to stable fracture patterns proximal to the coronoid tip that are not at risk for sigmoid notch compression.[20]
- Tension bands convert the dorsal distraction force of the triceps muscle into articular surface compression forces[21] via a figure-of-eight wire loop (Figure 8–6). This type of fixation is contraindicated in extensively comminuted fractures, which are best addressed with plate-and-screw constructs.
- Centrally compressed fragments must be elevated, and small amounts of cancellous graft may be used to reinstate a smooth trochlear notch.
- The emphasis remains on articular congruity, and small central areas of comminution may be discarded as long as the overall architecture of the trochlear curve is preserved.[2]

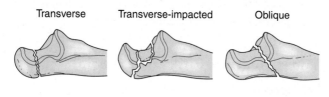

Transverse   Transverse-impacted   Oblique

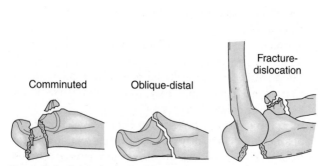

Comminuted   Oblique-distal   Fracture-dislocation

Figure 8–3: **Schatzker's classification system.**

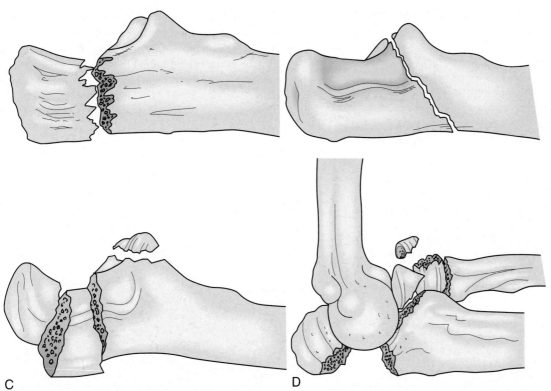

Figure 8–4: A modified version of Schatzker's classification provides the surgeon with a treatment-based system and clinical pearls. **A,** Transverse fractures: Tension-band wire in conjunction with Kirschner wires (K-wires) or an intramedullary screw. If they are used, the K-wires should engage the volar cortex. **B,** Oblique fractures: Lag screws find their primary application in the treatment of intraarticular epiphyseal fractures and metaphyseal fractures. If the screw is not inserted perpendicular to the fracture plane, shear force is introduced as the screw is tightened, and the fragments can displace. **C,** Comminuted fractures: In this scenario, it may be necessary to use a bridge plate to maintain length and alignment. This type of plate fixation is not stable; therefore, meticulous surgical dissection is required to minimize periosteal stripping, and every effort should be made to avoid the devitalization of individual bony fragments. Both plate ends must be solidly fixed to their corresponding ends of the bone. Increased plate length is desirable in this situation. **D,** Fracture-dislocations: The coronoid and the radial buttress must be reconstructed to prevent posterior subluxation or the dislocation of the joint.

- After adequate provisional reduction has been achieved, meticulous technique is required to provide stable fixation and to avoid hardware-related complications, which have been reported in up to 71% of patients treated with this method.[22]
- Parallel 1.6-mm or 2-mm K-wires should be inserted obliquely from the olecranon tip into the anterior cortex at the base of the coronoid.
- Ideal wire placement runs just posterior to the subchondral bone.
- A common error is to start too proximal (Figure 8–7). Intramedullary placement triples the risk of K-wire pullout and provides significantly less resistance to tensile forces.[23,24]
- K-wires (18-gauge or 22-gauge) may be used to create the tension band.
- Braided cable has been shown to be superior to monofilament wire in biomechanical studies.[24]

- The distal drill hole should be placed dorsal to the long axis of the ulna.[25–27] However, care must be taken to ensure that the hole placement is sufficiently volar, so that cutout and resultant construct failure are prevented.
- Both the ulnar and radial limbs of the figure-of-eight loop should be tensioned simultaneously to improve rigidity and to equalize medial and lateral compressive forces. Two knots generate greater construct rigidity than does one knot.[28]
- In osteoporotic bone, proximal and distal overlapping wires may be used to distribute forces and provide multivector compression.
- In the doubled construct, the proximal wire is tightened directly over the K-wires before the more distally based wire is threaded through the triceps tendon directly against the dorsal olecranon surface.
- Subperiosteal positioning is facilitated by feeding the wire through a 14-gauge angiocatheterization needle.

CLASSIFICATION OF OLECRANON BONE FRACTURES

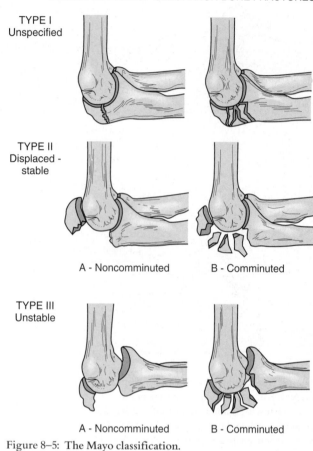

TYPE I
Unspecified

TYPE II
Displaced -
stable

A - Noncomminuted   B - Comminuted

TYPE III
Unstable

A - Noncomminuted   B - Comminuted

Figure 8–5: The Mayo classification.

- Triceps tendon necrosis may occur if the wire is placed proximally in the substance of the tendon.
- Ulnar nerve entrapment by free fragments or orthopedic hardware in the cubital tunnel must be ruled out by direct visualization or fluoroscopic assessment before wound closure.[29]

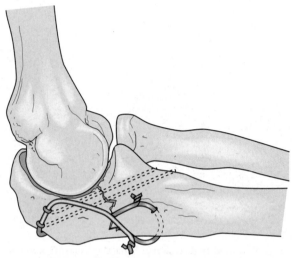

Figure 8–7: Illustration of tension-band construct: The figure-of-eight loop should be placed beneath the triceps tendon to prevent tissue necrosis, and the wire must be tightened separately to produce symmetrical tension.

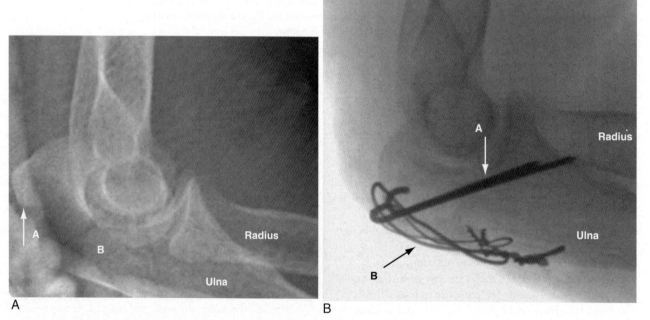

Figure 8–6: **A,** This figure depicts a transverse fracture that has been displaced by the unopposed pull of the triceps tendon. **B,** The fracture is first reduced with a bone forceps, after which the tension band construct is used to absorb the tensile forces and convert them into compressive forces.

Technique-Tension Band Fixation

- The patient is positioned in the lateral decubitus position with the arm draped over a post. A large C-arm is positioned behind the patient with the screen at the patient's feet. A well-padded tourniquet is placed high up on the arm.
- A small midline posterior incision is made starting just proximal to the olecranon tip. Care is taken to avoid violation of the triceps expansion with deep exposure. A broad elevator may be used to clear the subcutaneous tissues laterally from the extensor musculature.
- Medial exposure is undertaken cautiously to avoid injury to the ulnar nerve. The fracture site is explored, and the edges are cleared of soft tissue so that accurate reduction can be verified. A pointed reduction clamp is used to achieve provisional reduction.
- A 2-mm drill hole may be used to gain purchase for the clamp in the ulnar diaphyseal bone, if necessary.
- The accuracy of the reduction is established by visual inspection of the dorsal ulnar surface and is then confirmed fluoroscopically.
- A single 1.6-mm smooth K-wire is inserted obliquely from the olecranon tip into the anterior cortex at the base of the coronoid. Correct wire placement is confirmed fluoroscopically. A second wire is placed parallel to the first, and two small longitudinal nicks are made in line with each K-wire.
- Two transverse drill holes are made in the ulnar diaphysis distal to the fracture site. The holes are made approximately 1 cm anterior to the dorsal ulnar surface.
- A 22-gauge wire is threaded through the proximal hole and is tightened symmetrically over the K-wires.
- A 14-gauge angiocatheter is then passed from medial to lateral under the triceps tendon juxtaposed to the bony surface.
- An 18-gauge wire is then passed through the distal ulnar hole and is twisted into a figure-of-eight wire loop with the free limbs on the medial side. The wire is passed from lateral to medial through the angiocatheter, which is then removed. This second wire is also tightened symmetrically, and the reduction is again confirmed fluoroscopically throughout the full range of motion.
- The wire knots are clipped short and are buried anteriorly in the soft tissues.
- The two K-wires are backed out slightly from their purchase points in the anterior cortex. The wires are bent at their tips and impacted into place. Care is taken to orient the hooked wire ends to capture the figure-of-eight wire loop.
- Absorbable suture is then used to close the defects in the triceps tendon over the wire ends to further resist back out. The arm is immobilized in 90 degrees of flexion and neutral rotation in a well-padded splint. A drain is not routinely used.

Resection

- First described by Foille in 1918,[30] this method later gained wide acceptance after its description was published in the English literature by Dunn in 1939.[31] It has remained a part of the treatment armamentarium since that time.[32]
- This technique offers several advantages, primarily that of avoiding the problems inherent in open reduction and internal fixation (ORIF), such as loss of fixation and nonunion, hardware prominence, and the need for subsequent removal and imperfect articular surface reduction.
- It also offers inherent advantages, such as relative ease of surgery, and it eliminates the need for a bony union.
- These factors combine to make this the ideal surgery for older patients with osteoporotic bone, particularly in patients with proximal comminution.
- Before this procedure is performed, the integrity of the coronoid, the distal radioulnar joint, the interosseous membrane, and the MCL must be established to prevent resultant instability.[33]
- The triceps must be securely reattached with nonabsorbable sutures or suture anchors.
- Placement adjacent to the remaining articular surface provides a smooth transition between the remaining olecranon and the triceps tendon.[2] It may be argued that this is at the expense of power with a more dorsal reattachment site.[34,35]
- In their series of 107 patients, Gartsman and others[36] recorded equivalent isometric strength and functional ratings in patients treated with resection and triceps advancement and in those treated with ORIF.
- Some authors have expressed concern that a decreased articular surface area will result in increased contact pressures.[35]
- Increased rates of osteoarthritis were not seen in Gartsman's review.[36] However, in that article, patient follow-up averaged only 3.6 years with a 2-year minimum. Longer follow-up is needed to answer this question definitively.
- McKeever and Buck[37] reported good results with excisions of up to 80% of the trochlear notch.
- An and others[38] noted a linear loss of stability proportional to the amount of resection. Their recommendation to limit resection to no more than 50% of the articular surface is widely followed. Overall, in a select group of patients, the efficacy of this treatment modality has been confirmed by multiple authors.[32,36,39,40] We advocate its use for older patients and in certain revision settings for painful nonunions of the proximal ulna.

Oblique Fractures

- In the treatment of oblique fractures, ulnar length must be restored.
- If the fracture involves the ulnohumeral joint, then shortening could result in narrowing of the greater sigmoid notch and joint incongruity.
- To avoid this, we recommend provisional fixation with threaded K-wires or lag screws if the bone will accept them.

- Oblique fractures distal to the coronoid are usually more amenable to treatment with lag screws because the diaphyseal bone better accepts the screws.
- The metaphyseal portion of the olecranon is best treated with cancellous screws or threaded K-wires because lag screws can overcompress the softer bone in that region.
- We will often place a precontoured dorsal plate after preliminary fixation of the oblique fracture. This is always the case if the fracture line extends distal to the coronoid process. Recall that with respect to the sigmoid notch, the ulnar shaft lies in 4 degrees of valgus.
- A second option is to place a long intramedullary (IM) 6.5- or 7.3-mm partially threaded cancellous screw and tension band (Figure 8–8).
- A typical error with this technique involves the translational poor reduction of the fragments. This can be avoided by sequential drilling and distal tapping after provisionally reducing the fracture. The hole for the screw can be enlarged proximally to allow for distal alignment.
- Coonrad and Morrey[41] recommend that a screw of 10 to 12 cm in length (or at least 7 cm past the fracture site) be used to ensure adequate fixation.
- Screws longer than this may cause distal cortical penetration because of the proximal ulnar bow.[42]
- Increased torque while the screw is engaged distally can be mistaken for fracture compression. Conversely, poor purchase in a larger canal can be avoided by using screws of sufficient length and diameter.
- Fluoroscopic assessment of screw placement and confirmation of stability with range of motion have been recommended.[42]

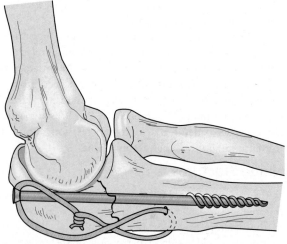

Figure 8–8: **An alternative technique for the treatment of oblique or transverse fractures consists of placing a long intramedullary 6.5 or 7.3 partially threaded cancellous screw and tension band.**

Comminuted Fractures

- In comminuted fractures, the principles remain the same as those used in simpler fracture patterns but must be adhered to more rigorously to optimize outcomes.
- The surgeon's goal remains that of reestablishing the olecranon and coronoid articular facets without altering the contour and dimensions of the trochlear notch.
- Small fragments may be absent or impacted, and the surgical strategy should emphasize realignment of the dorsal cortex.
- The trochlea can be used as a template to reconstitute the proximal ulna.
- In cases of severe comminution, it may be reasonable to use an external fixator or bridge plate and perform definitive fixation with corticocancellous grafting after the soft tissues have stabilized.

Anterior Fracture-Dislocations

- Strictly speaking, fracture-dislocations of the radial head differ from Monteggia fractures in that the proximal radioulnar joint remains intact in the former. Lack of clarity regarding this concept has led to some confusion in the literature.[43]
- Bado's initial classification scheme included Monteggia-equivalent fractures that did not involve the proximal radioulnar joint and consequently may have contributed to some of the confusion regarding this distinct entity.[44]
- This distinction is most clear in the anterior or so-called transolecranon fracture-dislocation[45,46] (Figure 8–9). These fractures, which include type III coronoid fragments, may extend into the diaphyseal portion of the ulna.
- Exposure and fixation of anterior fragments may be facilitated by working posteriorly through the fracture plane itself.
- Fractures of the radial head in this injury pattern are uncommon, and stability is usually restored by addressing the trochlear architecture.[47]

Posterior Fracture-Dislocations

- Posterior fracture-dislocations are often associated with radial head fractures (Figure 8–10).
- The key to treating these injuries is to use a posterior approach.
- The surgeon must work through the fracture defect in the proximal ulna.
- The olecranon and triceps are elevated.
- The radial head is then easily accessed through the fracture site and is either repaired or replaced.
- The coronoid is reduced with pointed reduction forceps.
- Temporary fixation is obtained with a K-wire or with a lag screw (Figure 8–11). The olecranon can then be reduced, and a precontoured plate is applied to the dorsal cortex (Figure 8–12).

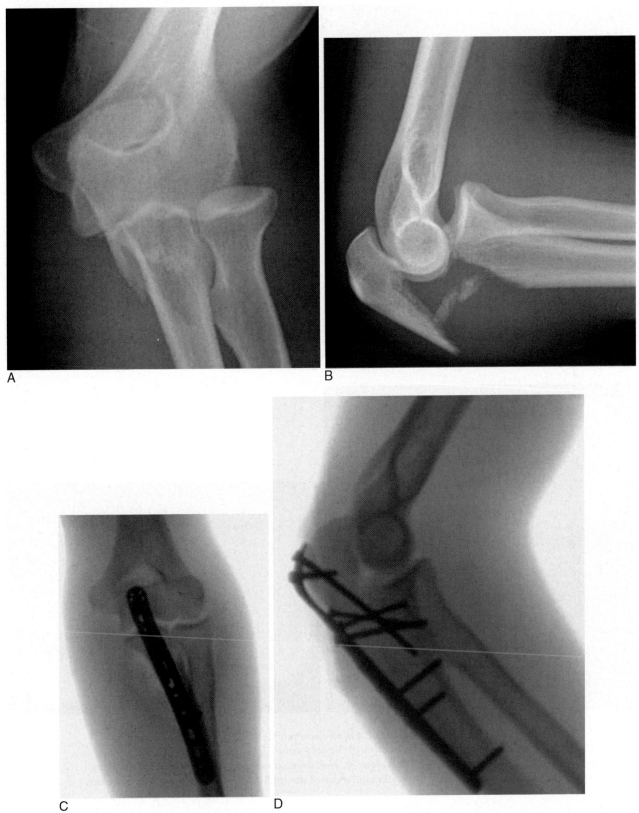

Figure 8–9: **A, B,** Transolecranon fracture–dislocation. Fracture of the olecranon and anterior displacement of the radius and ulna. **C, D,** Postoperative radiographs depict a lag screw combined with a precontoured dorsal plate.

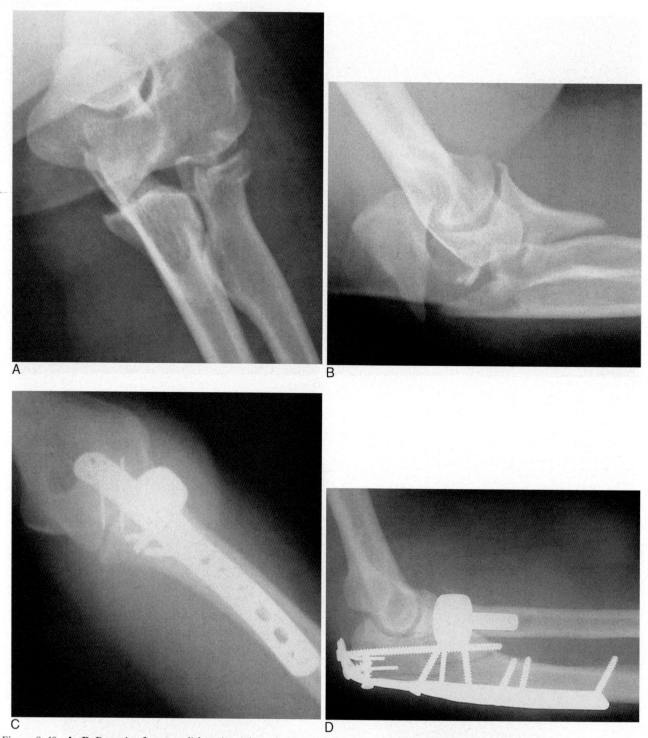

Figure 8–10: **A, B,** Posterior fracture-dislocation: The radial head is comminuted, and the coronoid fracture is displaced. **C, D,** The key to reconstruction is to work through the defect caused by the fracture. The radial head is always addressed first. In this case, the radial head was replaced. The coronoid was then reduced with a bone forceps, and Kirschner wires were provisionally placed. Final fixation required the application of a precontoured dorsal plate.

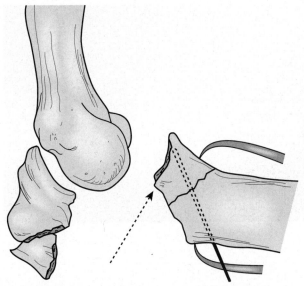

Figure 8–11: Temporary fixation is achieved by the reduction of the coronoid with a bone forceps and the placement of a provisional Kirschner wire (K-wire). Placing a lag screw perpendicular to the fracture line is another option.

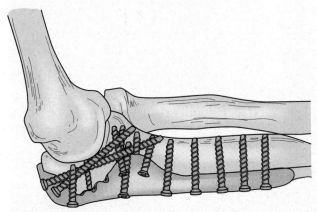

Figure 8–12: Precontoured plates are useful in the treatment of these fractures. Often, screws directed from the most proximal aspect of the plate into the volar cortex will enable a more stable construct.

Terrible Triad

- Dubbed the terrible triad by Hotchkiss,[8] fracture-dislocations that involve the radial head, coronoid, and ligamentous stabilizers of the elbow (Figure 8–13) are notoriously difficult to treat.[8,48-51]
- We believe that a careful stepwise approach that addresses each of the components of this challenging injury can yield consistent and reliable results.

Terrible Triad (Preferred Method of Fixation)

- A direct lateral approach is the preferred method for the terrible triad because the MCL tends to heal physiologically if the ulnohumeral joint is reduced.

- Formal repair is not necessary unless medial instability persists after coronoid, lateral ulnar collateral ligament (LUCL), and radial head pathologic conditions have been addressed.[50]
- If required, an accessory medial incision can be made to address the MCL.
- The patient is positioned supine with the arm extended at the side on the arm board. A tourniquet is applied. The lateral epicondyle and ulnar border are used as guides to plan a proximal Kocher incision centered over the lateral epicondyle.
- Because of soft-tissue swelling and fracture, the traditional superficial landmarks of the anconeus-ECU interval and the radial head are not reliably discernable. As a general rule, the distal portion of the incision should be directed to a point 5 cm distal to the tip of the olecranon along the ulnar border.
- Considerable soft-tissue disruption results from these injuries. Most patients exhibit a disruption of all or part of the common extensor origin.[52]
- An excellent point of reference from which to begin the dissection is the lateral supracondylar ridge. Staying anterior to this line ensures that no further damage is done to the lateral ligament complex.
- The anconeus-ECU interval can be most readily identified by a fat stripe or raphe in its distal portion. The radial extensors and brachioradialis are elevated and tagged with a Krakow stitch for later repair. The joint is entered through any capsular disruption created by the injury.
- The lateral ligamentous complex is identified, and a grasping stitch is placed with a 1-mm cottony Dacron suture.
- The most common injury is an avulsion of the lateral collateral ligament complex from the humerus, which leaves a typical bare spot on the posterolateral aspect of the lateral condyle.[52]
- The LUCL itself may be found as a relatively discrete structure deep to the anconeus, or the LUCL may blend with the capsular fibers and fascia of the anconeus and is palpable only as a capsular thickening.
- The most medial structure is addressed first.
- In our experience, most cases have a type I coronoid fracture. These fractures are fixed by placing a locked loop around the fragment with FiberWire and then threading the suture into an anchor. The anchor is inserted into the coronoid base. The fragment is then docked into position by pulling the nonlocked suture limb.
- We do not recommend definitive repair of the fragment until all radial head pathologic conditions have been addressed. It is difficult to insert a radial head prosthesis after definitive repair of the small coronoid fragment and anterior capsule.
- Large coronoid fractures are fixed with one or two self-compressing screws, which are directed from anterior to posterior.

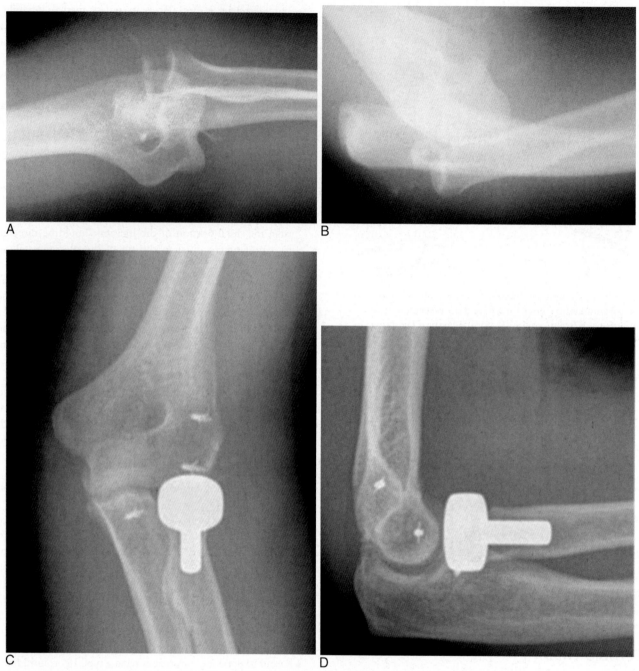

Figure 8–13: **A, B,** The "Terrible Triad" involves the fracture of both the radial head and the coronoid, and the disruption of the ligamentous stabilizers of the elbow. **C, D,** The elbow is stabilized by addressing all three facets of this injury. In this case, the radial head was replaced and the coronoid was fixed with a suture lasso technique. Finally, a Krakow stitch was placed in the lateral ulnar collateral ligament, and this was repaired through drill holes. In such cases, the radial head should never be excised.

- Another option is to use lag screws, which may be directed either from anterior to posterior or from the posterior surface of the ulna to engage the coronoid fracture fragment. Screw placement is determined at the time of surgery and is based on exposure and the ability to achieve an acceptable screw trajectory.

- The radial head is then addressed. The primary goal is to provide a stable anterior buttress and to resist valgus forces, given that the MCL is often compromised.
- The radial head is fixed with headless or 3-mm screws that engage the head and are directed distally into the shaft. If there is a displaced radial neck fracture, a precontoured

plate can be applied. The plate should be applied directly lateral with the forearm in neutral to prevent impingement in the lesser sigmoid notch.[53]

- If there are three or more fragments, the risk of complications from internal fixation increases.[54]
- If stable fixation is not possible, the radial head is replaced with a metallic prosthesis. Care sure should be taken to avoid overstuffing the joint.[55]
- A modular radial head prosthesis allows the surgeon to adjust the height, and the lesser sigmoid notch provides an excellent anatomic landmark. The radial head should not sit proud with respect to this structure. Valgus stress facilitates exposure.
- Trial components are inserted, and the elbow is ranged under fluoroscopy. The appropriate final implant is then seated.
- After insertion or fixation of the radial head, the elbow is repaired in a stepwise medial-to-lateral progression.
- If the coronoid fragment was fixed with a suture anchor or through drill holes, the fragment is reduced and the sutures are tied while the arm is held in 90 degrees of flexion.
- The LUCL is then repaired back to the lateral condyle at the center of rotation of the elbow. The ligament is repaired through drill holes in conjunction with an anchor placed just proximal to the center of rotation to create a broader surface area for healing. The arm is pronated and held in 45 degrees of flexion while the LUCL complex is secured. The extensors are then repaired back to the lateral column through drill holes.
- The elbow is again ranged and assessed for stability, both clinically and fluoroscopically. If significant instability remains, consideration must be given to repairing or reconstructing the MCL through a separate medial incision.
- Another option is the application of a hinged external fixator. A deep drain is not routinely used.
- The wound is closed in the routine fashion, and the elbow is splinted in 90 degrees of flexion and neutral rotation. We remove the splint at the first postoperative visit and place the patient in a range of motion brace locked at 45 to 135 degrees.

Complications

- As a general rule, the rate and severity of complications are proportional to the energy absorbed by the bone and soft tissues at the time of injury.
- Patient factors, such as age, nutritional and health status, compliance, and tobacco use, may play a role in complication risk.
- The consequence of the olecranon as a relatively superficial structure and the complex and highly conforming nature of the ulnohumeral, radiocapitellar, and proximal radioulnar joints cannot be overemphasized.

- Significant complications in this instance include posttraumatic arthritis, instability caused by initial or iatrogenic trauma, ulnar neuropathy and neuritis, restricted motion, heterotopic ossification, deep infection, and nonunion.
- When all complications are considered, hardware-related complications dominate the literature as those that occur most frequently and are most often discussed.[41]
- Reported in 3% to 80% of cases and historically approaching an incidence of 100%,[52–54] hardware-related complications most frequently occur with the use of tension-band type constructs in which symptomatic or unstable K-wires require a second operation for hardware removal.[56–58]
- These complications should be routinely discussed and emphasized with patients before surgery.
- Care in wire placement as discussed in the technique portion of this chapter can help reduce (although not eliminate) this problem.
- Romero and colleagues[22] have reported that hardware removal was required in 33 of 46 patients at a median of 8.5-months' follow-up. In that study, however, only 65% of patients with symptomatic hardware had objective evidence of hardware prominence.
- Ultimately, it appears that hardware-related problems are related to the essentially subcutaneous nature of the implant and may therefore be unavoidable, particularly in thinner patients.
- Motion loss, particularly in extension, is commonly seen in this patient group. Restriction is typically 10 degrees to 15 degrees.[59]
- Functional impairment with loss of more than 30 degrees is uncommon and occurs with greater frequency in fracture-dislocations and complex high-energy injuries.[44]
- Coonrad and Morrey[41] have stated that the degree of motion loss is almost directly proportional to the period of immobilization and the extent of edema or swelling around the joint.
- With an incidence of approximately 13%, heterotopic ossification is rarely a significant complication in simple olecranon fractures; it develops more often as a result of associated radial head dislocations, complex fracture types, and neurologic injuries secondary to head trauma.[58,60]
- In unstable fracture patterns, Ilahi and others[61] reported a 33% incidence of heterotopic ossification when surgical treatment was delayed for more than 48 hours. However in that study, the incidence of grade II, III, or IV heterotopic ossification dropped to 0% when surgery was performed within 48 hours of the initial injury.
- Treatment with indomethacin or radiation prophylaxis may be used in complex fracture types when treatment is delayed or a patient is deemed at risk for that complication.
- Ulnar neuropathy has been reported in 2% to 10% of patients.[22,29,60,62-68]
- Prominent hardware placement and the assessment of nerve subluxation may indicate the need for anterior

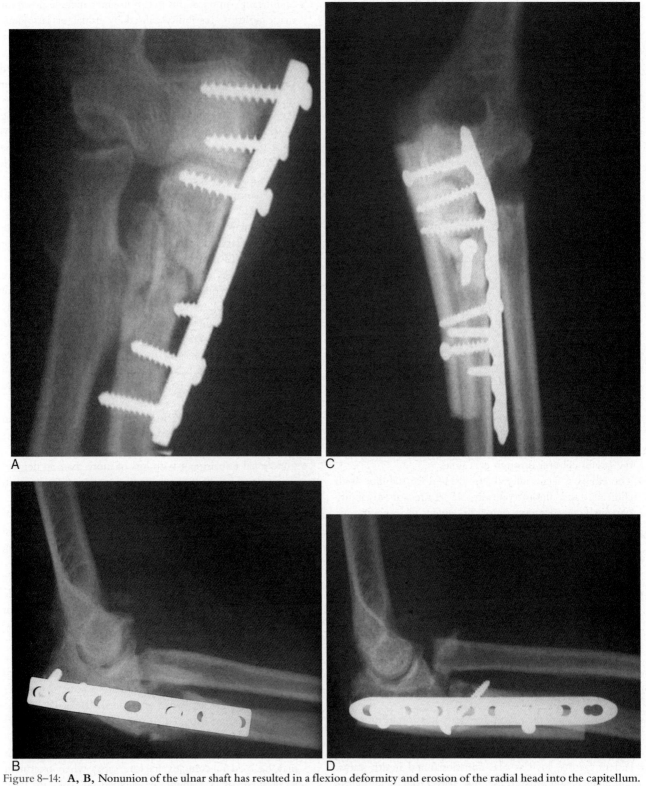

A

B

C

D

Figure 8–14: **A, B,** Nonunion of the ulnar shaft has resulted in a flexion deformity and erosion of the radial head into the capitellum. **C, D,** The deformity is corrected, and the fracture is reduced. The reduction is held with a lag screw followed by an allograft strut placed medially and a precontoured plate placed laterally.

subcutaneous transposition. Late neurolysis or transposition may occasionally be required.

- Ishigaki and others[65] retrospectively reviewed 18 cases of surgically treated olecranon fractures and identified 4 cases of ulnar nerve palsy. Three of those cases were noted to have a fair or poor reduction, and one case was noted to have medial side osteoarthritic changes. Those authors recommended careful intraoperative radiographic assessment that emphasized AP and cubital tunnel views to enable the visualization of displaced fracture fragments that disrupted or were within the cubital tunnel itself.

- Although radiographic evidence of posttraumatic arthritis is seen in 20% to 35% of patients, symptoms related to that condition are far less common.

- Articular surface changes correlate with the severity of the initial injury and with the quality of the reduction.[68]

- Gartsman and others[36] found a 20% rate of arthritis, regardless of whether patients were treated with open reduction and internal fixation or olecranonectomy.

- Instability after excision has rarely been reported in the literature. Inhofe and others[32] had one incident in their series, and Gartsman et al[36] reported no instances of subluxation in their series.

- Stability is linearly proportional to the amount of olecranon resected, and the current recommendation is that 50% of

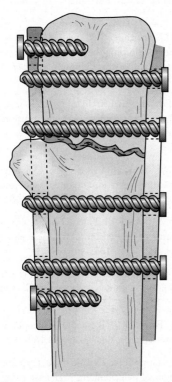

Figure 8–15: Illustration of a tibial strut used as a bone plate. The fracture is first reduced and is held with a lag screw when possible. The strut is then placed and is secured to the bone with cancellous screws. A 3.5-mm plate is then applied to the opposite cortex, and the screws are directed into the strut for enhanced fixation.

this joint can be removed without adversely affecting stability.[4] Extension strength is surprisingly well maintained in the postresection state, and no significant difference is seen when compared with the results of ORIF.[36]

- In a 1978 study, Mayer and Evarts[69] reported a 5% incidence of olecranon nonunion. With improvements in hardware design and dissemination of improved techniques, that number has now decreased, with one study reporting <1% incidence of olecranon nonunion.[70]

- Nonunion is often defined as cessation of all evidence of fracture healing after 6 months of conservative treatment (Figure 8–14).

- Clinically, false motion, pain, and tenderness are common presenting complaints.

- Options for treatment in symptomatic patients are resection, revision fixation, and either intramedullary or onlay bone-grafting techniques (Figure 8–15).

- Late revision for unsalvageable articular distortion may be performed with total elbow arthroplasty (TEA) or allograft replacement.

- Rarely, arthrodesis may be indicated in the treatment of young manual laborers who require maximum power and a stable joint.

Annotated References

1. An KN, Morrey BF: Biomechanics of the elbow. In: Morrey BF, editor: *The elbow and its disorders,* ed 2, Philadelphia, 1993, W. B. Saunders.

2. Cabanela ME, Morrey BF: Fractures of the proximal ulna and olecranon. In: Morrey BF, editor: *The elbow and its disorders,* ed 2, Philadelphia, 1993, W. B. Saunders.

3. Kapandji IA: *The physiology of the joints,* Edinburgh, 1982, Churchill Livingstone.
This book uses the visual approach and illustrates the anatomy, physiology, and mechanics of the joints by means of clear and simple diagrams and a minimum of text.

4. Morrey BF, An KN: Articular and ligamentous contributions to the stability of the elbow joint, *Am J Sports Med* 11:315–319, 1983.

5. Safran MR, Baillargeon D, Soft-tissue stabilizers of the elbow, *J Shoulder Elbow Surg* 14(1 Suppl S):179S-185S, 2005.

6. Morrey BF, An KN: Stability of the elbow: osseous constraints, *J Shoulder Elbow Surg* 14(1 Suppl S):174S-178S, 2005.

7. Hotchkiss RN: Displaced fractures of the radial head: internal fixation or excision? *J Am Acad Orthop Surg* 5:1-10, 1997.

8. Hotchkiss RN: Fractures and dislocations of the elbow. In: Rockwood CA Jr, Green DP, Bucholz RW, et al, editors: *Rockwood and Green's fractures in adults,* ed 4, vol 1, Philadelphia, 1996, Lippincott-Raven.

9. Baratz ME, Shanahan JF: Fractures of the olecranon, *J South Orthop Assoc* 4:283-289, 1995.

The authors discuss the applied surgical anatomy of the proximal ulna. The dorsal surface of the olecranon is a cortical shell of bone only 1 to 2 mm in thickness. The cortex thickens to 3.5 mm distal to the coronoid process. It is necessary to gain purchase in the anterior cortex of the base of the coronoid to obtain rigid fixation in the majority of olecranon fractures.

10. Cage DJ, Abrams RA, Callahan JJ, et al: Soft tissue attachments of the ulnar coronoid process: an anatomic study with radiographic correlation, *Clin Orthop Relat Res* 320:154-158, 1995.

11. Callaway GH, Field LD, Deng XH, et al: Biomechanical evaluation of the medial collateral ligament of the elbow, *J Bone Joint Surg Am* 79:1223-1231, 1997.

12. O'Donoghue DH, Sell LS: Persistent olecranon epiphysis in adults, *J Bone Joint Surg* 24:677, 1942.

13. Kohler A, Zimmer EA: *Borderlands of the normal and early pathologic in skeletal roentgenology,* New York, 1968, Grune & Stratton.

14. Colton CL: Fractures of the olecranon in adults: classification and management, *Injury* 5:121-129, 1973.

15. Morrey BF: Current concepts in the treatment of fractures of the radial head, the olecranon, and the coronoid. *Instr Course Lect* 44:175-185, 1995.

16. Muller ME, Allgower M, Schneider R, et al, editors: *Manual of internal fixation: Techniques recommended by the AO-ASIF group,* ed 3, Berlin, 1991, Springer-Verlag.
The tension-band technique converts the forces generated by the triceps extensor musculature into a dynamic compressive force at the articular surface.

17. Schatzker J: Fractures of the olecranon. In: Schatzker J, Title M, editors: *The rationale of operative fracture care,* Berlin, 1987, Springer-Verlag.

18. Murphy DF, Greene WB, Gilbert JA, et al: Displaced olecranon fractures in adults: biomechanical analysis of fixation methods, *Clin Orthop Relat Res* 224:210-214, 1987.

19. Eliot E: Fractures of the olecranon, *Surg Clin of North Am* 14:487-492, 1934.

20. Finsen V, Lingaas PS, Storro S: AO tension-band osteosynthesis of displaced olecranon fractures, *Orthopedics* 10:1069-1072, 2000.

21. Jupiter JB, Mehne DK: Fractures of the distal humerus, *Orthopedics* 15:825-833, 1992.

22. Romero JM, Miran A, Jensen CH: Complications and re-operation rate after tension-band wiring of olecranon fractures, *J Orthop Sci* 5:318-320, 2000.

23. Mullett JH, Shannon F, Noel J, et al: K-wire position in tension band wiring of the olecranon—a comparison of two techniques, *Injury* 31:427-431, 2000.

24. Prayson MJ, Williams JL, Marshall MP, et al: Biomechanical comparison of fixation methods in transverse olecranon fractures: A cadaveric study, *J Orthop Trauma* 11:565-572, 1997.

25. Paremain GP, Novak VP, Jinnah RH, et al: Biomechanical evaluation of tension band placement for the repair of olecranon fractures, *Clin Orthop Relat Res* 335:325-330, 1997.

26. Roe SC: Tension band wiring of olecranon fractures: a modification of the AO technique, *Clin Orthop Relat Res* 308:284-286, 1994.

27. Rowland SA, Burkhart SS: Tension band wiring of olecranon fractures. A modification of the AO technique, *Clin Orthop Relat Res* 277:238-242, 1992.

28. Fyfe IS, Mossad MM, Holdsworth BJ: Methods of fixation of olecranon fractures: an experimental mechanical study, *J Bone Joint Surg Br* 67:367-372, 1985.

29. Horne JG, Tanzer TL: Olecranon fractures: a review of 100 cases, *J Trauma* 21:469-472, 1981.

30. Foille DJ: [Note Les Fractures De Folecrane Par Projectiles De Guerre.] *Marsielle Med* 55:241-245, 1918.

31. Dunn N: Operation for fracture of the olecranon, *BMJ* 1:248-268, 1939.

32. Inhofe PD, Howard TC: The treatment of olecranon fractures by excision or fragments and repair of the extensor mechanism: historical review and report of 12 fractures, *Orthopedics* 16:1313-1317, 1993.

33. Teasdall R, Savoie FH, Hughes JL: Comminuted fractures of the proximal radius and ulna, *Clin Orthop Relat Res* 292:37-47, 1993.

34. Didonna ML, Fernandez JJ, Lim TH, et al: Partial olecranon excision: the relationship between triceps insertion site and extension strength of the elbow, *J Hand Surg (Am)* 28:117-122, 2003.

35. Moed BR, Ede DE, Brown TD: Fractures of the olecranon: an in vitro study of elbow joint stresses after tension-band wire fixation versus proximal fracture fragment excision, *J Trauma* 53:1088-1093, 2002.

36. Gartsman GM, Sculco TP, Otis JC: Operative treatment of olecranon fractures: excision or open reduction with internal fixation, *J Bone Joint Surg Am* 63:718-721, 1981.

37. McKeever FM, Buck RM: Fracture of the olecranon process of the ulna: treatment by excision of fragment and repair of triceps tendon, *J Am Med Assoc* 135:1-5, 1947.

38. An KN, Morrey BF, Chao EY: The effect of partial removal of proximal ulna on elbow constraint, *Clin Orthop Relat Res* 209:270-279, 1986.

39. Compton R, Bucknell A: Resection arthroplasty for comminuted olecranon fractures, *Orthop Rev* 18:189-192, 1989.

40. Rettig AC, Waugh TR, Evanski PM: Fracture of the olecranon: a problem of management, *J Trauma* 19:23-28, 1979.

41. Coonrad RW, Morrey BF: Management of olecranon fractures and nonunion. In: Morrey BF, editor: *The elbow: Masters techniques in orthopaedic surgery,* ed 2, Philadelphia, 2002, Lippincott, Williams and Wilkins.

42. Boyer MI, Galatz LM, Borrelli J Jr, et al: Intra-articular fractures of the upper extremity: new concepts in surgical treatment, *Instr Course Lect* 52:591–605, 2003.

43. Bell Tawse AJ: The treatment of malunited anterior Monteggia fractures in children, *J Bone Joint Surg Br* 47:718-723, 1965.

44. Bado JL: The Monteggia lesion, *Clin Orthop Relat Res* 50: 71-86, 1967.

45. Biga N, Thomine JM: Trans-olecranal dislocations of the elbow, *Rev Chir Orthop Reparatrice Appar Mot* 60:557-567, 1974.

46. Ring D, Jupiter JB, Sanders RW, et al: Transolecranon fracture-dislocation of the elbow, *J Orthop Trauma* 11:545-550, 1997.

In this study, 17 patients were identified with transolecranon fracture-dislocations. Patients underwent open reduction and internal fixation. The Broberg and Morrey performance rating was used to evaluate outcome. There were seven excellent results, eight good results, and two fair results. The critical point in this study is to recognize that in a transolecranon fracture-dislocation, the proximal radioulnar joint is not disrupted. The key to optimal treatment is the restoration of the contour and dimensions of the trochlear notch.

47. Mouhsine E, Akiki A, Castagna A, et al: Transolecranon anterior fracture dislocation, *J Shoulder Elbow Surg* 16:352-357, 2007.

48. McKee MD, Jupiter JB: Trauma to the adult elbow. In: Browner BD, Jupiter JB, Levine AM, et al, editors: *Skeletal trauma*, ed 3, vol 2, Philadelphia, 2003, W. B. Saunders.

49. McKee MD, Bowden SH, King GJ, et al: Management of recurrent, complex instability of the elbow with a hinged external fixator, *J Bone Joint Surg Br* 80:1031-1036, 1998.

50. O'Driscoll SW, Jupiter JB, King GJ, et al: The unstable elbow, *Instr Course Lect* 50:89-102, 2001.

51. Ring D, Jupiter JB, Zilberfarb J: Posterior dislocation of the elbow with fractures of the radial head and coronoid, *J Bone Joint Surg Am* 84-A:547-551, 2002.

52. McKee MD, Schemitsch EH, Sala MJ, et al: The pathoanatomy of lateral ligamentous disruption in complex elbow instability, *J Shoulder Elbow Surg* 12:391-396, 2003.

53. Soyer AD, Nowotarski PJ, Kelso TB, et al: Optimal position for plate fixation of complex fractures of the proximal radius, *J Orthop Trauma* 12:291-293, 1998.

54. Ring D, Quintero J, Jupiter JB: Open reduction and internal fixation of fractures of the radial head, *J Bone Joint Surg Am* 84-A:1811-1815, 2002.

55. Van Glabbeck F, Van Riet RP, Baumfeld JA, et al: Detrimental effects of overstuffing or understuffing with a radial head replacement in the medial collateral-ligament deficient elbow, *J Bone Joint Surg Am* 86:2629-2635, 2004.

56. Mathewson MH, McCreath SW: Tension band wiring in the treatment of olecranon fractures, *J Bone Joint Surg* 57B:399, 1975.

57. Murphy DF, Greene WB, Dameron TB Jr. Displaced olecranon fractures in adults. Clinical evaluation, *Clin Orthop Relat Res* 224:215-223, 1987.

58. Simpson NS, Goodman LA, Jupiter JB. Contoured LCDC plating of the proximal ulna, *Injury* 27:411-417, 1996.

Dorsal application of a 3.5-mm limited-contact dynamic-compression plate was performed in 13 complex proximal ulnar fractures and 24 Monteggia fracture dislocations. Plate fixation is recommended for fracture patterns that extend into the diaphysis or if there is involvement of the coronoid. The ideal olecranon plate is one that allows the surgeon to direct screw placement can be easily contoured and is low in profile.

59. Ates Y, Atlihan D, Yildirim H: Current concepts in the treatment of fractures of the radial head, the olecranon and the coronoid, *J Bone Joint Surg Am* 78:969, 1996.

60. Wolfgang G, Burke F, Bush D, et al: Surgical treatment of displaced olecranon fractures by tension band wiring technique, *Clin Orthop Relat Res* 224:192-204, 1987.

The authors treated 45 fractures with tension-band wiring. They reported good-to-excellent results in 98% of cases. Recommendations for this technique included engagement of the Kirshner wires through the anterior cortex of the proximal ulna and use of a double looped 18-gauge figure-of-eight wire for all simple transverse fractures.

61. Ilahi OA, Strausser DW, Gabel GT: Post-traumatic heterotopic ossification about the elbow, *Orthopedics* 21:265-268, 1998.

62. Bakalim G, Wilppula E: Fractures of the olecranon. I. Analysis of 109 consecutive cases, *Ann Chir Gynaecol Fenn* 60:95-101, 1971.

63. Helm RH, Hornby R, Miller SW: The complications of surgical treatment of displaced fractures of the olecranon, *Injury* 18:48-50, 1987.

64. Hume MC, Wiss DA: Olecranon fractures: a clinical and radiographic comparison of tension band wiring and plate fixation, *Clin Orthop Relat Res* 285:229-235, 1992.

Forty-one adult patients with displaced olecranon fractures were treated with open reduction and internal fixation (ORIF) in a prospective randomized study comparing tension band wiring and plate fixation. Range of motion at 6 months did not differ between the two groups. Tension-band wiring resulted in 37% good clinical and 47% good radiographic results, compared with plate fixation, which resulted in 63% good clinical and 88% good radiographic results. Loss of reduction and articular incongruity were most commonly seen in those patients who underwent tension-band wiring for oblique or comminuted fractures. The authors conclude that tension-band wiring is best reserved for simple transverse fractures and that plating is superior for comminuted fractures of the proximal ulna.

65. Ishigaki N, Uchiyama S, Nakagawa H, et al: Ulnar nerve palsy at the elbow after surgical treatment for fractures of the olecranon, *J Shoulder Elbow Surg* 13:60-65, 2004.

66. Kiviluoto O, Santavirta S: Fractures of the olecranon. Analysis of 37 consecutive cases. *Acta Orthop Scand* 49:28-31, 1978.

67. Macko D, Szabo RM: Complications of tension-band wiring of olecranon fractures, *J Bone Joint Surg Am* 67:1396-1401, 1985.

68. van Kloot JF: Results of treatment of fractures of the olecranon. *Arch Chir Neerl* 16:237-249, 1964.

69. Mayer PJ, Evarts CM: Nonunion, delayed union, malunion and avascular necrosis. In: Epps CH Jr, editor: Complications in orthopaedic surgery vol 1, Philadelphia, 1978, JB Lippincott, 59-175.

70. Papagelopoulos PJ, Morrey BF: Treatment of nonunion of olecranon fractures, *J Bone Joint Surg Br* 76B:627-635, 1994.

Diaphyseal Forearm Fractures

Frank A. Liporace, MD

- In 1998, 650,000 radius or ulna fractures occurred in the United States.[1]
- Common mechanisms of injury include motor vehicle accidents, falls, direct trauma, gunshot wounds, and athletic injuries. There is a bimodal age distribution, with the majority occuring in patients between 5 and 14 years of age or older than 65 years of age.[1]
- Femoral neck bone mineral density, height loss, calcium intake, and a history of falls have all been cited as risk factors in the elderly.[2]
- Significant potential for limitations in forearm rotation and hand function have been cited after these injuries.[3–5]
- The introduction of internal fixation has proven to be of greatest importance in improving results when treating these fractures.[6,7]

Anatomy

- The relationship of the radius and ulna with their soft-tissue connections represent a ring. A disruption of this ring leads to potential complications and associated injuries at the distal and proximal articulations.
- The ulna acts as a central axis for the radius. Disruption of this relation can lead to limited rotation and grip strength.[4]
- The site of maximum bowing of the radius is at (measuring from distally to proximally) 60% of the length of the radius. The value of maximum bending does not exceed 10% of the total length of the radius.[8]
- The Orthopaedic Trauma Association (OTA) classification is frequently used to describe the fracture pattern.
- Location of the fracture depending on which third of the forearm can determine deforming forces:
  - The proximal third has the radial tuberosity and beginning third of radial bow.
  - The middle third includes the radial bow until the point of straightening distally.
  - The distal third is straight.

- The interosseous membrane (proximal on radius/distal on ulna in the posterior plane)[9] has a central band of collagenous tissue that is twice as thick as the remaining membrane.[10] This thickened area is consistently located at a distance from the radial styloid of about 62% of the length of the radial shaft.[11] Sectioning results in 71% decreased stability.[10]
- Disruption of the interosseous membrane affects proximal and distal load bearing at the elbow and wrist joints, respectively. Normally the radius bears 80% of load at the wrist[12] and 57% of the load at the elbow.[13] The greatest force is transmitted from the wrist to the radial head when the elbow is in extension and the forearm in pronation.[14]
- The radius and ulna are also connected distally by the triangular fibrocartilage complex (TFCC)[12] and proximally by the annular and quadrate ligaments.
- Fracture location affects deformity:
  - Radius fractures distal to the supinator insertion but proximal to the pronator teres result in proximal fragment supination.
  - Radius fractures distal to both the supinator and pronator teres insertions result in neutral rotation.

Evaluation

- A careful neurovascular examination is paramount. Specific testing of the radial, ulna, median, anterior interosseus nerve (AIN), posterior interosseus nerve (PIN), and lateral antebrachial cutaneous nerves are essential.
- Pain with passive stretch of the fingers that is disproportional, accompanied by a tense forearm should lead to suspicion of compartment syndrome, and the potential for compartment pressure monitoring and possible fasciotomy must be considered.
- Radiographically, anteroposterior (AP) and lateral views of the forearm should be obtained. Also, orthogonal views of the wrist should be done. At times a comparison contralateral wrist radiograph may be useful to evaluate distal radial-ulna joint relationship.

Monteggia Fractures

- These are proximal ulna fractures associated with a radial head dislocation. In adults, posterior dislocations are most common[15] (Figure 9–1 *A-C*)
- The Bado classification is most frequently used to describe these injuries. It is based on the direction of radial head displacement. Types 1, 2, and 3 have anterior, lateral, and posterior displacements, respectively. Type 4 involves radio-capitellar instability with fracture of both the proximal ulna and radius.[15] Types 1 and 2 more commonly occur in younger patients, whereas type 3 occurs most commonly in middle-aged and elderly adults.[15–18]
- Anatomic ulna reductions usually result in radial head relocation. If there is an anatomic ulna reduction and the radial head is not reduced, an open reduction of the radial head is required.[19] Stable fixation with a 3.5-mm plate will allow for early motion and generally good results.[16] If there is an associated interosseous membrane injury with an irreconstructable radial head fracture, a radial head replacement is warranted to avoid inadvertent proximal migration of the radius.[15]
- Concomitant coronoid fractures can increase instability and must be addressed at the time of operative fixation.[16]
- Intraoperatively, the elbow should be tested for posterolateral rotatory instability, which may require lateral ligamentous repair or postoperative immobilization in pronation while allowing flexion and extension of the elbow.[20]
- With transolecranon-fracture-dislocations of the elbow, the entire forearm distal to the olecranon fracture is anteriorly dislocated relative to the distal humerus, requiring plate fixation of the olecranon.[21]
- A recent series of 17 transolecranon-fracture-dislocations of the elbow yielded 15 good-to-excellent results with plate fixation. Large coronoid fragments and extensive comminution of the trochlea notch did not preclude good results, even with stable fixation[21] (Figure 9-2 *A-D*).

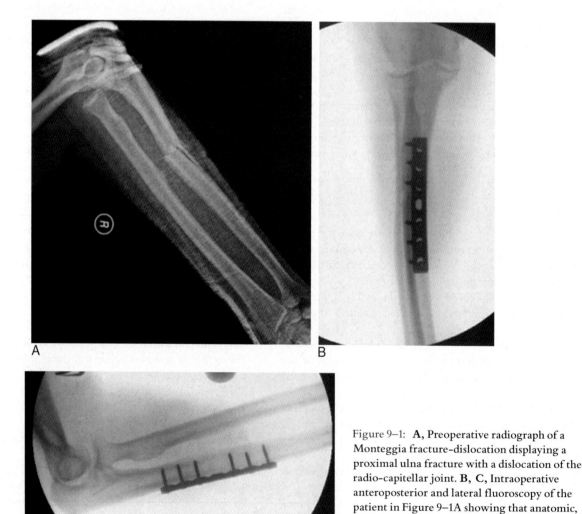

A

B

C

Figure 9–1: **A,** Preoperative radiograph of a Monteggia fracture-dislocation displaying a proximal ulna fracture with a dislocation of the radio-capitellar joint. **B, C,** Intraoperative anteroposterior and lateral fluoroscopy of the patient in Figure 9–1A showing that anatomic, stable fixation of the ulna fracture resulted in radio-capitellar joint reduction.

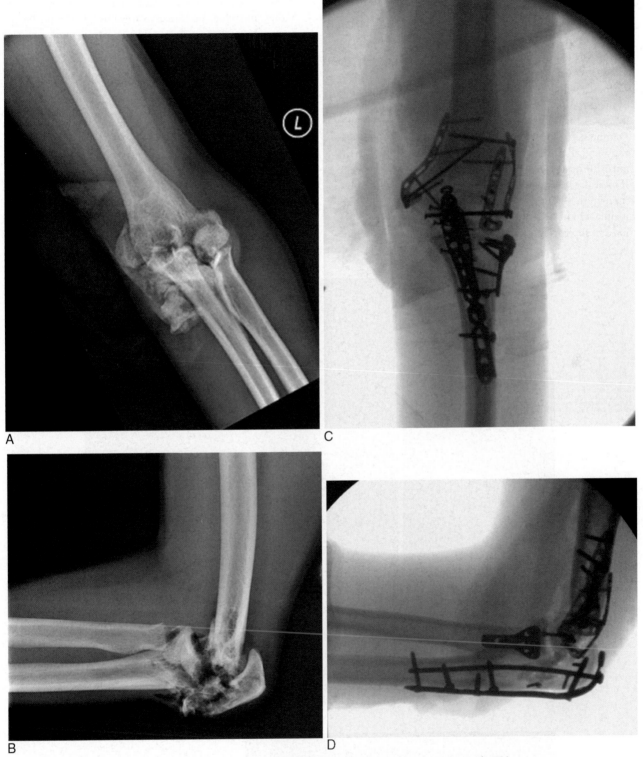

Figure 9–2: **A, B,** Preoperative radiograph of a 30-year-old man who fell 50 feet and sustained a grade IIIA transolecranon-fracture-dislocation of the left elbow with a concomitant distal humerus fracture. Note the missing area of articular surface from the olecranon, which was not recovered at the scene. **C, D,** Anteroposterior and lateral radiographs of the patient in Figure 9–2A, **B,** with plate fixation of the olecranon, radial neck, and distal humerus fractures with calcium sulfate, impregnated with antibiotics, filling the olecranon defect.

Galeazzi Fractures

- These are radial shaft fractures, most commonly at the middle and distal third junction (Figure 9–3 A-C). Frequently, distal radio-ulna joint (DRUJ) instability and interosseous injury accompany these.
- Clinically, the interosseous membrane integrity can be evaluated. When attempting to pull the radius proximally, if greater than 3 mm instability is present, the interosseous membrane is disrupted. If greater than 6 mm of instability is present, both the interosseous membrane and the triangular fibrocartilage complex (TFCC) are disrupted.[22]
- If interosseous instability is present, attempted reduction in supination should be done. If reduction is obtained and maintained in supination, then the patient can be immobilized in supination for approximately 6 weeks. If instability persists with attempted supination, then pinning across the radius and ulna, proximal to the DRUJ, should be performed after reduction is achieved. At 6 weeks, this pin can be removed. A recent case report sites the extensor carpi ulnaris (ECU) tendon as a potential block to DRUJ reduction, and if closed reduction cannot be obtained, then exploration of this joint may be required.[23]
- Location of the radial shaft fracture may lead to suspicion of a DRUJ injury. In one study, 55% of patients with a radial shaft fracture less than 7.5 cm from the distal radial articular surface exhibited instability whereas only 6% of patients with fractures greater than 7.5 cm from the distal radial articular surface had similar findings.[24]
- Additional factors to suggest DRUJ instability include[25,26]:
  - Ulna styloid fracture at the base.
  - Widening of the DRUJ on an AP radiograph.

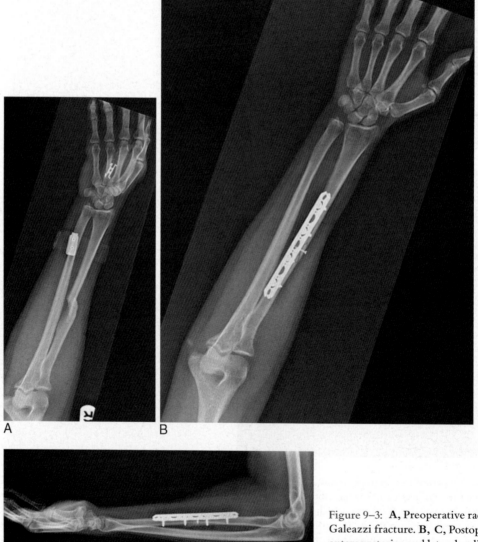

Figure 9–3: **A,** Preoperative radiograph of a Galeazzi fracture. **B, C,** Postoperative anteroposterior and lateral radiographs of an internally fixed Galeazzi fracture. Note the reduced distal radio-ulna joint (DRUJ).

- Dislocation of the DRUJ on a true lateral radiograph.
- Shortening of the radius greater than 5 mm relative to the distal ulna.

Distal-Third Fractures

- Displaced distal-third fractures at the meta-diaphyseal junction are potentially unstable and allow for limited fixation dependent on how distal the fracture lies.
- Smaller plates with or without locked screws, 90:90 minifragment plates, or intramedullary fixation may be needed to acquire adequate stability in these fractures (Figure 9–4 *A-D*).

Nonoperative Treatment Indications

- Only with a completely nondisplaced both bones fracture can nonoperative long arm casting be considered. Such instances require frequent clinical and radiographic follow-up. Any unacceptable displacement or angulation requires operative intervention.
- With isolated ulna shaft, "night stick" fractures, up to 50% displacement of the shaft width and 10 degrees of angulation can be considered for nonoperative treatment[27] (Figure 9-5 *A-D*).
- A recent review compared long arm casting with bracing. In patients being treated nonoperatively for isolated ulna diaphyseal fractures, casting and bracing exhibited similar times before union. However, those patients who received bracing had greater satisfaction and were able to return to work sooner.

Operative Treatment Indications

- Since the use of stable internal fixation for displaced forearm fractures has become the gold standard of treatment, studies have shown greater than 92% union rate.[29–31]
- Displaced fractures of the forearm diaphysis warrant operative intervention. Typically, open reduction and internal fixation (ORIF) with standard (3.5-mm limited-contact dynamic compression plating) or locked plating has been conducted. Intramedullary nailing has also been suggested as an alternative treatment method.[32–34]
- Early operative treatment allows decompression of fracture hematoma and ease of reduction, resulting in decreased soft-tissue trauma.[35]
- Early stable fixation allows for earlier range of motion of joints and maintenance of muscle strength.[36]

Operative Procedures

- Traditionally, fractures can be fixed with the patient in the supine position with an armboard or hand table extension for the operative extremity.

- The ulna is approached with the elbow flexed whereas the radius is usually approached with the elbow extended and the forearm supinated.
- A tourniquet may be used at the surgeon's discretion.
- Open fractures should undergo thorough debridement of any necrotic, nonviable, or heavily contaminated skin, subcutaneous tissue, muscle, fascia, and bone. Definitive internal fixation for type I to IIIA open fractures can be conducted acutely with good results, provided that adequate and complete debridement with appropriate soft-tissue coverage is possible.[37,38]
- Temporary external fixation may be needed for vascular injury, severely contaminated injuries requiring serial debridements, or definitive soft tissue coverage.
- When applying definitive internal fixation, using separate radius and ulna incisions may decrease the incidence of synostosis, which occurs in 5% to 10% of patients. Other predisposing factors include severity of trauma, multiple trauma, and closed head injury.[39,40]
- Fixation usually commences with the less comminuted bone to allow for appropriate restoration of length and rotation of the forearm.
- The volar Henry approach[41] is often used for radial shaft fractures. This approach is extensile, allowing for extension across the elbow or into the hand. It also allows fasciotomies of the superficial and deep volar compartments as well as releases of the pronator quadratus fascia and the carpal tunnel.
- The dorsal Thompson approach[42] may be used in select cases and allows plate application along the tension side of the bone. The proximal radius can also be easily addressed without confronting the same neurovascular structures encountered with a volar approach.
- The ulna can be approached along its subcutaneous border between the ECU and the FCU.
- Distally, the dorsal sensory branch of the ulna nerve crosses the field approximately 7 cm proximal to the ulna styloid.
- Care must be taken to preserve periosteum not disrupted by the initial trauma, allowing adequate vascularity for bone healing. Especially with extensive comminution, restoration of length and alignment via indirect reduction supersedes stripping each fragment of its vascularity. The concept of bridge plating allows these multiple comminuted fragments to function as vascularized grafts to allow for healing.[43]
- At the conclusion of internal fixation, the tourniquet should be released; with the elbow at 90 degrees, passive, pronation and supination should be symmetric to the contralateral extremity.
- After completion of fixation, intraoperative orthogonal fluoroscopy of the wrist and elbow should show a similar ulna variance to the uninjured extremity and anatomically reduced ulna-trochlea and radial-capitellar

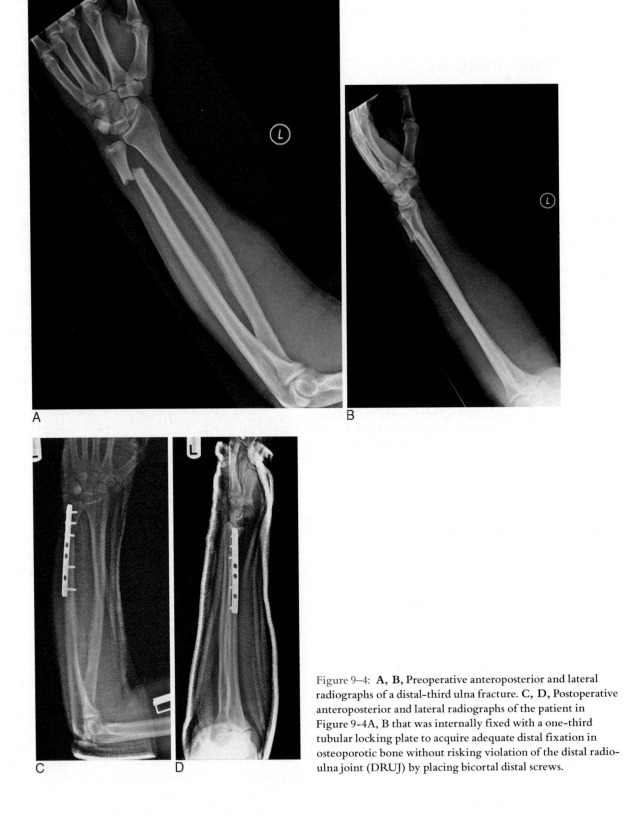

Figure 9–4: **A, B,** Preoperative anteroposterior and lateral radiographs of a distal-third ulna fracture. **C, D,** Postoperative anteroposterior and lateral radiographs of the patient in Figure 9-4A, B that was internally fixed with a one-third tubular locking plate to acquire adequate distal fixation in osteoporotic bone without risking violation of the distal radio-ulna joint (DRUJ) by placing bicortal distal screws.

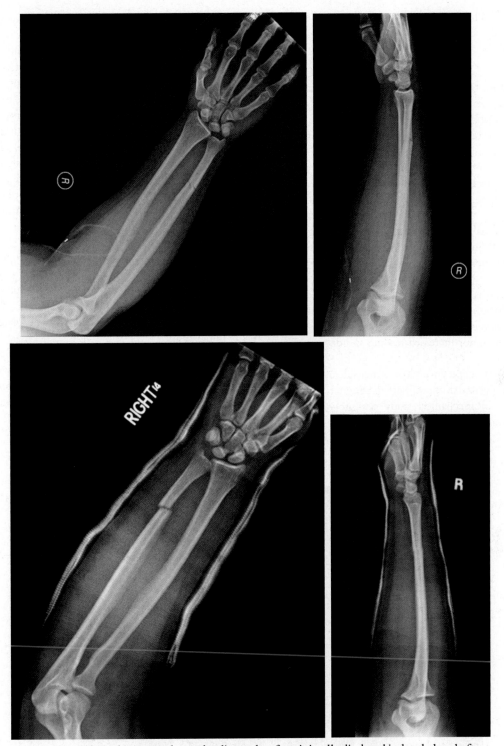

Figure 9–5: Anteroposterior and lateral injury and casted radiographs of a minimally displaced isolated ulna shaft fracture.

articulations. The radial styloid should be 180 degrees away from the bicipital tuberosity as well.

Plating

- When plating, if the fracture pattern allows, lag screw fixation can be acquired either through the plate or outside the plate.
- With simple transverse fractures that do not allow for lag screw fixation, a plate can be applied in compression mode.
- With severe comminution, bridge plating with attention to restoring mechanical axis and rotation is more advisable than extensively stripping soft tissue and reapproximating each fragment[43] (Figure 9–6 A-C).
- Although initial stiffness with bridge plating is less than seen with initial cortical contact, that callus from secondary bone healing ultimately provides greater stability overall.[44–46]
- Bridge plating is preferably done with a standard limited contact or locking plate. By decreasing plate-bone contact and potential periosteal strangulation, more biology is preserved, allowing for increased healing and decreased nonunion risk.
- Previously six to eight cortices on either side of the fracture have been suggested as appropriate fixation when plating.[47]
- Recently, a biomechanical study has shown that plate length is more important in contributing to bending

strength of the construct as opposed to the number of screws in the plate.[48]
- Longer plates with two screws on either side of the fracture ("near-near"/"far-far") are more effective than shorter plates with every screw hole filled[48] (Figure 9–7 A-D).
- The use of locking compression plates has been shown biomechanically to demonstrate similar if not subtly greater mechanical superiority to standard plating of the radial shaft.[49] In a prospective, randomized trial of 125 fractures, comparing limited contact dynamic compression plating with locked plating, no significant difference between the two groups could be found with respect to operative time, time to union, pain, or functional outcome.[50]
- With severe comminution, consideration for acute bone grafting can be made.[51]
- However, there is evidence that with appropriate stabilization and soft-tissue preserving techniques, bone grafting may not significantly increase union rates[4,52,53] (Figure 9–6A-C).
- With ulna plating, contouring of the plate is frequently unnecessary.
- When approaching the radius volarly, if the plate is over-contoured in an attempt to create a dorsal bow, gapping of the dorsal cortex may occur; frequently no plate contouring or minimal plate contouring is necessary, allowing for dorsal bony apposition.

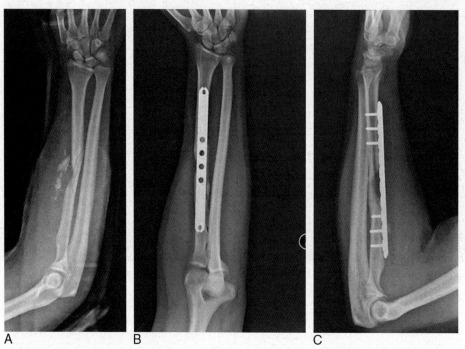

Figure 9–6: **A,** Anteroposterior and lateral radiographs of a patient who sustained 17 gunshots and had a severely comminuted left radial shaft fracture with an open contaminated wound. **B, C,** Anteroposterior and lateral radiographs of the patient from Figure 9–6A at 3 months postoperatively. He was bridge-plated with soft-tissue preserving technique that resulted in bridging of the defect. The patient has nearly full range of motion and is asymptomatic.

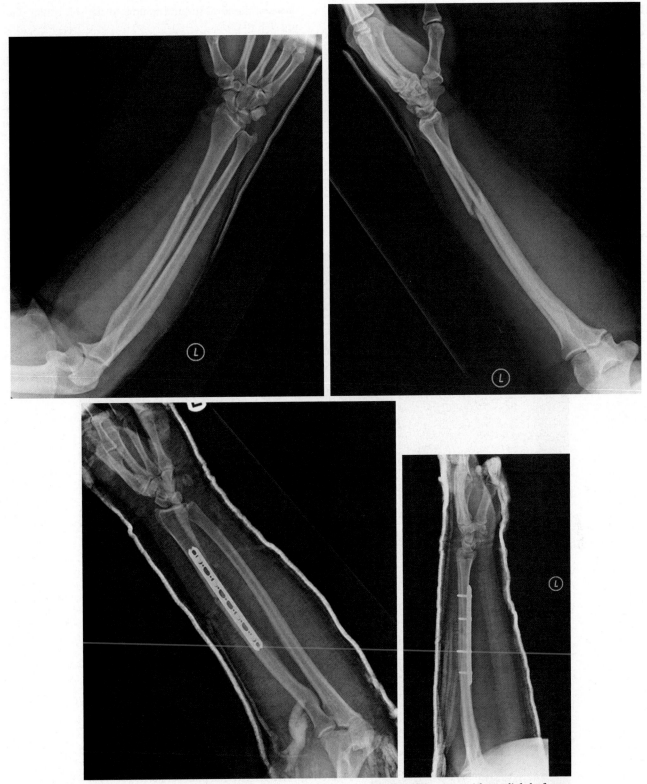

Figure 9–7: Preoperative and postoperative anteroposterior and lateral radiographs of a patient with a radial shaft fracture treated with an eight-hole 3.5-low contact dynamic compression plate (LCDCP) plate with "near-near"/ "far-far" screw configuration.

Intramedullary Fixation

- Alternatively, intramedullary fixation with flexible or contoured locked nails can be used.
- With extensive comminution of one bone and a simple fracture of the other (e.g., gun shot wound) fixation of the bone with the simple fracture pattern to restore length and rotation of the extremity and subsequent intramedullary nailing of the comminuted bone may decrease the local surgical trauma to the soft tissues (Figure 9–8 *A-C*).
- Interlocking nails offer the ability for rotational control. At times, impaction of the pointed distal tip of the nail near the subchondral bone allows for adequate interference fit. Therefore locking at the far end of the nail may not be needed. The forearm should be taken through full pronation/supination under live fluoroscopy to confirm that rotational stability is maintained (Figure 9-9, *A-E*).

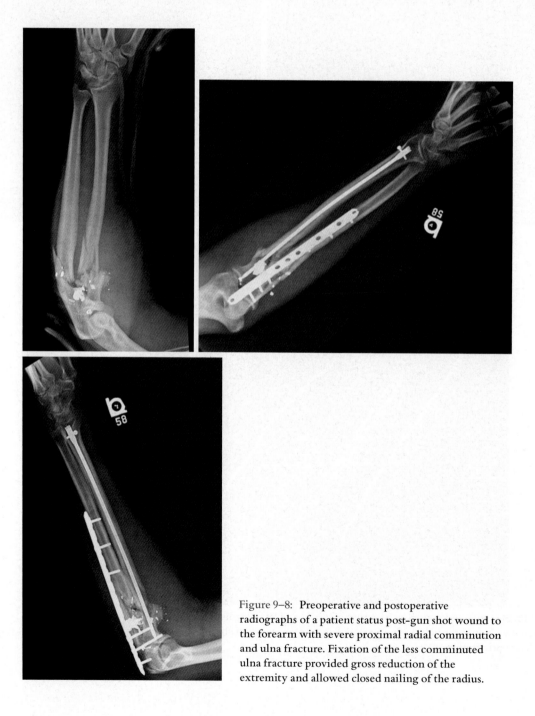

Figure 9–8: Preoperative and postoperative radiographs of a patient status post-gun shot wound to the forearm with severe proximal radial comminution and ulna fracture. Fixation of the less comminuted ulna fracture provided gross reduction of the extremity and allowed closed nailing of the radius.

- It is imperative to template the contralateral extremity so nail contour can match the anatomic dorso-radial bow of the radius to preserve pronation and supination.
- When using radial interlocking nails, a limited approach and entry point dorsally, just distal to Lister's tubercle, allows access to the intramedullary canal.

- Passage of hand reamers through the main distal and proximal fragments when held reduced allows "machining" of the intramedullary canal for subsequent nail passage.
- One may use a limited open approach at the fracture site to hold gross reduction but this may increase potentially increasing time to union from an average of 10 weeks to

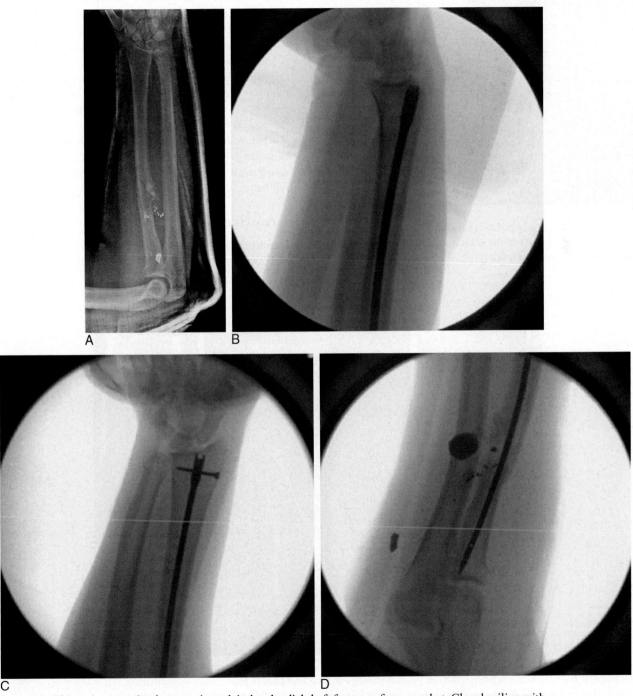

Figure 9–9: This patient sustained a comminuted, isolated radial shaft fracture after a gunshot. Closed nailing with the use of a sterile tourniquet to aid reduction was possible with impaction of the nail in the proximal radius providing an adequate interference fit, precluding the need for an interlocking screw.

(Continued)

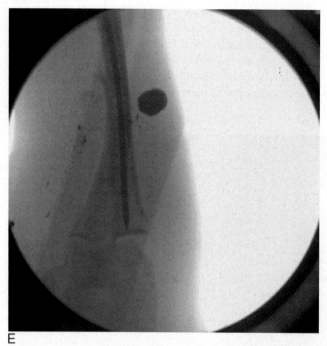

E

Figure 9–9, cont'd: D and E show that after release of the tourniquet, maintenance of the reduction remained throughout passive pronation and supination.

an average of 15 weeks.[32] Alternatively, a sterile tourniquet can be applied, centered at the fracture site, to help maintain closed reduction.

- Once the nail is passed across the fracture site, an interlocking screw can be passed through the proximal aspect of the nail via the jig attached to the nail.
- With a standard freehand technique, through a limited open approach to protect neurovascular structures, a bicortical interlocking screw can be applied at the distal aspect of the nail to prevent shortening and aid in rotational control across the fracture (Figure 9-10 *A-C*).
- A similar technique is used for the ulna, except the nail is introduced proximally into the canal with a 2-cm incision over the proximal ulna and subsequent inline splitting of the triceps, which can be repaired at the completion of the procedure.
- Recent studies show union rates (94% to 100%) and time to union (average 10 weeks with closed nailing versus 15 weeks with open nailing), which are comparable to open reduction with plating.[32–34]

Complications

- Refracture after plate removal has been cited between 4% and 25%.[29,54,55] The use of large fragment plates causing

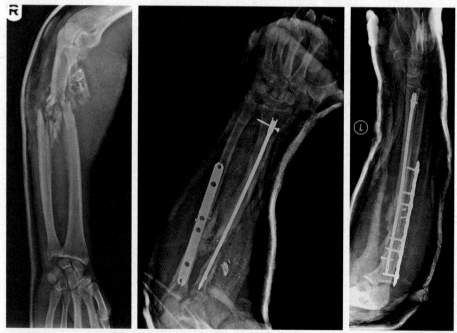

Figure 9–10: This patient sustained a gunshot wound with extensive comminution. Attempt at closed nailing with subchondral impaction was made but did not provide stability throughout passive pronation and supination. A limited open approach for the application of an interlocking screw was done, and a previously unrecognized coronal split was appreciated in the proximal radius. After overdrilling the near cortex, an interlocking screw was placed to lag the coronal split in the proximal fragment and provide rotational stability to the radius.

stress shielding and decreased bone mineral density under the plate has been suggested as a source of refracture.[29] Also, incomplete healing with early plate removal has been thought to contribute to refracture.[56] Propagation of stresses with resultant fracture through previous screw holes has been thought to contribute as well.[29,56] Recently, Perren and others[57] have suggested that the porosity under the plate is caused by a local circulatory disturbance and necrosis by the compression of the plate against the periosteal blood supply. This may support the use of limited contact plates and possibly locked plates that do not compress the intact periosteum.

- The use of small-fragment implants[58,59] and waiting more than 16 months, preferably more than 21 months, postfixation[56,60] before hardware removal have been shown to decrease refracture rates.

- Synostosis decreases forearm motion and is more common with more proximal fractures, high-energy trauma, open fractures, infection, concomitant head injuries, and delayed internal fixation.[61,62] Treatment options include resection of synostosis with fat interposition,[62,63] with or without postoperative single dose radiation or indomethacin prophylaxis.[62,64] For inoperable proximal synostosis, resection of a 1-cm portion of the radial shaft distal to the site of synostosis has been suggested.[61]

- Nerve injuries, aside from those iatrogenically caused with surgical fixation, most commonly occur with blast injuries (i.e., gunshot wounds) or posterior interosseous nerve injuries with Monteggia fractures.[65-67] Early exploration is not recommended because it is rare that the nerve is entrapped in the fracture site.

- Before adequate internal fixation techniques, nonunion was much more frequent.[5,68] Currently, nonunion rates are less than 2% in compliant patients with closed fractures.[29]

- Poor rotation can result in decreased rotation, especially pronation, and decreased grip strength, leading to worse patient outcomes.[3] Restoration of the normal radial bow in relation to the contralateral side is related to functional outcome and recovery of grip strength. Failure to restore the location and magnitude of the radial bow to within 4% to 5% of the uninjured extremity results in greater than 20% loss of forearm rotation.[4]

- A recent cadaveric study analyzing the effects of ulnar rotational malunions showed that they do not lead to a significant change in the total arc of forearm rotation. Instead, loss of motion in one direction is accompanied by an increase in motion in the opposite direction. Up to 45 degrees of ulnar malrotation did not decrease forearm rotation more than 20 degrees.[69]

- Infection with closed forearm fractures ranges from 1% to 7%. With open fractures, infection rates are from 1.2% to 20%.[70,71] Superficial infections often can be treated with antibiotics. Deeper infections require adequate debridement with resection of affected tissue. Often hardware

can be maintained unless severe osteomyelitis with the need for significant soft-tissue and segmental bone resection exists. These cases will require staged soft tissue and bony reconstructions.

Conclusions

- Forearm fractures are relatively common injuries.
- In the adult, they frequently require operative intervention.
- Anatomic restoration of length, alignment, and rotation are imperative.
- Poor rotation and angular deformities significantly affect range of motion, strength, and functional outcomes.
- Plating remains the gold standard, but intramedullary fixation with maintenance of anatomy has shown promising results.

Annotated References

1. Chung KC, Spilson SV: The frequency and epidemiology of hand and forearm fractures in the United States, *J Hand Surg Am* 26:908-915, 2001.

This study evaluated the frequency and described the epidemiology of hand and forearm fractures in the United States in 1998.

2. Nguyen TV, Center JR, Sambrook PN, et al: Risk factors for proximal humerus, forearm, and wrist fractures in elderly men and women: The Dubbo Osteoporosis Epidemiology Study. *Am J Epidemiol* 153:587-595, 2001.

This study evaluated risk factors for sustaining proximal humerus, forearm, and wrist fractures in 739 men and 1105 women greater than 60 years of age. Bone mineral density, height loss, and a history of falls all increased the relative risk.

3. Goldfarb CA, Ricci WM, Tull F, et al: Functional outcome after fracture of both bones of the forearm, *J Bone Joint Surg Br* 87:374-379, 2005.

The authors correlated health status with objective (disabilities of arm, shoulder, and hand [DASH] and musculoskeletal functional assessment [MFA] scores) and radiologic outcomes in 23 patients treated with open reduction and internal fixation of both bones forearm fractures. Deficiencies in pronation and grip and pinch strength correlated with poorer subjective outcomes.

4. Schemitsch EH, Richards RR: The effect of malunion on functional outcome after plate fixation of fractures of both bones of the forearm in adults, *J Bone Joint Surg Am* 74: 1068-1078, 1992.

This study evaluated 55 adults with both bones forearm fractures treated with plating with a mean follow-up of 6 years. Bone grafting did not affect union. A good functional result, grip strength, and forearm rotation were correlated with restoration of the quantity and location of the radial bow relative to the contralateral side.

5. Bolton H, Quinlan AG: The conservative treatment of fractures of the shaft of the radius and ulna in adults, *Lancet* 2:700-705, 1952.

This study reported on nonoperative results in patients with diaphyseal both bones fractures. There was a significant rate of malunion, nonunion, and functional limitation.

6. Burwell HN, Charnley AD Treatment of forearm fractures in adults with particular reference to plate fixation, *J Bone Joint Surg Br* 46:404-425, 1964.

The authors report their promising results with using rigid plate fixation for treating forearm fractures compared to the inferior results of nonoperative treatment in prior series. They suggest using a minimum of a 3 1/2-inch-long plate with three screws on either side of the fracture and beginning early mobilization postoperatively to achieve good results.

7. Anderson LD, Sisk D, Tooms RE, et al: Compression-plate fixation in acute diaphyseal fractures of the radius and ulna, *J Bone Joint Surg Am* 57:287-287, 1975.

This is one of the earliest and one of the largest series evaluating compression-plate fixation of diaphyseal forearm fractures. A total of 330 fractures were treated with compression plating for a greater than 96% union rate of the radius and ulna, which far surpasses any previous treatment recommendations.

8. Firl M, Wunsch L: Measurement of bowing of the radius, *J Bone Joint Surg Br* 86:1047-1049, 2004.

Using the technique of Schemitsch and Richards, the authors calculated that the maximal bowing of the radius was 10% of the length of the radius and was located at an average of 60.39% of the length of the radius measuring from the distal articular surface.

9. Poitevin LA: Anatomy and biomechanics of the interosseous membrane: its importance in the longitudinal stability of the forearm, *Hand Clin* 17:97-110, 2001.

This cadaveric study described the anatomy and biomechanical contributions of the components of the interosseous membrane of the forearm.

10. Hotchkiss RN, An KN, Sowa DT, et al: An anatomic and mechanical study of the interosseous membrane of the forearm: pathomechanics of proximal migration of the radius, *J Hand Surg Am* 142 Pt 1256-261, 1989.

Twelve fresh cadaver forearms were anatomically and mechanically tested to better understand the role of the interosseous membrane in stabilization of the radius after radial head excision. The central band was responsible for 71% of the longitudinal stiffness of the interosseous membrane after radial head excision. The triangular fibrocartilage complex (TFCC) contributed 8%.

11. McGinley JC, Kozin SH Interosseous membrane anatomy and functional mechanics, *Clin Orthop Relat Res* 383:108-122, 2001.

The authors anatomically describe the function of the interosseous membrane and the impact of disruption of this membrane on forearm mechanics.

12. Palmer AK, Werner FW: Biomechanics of the distal radioulnar joint, *Clin Orthop Relat Res* 187:26-35, 1984.

This study reviews the biomechanics and anatomical relationship of the distal radioulnar joint.

13. Halls AA, Travill A: Transmission of pressures across the elbow joint, *Anat Rec* 150:243-247, 1964.

This anatomic study identifies the ratio of pressures transmitted across the elbow along the radial and ulna columns.

14. Morrey BF, Askew L, Chao EY: Silastic prosthetic replacement of the radial head, *J Bone Joint Surg Am* 63:454-458, 1981.

The authors report on a high failure rate (>50%) of silicone radial head prosthesis in the treatment of fractures.

15. Bado JL: The Monteggia lesion, *Clin Orthop Relat Res* 50:71-86, 1967.

This article identifies the constellation of injuries associated with the Monteggia lesion and outlines a classification of these injuries.

16. Jupiter JB, Leibovic SJ, Ribbans W, et al: The posterior Monteggia lesion, *J Orthop Trauma* 5:395-402, 1991.

Thirteen patients with posterior Monteggia fracture dislocations were treated with ulna plate fixation + radial head resection/replacement. In four patients who had nonanatomic ulna reductions with persistent radiocapitellar subluxation there was loss of forearm supination.

17. Pavel A, Pitman JM, Lance EM, et al: The posterior Monteggia fracture: a clinical study, *J Trauma* 12:185-199, 1965.

18. Penrose JH: The Monteggia fracture with posterior dislocation of the radial head, *J Bone Joint Surg Br* 33-B:65-73, 1951.

This report of 10 patients with Monteggia injuries identified that associated posterior radial head dislocation was more prevalent than previously thought, 70% in this series. As well, the patients were all treated with operative stabilization (cerclage wiring + intramedullary screw or rod fixation). The authors report, "the functional results after operation are excellent, but some slight permanent restriction of movement is to respected."

19. Ring D, Jupiter JB, Simpson NS: Monteggia fractures in adults, *J Bone Joint Surg Am* 80:1733-1744, 1998.

This study evaluated 48 patients with Monteggia fractures and identified factors that affected results. Fair and poor results were related to malunited coronoid process, synostosis, malunion of the ulna, and concomitant radial head fracture.

20. Ring D, Jupiter JB, Waters PM: Monteggia fractures in children and adults, *J Am Acad Orthop Surg* 6:215-224, 1998.

21. Ring D, Jupiter JB, Sanders RW, et al: Transolecranon fracture-dislocation of the elbow, *J Orthop Trauma* 11:545-550, 1997.

This retrospective case series evaluated 17 patients with transolecranon fracture-dislocations of the elbow. It was concluded that stable plate fixation was required when treating these injuries.

22. Smith AM, Urbanosky LR, Castle JA, et al: Radius pull test: predictor of longitudinal forearm instability, *J Bone Joint Surg Am* 84-A:1970-1976, 2002.

This cadaveric study evaluated 12 specimens with radial head resection. One group had sequential transection of the triangular fibrocartilage complex (TFCC) and the interosseous membrane, whereas the other group had sequential transection in the opposite order. The models were used to determine a clinical examination test for evaluating longitudinal forearm instability.

23. Budgen A, Lim P, Templeton P, et al: Irreducible Galeazzi injury, *Arch Orthop Trauma Surg* 118:176-178, 1998.

This is a case report of a Galeazzi injury with an irreducible distal radio-ulna joint (DRUJ) until open reduction and removal of the extensor carpi ulnaris (ECU) tendon was performed.

24. Rettig ME, Raskin KB: Galeazzi fracture-dislocation: a new treatment-oriented classification, *J Hand Surg Am* 26:908-915, 2001.

This study evaluated the location of radius fractures to help determine the likelihood of concomitant distal radio-ulna joint (DRUJ) injury.

25. Alexander AH, Lichtman DM: Irreducible distal radioulnar joint occurring in a Galeazzi fracture: case report, *J Hand Surg Am* 6:258-261, 1981.

This case report first sited the extensor carpi ulnaris (ECU) as a potential block to acquiring a closed reduction of the distal radio-ulna joint (DRUJ).

26. Bruckner JD, Lichtman DM, Alexander AH: Complex dislocations of the distal radioulnar joint: recognition and management, *Clin Orthop Relat Res* 275:90-103, 1992.

This case series of 11 patients stresses the importance of recognizing DRUJ instability in association with forearm fractures and defines a management algorithm. Three of the patients even required open reduction of the distal radio-ulna joint (DRUJ), which had concomitant extensor carpi ulnaris (ECU) subluxation volar to the ulna.

27. Sarmiento A, Cooper JS, Sinclair WF: Forearm fractures. Early functional bracing: a preliminary report, *J Bone Joint Surg Am* 57:297-304, 1975.

This series reviewed 45 forearm fractures that were candidates for nonoperative treatment. a forearm fracture brace that allowed full flexion-extension but limited pronation supination was used for 3 to 42 days. There was only one nonunion and "minimum impairment of function in an overwhelming majority of cases."

28. Handoll HH, Pearce PK Interventions for isolated diaphyseal fractures of the ulna in adults, *Cochrane Database Syst Rev* 2: CD000523, 2004.

This metaanalysis of randomized or quasi-randomized trials comparing nonsurgical and surgical treatment of isolated ulna fractures concluded that there is insufficient evidence to determine the most appropriate method of treatment for isolated fractures of the ulna although greater patient satisfaction and sooner return to work resulted in the nonsurgical patients treated with bracing as opposed to casting.

29. Chapman MW, Gordon JE, Zissimos JG: Compression-plate fixation of acute fractures of the diaphysis of the radius and ulna, *J Bone Joint Surg Am* 71:159-169, 1989.

This is a retrospective series of 129 patients plated for both bones forearm fractures. There was a 98% union rate with 92% excellent and good results. The only refractures after plate removal was with 4.5-mm plating. All 3.5-mm plates removed did not have subsequent refracture.

30. Hicks JH: Fractures of the forearm treated by rigid fixation, *J Bone Joint Surg Br* 43-B:680-687, 1961.

The authors report on 66 forearm fractures treated with internal fixation using smaller screws and a 3-inch plate. They outline the technique and had a nonunion rate of 6%. Their results were superior to their contemporaries that used nonoperative treatment.

31. Ross ER, Gourevitch D, Hastings GW, et al: Retrospective analysis of plate fixation of diaphyseal fractures of the forearm bones, *Injury* 20:211-214, 1989.

In a retrospective review of 133 forearm fractures there was a 94.7% union rate with plate fixation, and it was determined that technical error is the main cause of nonunion.

32. Gao H, Luo CF, Zhang CQ, et al: Internal fixation of diaphyseal fractures of the forearm by interlocking intramedullary nail: short-term results in eighteen patients, *J Orthop Trauma* 19:384-391, 2005.

This retrospective study evaluated time to union, functional recovery, and the incidence of complications in eighteen patients with diaphyseal forearm fractures treated with an interlocking intramedullary nail. Time to union averaged 10 weeks with closed nailing and 15 weeks with open nailing. There was a 22% incidence of complications. When using the Grace and Eversmann rating scale, 13 patients had excellent, 3 patients had acceptable, and 2 patients had unacceptable results.

33. Moerman J, Lenaert A, De Coninck D, et al: Intramedullary fixation of forearm fractures in adults, *Acta Orthop Belg* 62:34-40, 1996.

This retrospective study of 70 diaphyseal forearm fractures treated with intramedullary fixation had a 94% union rate at an average of 73 days.

34. De Pedro JA, Garcia-Navarrete F, Garcia De Lucas F, et al: Internal fixation of ulnar fractures by locking nail, *Clin Orthop Relat Res* 283:81-85, 1992.

This study evaluated 20 forearm fracture patients treated with an intramedullary locked nail. The healing time for fractures that involved both forearm bones averaged 15 weeks. The healing time for isolated ulna fractures averaged 10 weeks.

35. Gelberman RH, Zakaib GS, Mubarak SJ, et al: Decompression of forearm compartment syndromes, *Clin Orthop Relat Res* 134:225-229, 1978.

This study outlined the method of compartment pressure measurement and the indications and choice of surgical incision to treat forearm compartment syndrome.

36. Grace TG, Eversmann WW Jr: Forearm fractures: treatment by rigid fixation with early motion, *J Bone Joint Surg Am* 62:433-438, 1980.

This review of 64 patients with forearm fractures concluded that in those with both bone forearm fractures, early motion without postoperative immobilization significantly increased the ultimate range of motion.

37. Duncan R, Geissler W, Freeland AE, et al: Immediate internal fixation of open fractures of the diaphysis of the forearm, *J Orthop Trauma* 6:25-31, 1992.

This study evaluates the immediate fixation of open forearm diaphyseal fractures. Of the 54 patients with grades I to IIIA injuries, immediate fixation resulted in acceptable results. Complication rate was significantly increased in IIIB and IIIC injuries treated with definitive fixation, and it is unclear whether these fractures should receive immediate fixation.

38. Jones JA: Immediate internal fixation of high-energy open forearm fractures, *J Orthop Trauma* 5:272-279, 1991.

Eighteen patients with open bones fractures treated with immediate internal fixation were evaluated. Even with grade III fractures and aggressive debridement, 66% of these patients had good or excellent results. It was determined that immediate internal fixation was acceptable.

39. Langkamer VG, Ackroyd CE: Internal fixation of forearm fractures in the 1980s: lessons to be learnt, *Injury* 22:97-102, 1991.

This review of 156 patients operatively treated for forearm fractures showed that accurate reduction, correct use of interfragmentary screw fixation, and rigid fixation were the most important factors to correlate with an acceptable result.

40. Stern PJ, Drury WJ: Complications of plate fixation of forearm fractures, *Clin Orthop Relat Res* 175:25-29, 1983.

The authors reviewed the complications of 64 adult patients with 87 diaphyseal forearm fractures treated with plate fixation. The authors reported on nonunion rate and synostosis formation. Nonunions occurred four times more in patients treated with a total of only four screws. They emphasized the importance of using long enough plates and cited important factors leading to synostosis as polytrauma and head injury.

41. Henry WA: *Extensile exposures*, ed 2, New York, 1973, Churchill Livingstone.

42. Thompson JE: Anatomical methods of approach in operations on the long bones of the extremities, *Ann Surg* 68:309-329, 1918.

43. Mast J, Jakob R, Ganz R: *Planning and reduction techniques in fracture surgery*, New York, 1989, Springer-Verlag.

44. Gerber C, Mast JW, Ganz R: Biological internal fixation of fractures, *Arch Orthop Trauma Surg* 109:295-303, 1990.

The authors stress the importance of using meticulous soft-tissue techniques when treating fractures, especially those with severe soft-tissue injury. They recommend stressing alignment rather than anatomical reduction of extraarticular fractures in an effort to preserve vascular supply.

45. Heitemeyer U, Claes L, Hierholzer G, et al: Significance of postoperative stability for bony reparation of comminuted fractures: an experimental study, *Arch Orthop Trauma Surg* 109:144-149, 1990.

This animal model evaluated four methods of fracture fixation and the immediate mechanical stability and ultimate course of bone reparation. Although plate osteosynthesis with interfragmentary lag screws gave the best initial biomechanical strength, bridging stabilization gave better bone regeneration.

46. Baumgaertel F, Buhl M, Rahn BA: Fracture healing in biological plate osteosynthesis, *Injury* 29Suppl 3C3-C6, 1998.

In this study it was shown that bony bridging of the fracture gap and mineralization of callus occurred faster and more efficiently after indirect (beginning in the second to third week), rather than direct (beginning in the sixth week), reduction and stabilization.

47. Browner BD, Jupiter JB, Levine AM, et al: *Skeletal trauma*, ed 2, Philadelphia, 1998, W. B. Saunders.

48. Sanders R, Haidukewych GJ, Milne T, et al: Minimal versus maximal plate fixation techniques of the ulna: the biomechanical effect of number of screws and plate length, *J Orthop Trauma* 16:166-171, 2002.

This in vitro study evaluated the significance of plate length and number of screws on the strength of fixation of ulna fractures fixed with 6-, 8-, or 10-hole plates. All the specimens fixed with longer plates with minimum ("near-near"/"far-far") screws were stronger than those fixed with six-hole plates with six screws when tested with four-point bending in the anteroposterior and medial-lateral planes.

49. Gardner MJ, Brophy RH, Campbell D, et al: The mechanical behavior of locking compression plates compared with dynamic compression plates in a cadaver radius model, *J Orthop Trauma* 19:597-603, 2005.

This cadaveric study compared the mechanical behavior in anteroposterior bending, mediolateral bending, and torsion of a locked compression plate and a dynamic compression plate when fixing a radial forearm fracture with a 5-mm gap. The authors concluded that with cyclical testing, the locking plate constructs demonstrated subtle mechanical superiority.

50. Leung F, Chow SP: A prospective, randomized trial comparing the limited contact dynamic compression plate with the point contact fixator for forearm fractures, *J Bone Joint Surg Am* 85-A:2343-2348, 2003.

This trial randomized 125 forearm fractures to treatment with either the point contact fixator (PC-fix) or a standard low contact dynamic compression plate (LCDCP) plate. There was no significant difference between the groups in terms of operative time, time to union, callus formation, pain, or functional outcome.

51. Browner BD, Jupiter JB, Levine AM, et al: *Skeletal trauma*, ed 2, Philadelphia, 1998, W. B. Saunders.

52. Ring D, Rhim R, Carpenter C, et al: Comminuted diaphyseal fractures of the radius and ulna: does bone grafting affect nonunion rate? *J Trauma* 59:438-441, 2005.

This study examined factors related to nonunion of comminuted diaphyseal both bones fractures over 15 years and the influence of acute bone grafting. They found that bone grafting was not associated with a higher union rate.

53. Wei SY, Born CT, Abene A, et al: Diaphyseal forearm fractures treated with and without bone graft, *J Trauma* 46:1045-1048, 1999.

This study determined whether acute bone grafting of diaphyseal forearm fractures decreased the incidence of nonunion or reduced the time to union. Fifty six fractures treated without bone graft were followed for at least 1 year beyond clinical and radiographic union with a 98% union rate and 95% with union at a mean of 50 days.

54. Dodge HS, Cady GW: Treatment of fractures of the radius and ulna with compression plates, *J Bone Joint Surg Am* 54:1167-1176, 1972.

55. Labosky DA, Cermak MB, Waggy CA: Forearm fracture plates: to remove or not to remove, *J Hand Surg Am* 15:294-301, 1990.

The authors discuss the pros and cons of removing forearm plates used to treat fractures and determined that in young patients, consideration should be given to removal of plates.

56. Rosson JW, Shearer JR: Refracture after the removal of plates from the forearm: an avoidable complication, *J Bone Joint Surg Br* 73:415-417, 1991.

This study evaluated 80 patients with forearm fractures that had subsequent plate removal. Premature plate removal and the use of large fragment plates were identified as causes that increase the rate of refracture.

57. Perren SM, Cordey J, Rahn BA, et al: Early temporary porosis of bone induced by internal fixation implants: a reaction to necrosis, not stress protection? *Clin Orthop Relat Res* 232:139-151, 1988.
This study helped define what the cause of bone loss in the vicinity of implants was attributed to. The authors concluded that the localized bone loss was secondary to necrosis, more so than unloading.

58. Hidaka S, Gustilo RB: Refracture of bones of the forearm after plate removal, *J Bone Joint Surg Am* 66:1241-1243, 1984.
This study reviewed 32 forearm fractures that had plates removed and the resultant refractures that occurred. Seven refractures all occurred within 40 weeks of plate removal. There were no refractures greater than 40 weeks after plate removal.

59. Deluca PA, Lindsey RW, Ruwe PA: Refracture of bones of the forearm after the removal of compression plates, *J Bone Joint Surg Am* 70:1372-1376, 1988.
After 62 forearm plates were removed, there were 7 refractures in this series. Refracture occurred between 42 and 121 days after plate removal. In retrospect, there was radiolucency at the site of the original fracture at the time of plate removal in most patients that refractured.

60. Rosson JW, Petley GW, Shearer JR: Bone structure after removal of internal fixation plates, *J Bone Joint Surg Br* 73:65-67, 1991.
With the use of single-photon absorptiometry, 14 patients with forearm fractures after plate removal were evaluated. Premature plate removal before 16 months resulted in cortical atrophy. The authors suggested plates should be retained for at least 21 months to allow bone density to return to prefracture levels.

61. Kamineni S, Maritz NG, Morrey BF: Proximal radial resection for posttraumatic radioulnar synostosis: a new technique to improve forearm rotation, *J Bone Joint Surg Am* 84-A:745-751, 2002.
The authors treated proximal forearm synostosis in seven patients with resection of a 1-cm thick section of radial shaft just distal to the area of synostosis. Patients retained an average arc of motion of 98 degrees.

62. Jupiter JB, Ring D: Operative treatment of post-traumatic proximal radioulnar synostosis, *J Bone Joint Surg Am* 80:248-257, 1998.
This study describes eighteen limbs in which proximal radioulnar synostosis was resected at an average of 19 months post-injury. Seventeen limbs did not have a recurrence and regained an average of 139 degrees of rotation at an average 34-month follow-up. No postresection prophylaxis was used.

63. Failla JM, Amadio PC, Morrey BF: Post-traumatic proximal radio-ulnar synostosis: results of surgical treatment, *J Bone Joint Surg Am* 71:1208-1213, 1989.
This study evaluated 20 patients with proximal radioulnar synostosis that underwent resection at a mean of 18 months after injury and were followed up at a mean of 40 months post-excision. At the most recent follow-ups patients averaged 55 degrees of active rotation. The authors concluded that outcome of excision varies

with approximately half of the patients receiving significant benefit.

64. Beingessner DM, Patterson SD, King GJ: Early excision of heterotopic bone in the forearm, *J Hand Surg Am* 25:483-488, 2000.
This study evaluated five patients who had early excision (4 months) of heterotopic bone in the forearm and postexcision radiotherapy and indomethacin prophylaxis. At an average of 37 months after excision, patients averaged 136 degrees of forearm rotation.

65. Jessing P: Monteggia lesions and their complicating nerve damage, *Acta Orthop Scand* 46:601-609, 1975.
This study reviewed 14 cases of Monteggia fractures treated over a 10-year period and identified common concomitant nerve injuries. The authors recommended clinical follow-up for the initial 8 weeks if a nerve injury is identified because most of the injuries do not have disruption of nerve continuity.

66. Spinner M, Freundlich BD, Teicher J: Posterior interosseous nerve palsy as a complication of Monteggia fractures in children, *Clin Orthop Relat Res* 58:141-145, 1968. 1968
This is one of the first reports on the association of posterior interosseous nerve injuries seen with Monteggia fractures.

67. Stein F, Grabias SL, Deffer PA: Nerve injuries complicating Monteggia lesions, *J Bone Joint Surg Am* 53:1432-1436, 1971.
This study identified common nerve injuries associated with Monteggia lesions and stressed the importance of identifying them.

68. Brakenbury PH, Corea JR, Blakemore ME: Non-union of the isolated fracture of the ulnar shaft in adults, *Injury* 12:371-375, 1981.
The authors evaluated 21 cases of nonunion in isolated ulna shaft fractures. Location of fracture, initial displacement, comminution, multiple injuries, and early mobilization were all mentioned as predisposing factors. Although plating decreased the nonunion rate, it did not decrease the delayed union rate.

69. Tynan MC, Fornalski S, McMahon PJ, et al: The effects of ulnar axial malalignment on supination and pronation, *J Bone Joint Surg Am* 82-A:1726-1731, 2000.
The objective of this study was to quantify the loss of forearm rotation with malrotation of the ulna in an in vitro model. In all trials, a decrease in forearm rotation after fixation of a poorly rotated ulna was accompanied by an increase in rotation in the opposite direction.

70. Haas N, Hauke C, Schutz M, et al: Treatment of diaphyseal fractures of the forearm using the Point Contact Fixator (PC-Fix): results of 387 fractures of a prospective multicentric study (PC-Fix II), *Injury* 32Suppl 2B51-B62, 2001.
This prospective multicenter study evaluated 387 diaphyseal forearm fractures treated with the point contact fixator (PC-fix II) and concluded that the internal fixator resulted in shorter surgical time and a lower complication rate when compared with data reported in the literature on conventional plating techniques in similar fractures.

71. Hertel R, Eijer H, Meisser A, et al: Biomechanical and biological considerations relating to the clinical use of the Point Contact-Fixator-evaluation of the device handling test in the

treatment of diaphyseal fractures of the radius and/or ulna, *Injury* 32Suppl 2B10-B14, 2001.

This multicenter study evaluated the handling ability, technique of reduction, and type of healing that occurred using the point contact fixator (PC-fix). Fractures healed with callus and it was recommended that three screws be placed on each side of the fracture. Also, early plate removal resulted in a greater rate of refractures than experienced with an early in vivo animal experiment.

CHAPTER 10

Fractures of the Distal Radius

Alfred V. Hess, MD

- The management of distal radius fractures has changed much over the last 25 years. Operative intervention has become more appealing with advances in technique and technology.
- Distal radius fractures have been recognized as a diverse group of injuries with the development of variable treatment options dependent on the particular injury pattern and the patient's overall health.
- Fractures of the distal radius are one of the most common injuries that are seen in emergency departments (EDs) and urgent care centers.
- Distal radius fractures occur in three different population groups: children and adolescents, young adults, and the elderly.
- Children's fractures tend to be extraarticular or involve the distal radius growth plate. Most pediatric fractures do well with reduction and casting given their potential for remodeling.
- Young adults tend toward high-energy mechanisms, such as sport or motor vehicle injuries, and consequently have a higher degree of intraarticular involvement.
- Elderly patients, especially women over 60, tend to require less energy to sustain distal radius fractures as a result of osteoporotic bone. This poor bone quality is detrimental to the maintenance of closed reduction.
- An understanding of the stability of certain fracture patterns and the efficiency of the various treatment options is requisite for those who manage these injuries.
- The outcome of treatment is dependent on the patient's ability to maintain grip strength with minimal pain and deformity.
- This chapter reviews the anatomy, classification, and treatment options for fractures of the distal radius.

Anatomy

- The articular surface of the distal radius is composed of the scaphoid fossa, the lunate fossa, and the sigmoid notch.

The scaphoid and lunate fossa articulates with the carpus. The sigmoid notch articulates with the ulnar head (Figure 10–1).
- The dorsal cortical surface is thin and convexed. The extensor tendons lie in intimate contact with this surface. Lister's tubercle is a midline prominence around which the extensor pollicis longus tendon travels.
- The volar surface of the distal radius is a concaved surface that slopes away from the center point of the distal radius as it proceeds distally up to the watershed line. This flattened area constitutes the area of attachment of the strong palmar wrist capsule (Figure 10–2).
- The hand and the distal radius act as a unit in supination and pronation rotating around the ulnar head. This relationship is stabilized by an ulnar group of ligaments called the triangular fibrocartilage complex (TFCC).
- The distal articular surface of the radius has an average 23-degree (23.6 ± 2.5) radial inclination and 11-degree (11.2 ± 4.6) palmar tilt (Figures 10–3 and 10–4; Box 10–1).

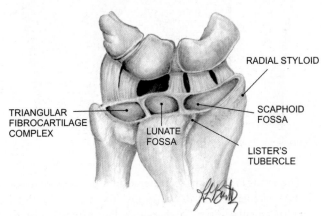

Figure 10–1: **Line diagram of dorsal view of the distal radial articular surface.**

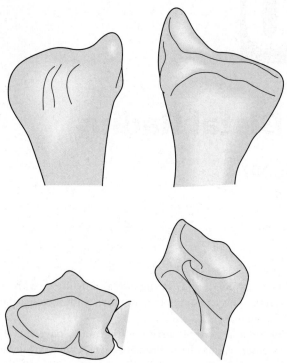

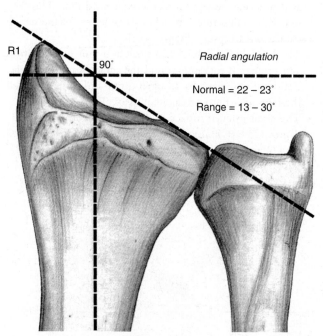

Figure 10–2: **Variable views depicting the surfaces of the distal radius.**

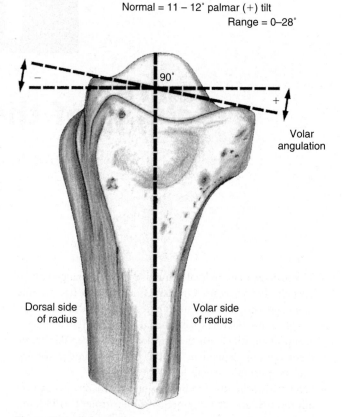

Normal = 11 – 12° palmar (+) tilt
Range = 0–28°

Volar angulation

Dorsal side of radius

Volar side of radius

Figure 10–4: **Palmar tilt.**

R1

90°

Radial angulation

Normal = 22 – 23°
Range = 13 – 30°

Figure 10–3: **Radial inclination.**

The radial inclination is measured in a posterior-anterior (PA) radiograph by drawing one line across the distal radial articular surface and another line perpendicular to the longitudinal axis of the distal radial shaft. The palmar tilt is measured in a lateral radiograph by the angle

Box 10–1   Radiographic Parameters

- Radial inclination 23
- Palmar tilt 11
- Radial length 12 mm
- Ulnar variance <2 mm

between the plane of the articular surface and the line perpendicular to the longitudinal axis.

- The restoration of the normal anatomic architecture is the ultimate goal, which will lead to the most optimal outcome when treating distal radius fractures. Several radiographic parameters help to determine the need for surgery and to predict the ultimate outcome.[1]
- Failure to reduce the palmar tilt to at least −5 degrees can result in an abnormal adaptive carpal malalignment (Figure 10–5). This compensatory dorsal intercolated segmental instability (DISI) pattern leads to abnormal carpal kinematics and progressive instability.
- Congruous articular surfaces of the scaphoid fossa and lunate fossa permit the normal transfer of forces across the wrist and allow for fluid motion of the radiocarpal joint. Knirk and Jupiter[2] were the first to emphasize the importance of this articular congruity. Greater than

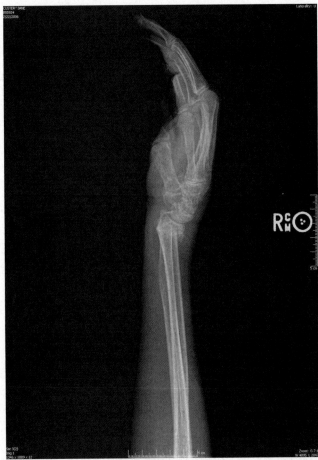

Figure 10–5: Lateral radiograph showing malalignment of the carpus resulting in a compensatory dorsal intercolated segmental instability pattern of carpal alignment. DISI, dorsal intercolated segmental instability.

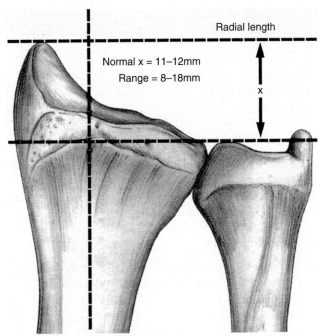

Figure 10–6: Radial height.

2 mm of articular step-off on plain radiographs show a high probability of developing degenerative arthritis. Articular incongruity identified in postreduction films is one of the most significant factors indicating the need for more aggressive surgical treatment.

- The concave articular surface of the sigmoid notch, with its well-defined palmar and dorsal ridges, assist in containing the ulnar head and stabilizing the distal radioulnar joint (DRUJ). Widening or displacement of the sigmoid notch can lead to instability and degenerative arthritis of the DRUJ.

- Radial shortening is the shortening of the distal radius' overall length, which often occurs with metaphyseal comminution and collapse (Figure 10–6). Radial height is measured by drawing a line perpendicular to the radial styloid tip and a line parallel to the distal articular surface of the ulnar head (average 12 mm). The ulnar variance is the difference in height between the articular surface of the lunate fossa and the distal articular surface of the ulnar head. Where the radial length shortens with fracture and the ulnar length remains intact a more positive ulnar

variance is produced. Assessment of ulnar variance depends on a properly positioned PA radiograph with the forearm in neutral rotation and should be compared to the contralateral wrist.

- Radial shortening and increased ulnar variance results in the ulnar head protruding beyond the articular surface of the distal radius, resulting in ulnar head impaction against the ulnar corner of the lunate and possible disruption of the TFCC and the ligamentous support of the DRUJ. Restoration and maintenance of radial height is therefore a primary goal of treatment.

Classification

- Classification systems are used to effectively communicate and exchange ideas regarding fracture treatment. Ideally, a classification system should allow the users to describe the anatomy of the fractures, be highly reproducible among multiple users, include associated soft-tissue injuries, and guide treatment.

- Historically, many classification systems have been proposed for the distal radius fractures. As these classification systems have become more complex, they have been able to more fully differentiate between various fracture patterns and lend themselves more toward the differentiation in treatment options. Unfortunately, the ability of different physicians to agree on the reproducibility of these systems lessens as they become more complex.

- There are several commonly used eponyms of fracture patterns, which should be known by all who study and treat these fractures (Box 10–2).

Box 10–2	Fracture Eponyms

- Colles'
- Smith's
- Barton's
- Chauffeur's
- Die punch

Colles Fractures

- First described by Abraham Colles in 1814, this is an extraarticular fracture of the distal radius with dorsal angulation, dorsal cortical comminution, and radial shortening are also usually part of this pattern (Figure 10–7).

Smith's Fracture

- This eponym is usually used in reference to the reverse of a Colles fracture with volar angulation (Figure 10–8).

Barton's Fracture

- This fracture pattern is usually described as either a dorsal or volar Barton's fracture. These intraarticular fractures involve the dorsal or volar lip of the articular surface of the distal radius with subsequent volar or radial subluxation of the carpus (Figure 10–9).

Chauffeur's Fracture

- This fracture pattern was originally described as the result of back firing of the crank used to start early model automobiles. It is an intraarticular fracture of the radial styloid (Figure 10–10).

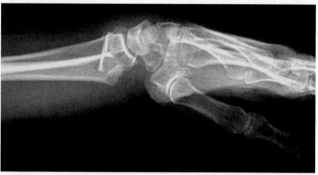

Figure 10–7: **Colles' fracture.**

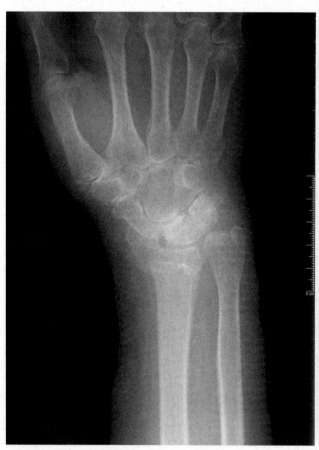

Figure 10–8: **Smith's fracture.**

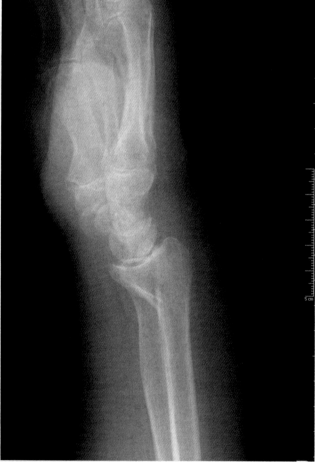

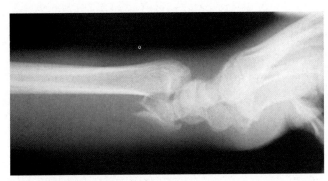

Figure 10–9: **Volar Barton's fracture.**

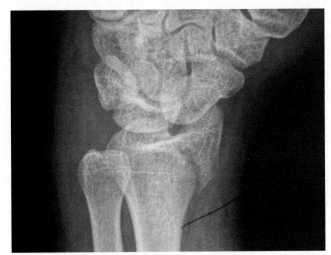

Figure 10–10: **Chauffeur's fracture.**

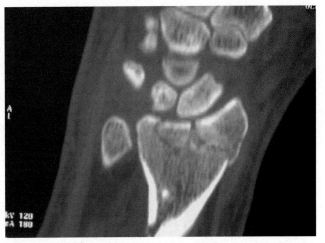

Figure 10–11: **Computed tomography scan demonstrating a die-punch fragment.**

Die-Punch Fracture

- This eponym is typically used to describe a fracture pattern with a depressed lunate fossa fragment. It is also commonly used to describe centrally depressed articular segment, which is often overlooked on plane radiograph and is best diagnosed by computed tomograph (CT) scan (Figure 10–11).

Classification Systems

- The Frykman classification is an early system that separated fracture patterns by differentiating extraarticular and intraarticular fractures of both the radiocarpal joint and the DRUJ. It further separated these patterns by whether or not there was involvement of the radial styloid (Figure 10–12).
- Classifications were subsequently proposed to aid in the differentiation of fracture stability, amount of displacement, and need for surgery. The AO classification is still widely used in publication because of its universal acceptance[3] (Figure 10–13).
  1. The three major types are: type A (extraarticular), type B (partial articular), and type C (complete articular).

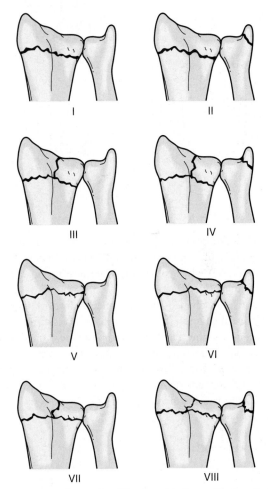

Figure 10–12: **Frykman classification.** (Frykman G: *Acta Orthop Scand* 108:1-155, 1967.)

2. These are further subgrouped to produce 27 different fracture patterns.
3. As each pattern is further broken down, there is less interobserver reproducibility.

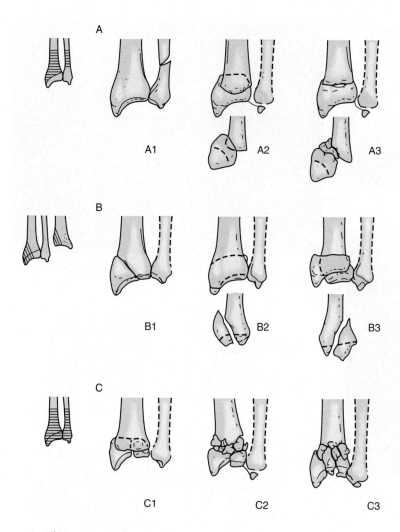

Figure 10–13: AO classification of distal radius fractures. (Muller ME, Allgower M, Schneider R, et al: *Manual of internal fixation: techniques recommended by the AO-ASIF Group,* ed 3, Berlin, 1991, Springer-Verlag.)

4. This system takes into account the severity of the intraarticular involvement and the metaphyseal comminution, which obviously have bearing on the need for operative intervention.

- Medoff[4] has divided the intraarticular fracture fragments into five fragments. This system has advanced the understanding of the radiographic appearance of displaced intraarticular fractures. It is a treatment-oriented classification that lends itself toward the use of fragment specific modular implants (Figure 10–14).

- The five main fragment types are the:
  1. radial styloid.
  2. volar lip.
  3. articular surface.
  4. dorsal wall.
  5. ulnar corner.

- Fernandez[5] proposed a classification system based on the mechanism of injury (Figure 10–15). He has divided this system into five major types, including:
  1. Type I—bending fractures of the metaphysis.
  2. Type II—shearing fractures of the joint surface.
  3. Type III—compression fractures of the joint surface.
  4. Type IV—avulsion fractures of the ligament attachments.

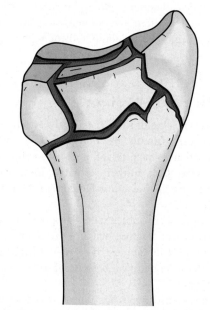

Figure 10–14: **Fragment specific view of distal radius.**

Fracture types (adults) Based on the mechanism of injury	Children fracture equivalent	Stability/instability: high risk of secondary displacement after initial adequate reduction	Displacement pattern	Number of fragments	Associated lesions carpal ligament, fractures, median, ulnar nerve, tendons, ipsilat. fx upper extremity compartment syndrome	Recommended treatment
Type 1 Bending fracture of the metaphysis 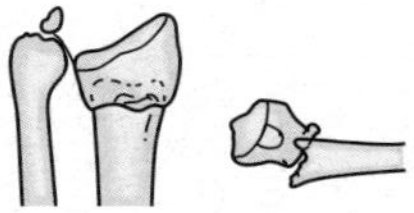	Distal forearm fracture Salter II	Stable Unstable	Nondisplaced Dorsally Colles, Volarly Smith, Proximal Combined	Always 2 main fragments + Varying degree of metaphyseal comminution (instability)	Uncommon	Conservative (stable fxs) Percutaneous pinning (extra- or intrafocal) External fixation (exceptionally bone graft)
Type II Shearing fracture of the joint surface 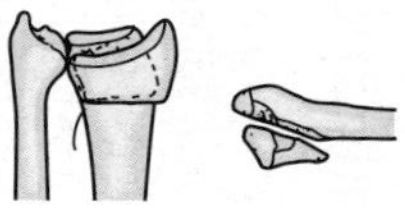	Salter IV	Unstable	Dorsal Barton, Radial chauffeur, Volar rev. Barton, Combined	Two-part Three-part Comminuted	Less uncommon	Open reduction Screw/plate fixation
Type III Compression fracture of the joint surface 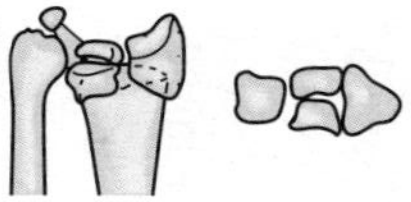	Salter III, IV, V	Stable Unstable	Nondisplaced Dorsal Radial Volar Proximal Combined	Two part Three part Four part Comminuted	Common	Conservative Closed, Limited, arthroscopic assisted or extensile open reduction Percutaneous pins External fixation Internal fixation Plate, bone graft
Type IV Avulsion fractures, radiocarpal fracture dislocation 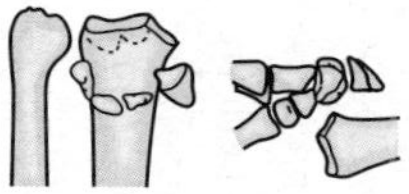	Very rare	Unstable	Dorsal Radial Volar Proximal Combined	Two part (radial styloid ulnar styloid) Three part (volar, dorsal margin) Comminuted	Frequent	Closed or open reduction Pin or screw fixation Tension wiring
Type V Combined fractures I, II, III, IVI High-velocity injury 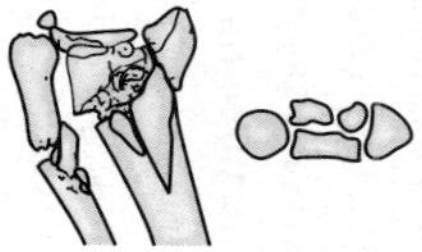	Very rare	Unstable	Dorsal Radial Volar Proximal Combined	Comminuted and/or bone loss (frequently intra-articular, open, seldom extra-articular)	Always present	Combined method

Figure 10–15: Fernandez classification of distal radius fractures. Jupiter JB, Fernandez DL.: *J Hand Surg Am* 22:563–571, 1997.

5. Type V—high-velocity injuries that involve combinations of bending, compression, shearing, and avulsion mechanisms.

- In this classification there are pediatric equivalents, probability of associated soft-tissue injuries and recommended treatment. He has also combined this with a classification of associated DRUJ injuries.

Initial Evaluation

- Before treatment, the wrist deformity should be observed and documented. The presence or absence of an open injury requires full inspection of the wrist by taking down the initial splint often applied to check for skin problems.
- Documentation of neurological (sensation) and vascular status (capillary refill, pulses, and swelling) is also done.

Radiology

- The initial radiographs should at least include a PA view and lateral view (Figure 10–16).
- A 10-degree lateral projection is taken with the wrist in neutral rotation and the wrist elevated 10 degrees off the film plane. This lateral view more clearly delineates the articular surface and can aid in delineating the palmar tilt (Figure 10–17).
- CT scans can be helpful in evaluating articular congruity if warranted, but they should not cause a delay in treatment.

Treatment of Nondisplaced Acute Distal Radius Fractures

- Nondisplaced fractures are treated with an initial sugar tong splint (Figure 10–18).
- This splint is changed to a short arm cast at 2 to 3 weeks post-injury.
- At 6 weeks, the cast is removed and wrist range-of-motion exercises are started.
- Patients often benefit from a removable wrist splint after casting so they can wean themselves out of it over a 3-week period. Wrist range of motion can be started by removing the splint three times daily to perform exercises.
- Finger range of motion is encouraged as soon as the initial sugar tong splint is applied. Shoulder and elbow range of motion is also encouraged to prevent stiffness.
- Splints should not unnecessarily restrict finger range of motion.

Closed Reduction Method

Anesthesia

- A hematoma block using 1% lidocaine without epinephrine is used in acute fractures. An 18-gauge to 20-gauge needle is used with a volar entrance into the fracture site.

- Conscious sedation can be used in an ED setting, especially for pediatric patients.
- Axillary blocks are used in late initial reductions or late remanipulation.
- General anesthesia is reserved for open fractures and those fractures that require operative intervention.

Reduction Techniques

Manual Reduction

- An assistant or finger traps provides longitudinal traction.
- The surgeon places himself in the supine patient's axilla.
- The fracture deformity is first increased to unlock the fragments.
- Then, while longitudinal traction is applied by an assistant, the surgeon manipulates the distal fragment in a volar and ulnar direction (in the case of Colles' fracture), with the forearm in pronation.
- This fracture reduction is completed with a volar directed force from the surgeon's thumbs.
- A Smith's type fracture requires a dorsal directed force with the forearm in supination

Longitudinal Traction

- Longitudinal traction can be applied by placing the patient's thumb, index, and middle fingers in finger traps and hanging them from an intravenous (IV) pole (Figure 10–19).
- Counter weights, 5 to 15 pounds, are hung from the patient's upper arm, with the elbow flexed 90 degrees. Commercially available traction devices are used in many EDs and operating rooms (ORs).
- Hanging the hand for 5 to 10 minutes before reduction assists in disimpacting the fragments and relaxing the patient's musculature.
- The reduction technique is similar with dorsal to volar pressure from the surgeon's thumb to lock in the fragments.
- The finger trap method allows for continued traction while placing and molding the splints.

Immobilization

- The preferred method of immobilization is a well-molded sugar tong splint.
  1. A dorsal mold is applied directly over the midcarpus.
  2. A volar mold is applied just proximal to the fracture line.
  3. A more proximal dorsal mold over the forearm is applied for a firm three-point fixation.
- A slight ulna deviation and pronation position is maintained in Colles' type fractures to realign the distal radius fragment with the radial shaft and ulna. Acute flexion of the wrist, the so-called "Cotton Loader" position, should be avoided.[6] This places undue pressure on the median nerve and has been associated with chronic regional pain syndrome.

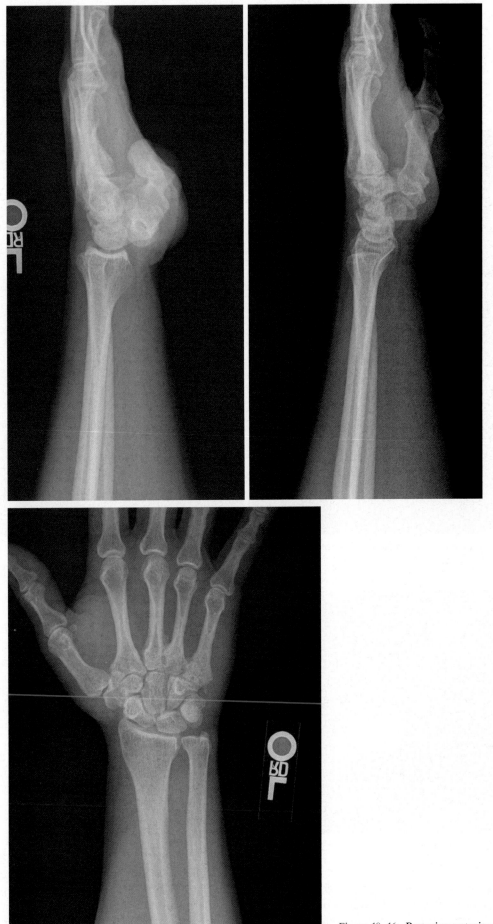

Figure 10–16: Posterior-anterior, lateral, and 10-degree lateral views of a normal wrist.

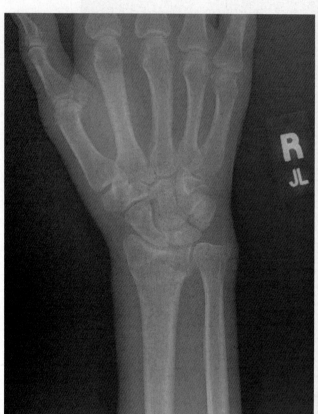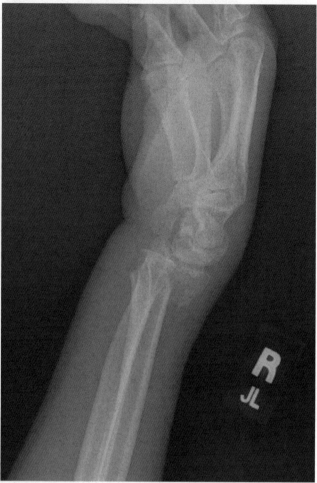

Figure 10–17: **Posterior-anterior and lateral views of a fractured distal radius.**

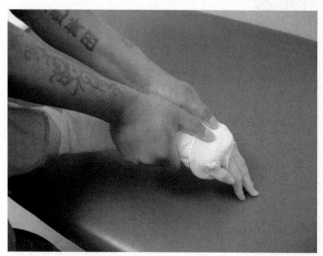

Figure 10–18: **Sugar tong splint.**

- The ideal position to maintain Colles' type fractures is 15 degrees of palmar flexion, 10 to 15 degrees of ulnar deviation and 25 degrees of pronation. If this position cannot

maintain alignment, then other means of fixation are indicated.

- Stable fractures are maintained in the initial splint for 2 to 3 weeks with weekly radiographs to check alignment. The splint can be rewrapped if it becomes loose.
- The splint is changed to a short arm cast for the final 2 to 4 weeks for a total of 6 weeks immobilization.
- The patient is encouraged to begin finger range-of-motion exercises immediately after reduction and continue throughout treatment.
- A removable wristlet splint is given to the patient at 6 weeks with instruction to remove it and do range-of-motion exercises at least three times a day and to wean out of the brace over 3 weeks.

Unstable Distal Radius Fractures

- Although an initial attempt at closed reduction should be made for most distal radius fractures, unstable fractures require further intervention to achieve and maintain correction.

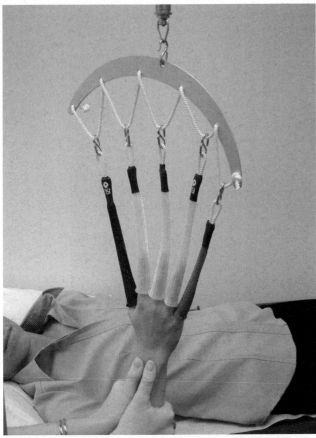

Figure 10–19: **Picture of hand in finger traps and traction reduction technique.**

- Fractures with an initial high degree of comminution, initial displacement, and those in patients over 60 are considered potentially unstable (Box 10–3).

Displaced Distal Radius Fractures

- A distal radius fracture with greater than 1 mm of articular step-off, loss of more than 20 degrees of palmar tilt, loss greater than 5 degrees of radial inclination, or greater than 3 mm of radial shortening is by definition displaced, and an attempt at reduction should be made.[7–9]
- Displaced distal radius fractures are treated with initial closed reduction and splinting.

Box 10–3 Factor Affecting Stability
• Degree of comminution
• Degree of initial displacement
• Initial dorsal angulation >20 degrees
• Intraarticular involvement
• Significant radial shortening
• Age >60

- Initial closed reduction should be done expeditiously. Fresh fractures are much easier to reduce before consolidation of the fracture hematoma that always occurs.
- Significantly displaced fractures can put continued pressure on the median nerve and vascular structures and therefore should be treated with initial reduction as soon as possible.

Operative Treatment of Unstable Distal Radius Fractures

Closed Reduction and Percutaneous Pinning

- Kirschner wires (K-wires; 1 mm or 0.625 inches) can be placed percutaneously to aid and maintain reduction (Figure 10–20; Boxes 10–4 and 10–5).
- These pins can be placed mainly through the radial styloid and into the proximal fragments' ulnar cortex to help maintain reduction of unstable fractures.[10]
- Pins are placed through small incisions with the use of a drill guide on bone to prevent cutaneous nerve injury and painful neuromas.
- The Kapandji technique uses these pins as levers throughout the fracture to help reduce and maintain length, radial inclination, and volar tilt.[11,12]
- The pins can also be placed throughout the ulna to help maintain length. The wrist is maintained in a splint or cast.
- The pins are capped and left out of the skin to be pulled at 4 to 5 weeks. After pulling pins, the wrist is usually casted for an additional 2 weeks.
- This technique is best reserved for simpler extraarticular fractures and does not impart significant stability to elderly patients.[13]
- Incisions and the use of drill sleeves lessen the chances of cutaneous nerve injury.
- The pins are placed under image intensification with the hand suspended in finger traps.

External Fixation

- External fixation has been used with success by applying and maintaining traction across the wrist while the fracture heals (Figure 10–21). This technique relies on ligamentotaxis to reduce and constrain the fracture while healing occurs, eliminating the joint reactive forces across the wrist.
- Excessive traction causes joint stiffness and median nerve dysfunction.[14]

Technique of External Fixation

- A brachial plexus block or general anesthesia and a tourniquet are used when applying an external fixator (Figure 10–22).

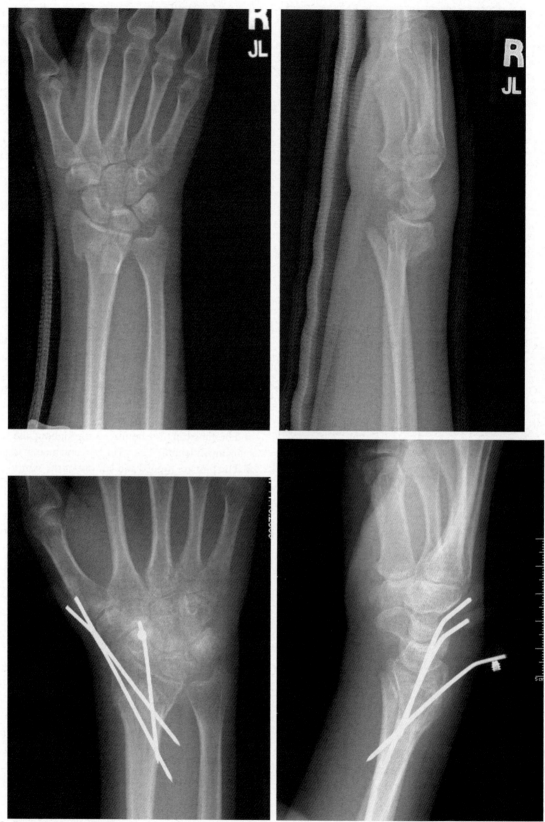

Figure 10–20: **Preoperative and postoperative views of a fracture treated with Kirschner wire fixation.**

| | |
| Box 10–4 | **Treatment Goals** |

- Restore and maintain length
- Restore radial tilt and inclination
- Reduce articular step off
- Restore distal radioulnar joint (DRUJ) stability
- Identify and treat associated injuries

| | |
| Box 10–5 | **Operative Treatment of Unstable Distal Radius Fractures** |

- Closed reduction and percutaneous pinning
- External fixation
- External fixation and percutaneous pinning
- External fixation with open reduction and internal fixation (ORIF)
- ORIF
  - Dorsal plating
  - Volar plating
  - Fragment specific fixation
- Arthroscopic assisted reduction and internal fixation

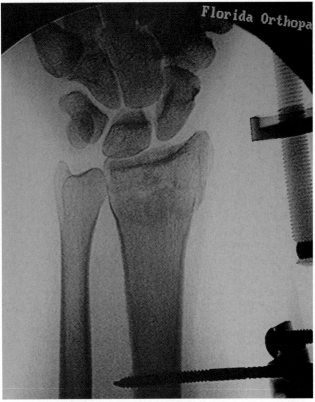

Figure 10–22: **Posterior-anterior radiograph of the previous wrist demonstrating a reduced distal radius fracture treated by external fixation.**

- Sterile finger traps can be used to apply traction with the hand suspended or by applying the traction over the end of the hand table.
- The C-arm fluoroscope is used to assist in pin placement and to judge reduction.
- Many external fixators are available, which have been designed for use across the wrist. These designs incorporate 3-mm half pins, with two placed in the second metacarpal and two in the radial shaft, proximal to the fracture.
- Using the C-arm to help guide pin placement, two small skin incisions are placed over the dorsoradial aspect of the second metacarpal. Blunt dissection is carried down

to bone to avoid tendon and cutaneous nerve injury. A double pin guide is used to place the self-tapping half pins in a bicortical fashion.

- A single 3- to 4-cm incision is then placed over the dorsoradial aspect of the radius shaft. Blunt dissection is carried down to the bone, finding and protecting the dorsal

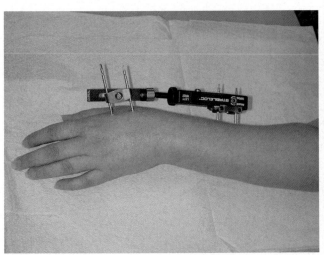 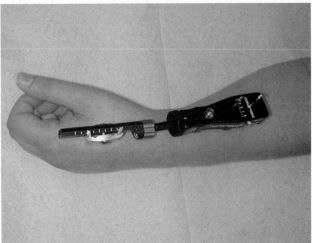

Figure 10–21: **Pictures of a hand and wrist with an external fixator in place.**

sensory branch of the radial nerve. The half pins are again placed in a bicortical fashion and checked with the C-arm.

- The proximal incision is closed and the frame is assembled. Newer universal pin clamps allow for three-dimensional (3D) adjustments of pins relative to the frame. This allows for greater flexibility in adjustment of the frame and less rigidly precise pin placement.
- Fine tuning adjustments are made to the frame using the C-arm to judge final reduction.
- Avoidance of overdistraction is judged by observing full passive range of motion of the fingers and observance of the intercarpal distraction.
- If a nonbridging external fixator is used, the distal pins are placed ulnarly between the fourth and fifth dorsal compartments and radially between the first and second dorsal compartments.
- Percutaneous pinning with 0.045- or 0.065-inch K-wires can be used as an adjunct to external fixation. One or two pins are placed through the radial styloid, and one pin is placed through the dorsomedial portion of the distal radius.
- External fixation can also be used in conjunction with open reduction and internal fixation (ORIF), with bone grafting, and with arthroscopically assisted reduction of intraarticular displacement.[15]

Dorsal Distraction Plate

- An excellent method for the treatment of highly comminuted fractures of the distal radial diaphysis is the use of a dorsal plate, which is fixed to the third metacarpal and the proximal radial diaphysis (Figure 10–23). A rigid 3.5-mm-long plate is used. Three bicortical screws are placed in the third metacarpal. The plate is then pushed distally and secured to the radius proximal to the fracture. Bone graft is often used to fill the defect.[16–18]
- The plate is left in until there is radiographic union, an average of 3 months.
- After removal, range-of-motion exercise is started.
- This technique is used in high-energy injuries, which are highly unstable as a result of the extensive comminution and can be used with supplemental K-wire fixation to restore articular congruity.

Arthroscopic Assisted Reduction of Distal Radius Fracture

- As more surgeons have become adept at wrist arthroscopy, the use of the arthroscope for the treatment of distal radius fractures has become more popular.[19]
- Arthroscopic-assisted reduction and pinning can be used in conjunction with an external fixator to achieve good results.
- The wrist is placed in a traction tower and percutaneous wires or small elevators are used to manipulate the articular fragments. The fragments are secured with pin fixation. An external fixator is applied to maintain some traction.
- This method is especially well suited for those injuries without excessive metaphyseal comminution.
- The use of the arthroscope to judge intraarticular reduction has been reported to be superior over fluoroscopy.

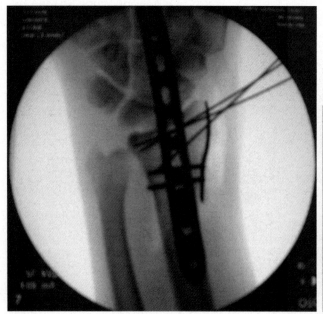
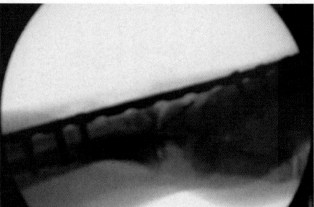

Figure 10–23: **Radiograph of a distal radius fracture treated with a dorsal spanning plate.**

Fragment-Specific Approach

- Medoff has developed an internal fixation system that uses small wireform and pin plate implants to stabilize intraarticular fracture of the distal radius.[20–23]
- This approach uses small incisions; utilizes dorsal, radial, and palmar implants; and provides secure fixation through the application of orthogonal internal constructs.
- The criticism of this system is its high learning curve and the need to remove irritation dorsal and radial implants.
- This design has been extended to develop multiple small radial and dorsal plates for fragment specific fixation (Figure 10–24).

Limited Open Reduction and Internal Fixation

- If there is still minimal displacement of an intraarticular fragment after closed reduction, a minimally invasive approach can be taken to achieve reduction. This is usually done for displaced volar or dorsal lunate fossa fracture fragments.
- The volar fragment can be reduced through a volar incision located proximal to the wrist crease and parallel to the flexor carpi ulnaris (FCU) tendon. Dissection is carried down radial to the ulnar artery to the wrist capsule. The pronator quadratus is elevated off its ulnar attachment, if necessary.
- The volar fragment is reduced and pinned through the dorsal cortex. The pin is pulled through the dorsal skin and left just through the volar cortex.
- The dorsal fragment is approached via a limited incision over and through the fifth dorsal compartment. The fragment is reduced under direct view and fixed with K-wires through the distal fragment and into the volar radial intact proximal cortex or through a wire placed through the radial styloid fragment and into the reduced dorsal ulnar fragment or both.
- A small arthrotomy can be made to visualize the lunate fossa.
- This fixation is best supplemented with external fixation or sugar tong splint.

Open Reduction and Internal Fixation

- Recent advances in internal fixation have improved both the ease of use and the rigidity of the internal fixation (Box 10–6). Specifically, the development of fragment specific fixation and fixed-angle plates allow for rigid fixation and early range of motion of intraarticular unstable fractures.[24–26]

Plate Design

- The advent of fixed angle plates has greatly improved the treatment of unstable distal radius fractures.[17]
- Screws or pegs that lock into the plate exert a blade plate type effect supporting the subchondral bone and preventing collapse and radial shortening.
- Fixed-angle devices lessen the need for bone graft; however, grafting of large metaphyseal defects is still recommended. Fixed-angle devices allow the application of a volarly placed plate to support the dorsal articular surface from collapse. This permits the thin and often highly comminuted dorsal cortex to consolidate out to length instead of collapsing under the joint reactive forces with the contracture of forearm musculature.[27]

Dorsal Plating

- Dorsal plating can be used with good results, but it has been abandoned by most surgeons in favor of volar plating as a result of the high incidence of extensor tendon irritation and rupture, but volar plates have been used with great success.[28–30]
- Dorsal plating is indicated in displaced dorsal rims or shear type fractures (Barton's).
- Smaller dorsal column plates, wireforms, or pin or plates are available to elevate and support dorsal die-punch lesions and ulnar column fragments. These devices can also be used as a dorsal buttress.
- Dorsal plates are in intimate contact with the extensor tendons and have been linked to late tendon rupture and pain secondary to tendonitis.
- If used, secondary plate removal is often needed.
- A retinacular flap to cover the plate and dorsal transposition of the extensor pollicis longus are done with closure to protect the tendons.
- Bone grafting is recommended.[31]

Advantages of Volar Plate Fixation

- Straightforward reduction of the volar cortex allows for restoration of the radial length and ulnar inclination[26] (Figure 10–25). Avoidance of dorsal dissection protects the periosteal sleeve and vascularity of the highly comminuted dorsal cortex.
- The concave anatomy of the volar cortex allows for a plate application that is deep and not in contact with the flexor tendons. The pronator quadratus muscle further protects these tendons.

Volar Fixed-Angled Plate Technique

- An 8- to 10-cm incision parallels the flexor carpi radialis (FCR) tendon (Figure 10–26).

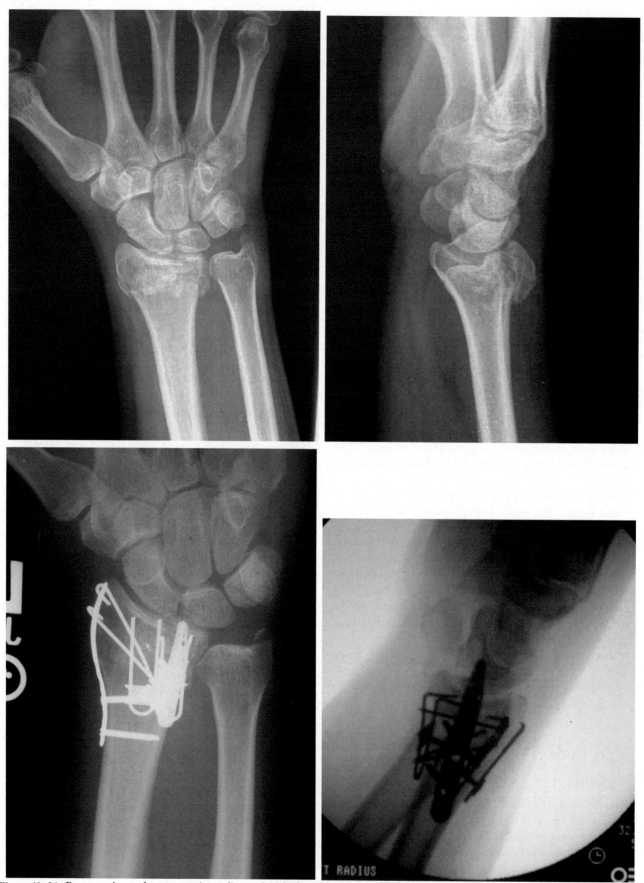

Figure 10–24: **Preoperative and postoperative radiographs of a fracture treated with fragment specific fixation.**

Box 10–6	Indications for Open Reduction and Internal Fixation

- Unstable extraarticular fractures
- Shear-type fractures (Barton's and volar Barton's type fracture)
- Intraarticular displacement greater the 2 mm
- Instability of the distal radioulnar joint
- Secondary to marginal fractures of the sigmoid notch
- Loss of initial reduction
- Fractures associated with carpal injuries
- Fractures associated with severe soft-tissue injuries (nerve, tendon, vessel compartment syndrome, or soft-tissue loss)
- Associated ipsilateral upper extremity fractures
- Associated multiple long-bone fractures

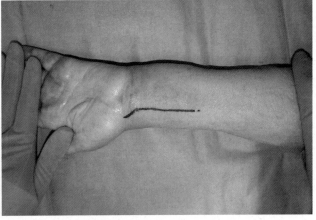

Figure 10–26: **Volar approach incision.**

- Dissection is carried down between the FCR and the radial artery to the pronator quadratus muscle (Figure 10–27).
- The pronator quadratus is detached from the radial border of the distal radius and elevated ulnarly.
- The brachioradialis is released with a step-cut incision near its distal insertion on the radial styloid so that it may be repaired later (Figure 10–28).
- The fracture is then reduced and temporary fixation is done with a K-wire in the radial styloid.

- A fixed-angle volar plate is then applied with a proximal shaft screw through the sliding hole.
- Flouroscopy is used to determine plate position.
- A 20-degree lateral projection is used to guide fixed-angle pin placement. Ideal pin placement is in the dorsal subcondral bone.
- Complete the plate fixation (Figure 10–29).
- Repairing the brachoradialis tendon allows its use as an anchor for the repair of the pronator quadratus over the plate.

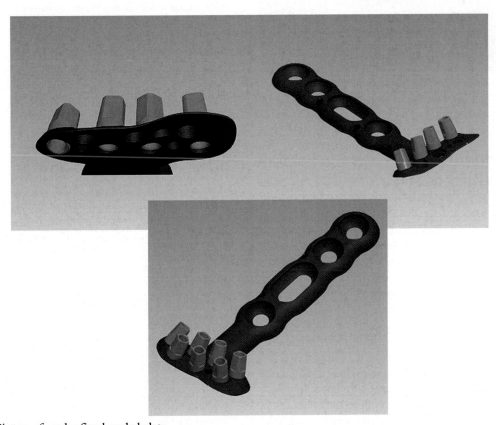

Figure 10–25: **Picture of a volar fixed angled plate.**

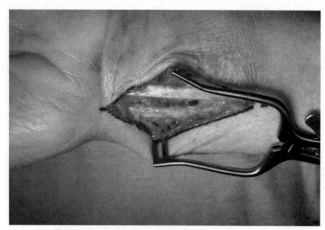

Figure 10–27: Interval between the flexor carpi radialis tendon and the radial artery.

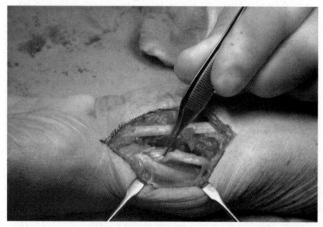

Figure 10–28: Brachioradialis is released from the radial styloid fragment.

Postoperative Care

- Apply volar splint for 10 to 14 days to allow for soft-tissue recovery.
- Begin finger motion immediately postoperatively.
- Start wrist range of motion after initial splint removal.
- A removable splint is used between range-of-motion exercises, after initial postoperative splint is removed for 4 to 6 weeks.
- Postoperative radiographs are obtained at 2 and 6 weeks.

Bone Grafting and Bone Graft Substitutes

- The distal radius lends itself to bone grafting as a result of the metaphyseal defects often caused by impacting fractures to this area. The recent development of multiple bone graft substitutes has increased the options available.

Fixed-angle plates have decreased the need for structural support provided by bone grafting.

- The decision to graft bone is based on the patient, the particular fracture pattern, and the fracture management technique used. Bone grafting can provide osteogenic precursors and osteoconductive, osteoinductive, and structural support.
- Autogenous bone graft, such as iliac crest bone graft, can provide the above advantages but carry with them the morbidity of harvesting. The use of allograft decreases morbidity and is usually sufficient in the treatment of metaphyseal defects.[26]
- The development of injectable cement, combined with limited internal fixation, has shown early functional return in multicenter studies.[33] This technique is limited by the material's lack of torsional and shear strength. Care must be exercised to not allow the cement to leak into surrounding soft tissue.

Distal Radioulnar Joint Instabilities

- DRUJ stability should be evaluated after stable fixation of the distal radius is achieved. Adequate reduction of the distal radius anatomy is an important aspect in achieving DRUJ stability. Widening or incomplete reduction of the sigmoid notch can lead to instability and pain.[34]
- Immobilizing the DRUJ in 45 to 90 degrees of supination for 6 weeks is often enough to restore stability. Transfixing the radial shaft to the ulnar shaft with two 0.065-inch K-wires proximal to the joint can also be used to achieve stability.
- When the ulnar styloid fragment includes the foveal insertion of the TFCC, internal fixation with tension band wiring, or ulnar pin plates may be indicated. An ulnar styloid fracture with significant displacement especially those with palmarly displaced styloid fragments should be treated with internal fixation.

Carpal Ligamentous Injuries

- Certain fracture patterns, such as radiocarpal fracture-dislocations and highly displaced radial styloid fractures, have a high incident of intercarpal ligament disruption. There is a 30% incidence of scapholunate and a 15% incidence of lunotriguetral ligament tears seen by both arthrography and arthroscopy in fractures of the distal radius.
- Those fractures that demonstrate dissociative type instability of the carpus should be addressed by open repair techniques at the time of fracture fixation, if possible.

Patients Who Are Elderly or Debilitated

- A less aggressive approach is taken for patients who are elderly or fragile as a result of poor health. Bone and soft-tissue quality does not lend itself to invasive treatments.

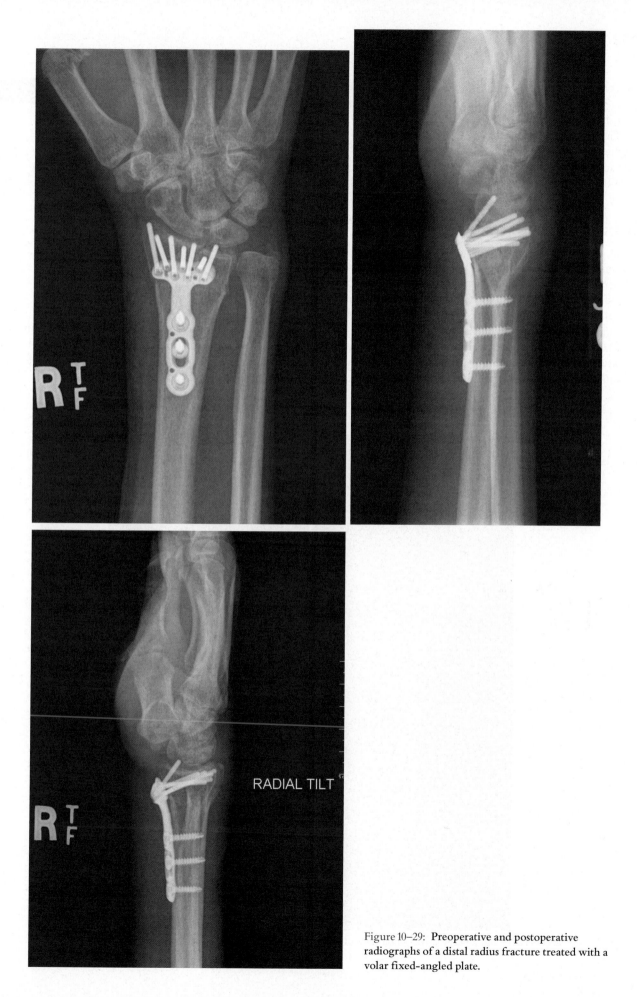

Figure 10–29: Preoperative and postoperative radiographs of a distal radius fracture treated with a volar fixed–angled plate.

- Treatment should proceed with initial closed reduction and placement in a well-padded sugar tong, followed by a short-arm cast at 2 to 3 weeks after reduction.
- The cast can be replaced by a removable splint at 6 to 8 weeks.
- Late deformity can be addressed by ulnar shortening only if the patient's symptoms warrant it.

Complications

- In contrast to the earlier reports, there is a significant complication rate and unsatisfactory results in distal radius fracture outcomes. Poor outcomes are associated with radiocarpal and radiulnar arthritis, malunion, nonunion, persistent neuropathy, late tendon ruptures, wrist and hand stiffness, and reflex sympathetic dystrophy[35–38] (Box 10–7)
- Malunions of the distal radius are still common despite advances in treatment. These malunions can result in significant deformity, pain, and loss of motion.

Box 10–7	Complications

- Malunion
- Nonunion
- Arthritis
- Persistent neuropathy
- Tendon rupture
- Stiffness
- Reflex sympathetic dystrophy (RSD)
- Infection
- Volkmann's ischemia
- Distal radioulnar joint (DRUJ) instability
- Carpal instability

- Malunions are successfully treated with both intraarticular and extraarticular osteotomies of the distal radius. Intraarticular osteotomies can be used to elevate missed Die-punch lesion of the radial articular surface.

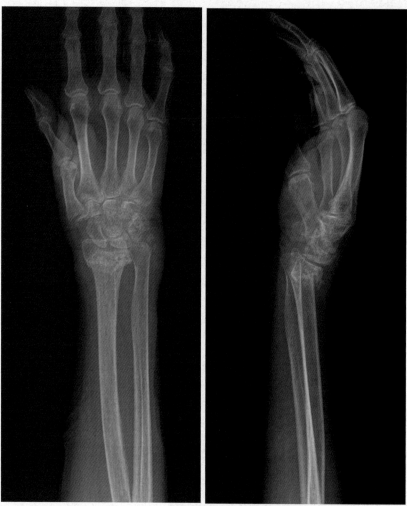

Figure 10–30: **Preoperative and postoperative radiographs of a malunion treated with a distal radius osteotomy.**

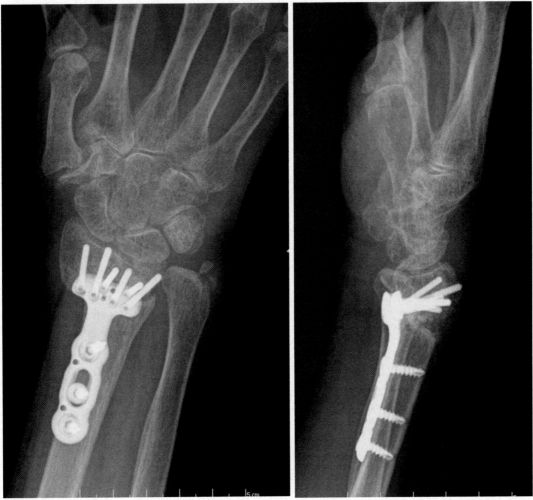

Figure 10–30, cont'd:

- Extraarticular osteotomies are used to correct radial length, palmar tilt, radial inclination, and rotational deformities of the distal radius.[39,40]
- The osteotomy and approach can be either dorsal or volar.
- I prefer a volar approach with the use of a fixed-angle volar plate for both Smith's and Colles' type deformities. Open wedge osteotomies are secured with the fixed angle plate, and the wedge is packed with cancellous bone graft (Figure 10–30).
- Protected wrist range of motion can be started 4 to 6 weeks after surgery, but the patient wears a removable splint and is warned against weight-bearing until radiographic consolidation occurs at the osteotomy site (usually by 3 months).
- Radial shortening without significant angular deformity of the radial articular surface can be treated with ulnar shortening osteotomies.

Conclusions

- Distal radius fractures are one of the most frequently encountered injuries seen in orthopaedic practices.
- There is a wide variety of fracture patterns and associated injuries that dictate the need for operative versus closed management.
- The multiple surgical approaches available allow the surgeon to vary his or her approach based on the patient's age, health, and concomitant injuries, and on the surgeon's own expertise.[41]
- Outcomes are not always satisfactory, especially in high-energy injuries and those that involve the articular surfaces.

Annotated References

1. Mackenney PJ, McQueen MM, Elton R: Prediction of instability in distal radial fractures, *J Bone Joint Surg Am* 88:1944-1951, 2006.

2. Knirk JL, Jupiter JB: Intra-articular fractures of the distal end of the radius in young adults, *J Bone Joint Surg Am* 68:647-659, 1986.

This oft-cited article established the idea that reduction of intraarticular step-offs to less than 2 mm is the most important factor in preventing arthritis.

3. Muller ME, Allgower M, Schneider R, et al: *Manual of internal fixation: techniques recommended by the AO-ASIF group*, ed 3, Berlin, 1970, Springer-Verlag.

4. Robert Medoff: Essential radiographic evaluation for distal radius fractures, *Hand Clin* 21:279-288, 2005.

A review of plain radiographs of the distal radius and how to interpret differences seen in distal radius fractures. An excellent explanation of the 10-degree lateral view.

5. Jupiter JB, Fernandez DL: Comparative classification for fractures of the distal end of the radius, *J Hand Surg Am* 22:563-571, 1997.

6. Cotton FJ: The pathology of fracture of the lower extremity of the radius, *Ann Surg* 32:194-218, 1900.

The author advocated a position of extreme flexion and ulnar deviation to immobilize distal radius fractures. Although this position may aid in providing ligamentotaxis to the dorsal and radial fragments, it is associated with a high incidence of median nerve compression and has been abandoned.

7. Trumble TE, Schmitt SR, Vedder NB: Internal fixation of pilon fractures of the distal radius, *Yale J Biol Med* 66:179-191, 1993.

Recommended supplemental fixation of fractures with greater than 2 mm of radial shortening and greater than 15 degrees of dorsal tilt after closed reduction.

8. Fernandez DL, Geissler WB: Treatment of displaced articular fractures of the radius, *J Hand Surg Am* 16:375-384, 1991.

A review of 40 articular fractures of the distal radius after percutaneous pinning or open reduction and internal fixation (ORIF). Over 90% had a less than 1 mm intraarticular step-off on follow-up, with less than 5% developing radiocarpal arthritis. These authors concluded that stable fixation and reduction of intraarticular malalignment to less than 1 mm should be the goal of operative intervention.

9. Wright TW, Horodyski M, Smith DW: Functional outcome of unstable distal radius fractures: ORIF with a volar fixed-angle time plate versus external fixation, *J Hand Surg Am* 30: 289-299, 2005.

A comparison study of open reduction and internal fixation (ORIF) with a fixed angle volar plate versus external fixation for the treatment of what the author termed unstable distal radius fractures. The PRWE and DASH scores were equivalent in both groups. The radiographic parameters of intraarticular step-ff, volar tilt, and radial length showed less complications in the ORIF group.

10. Kapandji IA: The Kapandji-Sauve operation: its techniques and indications in non rheumatoid diseases, *Ann Chir Main* 5: 181-193, 1986.

11. Trumble TE, Wagner W, Hanel, DP, et al: Intrafocal (Kapandji) pinning of distal radius fractures with and without external fixation, *J Hand Surg Am* 23:381-394, 1998.

12. Ruschel PH, Albertonin WM: Treatment of unstable extra-articular distal radius fractures by modified intrafocal Kapandji method, *Tech Hand Up Extrem Surg* 9:7-16, 2005.

13. Azzopardi T, Ehrendorfer S, Coulton, T, et al: Unstable extra-articular fractures of the distal radius: a prospective, randomized study of immobilization in a cast versus supplementary percutaneous pinning, *J Bone Joint Surg Br* 87:837-840, 2005.

14. Papadonikolakis A, Shen J, Garrett, JP, et al: The effect of the increasing distraction on digital motion after external fixation of the wrist, *J Hand Surg Am* 30:773-779, 2005.

15. Harley BJ, Scharfenberger A, Beaupre, LA, et al: Augmented external fixation versus percutaneous pinning and casting for unstable fractures of the distal radius: a prospective randomized trial, *J Hand Surg Am* 29:815-824, 2004.

16. Ruch DS, Ginn TA, Yang, CC, et al: Use of distraction plate for distal radial fractures with metaphyseal and diaphyseal comminution, *J Bone Joint Surg Am* 87:945-954, 2005.

The authors describe their experience with 22 patients using a 3.5-mm dorsal plate from the third metacarpal to the radial cortex proximal to the fracture. This plate acts as an internal distraction device and was removed on an average of three months after surgery. This technique is used on fractures with extensive diaphyseal comminution.

17. Wolf JC, Weil WM, Hanel DP, et al: A biomechanic comparison of an internal radiocarpal spanning 2.4 mm locking plate and external fixation in a model of distal radius fractures, *J Hand Surg Am* 31:1578-1586, 2006.

18. Ginn TA, Ruch DS, Yang CC, Hanel DP: Use of a distraction plate for distal radial fractures with metaphyseal and diaphyseal comminution: surgical technique, *J Bone Joint Surg Am* 88(Suppl 1 Pt 1):29-36, 2006.

19. Wiesler ER, Chloros GD, Mahirogullari M, et al: Arthroscopic management of distal radius fractures, *J Hand Surg Am* 31:1516-1526, 2006.

20. Bae DS, Koris MJ: Fragment-specific internal fixation of distal radius fractures, *Hand Clin* 21:355-362, 2005.

A review of a fragment specific approach to the distal radius with the use of the Trimed Wrist Fixation system (Trimed, Valencia, California). There is discussion of basic surgical technique and hardware design. The need for hardware removal continues to be a problem, but this system works well for high comminuted intra articular fractures of the distal radius in osteoporotic bone.

21. Dodds SD, Cornelissen S, Jossan S, et al: A biomechanical comparison of fragment specific fixation and augmented internal fixation for intra articular distal radius fractures, *J Hand Surg Am* 27:953-964, 2002.

22. Taylor KF, Parks BG, Segalman KA: Biomechanical stability of a fixed angle volar plate versus fragment specific system: cyclic testing in a C2-type distal radius cadaver fracture model, *J Hand Surg Am* 31:373-381, 2006.

This study compared the stability of the Trimed Fragment Specific system and a volar fixed angled plate in a cadaveric model. Both systems proved to be stable constructs. The fragment specific design was more stable only for ulnar fragment fixation.

23. Benson LS, Minihane KP, Stern LD, et al: The outcome of intra-articular distal radius fractures treated with fragment specific fixation, *J Hand Surg Am* 31:1333-1339, 2006.

A study of 85 patients treated with fragment-specific fixation of the distal radius. All fractures were intraarticular, and they obtained 61 excellent and 24 good results. They therefore concluded that fragment-specific fixation is a reasonable method of treatment. They emphasized the immediate institution of active and passive range of motion postoperatively.

24. Liporace FA, Gupta S, Jeong GK, et al: A biomechanical comparison of a dorsal 3.5 mm T plate and a volar fixed angle plate in a model of dorsally unstable distal radius fractures, *J Orthop Trauma* 19:187-191, 2005.

25. Smith DW, Henry MH: Volar fixed angle plating of the distal radius, *J Am Acad Orthop Surg* 13:28-36, 2005.

26. Orbay JL, Fernandez DL: Volar fixed angled plate fixation for unstable distal radius fractures in the elderly patient, *J Hand Surg Am* 29:96-102, 2004.

27. Blythe M, Stoffel K, Jarrett P, et al: Volar versus dorsal locking plates with and without radial styloid locking plates for the fixation of dorsally comminuted distal radius fractures: a biomechanical study in cadavers, *J Hand Surg Am* 31: 1587-1593, 2006.

A cadaveric comparison of a single fixed angle volar plate, a single fixed angle dorsal plate, and a volar plate with the addition of a radial styloid plate.

28. Nana AD, Joshi A, Lichtman DM: Plating of the distal radius, *J Am Acad Orthop Surg* 13:159-171, 2005.

29. Grewal R, Perey B, Wilmink M, et al: A randomized prospective study on the treatment of intra-articular distal radius fractures: open reduction and internal fixation with dorsal plating versus mini open reduction, percutaneous fixation, and external fixation, *J Hand Surg Am* 30:764-772, 2005.

30. Simic PM, Robison J, Gardner MJ, et al: Treatment of distal radius fractures with a low-profile dorsal plating system: an outcomes assessment, *J Hand Surg Am* 31:382-386, 2006.

31. Suckel A, Spies S, Munst P: Dorsal (AO/ASIF) pi-plate osteosynthesis in the treatment of distal intraarticular radius fractures, *J Hand Surg Br* 31:673-679, 2006.

33. Cassidy, C, Jupiter JB, Cohen M, et al: Norian SRS cement compared with conventional fixation in distal radius fractures: a randomized study, *J Bone Joint Surg Am* 85-A:2127-2137, 2003.

34. May MM, Lawton JN, Blazer PE: Ulnar styloid fractures associated with distal radius fractures: incidence and implications for distal radioulnar joint instability, *J Hand Surg Am* 27: 965-971, 2002.

A retrospective review of 166 distal radius fractures over 1 year. All distal radius fractures that had clinical evidence of distal radioulnar joint (DRUJ) instability had an associated ulnar styloid fracture. Fractures that included the base of the ulnar styloid and those with significant styloid displacement showed an increased risk of DRUJ instability.

35. Fernandez DL, Ring D, Jupiter JB: Surgical management of delayed union and nonunion of distal radius fractures, *J Hand Surg Am* 26:201-209, 2001.

36. Ruch DS: Fractures of the distal radius and ulna. In Rockwood & Green

An all-inclusive chapter that covers the rationale for treatment of the multiple fracture patterns well. A good reference source that should be available in all orthopaedic libraries.

37. Fernandez DJ, Palmer AK: Fractures of the distal radius. In *Green's operative hand surgery*, ed 4, vol 1.

An extensive study and review of the literature by two experts in the field of wrist surgery. The concise treatment protocol can be of valuable assistance to those new to the field. The authors cover the gamut of treatment options and rationale, while offering pearls on everyday management based on their years of experience.

38. Gutow AP: Avoidance and treatment of complications of distal radius fractures, *Hand Clin* 21:295-305, 2005.

39. Sharpe F, Stevanovic M: Extra articular distal radius fracture malunion, *Hand Clin* 21:469-487, 2005.

A review of the sequelae, indications for surgery, and surgical techniques for extraarticular malunions. This is an extensive review with a list of good references for those interested in this subject. There is discussion of the indications and use of ulnar-sided options, such as ulnar shortening osteotomy and the Barrack procedure.

40. Malone KJ, Magnell TD, Freeman DC, et al: Surgical correction of dorsally angulated distal radius malunions with fixed angle volar plating: a case series, *J Hand Surg Am* 31:366-372, 2006.

41. Gutow AP: Avoidance and treatment of complications of distal radius fractures, *Hand Clin* 21:295-305, 2005.

As with all *Hand Clinics*, this is an up-to-date collection of review articles covering many topics of distal radius fractures including the majority of treatment options. This is multiauthored by a collection of experts in this field of study.

Further Reading

32. Rajan GP, Fornaro J, Trentz O, et al: Cancellous allograft versus autologous bone grafting for repair of comminuted distal radius fractures: a prospective, randomized trial, *J Trauma* 60:1322-1329, 2006.

CHAPTER 11

Fractures of the Spine

Carlo Bellabarba, MD

- Fractures of the spine, particularly when associated with spinal cord injury (SCI), rank among the most costly to society.
- The treatment of spine fractures cannot be guided by a stringently generic approach because of the infinite number of fracture permutations, comorbidities, and associated patient factors that may influence treatment.
- The aim of this chapter is to provide an overview of the more established injury patterns throughout the spine, from occiput to sacrum, and to illustrate in general terms the salient features and preferred treatment options for these injuries.

Preliminary Evaluation

Clinical Evaluation

- The initial priority in patients with injury to the cervical spine (c-spine) is to establish an airway, restore ventilation as required, and maintain blood pressure.
- Normally, hypotensive trauma patients have insufficient blood volume and respond to fluid resuscitation and transfusion. In a patient with SCI this probable hypovolemia may be accompanied by neurogenic shock from loss of sympathetic tone, manifested as hypotension with bradycardia.
- It is imperative to normalize systemic blood pressure because spinal cord perfusion has lost its autoregulatory capabilities and is entirely dependent on mean arterial pressure (MAP). Maintaining adequate spinal cord perfusion may be a vital factor in minimizing the extent of SCI and in promoting greater functional recovery.
- Neurogenic shock usually responds to vasopressors, although atropine may be required if bradycardia is severe.
- After completing the primary survey, sensorimotor function of the extremities and the integrity of the spinal column are assessed in detail as part of the secondary survey.
- The neurologic examination includes documentation of the Frankel (American Spinal Injury Association [ASIA])

grade, level of neurologic injury, and ASIA motor score, which is based on manual muscle testing of five key muscle groups in both the upper and lower extremities (Figure 11–1).
- Sensation to pinprick and light touch in all dermatomes and vibration or position sense is elicited. Deep tendon reflexes in both arms and legs should be performed and pathologic responses recorded.
- Perineal function is assessed by evaluation of perianal pinprick sensation, voluntary anal sphincter contraction, and the bulbocavernosus reflex. Intact perianal function may be the only indication of an incomplete lesion and in addition to having significant prognostic value may influence the timing of surgical intervention. Perineal deficits may be the only indication of neurologic compromise in patients with conus medullaris or cauda equina injuries.
- Intravenous (IV) infusion of high-dose methylprednisolone for SCI is controversial. It is currently considered a treatment option rather than the standard of care and is not mandatory. It should be considered, according to institutional protocol, in patients with SCIs as a result of nonpenetrating trauma who are within 8 hours of injury.

Radiographic Evaluation and Cervical Spine Clearance

Asymptomatic Patients

- The clinical evaluation is often an important element in assessing for potential spine injury.
- Important elements of the clinical examination include the presence of a neurologic deficit, neck or back pain, or a palpable abnormality in spinal alignment.
- In alert patients with low-energy mechanisms and no distracting injuries, the absence of neck tenderness or pain through a physiologic range of motion is considered sufficient to clear the c-spine.

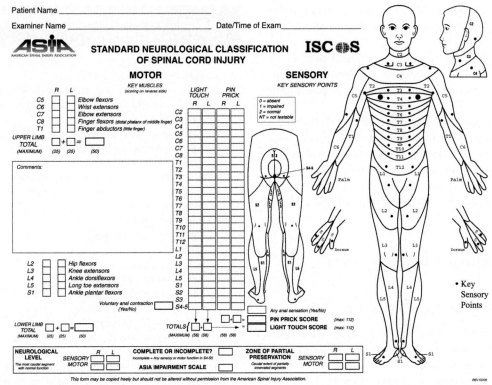

Figure 11–1: American Spinal Injury Association method of evaluating neurologic function. ASIA, American Spinal Injury Association.

Symptomatic and Obtunded Patients

- Patients who do not match the previous description require radiographic screening, which consists of any variety of institutionally standardized methods designed to exclude fracture and confirm anatomic cervical alignment.
- The question of how c-spine clearance should be undertaken in the comatose patient remains a matter of controversy.
- Radiographic evaluation consists of:
  - The cross-table lateral plain radiograph, which is widely available and has a relatively high specificity (94%) and sensitivity (96%) in most circumstances.
  - These radiographs must be evaluated for soft-tissue swelling, fractures, and abnormalities in alignment.
- Helical computed tomography (CT) evaluation
  - High sensitivity (95% to 99%) and specificity (93%) for detecting c-spine fractures.
  - Cost and efficiency are enhanced by combining the cervical CT with an already planned head CT.
- Dynamic radiographic evaluation
  - Dynamic lateral flexion and extension cervical radiographs are used to detect occult cervical instability, presumably as a result of radiographically invisible discoligamentous injury.
  - These can be either upright, patient-performed studies in the awake, alert patient, who complains of neck pain

but has negative preliminary imaging studies, or passive studies under live fluoroscopy in the obtunded patient.
- I caution against obtaining dynamic studies in the immediate postinjury period because the potential for severe muscle spasm and pain-mediated nuchal rigidity soon after the injury may preclude a satisfactory dynamic range of motion, which may mask pathologic instability.
- In the early postinjury setting, dynamic radiographs have been associated with neurologic injury resulting from vertebral subluxation.
- In lieu of immediate dynamic radiographs, I recommend 2-week-long period of external immobilization in a rigid cervical orthosis followed by evaluation with flexion-extension films.
- Dynamic evaluation of the c-spine with live fluoroscopy in unconscious patients is a controversial issue that has both proponents and detractors.
- Magnetic resonance imaging (MRI)
  - MRI is useful in defining vertebral column and spinal anatomy in patients with neurologic deficits and otherwise undetectable soft tissue injury that may influence treatment.
  - It is especially helpful in patients with progressive neurologic deficits or deficits that do not correspond to CT findings.
  - MRI findings that may not be obvious on CT include disc disruption or herniation and epidural abscess.

- Cord signal change on MRI may also shed light on the nature of a neurologic injury in the absence of osseoligamentous injury
- MRI also allows for prognostic assessment of SCI.
- MRI has excellent sensitivity but poor specificity, which makes its role in the screening of c-spine injuries uncertain.
- If neural imaging is desirable but MRI is unavailable or contraindicated, CT-myelography can be considered.
- Patients with high-energy mechanisms should receive routine imaging of the thoracic and lumbar spines, whether by plain radiographs, helical CT of the thoracic and lumbar spines, or reformatting of thoracic and abdominal CT.

Specific Injuries by Anatomic Region

Upper Cervical Spine (Occiput to C2)

- The craniocervical junction is a functional unit consisting of osseoligamentous and neurovascular structures that extend from the skull base to C2. It includes the occipitocervical and atlantoaxial articulations (Box 11–1).
- Stability of the craniocervical junction is established primarily by its unusual ligamentous anatomy rather than on intrinsic bony stability, which allows for considerable motion while still providing the stability that is necessary for protection of the vital traversing neurovascular structures.
- Patient outcome is often more dependent on associated intracranial injury than on the injury to the spine.

Injury Classification, Indications for Surgery, Outcomes, and Complications

Occipital Condyle Fractures

Classification

- Occipital condyle fractures (Box 11–2) may be highly unstable if they represent bony avulsion of major craniocervical stabilizers. Anderson described a classification system (Figure 11–2) consisting of three categories.
- Type I—stable, comminuted axial loading injuries.
- Type II—potentially unstable injuries caused by a shear mechanism that results in an oblique fracture extending from the condyle into the skull base.
- Type III—unstable alar ligament avulsion fractures that result in a transverse fracture line through the occipital condyle. A possible component of craniocervical dissociation.

Indications for Surgery

- Operative treatment is generally reserved for the type III injuries with craniocervical instability and consists of occipitocervical fusion.

Box 11–1	Common Craniocervical Injury Patterns

1. Occipital condyle fracture
   a. Type 1—axial loading injury
   b. Type 2—shear force with associated basilar skull fracture
   c. Type 3—occipital condyle (alar ligament) avulsion
2. Craniocervical injury
   a. Type 1—minimally displaced, stable
   b. Type 2—minimally displaced, unstable
   c. Type 3—displaced, unstable
3. Atlas fracture—stable versus unstable (transverse alar ligament [TAL] injury, lateral mass overhang >7 mm)
   a. Posterior arch fractures
   b. Lateral mass fractures
   c. Isolated anterior arch fractures
   d. Bursting type fractures.
4. Atlantoaxial instability
   a. Type A—rotational injuries
   b. Type B—translational injuries
      i. Type 1—TAL bony avulsion
      ii. Type 2—TAL disruption
   c. Type C—distraction injuries
5. Odontoid fracture
   a. Type I: bony avulsion of the alar ligament from the odontoid tip
   b. Type II: occurs at the odontoid waist, at the level of the TAL and above C1-C2
      i. Type II-A—segmentally comminuted fracture
   c. Type III: extends into the vertebral body
6. Traumatic spondylolisthesis of the axis (hangman's fracture)
   a. Type I: minimally displaced fracture of the pars interarticularis
      i. Type I-A: involves single pars and contralateral vertebral body
   b. Type II: displaced fracture of the pars interarticularis
      i. Type II-A: flexion-distraction injury with primarily kyphotic deformity
   c. Type III: pars interarticularis fractures with C2-C3 facet dislocation

---

Outcomes and Complications

- Complications depend on the presence or absence of symptomatic posttraumatic arthritis resulting in neck pain, occipital headaches, restricted craniocervical motion, and torticollis.
- Palsy of closely associated cranial nerves (IX, X, XI, XII) has also been described.
- If part of a craniocervical dissociation, prognosis is worse.

Craniocervical Dissociation

Classification

- Traynelis identified three craniocervical dissociation patterns according to the direction of displacement.
- The Harborview Classification system, which is based on the extent of displacement and instability, includes traction testing of minimally displaced injuries (<2 mm) and

Box 11–2	**Classification and Treatment of Occipital Condyle Fractures**	
INJURY TYPE	**DISTINGUISHING CHARACTERISTICS**	**SIGNIFICANCE**
I	Comminuted fracture of an occipital condyle	Stable injury treated with a cervical collar, possibly a halo for severe collapse, unless associated with craniocervical dissociation
II	Extension of a basilar skull fracture into an occipital condyle	Stable injury treated with a cervical collar unless associated with craniocervical dissociation
III	Avulsion fracture at alar ligament insertion	Labeled unstable in the original description, but commonly treated with halo unless associated with craniocervical dissociation

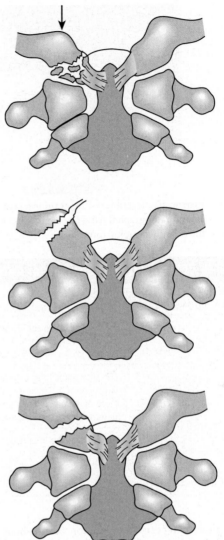

Figure 11–2: Anderson and Montesano classification of occipital condyle fractures. (From Bellabarba C, Mirza SK, Chapman JR: Injuries to the craniocervical junction. In Bucholz RW, Heckman JD, Court-Brown CM, editors: *Rockwood and Green's fractures in adults,* ed 6, Philadelphia, 2006, Lippincott Williams & Wilkins, Chapter 38, pp. 1435-1496. [Figure 38–10, p. 1448.])

may be more useful in guiding treatment and prognosis (Box 11–3).

Indications for Surgery

- If distance between the basion and tip of the dens (basion dens interval [BDI]) and between the basion and a line drawn along the posterior body of the axis (basion axis interval [BAI]) is greater than 12 mm, craniocervical dissociation is likely and should be investigated with MRI.
- Displacement of more than 2 mm at the atlanto-occipital joint, either on static imaging studies or with provocative traction testing (Figure 11–3, Box 11–3) or the presence of neurologic injury are indications for craniocervical stabilization.

Outcomes and Complications

- Most craniocervical dissociations are fatal.
- The outcome of survivors is dependent on:
  - The type and severity of associated injuries, particularly closed head injuries.
  - The severity of neurologic injury.
  - The timeliness with which the diagnosis of craniocervical dissociation is recognized and can be operatively stabilized.
- Delayed diagnosis is associated with secondary neurologic deterioration and possibly death in up to 75% of patients.
- Vertebral artery injury should be considered in any distractive upper cervical injury.

Fractures of the Atlas

Classification

- These fractures are classified as either stable or unstable based on the presence of transverse alar ligament (TAL) insufficiency (Box 11–4).

- TAL insufficiency can be diagnosed either by direct means, such as by identifying bony avulsion on CT scan or ligament rupture on MRI or indirectly by identifying widening of the lateral masses with greater than 7 mm lateral overhang relative to the lateral masses of C2.
- C1 fractures are also classified as: (1) posterior arch fractures (2) lateral mass fractures (3) isolated anterior arch fractures, and (4) Bursting type fractures.

Indications for Surgery

- Most C1 fractures are treated nonoperatively.
- Halo immobilization alone may be insufficient in unstable injuries. If upright radiographs in a halo show further lateral

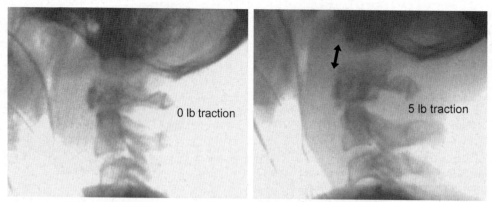

Figure 11–3: Provocative traction test for craniocervical instability. Resting lateral radiograph of the craniocervical junction and lateral radiograph during the application of 5 pounds of cranial tong traction shows pathologic widening of the atlanto–occipital joint.

Box 11–3	**Classification Treatment of Occipitocervical Junction Injuries**	
HARBORVIEW CLASSIFICATION	**DESCRIPTION OF INJURY**	**TREATMENT**
Stage 1	1. MRI shows hemorrhage or edema at the occipitocervical junction 2. Occipitocervical alignment is normal by Harris' lines 3. No distraction with provocative traction testing	Nonoperative Halo-vest versus C-collar
Stage 2	1. MRI shows hemorrhage or edema at the occipitocervical junction 2. Occipitocervical alignment is normal by Harris' lines 3. Provocative traction shows sufficient distraction to meet criteria for occipitocervical dissociation established by Harris' lines.	Posterior occipitocervical instrumented arthrodesis
Stage 3	Overt occipitocervical dissociation	Posterior occipitocervical instrumented arthrodesis

MRI, magnetic resonance imaging.

mass displacement or an anterior atlanto-dens interval (ADI) of greater than 3 mm, patients must be treated either with a period of recumbency in cranial tong traction or with posterior C1-C2 or occiput-C2 fixation.

- Surgical stabilization options consist of C1-C2 transarticular screws or segmental fixation with C1 lateral mass screws connected to C2 pedicle or laminar screws.

Outcomes and Complications

- Severe complications are rare.
- There is an 80% incidence of residual neck pain, possibly as a result of posttraumatic arthritis.
- There is a 17% nonunion rate.
- Severe malunion of unstable atlas fractures may result in painful torticollis, requiring realignment and occipitocervical fusion.

Atlanto-Axial Instability

Classification

- Three atlanto-axial instability patterns can occur and may coexist (Box 11–5).

- Type A injuries are rotationally displaced in the transverse plane. These deformities are usually nontraumatic in nature and will not be discussed.
- Type B injuries are translationally unstable in the sagittal plane as a result of TAL insufficiency.

Treatment

- Treatment of these injuries depends on distinguishing a ligamentous TAL tear (type I) from a bony avulsion fracture (type II; Figure 11–4).
  - Type C injuries are distractive injuries that represent a variant of craniocervical dissociation.

Diagnosis

- Type B—suspect if plain radiographs or CT show ADI greater than 3 mm.
- Type C—suspect if distraction is noted on imaging studies or if Harris' lines greater than 12 mm.

Indications for Surgery

- Type B—translational instability: posterior atlanto-axial arthrodesis.

Box 11–4	Classification and Treatment of C1 Fractures	
INJURY TYPE	DISTINGUISHING CHARACTERISTICS	TREATMENT
Stable	Posterior arch fracture	Rigid collar
	Anterior arch avulsion fracture	Rigid collar
	C1 ring fracture with < 7 mm of overall lateral mass displacement	Rigid collar or halo vest
	C1 ring fracture with > or = 7 mm of overall C1 lateral mass displacement	Traction followed by halo vest versus C1-C2 arthrodesis
Unstable	Anterior arch fracture with posterior displacement relative to the dens (plough fracture)	Halo vest versus C1-C2 arthrodesis

Box 11–5	Classification and Treatment of C1-C2 Dislocations	
INJURY TYPE	DISTINGUISHING CHARACTERISTICS	SIGNIFICANCE
A	Rotation centered on the dens, where the transverse atlantal ligament is normally intact	Treated with closed reduction and immobilization. Beware of associated fractures.
B	Translation between C1-C2, where transverse ligament is disrupted	Midsubstance transverse ligament tears (type I) are treated with C1-C2 arthrodesis. Bony avulsions (type II) may be treated with halo or C1-C2 arthrodesis. Treated with arthrodesis and internal fixation.
C	Distraction indicating craniocervical dissociation	

- Type C—distraction injuries: posterior atlanto-axial versus occipitocervical stabilization if greater than 2 mm of displacement.

Outcomes and Complications

- Acute TAL insufficiency is usually fatal.
- In survivors, profound neurologic deficits or head injury may be present.
- Syncope and vertigo may result from injury to the vertebrobasilar arterial system.
- Atlanto-axial distraction has a similar prognosis to craniocervical dissociation.

Odontoid Fractures

Classification

- Three-part classification of Anderson and D'Alonzo (Box 11–6; Figure 11–5).
  - Type I injuries are bony avulsions of the alar ligament and represent a component of a craniocervical dissociation.
  - Type II injuries occur at the odontoid waist and have the highest propensity for pseudarthrosis.
  - Type II-A subtype consists of a highly unstable, segmentally comminuted fracture.
  - Type III fractures extend into the cancellous vertebral body and have wider, well-vascularized cancellous fracture surfaces.

Indications for Surgery

- The treatment of type I odontoid fractures relates to their impact on craniocervical stability. Therefore indications for surgical management of these injuries are the same as those discussed for the treatment of craniocervical instability.
- Surgical indications remain controversial for type II odontoid fractures. I advocate surgical stabilization for irreducible fractures, fractures with distractive patterns of displacement, or fractures with associated SCI (Figure 11–6).
- Relative indications include patients with multiple injuries, associated closed head injury, initial displacement of greater than 4 mm, angulation greater than 10 degrees, delayed presentation (>2 weeks), multiple risk factors for nonunion, the inability to treat with a halo as a result of advanced age or body habitus, associated cranial or thoracoabdominal injury, other medical comorbidities, and the presence of associated upper cervical fractures.
- Noncomminuted fractures in patients with favorable bone quality and fracture obliquity and appropriate body habitus are ideal for anterior odontoid screw fixation.
- In patients with extensive fracture comminution, compromised bone quality, or with technical constraints to anterior odontoid screw trajectory, I favor posterior atlanto-axial fusion using either transarticular screw fixation or segmental C1-C2 fixation.
- Operative stabilization is not commonly required for type III odontoid fractures, but is warranted in patients with SCI or distractive instability patterns.
- Relative indications include highly displaced irreducible fractures, patients with displaced injuries who cannot be treated with a halo, and fractures with initial displacement of 5 mm or more, which have a high potential for nonunion.
- Delayed unions or pseudarthroses occur in up to 54% of nonoperatively treated patients and are also amenable to posterior C1-C2 fixation.
- Posterior C1-C2 arthrodesis is the surgical treatment method of choice because anterior odontoid screw fixation has a high failure rate with type III odontoid fractures.

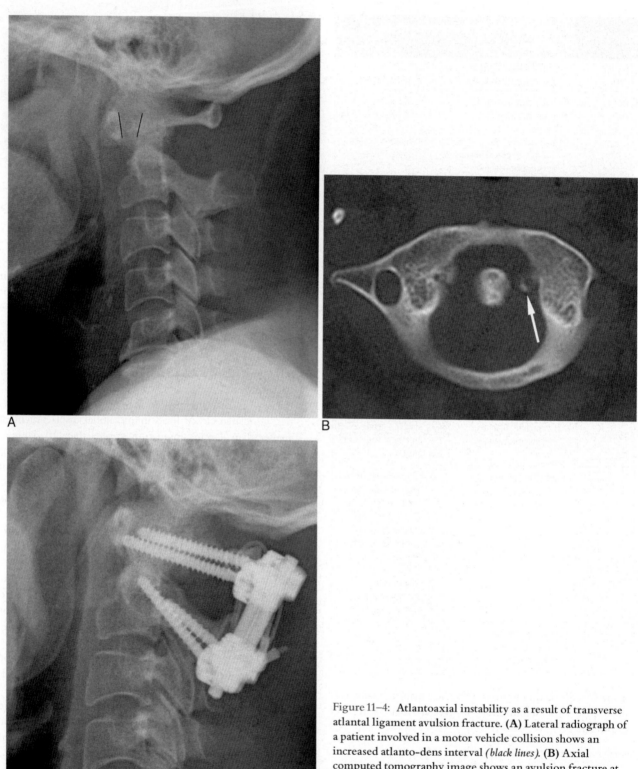

Figure 11–4: Atlantoaxial instability as a result of transverse atlantal ligament avulsion fracture. (A) Lateral radiograph of a patient involved in a motor vehicle collision shows an increased atlanto–dens interval (black lines). (B) Axial computed tomography image shows an avulsion fracture at the insertion of the transverse atlantal ligament onto the C1 lateral mass (arrow). (C) Postoperative lateral radiograph after reduction and posterior C1–C2 arthrodesis with segmental instrumentation.

Box 11–6	Classification and Treatment of Dens Fractures	
INJURY TYPE	**DISTINGUISHING CHARACTERISTICS**	**SIGNIFICANCE**
I	Avulsion injury at insertion of the alar ligament (cephalad to the transverse ligament)	Treated with halo or surgery if associated with craniocervical dissociation.
II	Fracture at the waist of the dens where it consists primarily of a ring of cortical bone surrounded by synovial capsule	High risk of nonunion. Usually treated with a halo initially but strong indication for surgery if widely displaced or if fracture shows continued movement despite halo immobilization.
III	Fracture extending into cancellous bone within the C2 vertebral body	Treated with a halo or brace.

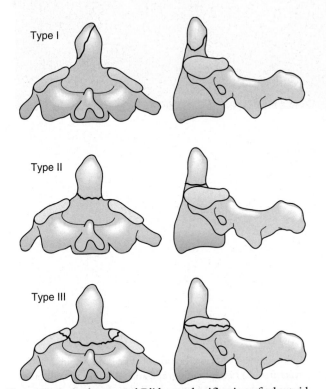

Figure 11–5: Anderson and D'Alonso classification of odontoid fractures. (From Bellabarba C, Mirza SK, Chapman JR: Injuries to the craniocervical junction. In Bucholz RW, Heckman JD, Court-Brown CM, editors: *Rockwood and Green's fractures in adults*, ed 6, Philadelphia, 2006, Lippincott Williams & Wilkins, Chapter 38, pp. 1435–1496. [Figure 38–14, p. 1451]).

Outcomes and Complications

- Odontoid fractures are associated with significant morbidity and mortality.
- Neurologic injury occurs in 18% to 25% of type II odontoid fractures and ranges in severity from isolated cranial nerve injury to complete quadriplegia.
- In-hospital mortality rates for elderly patients with type II odontoid fractures range from 27% to 42%.
- Fracture nonunion and missed injuries are the most common complications.
- Fracture displacement of greater than 4 mm has been the most consistently identified risk factor for nonunion. Other risk factors include age above 60 years, fracture angulation of 10 degrees or above, and delay in treatment.
- An overall perioperative complication rate of up to 28% and a nonunion rate of 10% has been described with odontoid screw fixation.
- C1-C2 fusions have reported nonunion rates of 4% or less using transarticular screw and wired structural bone-graft constructs.
- Nonoperative treatment of type III odontoid fractures in a halo is associated with pseudarthrosis rates from 9% to 13%.
  - Fracture displacement greater than 4 mm or angulation greater than 9 degrees have been associated with nonunion rates of 22% to 54%.
- If surgical stabilization of type III odontoid fractures is undertaken, it should consist of atlanto-axial fixation because excessively high failure rates (55%) have been reported for odontoid screw fixation.

Traumatic Spondylolisthesis of the Axis (Hangman's Fractures)

Classification

- Three primary injury types and two atypical subtypes exist (Box 11–7; Figure 11–7).
  - Type I are minimally displaced, relatively stable fractures of the pars interarticularis that result from hyperextension and axial loading.
  - Type I-A are atypical unstable lateral bending fractures that are obliquely displaced, with a fracture through one pars and more anteriorly into the body on the contralateral side.
  - Type II are displaced injuries that occur when a flexion force follows the initial hyperextension and axial loading insult.
  - Type II-A is an unstable injury with associated C2-C3 disc and interspinous ligament disruption caused by a flexion-distraction mechanism. Kyphosis is the prevailing deformity rather than translation (Figure 11–9).
  - Type III are highly unstable injuries in which the pars interarticularis fractures are associated with dislocation of the C2-C3 facet joints.

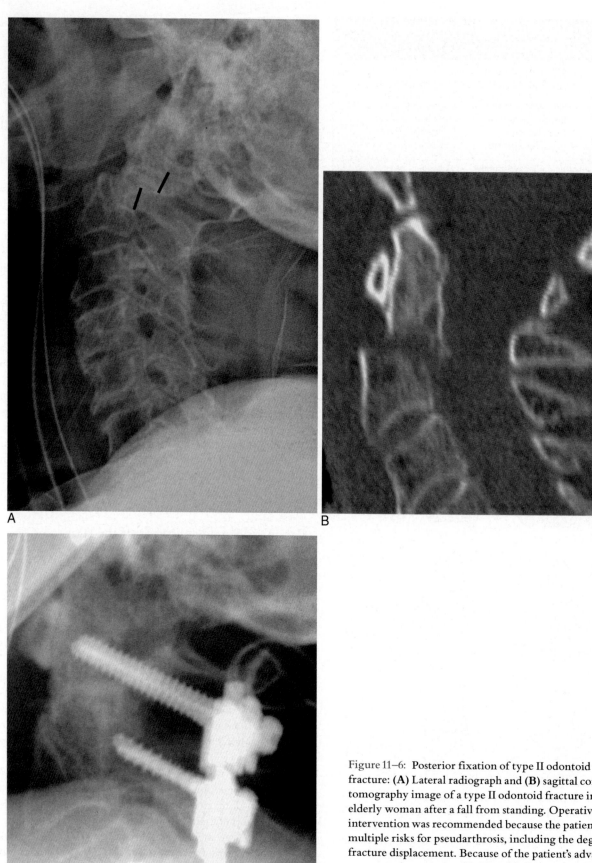

A

B

C

Figure 11–6: Posterior fixation of type II odontoid fracture: **(A)** Lateral radiograph and **(B)** sagittal computed tomography image of a type II odontoid fracture in an elderly woman after a fall from standing. Operative intervention was recommended because the patient had multiple risks for pseudarthrosis, including the degree of fracture displacement. Because of the patient's advanced osteoporosis, posterior C1-C2 arthrodesis was performed with segmental instrumentation, as shown on **(C)** the postoperative lateral radiograph.

Box 11-7 Classification and Treatment of Hangman's Fractures

INJURY TYPE	DISTINGUISHING CHARACTERISTICS	SIGNIFICANCE
I	Nondisplaced (displacement of <2 mm) fracture through the arch of C2	Treated with a collar, occasionally with halo
IA	Atypical fracture involving C2 arch on one side and vertebral body on contralateral side. Often extends into vertebral artery foramen	Displacement of these atypical fractures may result in considerable canal compromise and spinal cord injury. Usually treated with a halo. May require reduction and fixation if severely displaced or in the presence of spinal cord injury. Fixation options include C2-C3 anterior arthrodesis, posterior C1-C3 versus C2-C3 arthrodesis, or combined approach (usually reserved for spinal cord injuries)
II	Displaced fracture of C2 arch	Treated with a halo
IIA	Fracture of C2 arch associated with disruption of the C2-C3 intervertebral disc, showing angulation of C2-C3 endplates without anterior translation of C2 body on C3 body	Treated with a halo, and if markedly displaced, possibly direct fixation of fractured arch through a posterior approach, or by C2-C3 anterior arthrodesis
III	Fracture of the C2 arch associated with dislocation of the C2-C3 facet joints	Frequently associated with neurologic deficit. Requires open reduction and posterior arthrodesis.

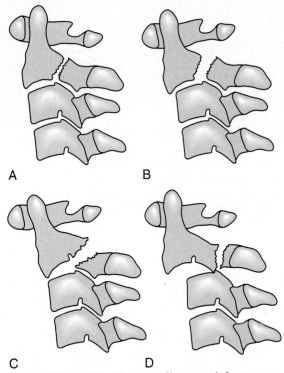

A   B

C   D

Figure 11-7: Effendi Classification of hangman's fractures as modified by Levine. (From Bellabarba C, Mirza SK, Chapman JR: Injuries to the craniocervical junction. In Bucholz RW, Heckman JD, Court-Brown CM, editors: *Rockwood and Green's fractures in adults*, ed 6, Philadelphia, 2006, Lippincott Williams & Wilkins, Chapter 38, pp. 1435-1496. [Figure 38-15, p. 1451]).

Indications for Surgery

- Operative stabilization is rarely indicated for traumatic spondylolisthesis of the axis.
- Most injuries can be treated with 12 weeks of external immobilization using a rigid collar for type I (and most type I-A) and a halo vest for most type II fractures.

- Type II-A injuries may be treated with halo immobilization if their alignment can be successfully maintained.
- Traction is contraindicated because it accentuates their kyphotic deformity.
- If the kyphosis cannot be controlled in a halo, surgery should be considered.
- A C2-C3 anterior cervical discectomy and fusion (ACDF) with plating allows for fusion across the least number of levels but requires compromising the anterior longitudinal ligament (ALL) and anterior annulus, the only intact major ligamentous structures at C2-C3.
- Posterior stabilization is more versatile and stable, but unless adequate purchase is achieved across the fractured C2 pars interarticularis, loss of atlanto-axial motion results from the need to extend fixation to C1 (Figure 11-8).
- Type III injuries are generally irreducible by traction and require operative reduction and stabilization. Stabilization options include:
  - Posterior C1-C3 fusion (see Figure 11-8).
  - Posterior C2-C3 fusion using lag screws across the fracture at C2.
  - Anterior C2-C3 ACDF (Figure 11-9) in the unusual event that reduction occurs by closed methods.

Outcomes and Complications

- Associated upper cervical (15%), subaxial (23%), or head injuries usually have a greater effect on prognosis than the C2 fracture itself.
- Neurologic injury has been identified in only 3% to 10% of patients but occurs in 60% of type III and 33% of type I-A fractures (Figure 11-10).
- Type I-A injuries also have a greater potential for vertebral artery injury because of common foramen transversarium involvement.

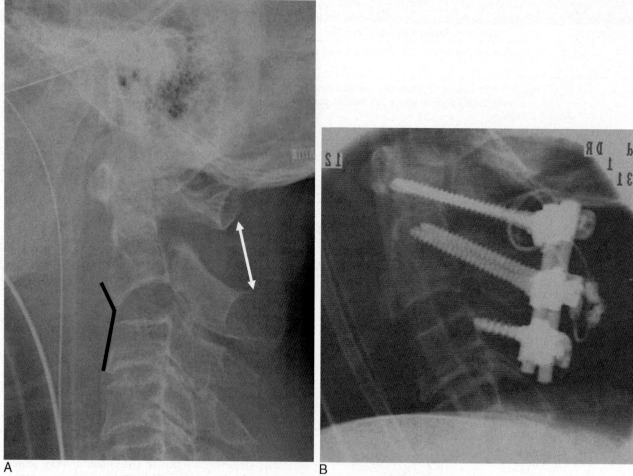

A

B

Figure 11–8: Type II-A hangman's fracture treated with posterior C1-C3 fixation. **(A)** Preoperative lateral cervical spine radiograph of an elderly male after a motor vehicle collision shows a type II-A hangman's fracture characterized by a flexion-distraction injury pattern with distraction of the posterior elements *(white arrow)* and a preponderance of kyphosis rather than translation as the anterior longitudinal ligament acts as a hinge *(black line)*, and the posterior elements are splayed apart *(white arrow)*. **(B)** Lateral radiograph after posterior C1-C3 arthrodesis with posterior segmental instrumentation.

- There is a 5% pseudarthrosis rate.
- Type I-A, type II-A, and type III fractures constitute a greater treatment challenge as a result of either their atypical fracture orientation or their associated ligamentous injury.

Subaxial Cervical Spine (Below C2)

Classification of Subaxial Cervical Spine Injuries

- There is no universally accepted classification system for fractures and dislocations of the subaxial c-spine.
- A mechanistic classification system was proposed by Allen and others in 1982. A modified version of this scheme will be used in this chapter (Box 11–8).
- Spine injuries will be categorized into nine injury types that are discussed in six categories.

- It is useful to consider the four "cardinal" force vectors to which the spine may be subjected—distraction, compression, extension, and flexion—and realize that most injuries will result from a combination of these forces (Figure 11–12).
- The injured spine can therefore be conceptualized as being subjected to four additional primary injury vectors corresponding to equal proportions of extension-distraction, extension-compression, flexion-compression, and flexion-distraction (Figure 11–12).

Categories of Injury

Extension-Type Injuries

- Extension-distraction, extension, and extension-compression mechanisms are considered together.
- Extension-type injuries usually result from a blow to the face or forehead.

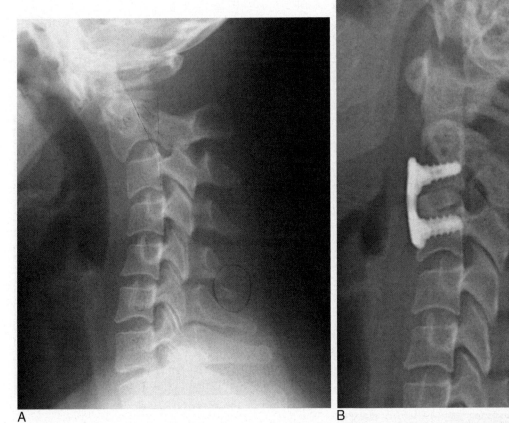

A B

Figure 11–9: C2-C3 anterior cervical discectomy and fusion for type III hangman's fracture with successful closed reduction an anterior fixation: **(A)** Upright lateral cervical spine radiograph showing a type III hangman's fracture characterized by minimally displaced pars interarticularis fractures and C2-C3 bilateral facet dislocation. A closed manipulative reduction was achieved, which made this injury amenable to anterior C2-C3 interbody arthrodesis, as shown on **(B)** the lateral postoperative radiograph. Because the C2 body is disconnected from the dislocated C2 facet joints, closed reduction is not normally considered feasible with type III hangman's fractures.

- The degree to which extension is combined with distraction or compression force vectors influences both the injury pattern and subsequent treatment.
- Extension injuries typically result from high-energy mechanisms in younger patients with nonspondylotic c-spines or from seemingly trivial injuries in older patients with spondylotic or ankylosed spines.
- They are broadly divided into injuries that result in obvious compromise of the osseoligamentous elements of the c-spine and those with SCI but no obvious radiographic evidence of musculoskeletal injury or spinal instability.
- Injuries with radiographic signs of a vertebral column lesion are classified broadly as (1) extension teardrop fractures, (2) disruptions to the anterior longitudinal ligament and intervertebral disc, (3) extension-distraction fracture-dislocations and (4) extension-compression fracture-dislocations.
- Injuries 1, 2, and 3 involve a distraction force that contributes variably to the primary extension vector, resulting in what has been defined by Allen and others as the distractive extension lesion.

- The fourth injury combines compression with extension and has many characteristics distinct from the extension-distraction injury.
- Cervical SCIs not accompanied by radiographic signs of osseoligamentous injury include central cord syndrome and spinal cord injury without radiographic abnormality (SCIWORA).

Extension-Distraction Injuries

Classification and General Considerations

- In extension-distraction injuries, the sequence of injury to the spinal column progresses from the anterior through the middle column to the posterior column.
- Simultaneous compressive forces across the posterior elements may result in fractures involving the neural arch, lateral masses, or pedicles
- Injuries with distractive components have been classified by Allen and others into two stages (Box 11–9, Figure 11–13):
  - Stage 1 injuries are characterized by failure of the anterior ligamentous complex (ALL and anterior annulus) or

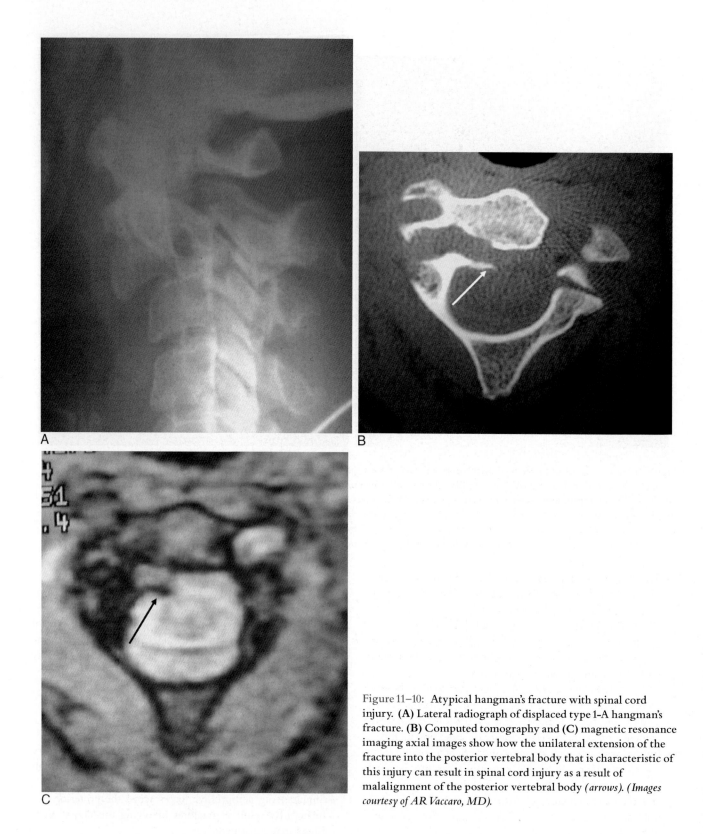

Figure 11–10: Atypical hangman's fracture with spinal cord injury. **(A)** Lateral radiograph of displaced type 1-A hangman's fracture. **(B)** Computed tomography and **(C)** magnetic resonance imaging axial images show how the unilateral extension of the fracture into the posterior vertebral body that is characteristic of this injury can result in spinal cord injury as a result of malalignment of the posterior vertebral body *(arrows). (Images courtesy of AR Vaccaro, MD).*

The NEXUS Low-Risk Criteria*

Cervical spine radiography is indicated for patients with trauma unless they meet all of the following criteria:
No posterior midline cervical-spine tenderness,[†]
No evidence of intoxication,[‡]
A normal level of alertness,[§]
No focal neurologic deficit,[¶] and
No painful distracting injuries.[¶]

*Criteria are from Hoffman and colleagues
[†]Midline posterior bony cervical-spine tenderness is present if the patient reports pain on palpitation of the posterior midline neck from the nuchal ridge to the prominence of the first thoracic vertebra or if the patient evinces pain with direct palpitation of any cervical spinous process.
[‡]Patients should be considered intoxicated if they have any of the following: a recent history provided by the patient or an observer of intoxication or intoxicating ingestion, evidence of intoxication on physical examination, such as an odor of alcohol, slurred speech, ataxia, dysmetria, or other cerebellar findings, or any behavior consistent with intoxication. Patients may also be considered to be intoxicated if tests of bodily secretions are positive for alcohol or drugs that affect the level of alertness.
[§]An altered level of alertness can include any of the following: a Glasgow Coma Scale score of 14 or less; disorientation to person, place, time, or events; an inability to remember three objects at 5 minutes; a delayed or inappropriate response to external stimuli; or other findings.
[¶]No precise definition of a painful distracting injury is possible. This category includes any condition thought by the clinician to be producing pain sufficient to distract the patient from a second (neck) injury. Such injuries may include, but are not limited to, any long-bone fracture; a visceral injury requiring surgical consultation; a large laceration, degloving injury, or crash injury; large burns; or any other injury causing acute functional impairment. Physicians may also classify any injury as distracting if it is thought to have the potential to impair the patient's ability to appreciate other injuries.
[¶]A focal neurologic deficit is any focal neurologic finding on motor or sensory examination.

A

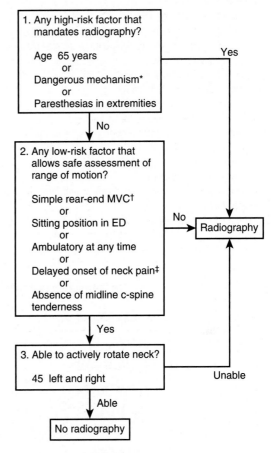

B

Figure 11–11: **Algorithms for clearing the cervical spine according to (A) the National Emergency X-Radiography Utilization Study Group and (B) the Canadian C-spine Rule.** (From [A] Hoffman JR, Mower WR, Wolfson AB, et al: *N Engl J Med* 343:94–99, 2000 and [B] Steill IG, Wells GA, Vandemheem KL, et al: *J Am Med Assoc* 286:1841–1848.)

Box 11–8	**Mechanistic Classification of Subaxial Cervical Spine Injuries**

1. Extension-type injuries
   a. Extension-distraction injuries
      i. Extension teardrop fractures
      ii. Disruption of anterior ligamentous complex (ALL) and intervertebral disc
      iii. Extension injuries in ankylosed spines
   b. Extension-compression injuries
   c. Extension injuries without radiographic abnormality
2. Vertical compression injuries (burst fractures)
3. Flexion-compression injuries (flexion teardrop fractures)
4. Flexion-distraction injuries
   a. Facet dislocations
   b. Facet fracture-dislocations
   c. Interspinous or supraspinous ligament and facet disruptions
5. Distraction injuries
6. Lateral compression injuries

transverse fracture through the vertebral body without retrolisthesis.

- Stage 2 injuries share the same basic features as stage 1 injuries but include retrolisthesis, with presumed disruption of the posterior longitudinal ligament (PLL) and possibly the posterior ligament complex.
- SCIs occur with high frequency in stage 2 injuries as a result of cord compression between the posteroinferior end plate of the posteriorly displaced vertebral body and the anterosuperior lamina of the next caudal vertebra.
- The aforementioned classification system and the subsequently described treatment guidelines can be applied to any extension injury with a distractive force vector, the most common of which are discussed here.

Extension teardrop fractures

- The extension teardrop fractures most commonly affect C2 and feature a malrotated avulsion fracture of the anterior inferior end plate.

MECHANISTIC CLASSIFICATION OF LOWER CERVICAL INJURIES

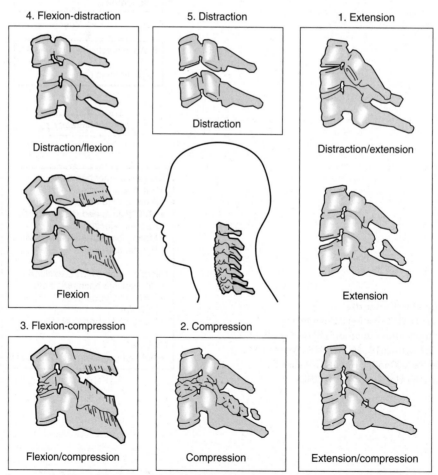

Figure 11–12: Schematic representation of the potential mechanisms of cervical spine injury. From Bellabarba C, Anderson PA: Injuries of the lower cervical spine. In Herkowitz HN, Garfin SR, Eismont FJ, Bell GR, Balderston RA, editors: *Rothman-Simeone: The spine,* Philadelphia, 2006, Elsevier. (Figure 68–3, p. 1103)

	ALLEN AND OTHERS'		
STAGE	**NOMENCLATURE**	**DESCRIPTION OF INJURY**	**TREATMENT**
1	DES1	Extension without retrolisthesis	Rigid immobilization versus anterior instrumented fusion
2	DES 2	Extension with retrolisthesis (posterior longitudinal ligament injury)	Anterior instrumented fusion

Box 11–9   Extension-Distraction Injuries of the Subaxial Cervical Spine

From Allen BL Jr, Ferguson RL, Lehmann TR, et al: *Spine* 7:1-7, 1982.

- They should be differentiated from the more severe flexion teardrop fracture.
- External immobilization of these fractures for 6 to 12 weeks is successful in the majority of patients.

Disruptions of the anterior longitudinal ligament and intervertebral disc

- These are purely discoligamentous injuries involving the ALL, intervertebral disc, and possibly the posterior ligaments.
- Lack of a visible fracture may present a diagnostic dilemma, particularly in injuries that reduce spontaneously on supine lateral radiographs.
- Retrolisthesis indicates a more unstable injury with compromise of the PLL.
- Anterior cervical discectomy and fusion with plating is effective as either a primary form of treatment or in patients with dynamic instability after nonoperative treatment.

Extension injuries in ankylosed spines

- Patients with ankylosed spines secondary to diffuse idiopathic skeletal hyperostosis (DISH) or seronegative inflammatory spondyloarthropathies, such as ankylosing spondylitis, have poor tolerance for even nominal extension forces.
- These fractures usually occur in the lower c-spine and may result in highly unstable fractures that appear to be trivial injuries.
- Less displaced injuries can be difficult to identify and are frequently missed, with potentially catastrophic neurological consequences (Figure 11–14).
- It is imperative that patients with ankylosing conditions affecting the c-spine who are diagnosed with neck pain

and no obvious acute injury on initial radiographic assessment be evaluated with a thorough imaging workup including CT and MRI.

- If a spine fracture is identified in this patient population, noncontiguous injuries should be sought with multiplanar CT or MRI imaging of the entire spine.
- Even when nondisplaced, the forces to which these fractures are subjected by the long adjacent lever arm often result in displacement.

Treatment of Extension-Distraction Injuries

- Stage 1: cervical orthosis versus ACDF
- Stage 2:
  - ACDF—unless severe osteoporosis, DISH or inflammatory ankylosing disorders.
  - With greater initial malalignment, secondary posterior instrumentation may be required if there are concerns about instability after initial anterior stabilization.
  - In patients whose injuries have a large translational component, realignment is likely to be less straightforward and would thus be more reliably achieved with posterior reduction and stabilization, possibly with secondary anterior fixation.
  - In patients with ankylosing conditions who sustain extension injuries and SCI, treatment should consist of urgent decompression of the spinal canal, which can usually be achieved through closed spinal realignment techniques.
  - Patients should not be placed in standard longitudinal tong traction, which would likely further extend and potentially distract these three-column injuries.

Direction of force

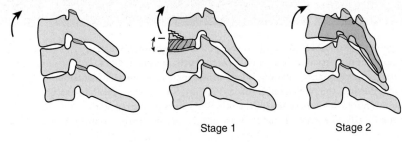

Stage 1   Stage 2

Figure 11–13: Classification and treatment of extension-distraction injuries of the subaxial cervical spine. From Bellabarba C, Anderson PA: Injuries of the lower cervical spine. In Herkowitz HN, Garfin SR, Eismont FJ, Bell GR, Balderston RA, editors: *Rothman-Simeone: The spine,* Philadelphia, 2006, Elsevier. (Figure 68–4, p. 1106)

- Provisional immobilization in a halo vest is recommended after gentle realignment of the spine to its native, usually kyphotic position.
- Resulting from their elevated risk of developing epidural hematoma, patients with ankylosing spondylitis should have an MRI of the c-spine at the earliest opportunity, particularly when they have neurologic deficits.
- Mortality rates greater than 30%, neurologic morbidity rates over 50%, and a high likelihood of pulmonary complications have been reported in patients with ankylosing spondylitis who sustain c-spine fractures.
- Because of the high complication rates in patients treated nonoperatively, an aggressive surgical approach is recommended.
- Canal decompression and stabilization is best achieved by posterior multisegmental instrumentation using plate or rod-screw systems.

- Anterior fixation alone is generally not recommended as a result of the difficulty with achieving adequate screw fixation in the usually osteoporotic vertebral bodies.

Extension-Compression Injuries

Classification and General Considerations

- Extension-compression injuries are also caused primarily by an extension moment but with simultaneous application of a compressive force across the posterior elements by axial loading of the extended spine.
- The resulting shear force on the posterior elements of the lower cervical vertebrae leads to a spectrum of injury severity that ranges from unilateral posterior element fracture to an oblique shear fracture across the three spinal columns with greater than 100% anterolisthesis (extension-compression fracture-dislocation).

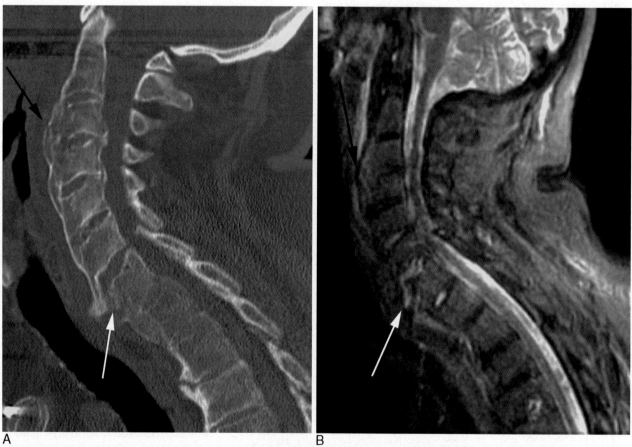

A   B

Figure 11–14: **Cervical spine extension injury in a patient with DISH.** (A) Sagittal computed tomography image in a patient with DISH who fell from standing is suspicious for disc space widening with osteophyte fracture at C6-C7 *(white arrow)* and C3-C4 *(black arrow)*. (B) Sagittal magnetic resonance imaging image shows increased short T1 inversion recovery (STIR) signal within the disc space that extends into the prevertebral soft tissues at C6-C7 *(white arrow)* and to a lesser degree, at C3-C4 *(black arrow)*. Although extension injuries in patients with ankylosed spines can occur with insignificanttrauma and be relatively subtle radiographically, as a general rule they are highly unstable three-column injuries that require operative stabilization.

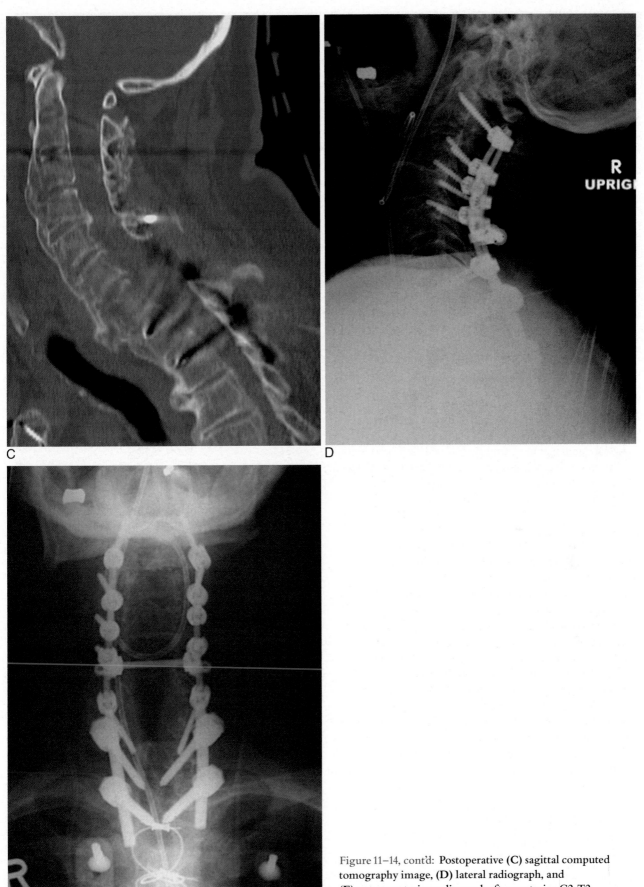

Figure 11–14, cont'd: Postoperative **(C)** sagittal computed tomography image, **(D)** lateral radiograph, and **(E)** anteroposterior radiograph after posterior C2-T2 instrumented arthrodesis.

	ALLEN AND OTHERS'		
Box 11–10		**Extension-Compression Injuries of the Subaxial Cervical Spine**	

STAGE	ALLEN AND OTHERS' NOMENCLATURE	DESCRIPTION OF INJURY	USUAL TREATMENT
1	CES1	Unilateral vertebral arch fracture Free-floating lateral mass may occur with simultaneous pedicle and lamina fracture, which may cause rotary listhesis	Rigid collar versus anterior instrumented arthrodesis (if floating facet with rotatory listhesis)
2	CES2	Bilateral vertebral arch fracture without compromise to stability of motion segment; may be multilevel	Rigid collar
3	CES3	Bilateral vertebral arch fracture with potential compromise to motion segment stability but without anterolisthesis	Rigid collar versus halo vest
4	CES4	Bilateral neural arch fractures and incomplete anterolisthesis of vertebral body	Posterior instrumented arthrodesis
5	CES5	Bilateral neural arch fractures and complete anterolisthesis of vertebral body	Posterior instrumented arthrodesis

From Allen BL Jr, Ferguson RL, Lehmann TR, et al: *Spine* 7:1-27, 1982.

- This broad range of injury severity consists of five specific extension-compression injury stages (Box 11–10; Figure 11–15).
- Stage 1 injuries are considered stable and include isolated spinous process fractures and unilateral laminar, pedicle or facet fractures.
  - The combination of laminar and pedicle fractures constitutes a fracture-separation of the lateral mass, which is typically unilateral
  - In the case of lateral mass separation, MRI is useful in assessing for annular disruption and disc injury, which negatively influences the success of nonoperative treatment.
- Stage 2 lesions are bilateral neural arch fractures without anterior injury, which may involve multiple levels.
- Stages 3–5 are more complex.
  - Additional extension-compression forces result in an oblique shearing force that extends anteroinferiorly, resulting in discoligamentous injury or vertebral body fracture.
- Radiographically, these appear as traumatic spondylolistheses with varying degrees of vertebral subluxation.
- Stage 3 has no vertebral body displacement.
- Stage 4 has partial vertebral body displacement.
- Stage 5 has 100% vertebral body displacement.
  - Despite a high likelihood of neurologic deficit in higher-stage injuries, a relative sparing of neurologic function has been noted as a consequence of the increased canal patency that results from separation of the anterior and posterior columns.

Treatment of Extension-Compression Injuries

- Stage 1 is treated with a cervical orthosis for 12 weeks
  - However, as a result of the extension mechanism, if the stage 1 injury involves tension failure of the ALL and

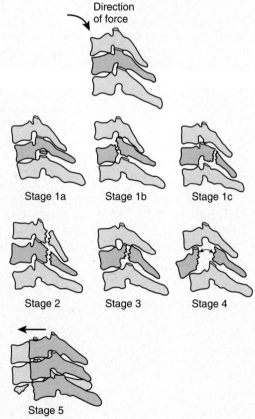

Figure 11–15: **Classification and treatment of extension-compression injuries of the subaxial cervical spine.** From Bellabarba C, Anderson PA: Injuries of the lower cervical spine. In Herkowitz HN, Garfin SR, Eismont FJ, Bell GR, Balderston RA, editors: *Rothman-Simeone: The spine,* Philadelphia, 2006, Elsevier. (Figure 68–9, p. 1111)

anterior annulus in addition to a disarticulated lateral mass, stabilization, usually with ACDF, is required.
- Stage 2 is treated with a cervical orthosis for 12 weeks.
- Stage 3 is treated with a halo vest posterior instrumented arthrodesis.
- Stage 4 and 5 are treated with open reduction, decompression as required, and multilevel instrumented arthrodesis through a posterior approach.
  - A secondary anterior approach can be performed if anterior column integrity is significantly compromised or if there are concerns about inadequate stability.

Extension Injuries without Radiographic Abnormality

Central Cord Syndrome

- Forced transient neck hyperextension causes infolding of the ligamentum flavum, posterior bulging of the intervertebral disc, and occasionally, retrolisthesis of the vertebral bodies.
- In patients with a narrow spinal canal, the spinal cord is compressed by a pincer effect, causing selective injury to the central aspect of the spinal cord.
- The resulting central cord syndrome is characterized by worse upper than lower extremity function.
- The prognosis for recovery is thought to be good, although patients frequently have significant residual hand dysfunction and spasticity.
- The treatment of patients with central cord syndrome remains controversial.

- Surgical intervention is appropriate in patients with ongoing compression who are not improving neurologically, patients who have plateaued neurologically, or in patients with cervical instability.
- Various surgical options are available, and the appropriate choice depends on the primary location of compression (e.g., anterior versus posterior), the number of levels involved, associated instability patterns, and preexisting diseases.

Vertical Compression Injuries: Burst Fractures

General Considerations

- Vertical compression injuries result from an axial load applied to the top of the head with the c-spine in a non-flexed position.
- It is an uncommon injury. C6 and C7 are most commonly affected.
- The fracture pattern, commonly referred to as a cervical burst fracture, is characterized by comminution that is evenly distributed between the anterior and middle columns and leads to a relatively symmetric loss of vertebral body height.
- Unlike with flexion-compression injuries, there is relatively little kyphosis or translational malalignment.
- Injury to the posterior ligament complex is uncommon.

Classification and Treatment

- Allen and others classified vertical compression fractures into three stages based on the severity of the vertebral body fracture (Box 11–11; Figure 11–16).

Box 11–11 Vertical Compression Injuries of the Subaxial Cervical Spine

STAGE	ALLEN AND OTHERS' NOMENCLATURE	DESCRIPTION OF INJURY	USUAL TREATMENT
1	VCS1	Fracture of superior *or* inferior endplate with cupping deformity and minimal loss of height or fracture displacement. Symmetric loss of anterior and posterior vertebral body height without gross angular or translational malalignment	Rigid collar
2	VCS2	Same as stage 1 but with fracture of superior *and* inferior endplate	Rigid collar versus halo vest
3	VCS3	Same as stage 2, with vertebral body fragmentation, greater fracture displacement, retropulsion, and loss of height. May have secondary posterior ligament injury	Corpectomy and anterior instrumented reconstruction versus halo vest

From Allen BL Jr, Ferguson RL, Lehmann TR, et al: *Spine* 7:1-27, 1982.

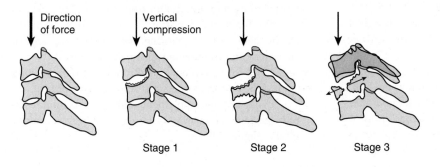

Figure 11–16: **Classification and treatment of vertical compression injuries of the subaxial cervical spine. From Bellabarba C, Anderson PA: Injuries of the lower cervical spine. In Herkowitz HN, Garfin SR, Eismont FJ, Bell GR, Balderston RA, editors: *Rothman-Simeone: The spine,* Philadelphia, 2006, Elsevier. (Figure 68–12, p. 1115)**

- Treatment is largely determined by the presence or absence of SCI, the degree of canal compromise, spinal alignment, and the integrity of posterior soft tissues.
- Stage 1 fracture has increased concavity of the superior or inferior vertebral endplates. Treatment consists of 12 weeks of immobilization with a rigid cervical orthosis.
- Stage 2 fracture extends through the endplate and into the vertebral body, yet remains relatively nondisplaced, with little or no bony retropulsion into the spinal canal and minimal kyphosis. Neurologic injury is uncommon. Treated with immobilization in a hard cervical collar, SOMI-type brace, or halo vest.
  - Corpectomy and anterior reconstruction for patients with neurologic deficits.
- Stage 3 fractures have a greater loss of vertebral body height with wider centrifugal fracture displacement, resulting in greater bony retropulsion into the spinal canal.
  - Neurologic deficits occur more frequently.
  - Anterior decompression and stabilization with corpectomy, interbody reconstruction, and plating is warranted.

Flexion-Compression Injuries: Flexion Teardrop Fractures

General Considerations

- The flexion-compression injury warrants a separate category because of several characteristic features relating to diagnosis, treatment, and prognosis that distinguish it from other flexion injuries and compression injuries.
- Also known as flexion teardrop fractures, flexion-compression injuries most frequently involve C5 but commonly involve C4 and C6.
- These injuries result from diving injuries, football spearing injuries, and motor vehicle collisions.
- They constitute axial loading injuries with an associated flexion force vector.
- They have a consistent injury pattern that ranges in severity over five stages.
  - Its more severe stages involve a pattern of injury in which the primary fracture line separates the anterior-inferior corner of the vertebral body (the so-called "teardrop"), which remains aligned with the caudal intervertebral disc and vertebra, from the remaining, posteriorly-displaced vertebral body.
  - Severe retrolisthesis and canal compromise may result, the severity of which correlates with the risk of SCI.
  - The axial compression results in an associated sagittal split through the vertebral body in up to two thirds of cases and bilaminar fracture.
- This combination of sagittal vertebral body split with neural arch fracture is usually associated with a severe SCI.
- The flexion-compression (flexion teardrop) fracture differs from the vertical compression (burst) fracture in that, although anterosuperior endplate compression is a component of the flexion compression injury, its primary fracture line extends from the anterior cortex inferiorly toward the intervertebral disc rather than extending axially into the vertebral body from the superior endplate.
- An important component of flexion-compression injuries is that the flexion component threatens the integrity of the posterior ligamentous structures.

Classification

- Flexion-compression injuries have been divided into five stages of severity by Allen and others based on the extent of vertebral body fracture and displacement (Box 11–12; Figure 11–17).
- Stage 1, 2 and 3 injuries have varying degrees of vertebral comminution without gross angular or translational malalignment. Twenty-five percent of stage 3 injuries have an associated SCI.
- Stage 4 injuries have 3 mm or less of retrolisthesis with a probable injury to the posterior ligament complex. Thirty-eight percent of stage 4 injuries have an associated SCI.
- Stage 5 injuries have more than 3 mm of retrolisthesis and associated posterior ligamentous instability. Ninety-one percent of stage 5 injures have an associated SCI, over half of which are complete.

Treatment

Patients without Neurological Deficit

- Attempts at nonoperative treatment are reasonable in the absence of neurologic deficits or posterior ligament disruption.
- The potential for progressive kyphosis and instability after nonoperative treatment is high and is normally associated with posterior ligamentous injury.
- Stages 1 and 2—Nonoperative treatment consisting of 12 weeks in a cervical orthosis or halo vest. Flexion-extension radiographs should be obtained after 12 weeks, when bracing is discontinued.
- Stage 3—Operative intervention is required with SCI or posterior ligament injury.
  - Radiographs and CT scan should be scrutinized for evidence of interspinous or facet widening, and MRI should be obtained to assess the status of the interspinous ligament, facet capsules, and ligamentum flavum
  - Corpectomy and anterior instrumentation are safe and effective for flexion teardrop fractures and are superior to the halo vest in restoring and maintaining sagittal alignment and minimizing treatment failures.
- Stages 4 and 5—Provisional stabilization with cranial tong traction followed by corpectomy and anterior plating.
  - These may require supplemental posterior fixation if stability remains a concern as a result of extensive posterior injury (Figure 11–18).

	Box 11–12	**Flexion-Compression Injuries of the Subaxial Cervical Spine**	

STAGE	ALLEN AND OTHERS' NOMENCLATURE	DESCRIPTION OF INJURY	USUAL TREATMENT
1	CFS1	Blunting of anterosuperior endplate. Intact posterior ligaments	Rigid collar
2	CFS2	Compression of anterosuperior and inferior endplates with anteroinferior "beaking." Intact posterior ligaments	Rigid collar
3	CFS3	Flexion teardrop fracture of anteroinferior body, without retrolisthesis. Posterior ligament injury is possible.	Halo vest versus corpectomy and anterior instrumented arthrodesis versus posterior instrumented arthrodesis
4	CFS4	Flexion teardrop fracture of anteroinferior body, with <3 mm of retrolisthesis. Posterior ligament injury is possible.	Corpectomy and anterior instrumented arthrodesis ± (occasionally) posterior instrumented arthrodesis
5	CFS5	Flexion teardrop fracture of anteroinferior body, with = 3 mm of retrolisthesis. Posterior ligament injury is probable.	Corpectomy and anterior instrumented arthrodesis ± (occasionally) posterior instrumented arthrodesis

From Allen BL Jr, Ferguson RL, Lehmann TR, et al: *Spine* 7:1-27, 1982.

Patients with Neurologic Injury

- Most patients with flexion-compression injuries sustain SCIs.
- Traction and a cervical bump are used to achieve at least partial realignment and provisional decompression of the cervical spine. Surgical decompression and stabilization should be performed when safely feasible.
- Anterior corpectomy and instrumented interbody arthrodesis allow for realignment and stabilization through a direct approach to the site of spinal cord compression.
- High fusion and functional neurologic recovery rates in patients with incomplete SCIs have been reported with anterior treatment of flexion-compression injuries, with few approach-related complications.

- Secondary posterior stabilization may be required in the presence of posterior ligamentous injury. However unless treatment of the injury requires multilevel corpectomy, supplemental posterior stabilization is usually not necessary.

Flexion-Distraction Injuries: Facet Dislocations versus Fracture-Dislocations

Classification and General Considerations

- All flexion-distraction injuries involve injury to the facet joints.
- The mechanism of injury usually involves a blow or fall onto the occiput or a deceleration mechanism usually associated with motor vehicle collision.

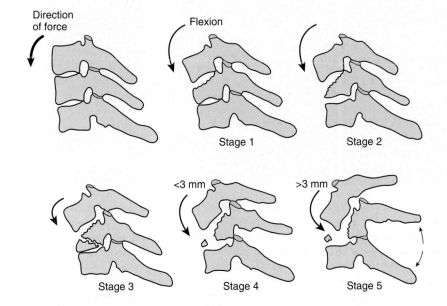

Figure 11–17: Classification and treatment of flexion-compression injuries of the subaxial cervical spine. From Bellabarba C, Anderson PA: Injuries of the lower cervical spine. In Herkowitz HN, Garfin SR, Eismont FJ, Bell GR, Balderston RA, editors: *Rothman-Simeone: The spine*, Philadelphia, 2006, Elsevier. (Figure 68–14, p. 1117).

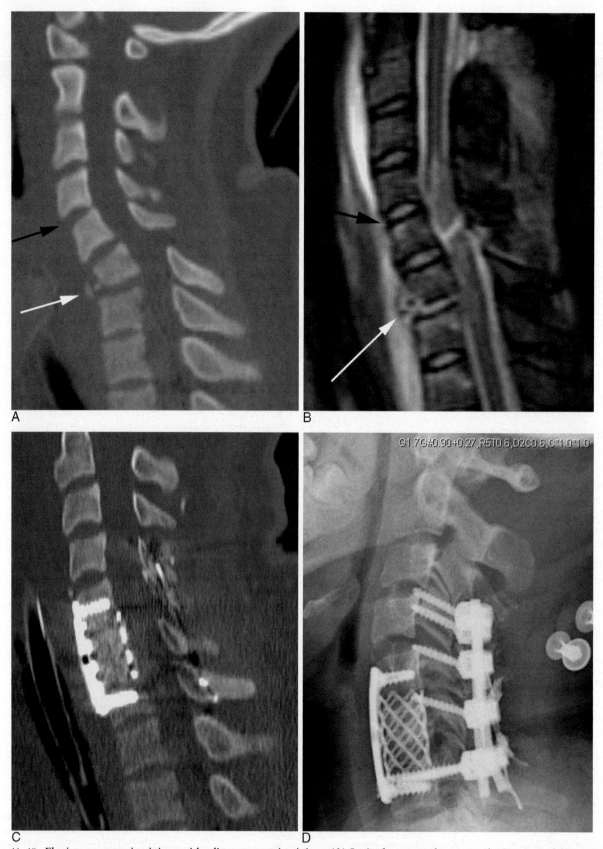

Figure 11–18: Flexion-compression injury with adjacent extension injury. **(A)** Sagittal computed tomography image, and **(B)** sagittal magnetic resonance image of a patient with a stage 5 flexion-compression injury at C6 *(white arrows)* and a C4 complete spinal cord injury following a motor vehicle collision. The patient was also noted to have hyperextension of the C4-C5 disc space on computed tomography, and disruption of the anterior longitudinal ligament (ALL) and anterior annulus of C4-C5 on magnetic resonance imaging *(black arrows)*. Note also the hyperextension posture of C4-C5 on the sagittal computed tomography image. As a result of the highly unstable nature of this injury, the patient was treated with a single-stage anterior and posterior procedure as shown on the **(C)** postoperative sagittal computed tomography image and **(D)** postoperative lateral radiograph. The anterior procedure spanned the C5 to C7 levels, whereas the injured C4-C5 level was also included in the posterior construct. Different injury types can often occur simultaneously, particularly with high-energy mechanisms.

- Purely ligamentous injuries occur when distractive forces across the posterior elements outweigh shear forces, whereas the propensity for facet fracture increases when the facet is subjected to relatively greater shear.
- The severity of flexion-distraction injuries ranges from attenuation of the posterior soft-tissue restraints with mild facet subluxation that can be successfully treated with external immobilization to complete dislocation of the facets with gross angular and translational malalignment and SCI that warrants surgical intervention.
- Based on this spectrum of injury severity, Allen and others have identified four stages of the "distractive flexion" injury (Box 11–13, Figure 11–19).
- Stage 1—Facet sprains. Slight widening of the facet joints and interspinous distance, causing mild focal kyphosis (<10 degrees). Facet widening with increased T2 signal intensity is the typical finding on MRI.
- Stage 2—Unilateral facet dislocations and fracture-dislocations. Their defining characteristic is a rotational deformity in the axial plane.

- The mechanism of injury involves a flexion injury with resulting distraction of the posterior elements, coupled with a rotational force.
- Because of the associated annular disruption, the potential for extrusion of the nucleus pulposus into the spinal canal may have important implications in the treatment of patients with unilateral facet injuries.
- The rotational deformity in unilateral facet injuries is manifested on the lateral radiograph as rotation of the right and left facet joints relative to each other ("bow tie" sign), with the appearance of 25% or less anterolisthesis of the affected vertebral body.
- Spinous process malalignment on the anteroposterior (AP) radiograph is the hallmark of the rotational deformity.
- Reversal of the position of the superior relative to the inferior facets provides the typical appearance of facet dislocation on axial and sagittal CT images.
- Facet fractures occur frequently with unilateral facet dislocations. They are best visualized on sagittal CT reformations.

| | **ALLEN AND OTHERS'** | | |
STAGE	**NOMENCLATURE**	**DESCRIPTION OF INJURY**	**USUAL TREATMENT**
1	DFS1	Facet sprain with widening of facet and interspinous distance in flexion and occasional blunting of anterosuperior endplate	Rigid collar
2	DFS2	Unilateral facet dislocation or fracture/dislocation	Anterior instrumented arthrodesis versus posterior instrumental arthrodesis
3	DFS3	Bilateral facet dislocation or fracture/dislocation with incomplete anterolisthesis	Anterior instrumented arthrodesis versus posterior instrumental arthrodesis
4	DFS4	Bilateral facet dislocation or fracture/dislocation with complete anterolisthesis	Posterior instrumental arthrodesis versus secondary anterior arthrodesis

Box 11–13 **Classification and Treatment of Flexion-Distraction Injuries of the Subaxial Cervical Spine**

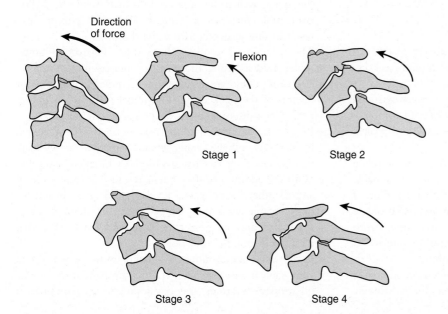

Stage 1

Stage 2

Stage 3

Stage 4

Figure 11–19: **Classification and treatment of flexion-distraction injuries of the subaxial cervical spine. From Bellabarba C, Anderson PA: Injuries of the lower cervical spine. In Herkowitz HN, Garfin SR, Eismont FJ, Bell GR, Balderston RA, editors:** *Rothman-Simeone: The spine,* **Philadelphia, 2006, Elsevier. (Figure 68–17, p. 1121).**

- Although similar to pure facet dislocations, reduction is generally easier to achieve in the presence of an associated facet fracture because less distraction is required to clear the fractured facet and achieve reduction. However, the reduction is also likely to be less stable once realigned as a result of loss of the buttressing effect of the intact facet.
- Stage 3 and 4 injuries are bilateral facet dislocations and fracture-dislocations.
- The severity of stage 3 ligamentous injuries of the facet joints ranges from facet subluxation to perched facets to facet dislocations.
- Full dislocation results in at least 50% anterior translation of the vertebral body and milder kyphosis and interspinous widening than is seen with perched facets.
- Rotational malalignment is not characteristic of bilateral facet injuries.
- An associated facet fracture may require that posterior fixation be extended to adjacent levels or may encourage the surgeon to more strongly consider an anterior surgical approach that would obviate the need to fuse adjacent levels.
- Because the injuries behave so differently, it is important that facet dislocation with shear or avulsion fracture patterns typical of flexion mechanisms be distinguished from posterior compressive fracture patterns and the "oblique shear" fracture pattern typical of fracture-dislocations secondary to extension-compression mechanisms.
- MRI illustrates the soft-tissue injury and degree of spinal cord compression and is likely to show disruption of the interspinous ligament and facet capsules, with at least partial intervertebral disc disruption in over 60% of cases.
- MRI findings of intervertebral disc herniation may profoundly influence treatment.
- MRI also plays a prognostic role in predicting the potential for functional recovery from SCI based on the appearance of the injured spinal cord.

The Role of Prereduction Magnetic Resonance Imaging in Facet Dislocations and Fracture-Dislocations

- Whether an MRI scan to identify disc herniations is required before closed reduction in patients with facet dislocations is a controversial matter.
- Spinal realignment in the presence of posteriorly extruded disc material can result in SCI as a result of cord compression from displacement of the disc material into the canal at the time of reduction.
- Regardless of the presence or absence of intervertebral disc extrusion, if a patient is awake, alert, and examinable for neurologic status, closed reduction with application of sequential weight and monitoring of interim neurologic status has been shown to be safe when done with the understanding that the procedure must be aborted at the first sign of any neurologic abnormality.
- Conversely, in any patient who is obtunded, anesthetized, or is otherwise not reliably examinable for neurologic

status during the course of reduction, an MRI scan should be obtained before any attempt at reduction. If the MRI were to demonstrate the presence of extruded disc material, anterior discectomy should be undertaken before spinal realignment and fixation.
- In addition to recognizing that neurologic worsening may occur during spinal realignment, an appropriate treatment algorithm must also acknowledge the potentially detrimental effects on neurologic recovery that may result from delays in spinal cord realignment, particularly in patients with incomplete SCIs.
- Immediate reduction in all examinable patients with neurologic deficits minimizes the risk of iatrogenic injury while acknowledging the importance of avoiding unfounded delays in spinal realignment.
- In unexaminable patients, MRI should be obtained before reduction. In the absence of significant disc extrusion on MRI, closed reduction can be performed at the earliest possibility. If the MRI shows disc extrusion, an anterior discectomy should precede reduction and stabilization.
- In patients who are neurologically intact or have limited nonprogressive deficits, such as mild radiculopathy, the need for urgent closed reduction before MRI is less convincing. However, closed reduction in an awake patient is appropriate and safe under these circumstances.

Treatment

Stage 1 Injuries

- Facet sprains generally require 6 to 12 weeks in a rigid orthosis.

Closed Reduction Technique: Stages 2, 3, and 4 Injuries

- Patients who are diagnosed with a unilateral (stage 2) or bilateral (stage 3 or 4) facet dislocation, particularly when associated with neurologic injury, should undergo an attempt at closed reduction at the earliest possibility.
- Stainless steel Gardner-Wells tongs are recommended for the initial reduction because deformation of the MRI-compatible materials at weights above 50 pounds may result in disengagement from the skull.
- The reduction is ideally performed in a fluoroscopy suite, under mild sedation, and with appropriate monitoring.
- Traction pulleys are arranged in a manner that allows for flexion of the neck during the initial phase of reduction to facilitate disengagement of the dislocated facet.
- Initial traction with 5 to 10 pounds should be followed by scrutiny of the craniocervical junction to evaluate for undetected injuries that may distract with minimal weight.
- With the addition of subsequent weight, the injured level and all other intervertebral levels should be evaluated for unacceptable distraction, which is normally defined as disc space widening of greater than one-and-a-half times that of adjacent uninjured levels.
- A thorough sensorimotor evaluation must be performed after each increase in weight, and the patient should be questioned regarding the development or evolution of

any neurologic symptoms. With any complaints of sensorimotor symptoms during the reduction, the procedure should be aborted in lieu of an open reduction.

- Weight is added in 5- to 10-pound increments until the dislocated facet appears to have cleared its more caudal counterpart. Increasing the extension vector of the traction by lowering the height of the traction pulley or placing an interscapular bump beneath the patient may facilitate the final phase of reduction.
- Once reduction has been achieved, traction weight is incrementally reduced under fluoroscopic evaluation to between 15 and 25 pounds, depending on which level is involved. Higher weights may be required if recurrence of subluxation occurs.
- Following reduction, MRI-compatible tongs are substituted for the stainless steel Gardner-Wells tongs while manual axial traction stabilizes the c-spine.
- An MRI of the c-spine is obtained at the earliest possibility, regardless of whether one was obtained before reduction, to evaluate the spinal cord and establish the presence of any compressive lesions.
- If an objective neurologic deficit occurs, the inciting event should be reversed, methylprednisolone should be administered according to institutional protocol, imaging studies should be obtained to assess for potential causes, and treatment should proceed accordingly.

Surgical Treatment: Stages 2, 3, and 4 Injuries

- Most stages 2, 3, and 4 flexion-distraction injuries require operative stabilization.
- In the absence of spinal cord or nerve root compression resulting from disc herniation on postreduction MRI, posterior stabilization is appropriate, and offers superior biomechanical properties to anterior fixation.
- However, even in the absence of disc herniation, ACDF remains an acceptable and sometimes preferable approach, particularly in patients with facet fractures that preclude lateral mass fixation at the injured level alone and would require fusion of adjacent segments if stabilized posteriorly.
- Although biomechanically inferior to the posterior approach, the clinical results with ACDF have been largely equivalent to those with posterior stabilization in the treatment of facet dislocations and fracture-dislocations, with fusion rates exceeding 90%.
- In the presence of significant disc herniation on postreduction MRI, ACDF is the most appropriate treatment.
- Although not often necessary after anterior stabilization, secondary posterior stabilization may be appropriate for highly unstable injuries involving the lower cervical levels or in patients otherwise prone to failure of fixation resulting from osteoporosis or other medical comorbi-dities.
- If the amount of distraction required to achieve a reasonable press-fit of the interbody graft is thought to be excessive during the anterior procedure, a looser press-fit should be accepted and followed by posterior stabilization.

- The inability to successful reduce a facet dislocation with closed techniques may complicate the choice of anterior versus posterior approach.
  - Traditionally, in the absence of disc herniation, unreduced flexion-distraction injuries have been realigned and stabilized through a posterior approach.
  - Conventional treatment for unreduced injuries with MRI evidence of disc herniation has been anterior discectomy followed by prone positioning and posterior reduction and stabilization, possibly followed by anterior interbody grafting.
  - If an anterior approach is warranted for unreduced dislocations, I prefer to complete the reduction and stabilization entirely from the anterior approach, when possible. Once the discectomy has been performed, reduction can safely be performed by various means, including the application of weight under lateral fluoroscopy or direct manipulation of the vertebral bodies with a lamina spreader or Caspar pins.
  - Surgical procedures requiring reduction are performed with spinal cord monitoring.

Distraction Injuries

- Distraction injuries of the c-spine are extremely unstable high-energy injuries that result in tension failure of all three columns (Figure 11–20).
- Discoligamentous injury with or without avulsion fracture is most common.
- In addition to resuscitation measures, early treatment should focus on the evaluation and treatment of spinal cord and vertebral artery injury.
- Surgical stabilization is invariably required, with posterior reduction and stabilization being the preferred method.
- Secondary anterior cervical discectomy and interbody fusion may be considered, but are not routinely necessary.

Lateral Compression Injuries

- Lateral compression (LC) injuries are unusual and occur mainly as a result of motor vehicle collisions and sports-related mechanisms.
- Two injury types have been identified (Box 11–14; Figure 11–21).
  - Stage 1 is unilateral arch fracture with lateral vertebral body compression.
  - Stage 2 is the same as stage 1 with associated contralateral posterior facet widening.
- SCI is unusual. Because of a mechanism involving violent lateral flexion of the neck, traction injuries of contralateral nerve roots and brachial plexus occur with relative frequency.
- Most stage 1 injuries can be treated with 12 weeks of rigid collar immobilization.
- Stage 2 injuries require realignment and posterior stabilization because of their greater coronal plane deformity and associated posterior ligamentous injuries.

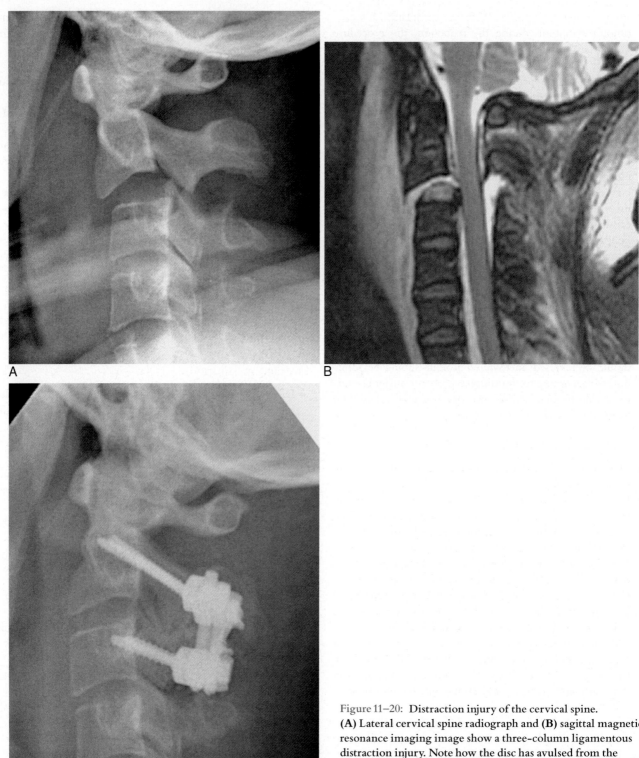

Figure 11–20: Distraction injury of the cervical spine.
(A) Lateral cervical spine radiograph and **(B)** sagittal magnetic resonance imaging image show a three-column ligamentous distraction injury. Note how the disc has avulsed from the inferior endplate of C2 but has remained otherwise intact.
(C) Postoperative lateral radiograph after posterior C2-C3 instrumented arthrodesis.

Box 11–14	Classification and Treatment of Lateral Compression Injuries			
STAGE	**ALLEN AND OTHERS' NOMENCLATURE**	**DESCRIPTION OF INJURY**		**USUAL TREATMENT**
1	LFS1	Asymmetric lateral compression of the body and nondisplaced ipsilateral vertebral arch fracture		Rigid collar
2	LFS2	Asymmetric lateral compression of the body and either displaced ipsilateral vertebral arch fracture or contralateral facet dislocation		Posterior instrumented arthrodesis

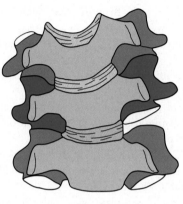

Stage 1

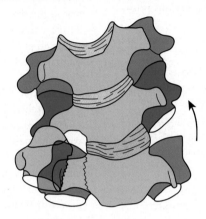

Stage 2

Figure 11–21: Classification and treatment of lateral compression injuries of the subaxial cervical spine. From Bellabarba C, Anderson PA: Injuries of the lower cervical spine. In Herkowitz HN, Garfin SR, Eismont FJ, Bell GR, Balderston RA, editors: *Rothman-Simeone: The spine,* Philadelphia, 2006, Elsevier. (Figure 68–20, p. 1127).

Cervicothoracic Junction

Introduction

- Cervicothoracic (C-T) injuries present unique diagnostic and therapeutic challenges.
- Limitations in plain radiographic visualization contribute to delays in diagnosis.
- Attempts at closed reduction of fracture-dislocations are frequently unsuccessful.
- Nonoperative treatment of unstable C-T injuries often results in progressive kyphosis.
- Anterior C-T exposure may be difficult and associated with high complication rates.
- Posterior instrumentation is complicated by the transitional C-T anatomy and by potential hardware prominence.

Anatomy

- The C-T junction extends between C6 and T2.
- It is an area of transition from cervical lordosis to thoracic kyphosis.
- The junction of the mobile subaxial cervical spine with the stiff upper thoracic spine (stabilized by upper ribcage) creates a fulcrum at the C-T junction.
- The combination of this stress-riser effect and the change in sagittal plane alignment increases the susceptibility of the C-T junction to injury.
- Anterior plate fixation in the vertebral bodies of the C-T junction may be suboptimal as a result of the relative

osteopenia of the upper thoracic vertebra, caused by the stress shielding effect of the upper ribcage.
- The C7 pedicles are more lateral than the upper thoracic pedicles, making posterior pedicle screw instrumentation across the C-T junction more challenging.
- The spinal cord occupies over 80% of the upper thoracic spinal canal, and the C7, C8, and T1 roots lie in close proximity to the medial wall of their respective pedicles, emphasizing the need for accurate pedicle screw placement.
- The esophagus, segmental vessels, and pleura and great vessels lie adjacent to the upper thoracic vertebrae in the upper thoracic spine, complicating anterior exposures and placing them at risk during pedicle screw placement.

Diagnosis

- Initial clinical and radiographic management is similar to that described for the cervical and thoracic spine.
- Because the C-T junction is obstructed by the shoulders, over one third of C-T injuries are missed with plain X-rays despite the use of oblique and swimmer's views.
- CT scan is far more sensitive and specific in evaluating the C-T junction.
- Specific injury types are largely equivalent to those described in the subaxial cervical spine and thoracic spine. The transitional nature of the C-T junction may complicate the diagnosis and treatment of injuries, thus warranting a separate C-T category.

Nonoperative Treatment

- C-T braces (e.g., Minerva) and halo vests are most commonly used for the nonoperative treatment of patients with C-T injuries.
- External immobilization of C-T injuries is difficult because of:
  - The high strain caused by transition between the mobile, lordotic cervical spine and the immobile, kyphotic, upper thoracic spine.
  - Difficulty in achieving a tight torso fit for various possible reasons including obesity.
  - The "snaking" phenomenon that may occur with halo vest immobilization.
- Closed reduction of burst fractures, facet dislocations, and fracture-dislocations can be performed emergently under fluoroscopic visualization with Gardner-Wells tongs.
- Closed reduction at the C-T junction is often complicated by the need for high traction weights (routinely up to 60% of body weight) and poor fluoroscopic visualization.

Surgical Approaches

- The choice of anterior, posterior, or circumferential approach is influenced by injury type, bone quality, body habitus, spinal alignment, the presence of multiple injuries, host physiologic factors, and surgeon preference.

Anterior Approach

- The Smith-Robinson approach can allow for exposure as low as T2.
  - Risks include injury to the recurrent laryngeal nerve, vascular structures, and thoracic duct and the potential for esophageal dysfunction.
  - Difficulty with exposure of the caudal C-T segments may hamper the decompression and impede optimal positioning of bone graft or instrumentation.
  - Screw purchase may be compromised in the upper thoracic vertebral bodies as a result of the relatively decreased bone density of these segments.
  - Correction of a traumatic spinal deformity, such as a facet dislocation, is more difficult from an anterior than a posterior approach.
- Alternatives to the Smith-Robinson approach to the anterior C-T junction consist of:
  - High transthoracic and transsternal exposure techniques.
  - Variations of conventional low anterior neck approaches that are extended caudally with clavicular or manubrial splitting techniques.
  - Sternal splitting approaches, which carry high (up to 40%) morbidity.
- Anterior approaches to the C-T junction are limited by their increased potential for marked morbidity.
- The possible advantages of anterior approaches, such as the potential for comprehensive ventral spinal canal decompression, restoration of the weight-bearing anterior column, and supine positioning, have to be weighed against their morbidity.

Posterior Approach

- This approach is more extensile in rostral and caudal directions than anterior approaches.
- It allows for direct reduction of facet injuries.
- It also offers multiple fixation points for a variety of posterior segmental fixation systems.
- Three-column pedicle screw fixation can safely be achieved at C7 and below.
- Lateral mass screw fixation is more desirable at C3 through C6.
- Preoperative CT is essential to evaluate the patient's specific vertebral anatomy.
- Direct visualization and palpation of the medial pedicle walls through a small laminotomy can provide additional guidance for safe C-T pedicle screw placement.
- The transposition of C7 and T1 screw fixation points in the coronal plane may pose considerable challenges with posterior fixation of the C-T junction.
- Specialized devices, such rod-plate and tapered rod devices and polyaxial screws, can accommodate these anatomic challenges and the smaller screw diameters required in the c-spine compared to the upper thoracic spine (Figure 11–22).

Summary

- Instability of the C-T junction remains a treatment challenge.
- Diagnosis by clinical examination and conventional radiographs can be difficult.
- CT and MRI are valuable diagnostic tools in identifying injuries in this region.
- The C-T junction is subject to marked biomechanical stresses, which can render external orthoses inadequate.
- Anterior approaches to the C-T junction are associated with high morbidity.
- Posterior segmental instrumentation and arthrodesis is recommended for C-T injuries.
- Secondary anterior procedures may be considered for highly unstable C-T injuries.
- For upper thoracic lesions below the T1 level, use of a costotransversectomy may be preferable to anterior procedures

Thoracic and Lumbar Spine

- This area is comprised of the thoracic region (T3-T10), thoracolumbar region (T11-L2), and lumbosacral region (L3-S1).
- These three regions differ with regard to biomechanical and neurologic factors.

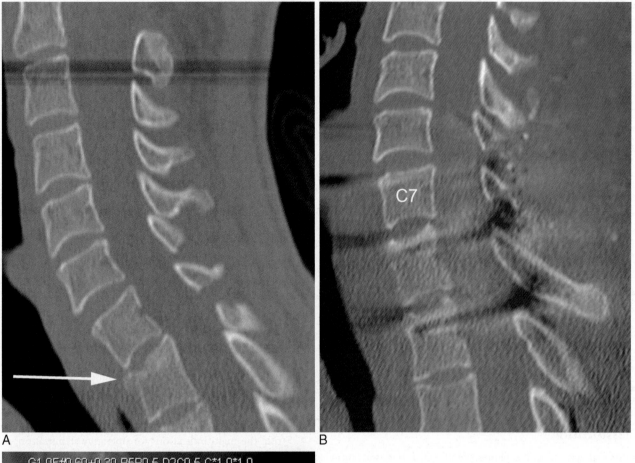

A

B

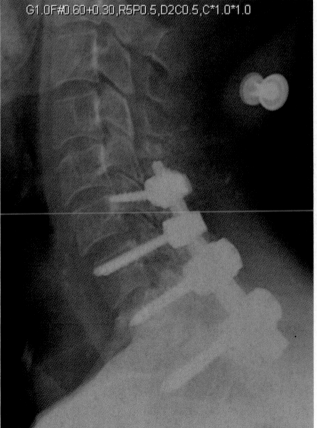

C

Figure 11–22: Posterior fixation of the cervicothoracic junction. **(A)** Sagittal computed tomography image of the cervical spine of a patient involved in a motorcycle collision shows a C7-T1 flexion-distraction injury characterized by tension failure of the posterior elements and compression failure of the anterior column. The posterior injury consists of C7 spinous process and lamina fracture involving the C7-T1 facet joints bilaterally and a C6 spinous process fracture. Magnetic resonance imaging scan also showed disruption of the ligamentum flavum at C7-T1 *(not shown)*. The anterior injury consists of a superior end plate fracture of T1 *(arrow)*. The transitional nature of the cervicothoracic junction makes it particularly susceptible to this type of injury and makes it difficult to prevent progressive kyphosis with external immobilization alone. Postoperative **(B)** sagittal computed tomography image and **(C)** lateral radiograph after posterior C6-T2 instrumented arthrodesis with a tapered rod construct show correction of the kyphotic malalignment.

- Injuries to the thoracic region:
  - Are negatively influenced by the kyphotic moment placed on the injury by the more anteriorly positioned weight-bearing line.
  - Are positively influenced by the stability imparted by the rib cage.
  - Occur at the spinal cord level, giving rise to the potential for severe neurological deficits even with limited amounts of canal compromise.
- Injuries to the thoracolumbar (T-L) region:
  - Are the most common as a result of their transitional location at the junction of the rigid thoracic spine and the mobile lumbar spine.
  - May be difficult to treat nonoperatively as a result of this transitional anatomy.
  - Occur at the conus medullaris level, with the potential for neurologic deficits ranging from complete paralysis to isolated bowel or bladder deficits.
- Injuries to the lumbosacral (L-S) region:
  - Are positively influenced by the more posteriorly located weight-bearing axis, which minimizes the kyphotic forces on the injury.
  - Occur at the level of the cauda equina, resulting in a high tolerance for canal compromise without neurologic injury.
- The discussion will focus primarily on injuries to the T-L region because they are most common.

Classification

- Several classification schemes exist for T-L fractures, most of which distinguish injuries based on which column is disrupted and the mechanism of injury.
- There are three general categories of injury: (1) axial loading injuries, such as compression fractures, stable burst fractures, and unstable burst fractures; (2) bending injuries, such as Chance fractures (bony and ligamentous) and flexion-distraction injuries; (3) shear or rotational injuries, such as fracture-dislocations. Extension injuries have been included in categories 2 and 3, depending on the preponderance of extension deformity versus extension and translational or rotational deformity.
- The classification described in Box 11–15 combines the principles behind the AO classification and the classification initially proposed by McAfee and others.[21]

Treatment

- Treatment of T-L fractures may be nonoperative or may involve operative treatment through either an anterior, posterior, or combined anterior and posterior approach.
- The need for operative intervention is determined largely on the integrity of the posterior column.
  - Most compression fractures and burst fractures can be treated nonoperatively, unless accompanied by loss of posterior column integrity.
  - Greater than 25 to 30 degrees of kyphosis and greater than 50% loss of vertebral body height are potential indicators of posterior column injury.

- Chance fractures that involve primarily bony injury can be treated nonoperatively.
- Bracing of these injuries consists of:
  - Cervicothoracolumbosacral orthosis (CTLSO) for injuries above T7.
  - Thoracolumbosacral orthosis (TLSO) for injuries from T7 to L3.
  - Hipthoracolumbosacral orthosis (HTLSO) for injuries below L3.
- Most other fractures with posterior column injury, such as three-column (unstable) burst fractures, fracture-dislocations, extension fractures, and flexion-distraction injuries, including ligamentous Chance injuries, are treated with operative intervention (Box 11–15).

Burst Fractures

- Burst fractures are the most controversial T-L fractures with respect to the need for operative intervention and the optimal operative approach
- Decompression and stabilization is advocated for T-L burst fractures with neurologic deficits.
- In neurologically intact patients, the indications are less concrete and depend on individual patient factors.
  - Three-column burst fracture, multiple associated injuries, the inability to effectively brace the patient (resulting from other injuries or body habitus), and the anticipated morbidity of prolonged recumbency constitute the main indications for operative stabilization.
- Kyphosis of 25 degrees or more and loss of more than 50% of vertebral body height are relative indications for operative intervention.
- Early stabilization ± decompression of these injuries:
  - Facilitates patient mobilization and nursing care of the patient with multiple injuries.
  - Offers the best environment for potential recovery of neurologic deficits.
  - Allows for restoration of spinal alignment and optimal canal decompression by both ligamentotaxis and direct ventral disimpaction of retropulsed fragments (Figure 11–23).

Posterior Approach

- The posterior approach offers an extensile, straightforward, and familiar means for realigning and stabilizing most T-L spine injuries with three-column fixation while allowing sufficient anterior access to effectively decompress the anterior spinal canal (Figure 11–23).
- In specific circumstances requiring anterior interbody support in the thoracic region, a costotransversectomy approach can be performed.
- Although surgical intervention is less commonly required in the L-S region, the ability to retract the neural elements facilitates decompression of the cauda equina.
- The posterior approach offers advantages in the patient population with multiple injuries as a result of the expeditious manner in which stability and decompression can be achieved while minimizing additional physiologic challenges.

Box 11–15	Classification and Preferred approach for Operative Treatment of Thoracolumbar Fractures

A. Axial Loading Injuries

1. Compression fracture
   Characteristics—Compression fracture of the anterior column only. No posterior ligamentous disruption.
   Treatment—6 to 12 weeks of brace immobilization.
2. Stable Burst fracture
   Characteristics—Fracture of the anterior and middle columns. No facet subluxation or posterior ligamentous disruption. Vertical lamina fractures do not constitute unstable posterior column injuries. Usually neurologically intact.
   Treatment—6 to 12 weeks of brace immobilization.
3. Unstable Burst fracture
   Characteristics—Fracture of the anterior and middle columns with facet subluxation. Unlike with flexion-distraction injury, mechanism is primarily axial loading rather than bending. Often neurologically compromised.
   Treatment—Posterior (short-segment versus multilevel) versus anterior versus combined approach

B. Bending Injuries

1. Chance fracture
   Characteristics—Tension failure of all three columns. Injury may be primarily through the bony elements (bony Chance) or the discoligamentous structures (ligamentous Chance).
   Treatment—Posterior approach, short-segment fixation. Possible hyperextension bracing for bony Chance fractures.
2. Flexion-Distraction injury
   Characteristics—Tension failure of the posterior column and compression fracture of the anterior column. The middle column may be fractured, in which case these injuries may be difficult to distinguish from unstable burst fractures but appear to have primarily a bending mechanism.
   Treatment—Posterior approach, short-segment fixation.
3. Extension injuries
   Characteristics—May fit into bending injury or fracture-dislocation category, depending on extent of preponderance of extension deformity alone versus extension and translational or rotational deformity. Extension deformity may be difficult to correct.
   Treatment—Posterior approach, multilevel fixation. Possible secondary anterior reconstruction if residual extension deformity leaves large anterior column defect.

C. Fracture-Dislocations (Translationally or Rotationally Unstable Injuries)

Characteristics—Failure of all three columns in shear or rotation, as evidenced by translational ± rotational malalignment. Posterior element injury may consist of ligamentous injury with pure facet dislocation but usually involves fracture of the facets or pars interarticularis. Canal compromise is primarily a result of translational malalignment. May have associated vertebral body comminution and bony retropulsion. This category also includes extension injuries with primarily rotational or translational instability patterns.
   Treatment—Posterior approach, multilevel fixation. Possible secondary anterior decompression and reconstruction.

- In patients with vertebral body compromise of sufficient severity to warrant a second-stage anterior procedure, anterior reconstruction can be performed on a delayed basis:
  - while the patient is fully mobilized as his or her physiologic status improves.
  - through less invasive means because supplemental anterior plating is not required.
- The concerns with posterior fixation of thoracolumbar burst fractures pertain to potential failure of fixation and loss of alignment, particularly with short-segment fixation. This problem can be minimized by avoiding postoperative kyphosis and by enhancing fixation by maximizing screw length, endplate purchase and triangulation.

Anterior Approach

Rationale

- Anterior surgery offers the opportunity for immediate restoration of the load-bearing capacity of the anterior spine (Figure 11–24).

- Proposed advantages of anterior surgery consist of:
  - Direct ventral canal decompression, possibly resulting in improved neurologic recovery in patients with incomplete SCI.
  - The chance to immediately restore a structurally contiguous weight-bearing anterior vertebral column, possibly minimizing the risk of progressive kyphosis.

Concerns regarding anterior column surgery pertain to:
- Increased blood loss.
- Proximity of anterior implants to large vessels.
- Insufficient biomechanical properties of anterior implants.
- Difficulty manipulating the spine and reducing translational deformities.
- Limited extensile properties.
- Surgical approach-related morbidity compared to posterior spinal surgery.
- There are three well-accepted indications for anterior fixation of T-L fractures:
  - Unstable burst fractures with neurologic impairment.

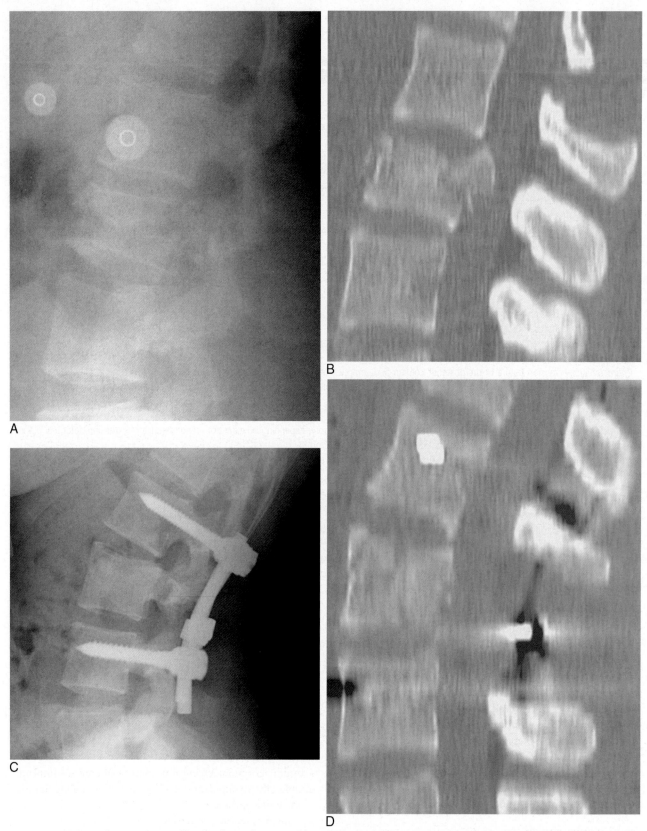

Figure 11–23: Posterior treatment of lumbar burst fracture with neurologic deficit. **(A)** Lateral radiograph and **(B)** sagittal computed tomography image of a woman who sustained an L2 burst fracture from a horseback riding accident show kyphosis, loss of vertebral body height, and severe canal compromise. This patient with multiple injuries had an incomplete cauda equina injury with profound lower extremity weakness and bowel and bladder dysfunction. She was treated with posterior decompression, kyphoreduction, and disimpaction of the retropulsed bony fragment from the posterior approach. The postoperative **(C)** lateral radiograph and **(D)** sagittal computed tomography image show restoration of physiologic alignment and spinal canal patency. This technique can successfully decompress the spinal canal, even if the compressive pathology is located anteriorly and may be better tolerated acutely than the anterior approach in patients with multiple injuries.

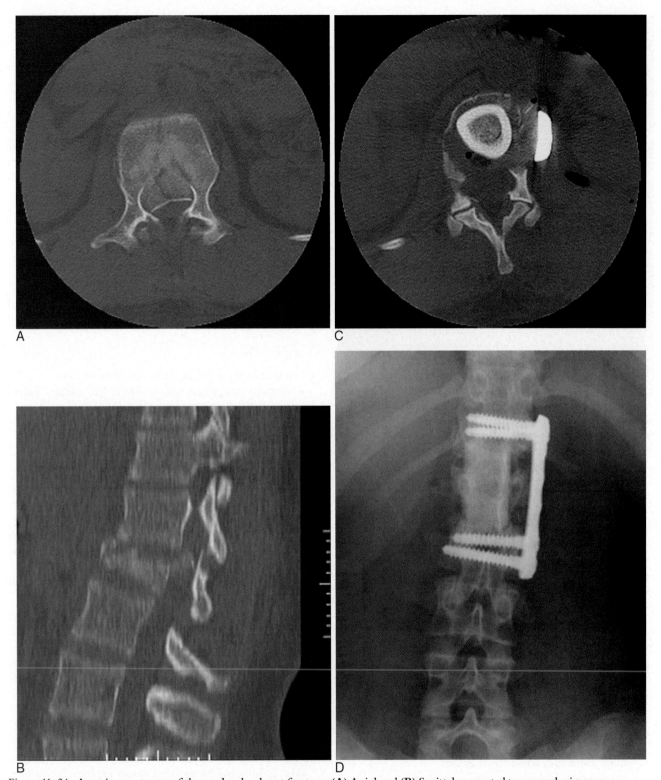

Figure 11–24: Anterior treatment of thoracolumbar burst fracture. **(A)** Axial and **(B)** Sagittal computed tomography images of a patient who sustained an isolated L1 burst fracture with severe canal compromise and an incomplete conus medullaris injury. Postoperative **(C)** axial computed tomography image, **(D)** anteroposterior, and

(Continued)

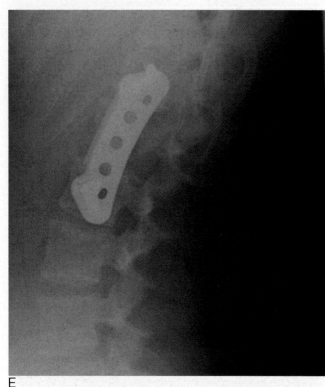

E

Figure 11–24 cont'd: (E) lateral radiographs after corpectomy and instrumented anterior thoracolumbar reconstruction with a structural tibial allograft show restoration of alignment and canal patency.

- Second-stage anterior reconstruction as a result of structural concerns or residual anterior compression after posterior stabilization.
- Correction of posttraumatic deformity
- Anterior procedures as stand-alone procedures are usually limited rostrally to the T6 level as a result of vertebral body size and the proximity of large vessels.

General Principles

- The sequence of events in the anterior treatment of T-L fractures consists of:
  - Adequately decompressing the neural elements.
  - Realigning the spinal column.
  - Can be achieved indirectly, such as by pushing on the posterior spinal elements, or directly with tools that allow distraction across the endplates.
  - Inserting a structural interbody graft or cage.
  - Endplate dissection with preservation of bony endplate, graft preparation, realignment of the spinal column, and graft insertion.
- If being done as a second-stage procedure after adequate posterior instrumentation, interbody support alone without anterior plating is generally sufficient.

- A thoracotomy is required for injuries between T2 and T12 and a retroperitoneal approach for injuries involving T12-L5 depending on variations in patient anatomy.
  - The T-L junction may be visualized by a combined thoracoabdominal approach through a thoracotomy with takedown of the diaphragm or a subdiaphragmatic exposure with partial takedown of the diaphragm but more limited exposure of T12.
- Thoracotomies for anterior spinal procedures in the upper thoracic and midthoracic spine are usually done from a right-sided approach to avoid cardiac structures. Lower thoracic and retroperitoneal approaches are preferably performed from the left (aortic) side as a result of the safer vascular dissection.
- Anterior treatment of an unstable thoracolumbar burst fracture generally requires full exposure of the lateral surface of the injured vertebral body.
- If anterior plating is required, the adjacent cranial and caudal segments are also fully exposed after obtaining surgical control of the associated segmental vessels.

Complications

- Complications occur in up to one third of cases.
  - Mortality associated with anterior T-L surgery ranges from 0.4% to 3.2%.
  - Postoperative paraplegia is reported in about 0.2% to 0.3% of patients.
  - The most common complications are pulmonary, especially in patients older than 60.
  - Other complications include high blood loss and transfusion requirements, aortic and cardiovascular injury requiring additional surgery, and neural or genitourinary injury.
- Sequential same-anesthetic anterior and posterior surgery, blood loss above 520 ml, and prolonged operative time have been associated with major complications.
  - Up to ≈15% of patients sustain vascular injury as a result of anterior T-L surgery.
- Intercostal thoracotomy may require sacrifice of one or more intercostal nerves or may impose significant retraction-induced trauma on these structures.
- Retroperitoneal exposure may be associated with neurologic sequelae, most commonly affecting the sympathetic chain or ilioinguinal, iliofemoral, and lateral femoral cutaneous nerves.
- Atony of the external oblique musculature following anterior thoracolumbar surgery may be mistaken for a postoperative incisional hernia.
- Mobilization and retraction of the psoas may adversely affect lumbar and lumbosacral plexus function, albeit usually to a transient degree.

Treatment Results

- To date there is no conclusive evidence to strongly support anterior over posterior or combined anterior and posterior treatment of T-L fractures.

- There is an 80% neurologic improvement in patients with T-L burst fractures, and incomplete neurologic deficits have been reported with both anterior and posterior procedures.

Fracture-Dislocations

- Fracture-dislocations are highly unstable three-column injuries resulting from shear and rotation forces
- Although unusual, true facet dislocations without fracture may occur in the T-L spine. More commonly fractures occur through the facets or pars interarticularis with translation or rotation about the axial plane.
- Canal compromise in these injuries is often primarily caused by rotational or translational displacement rather than by vertebral body comminution with bony retropulsion, although a combination of these factors may coexist.
- Operative stabilization is generally recommended for these highly unstable injury patterns, regardless of the patient's neurologic status.
  - A posterior approach to these injuries is advocated for several reasons.
  - They generally require multilevel instrumentation that cannot be easily achieved through a typical anterior approach (Figure 11–25).
  - The multiplanar pattern of displacement is more easily correctible through the posterior approach than through a more limited anterior exposure.
- Realignment will often result in decompression of the spinal canal, even in patients with associated vertebral body fractures, thus precluding the need for corpectomy.
- Most fracture-dislocations are diagnosed with anterolisthesis and kyphosis, with some degree of rotation and lateral listhesis.
- Kyphosis can be corrected by contouring the rods to the desired alignment.
- Anterolisthesis may be simultaneously corrected by ensuring that the final position of the pedicle screw heads relative to the vertebrae above the injury corresponds to that of the screws heads below the injury.
- Coronal-plane translation and rotation are corrected by sequential approximation of pedicle screws to the rod, initially on the convex side of the deformity, in a manner similar to that described for correction of nontraumatic scoliotic deformities using the so-called translational technique.
- The decompression achieved with reduction can be enhanced, if necessary, by laminectomy.
- If concerns remain about compression of the neural elements by anterior bony fragments, transpedicular or transforaminal decompression with ventral disimpaction of retropulsed fragments may be performed, as previously described.
- Postoperative CT scan can help determine the need for a second-stage anterior corpectomy and reconstruction, using an algorithm similar to that described in the treatment of unstable burst fractures.

Extension Injuries

- Extension injuries, also known as extension-distraction fracture-dislocations, are highly unstable three-column injuries that occur primarily in patients with ankylosing spinal conditions.
- These patients are thus often severely osteoporotic with premorbid kyphotic deformities, both of which are important considerations in their treatment.
- They constitute high-risk injuries because of their severe degree of instability and the advanced age and frequent comorbidities with which patients are diagnosed.
- Because of the extent of instability, I advocate operative stabilization of these injuries (Figure 11–26).
- Prone positioning on tables designed to correct the usual kyphosis and anterolisthesis deformities may accentuate hyperlordosis and retrolisthesis deformities. Alternative positioning techniques should therefore be considered, with the goal of restoring the patients' premorbid alignment rather than physiologic alignment.
- The posterior approach is favored in extension injuries for various reasons.
  - First, these injuries may present with severe malalignment, which is more easily addressed through a multilevel posterior exposure.
  - Second, the osteoporosis seen in these often metabolically compromised patients renders attempts to achieve meaningful fixation through shorter-segment anterior instrumentation fruitless and mandates the use of multilevel three-column instrumentation through a posterior approach.
- Correction of any remaining extension deformity can be achieved by overcontouring the rods into kyphosis, securing them loosely to the pedicle screws at an angle up to 180 degrees from their final orientation before finally rotating the rods into their correct position, thus introducing relative kyphosis and correcting the distraction of the anterior spine. Associated coronal plane deformities are corrected in a manner similar to that described for the more typical fracture-dislocations.

Flexion-Distraction Injuries and Chance Fractures

- Flexion-distraction and Chance fractures result from similar mechanisms that cause the posterior elements to fail in tension. Therefore in some classification systems they are designated as equivalent injuries. In my opinion, however, these are distinct injury patterns, and important nuances between them play an important role in determining the most favorable technique for stabilization.

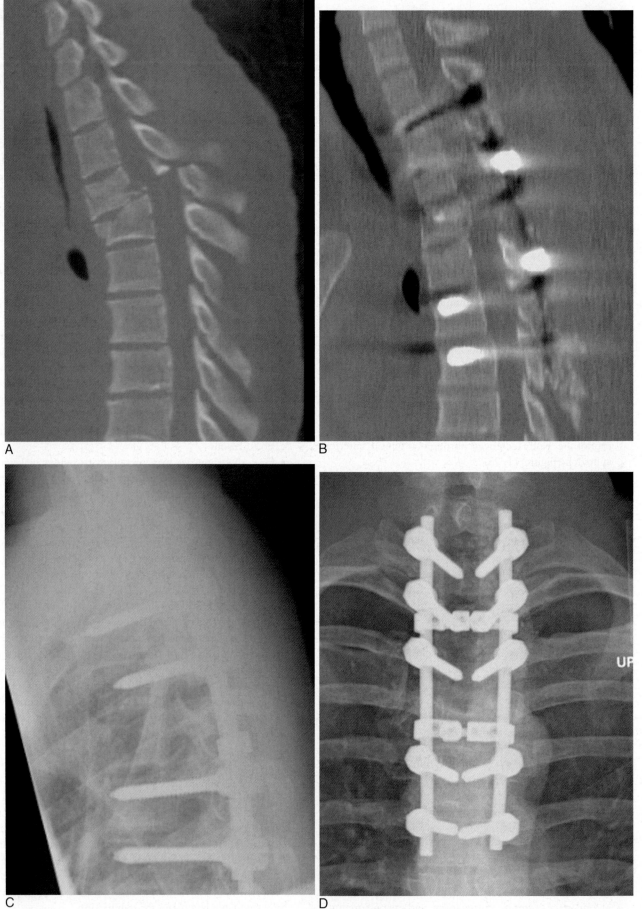

Figure 11–25: Posterior treatment of a thoracic spine fracture-dislocation. **(A)** Sagittal computed tomography image shows a fracture-dislocation at T3-T4 caused by a bicycling accident. The characteristic findings include a translational (shear) instability pattern and a three-column fracture that extends through the pars interarticularis bilaterally. The patient had an incomplete spinal cord injury from which he recovered after having undergone posterior realignment and decompression, followed by T1-T6 instrumented arthrodesis as shown on a **(B)** postoperative sagittal computed tomography image, **(C)** lateral radiograph, and **(D)** anteroposterior radiograph.

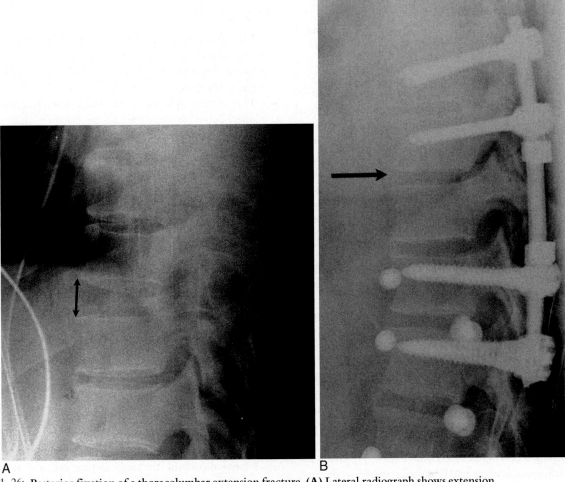

Figure 11–26: Posterior fixation of a thoracolumbar extension fracture. **(A)** Lateral radiograph shows extension injury at T9-T10 caused by a motor vehicle collision *(double arrow).* The extension deformity was corrected *(single arrow)* by contouring posterior rods to match the patient's preinjury alignment, as shown in a **(B)** lateral radiograph after posterior instrumented arthrodesis.

Chance Fractures and Their Variants

- Chance fractures and their variants involve tension failure of all three columns and may involve injury to bone, soft tissue, or both.
- The axis of rotation is therefore anterior to the vertebral body.
- Bony Chance fractures may be treated with closed manipulation and application of a hyperextension cast in neurologically intact patients, when not precluded by associated abdominal and thoracic injuries.
- Injuries that propagate through posterior ligaments or the intervertebral disc require operative stabilization in adults.
- A short-segment posterior compression construct is ideal and provides the best mechanical advantage for stabilization of these injuries.

- Redundant torn, or infolded ligamentum flavum is generally excised before reduction to prevent it from causing posterior canal compromise after reduction.
- In patients with an anterior injury that appears to propagate through the posterior annulus, MRI is useful in identifying associated disc herniation that may potentially result in neurologic injury at the time of posterior compression instrumentation.
- Although single-level pedicle screw fixation is generally sufficient, the number of levels that need to be spanned depends specifically on the pattern of injury.

Flexion-Distraction Injuries

- Certain important distinctions between flexion-distraction injuries and Chance fractures influence their treatment.

- A flexion-distraction injury has been defined by McAfee as an injury where the posterior column fails in tension but the anterior column fails in compression. The osseous component of the middle column often remains intact.
- The axis of rotation in these injuries is therefore presumably within the vertebral body rather than in the more anterior location described for Chance fractures. This distinction is important for two reasons.
  - When the tension failure of the posterior elements is unrecognized, these injuries may be mistakenly treated as stable compression or burst fractures based on the more obvious bony injury. Attempts to simply brace these injuries are likely to result in progressive kyphosis and the eventual need for a more complex late reconstruction.
  - The preserved bony integrity of the middle column allows it to act as a fulcrum, making the same short-segment posterior compression construct used with Chance fractures biomechanically ideal for the treatment of these injuries.
- Variants of these fractures exist, however, in which there is comminution of the middle column. These injuries must not be mistaken for burst fractures, because:
  - In my experience they respond less effectively to nonoperative treatment, which results in progressive kyphosis, and
  - They are less amenable to anterior fixation than are burst fractures because instead of neutralizing what would be a burst fracture's axial compressive forces from a mechanically advantageous interbody position, the fixation must counteract rotational forces from the mechanically disadvantaged position at their center of rotation.
- The potential for middle column comminution also sets flexion-distraction injuries apart from Chance type fractures. With compromise of the middle column, posterior compression instrumentation would result in shortening of the middle column and a worsening of bony retropulsion.
- In flexion-distraction injuries with fracture of the middle column, kyphoreduction must therefore by achieved without shortening the middle column, in a manner similar to that described for posterior stabilization of unstable burst fractures.

Postoperative Bracing

- A TLSO (CTLSO for injuries above T7 and HTLSO for injuries below L3) is generally prescribed to provide supplemental support for 3 months after surgery.
- Postoperative bracing is not routinely used in:
  - Patients with acceptable bone quality who had injury patterns (Chance fractures, flexion-distraction injuries with intact middle column) amenable to posterior compression instrumentation.
  - Patients who have undergone anterior and posterior surgery.
  - Patients who have a body habitus that precludes effective bracing.
- Patients who are extremely frail or unable to tolerate a brace because of associated pulmonary or skin conditions.

Sacrum

- The sacrum is crucial in maintaining pelvic and spinal column alignment.
- Sacral fractures vary from insufficiency to high-energy injury fractures.
- This section will focus on sacral fractures resulting in spino-pelvic dissociation. Sacral fractures that primarily destabilize the pelvic ring are discussed elsewhere.

Initial Evaluation

- These patients with multiple injuries require standard Advanced Trauma Life Support (ATLS) resuscitation.
- Pelvic sheets and femoral traction can be used to treat associated pelvic instability.
- Early determination of cauda equina function is essential.
  - Perianal sensation, anal sphincter tone, voluntary perianal contraction, and the integrity of the bulbocavernosus reflex arc should be evaluated.
- Rectal and vaginal examinations are important to identify open sacral fractures.
- The presence of cauda equina deficits or open fracture impacts treatment and prognosis.

Radiographic Evaluation

- Sacral fractures are commonly missed on the trauma AP pelvis radiograph.
- Careful scrutiny demonstrates abnormalities in the sacral foraminal contour, the sacral arcuate line, and the presence of a "paradoxical inlet" view of the sacrum.
- Use of the CT scan for routine initial assessment of abdominal and pelvic trauma has decreased the delay in diagnosis of sacral fractures.
- Detection of a sacral fracture warrants full radiographic evaluation with inlet and outlet pelvis views and a dedicated sacral CT with coronal and sagittal reformations

Fracture Classification

- Sacral fractures have been classified by Denis and others into the following categories (Box 11–16; Figure 11–27):
  - Zone I fractures involve only the sacral ala and have a 5.9% rate of neurologic injury.
  - Zone II fractures extend into the neuroforamina but not more medially into the sacral canal and have a 28% incidence of neurologic injury.
  - Zone III fractures extend into the sacral canal and have a 57% rate of neurologic injury, which consists most commonly of cauda equina syndrome (76%).
  - Whereas zone I injuries pertain mainly to posterior pelvic ring stability, some zone II and many zone III injuries affect both posterior pelvic ring and L-S stability.

Box 11–16	Classification of Sacral Fractures

1. Denis zone I—fracture involves the sacral ala only
2. Denis zone II—fracture involves the neuroforamina but not the spinal canal
   a. Isler type 1: fracture is lateral to L5-S1 facet—stable L-S junction
   b. Isler type 2: fracture involves L5-S1 facet—possibly unstable L-S junction
   c. Isler type 3: fracture medial to L5-S1 facet—unstable L-S junction
3. Denis zone II—Fracture involves sacral canal
   a. Roy-Camille type 1—sacral kyphosis without translation
   b. Roy-Camille type 2—sacral kyphosis retrolisthesis
   c. Roy-Camille type 3—sacral extension with anterolisthesis
   d. Strange-Vognsen type 4—upper sacral comminution

- Zone II fractures were categorized by Isler according to their effect on L-S stability.
  - Type I fractures extend lateral to L5-S1 facet joint, which is therefore connected to the stable component of the sacral fracture.
  - Type II fractures extend into the L5-S1 facet joint. Lumbosacral junction may be unstable.
  - Type III fractures extend medial to the L5-S1 facet joint, which is therefore associated with the unstable sacral fragment.
- Most sacral fractures with a transverse fracture component also have associated longitudinal or "vertical" injury components, usually in the form of bilateral transforaminal fractures, which produce the so-called sacral "U" fracture and its variants, the "H," "Y," and "λ" fractures.
  - All of these variants have a similar instability pattern, in which the central upper sacral segment to which the remainder of the spine is attached is dissociated from the pelvis and peripheral sacrum, resulting in "spino-pelvic dissociation" (Figure 11–28).

- The deforming forces cause the spine and upper sacral segment to displace anterocaudally, resulting in shortening and sacral kyphosis.
- Roy-Camille and Strange-Vognsen further subdivided zone III injuries with transverse fractures into four fracture types according to direction of transverse fracture angulation, displacement, and comminution:
  - Type I fractures are caused by a flexion moment, resulting in kyphosis without displacement.
  - Type II fractures are caused by a flexion moment, resulting in kyphosis with posterior translation of the upper fragment relative to the lower fracture fragment.
  - Type III fractures are caused by an extension moment, resulting in an extension deformity with anterocaudal translation of the upper sacrum relative to the lower fracture fragment.
  - Type IV fractures are caused by axial loading of the neutral spine, resulting in a segmentally comminuted fracture of the sacrum without significant translation or angulation.

Neurologic Injury

- Sacral root injury may manifest as monoradiculopathy, multiple unilateral radiculopathies, or incomplete and complete cauda equina syndrome.
- Gibbons proposed a grading scheme for severity of sacral root injuries (Box 11–17).

Treatment Options

- If left untreated, a sacral fracture with spino-pelvic dissociation can result in painful deformity or loss of neurologic function.
- Nonoperative treatment may be considered for patients with predominantly isolated, closed, osseous injuries with retained lumbosacral stability.
- In unstable injuries, particularly those with neurologic compromise, surgical realignment, and fixation of the

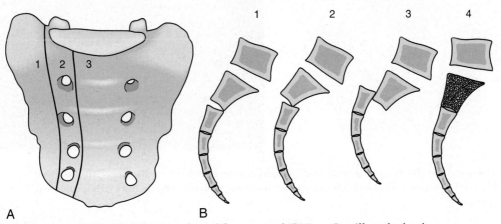

Figure 11–27: **(A)** Denis and coauthors' classification of sacral fractures and **(B)** Roy-Camille and others' subclassification of zone III sacral fractures.

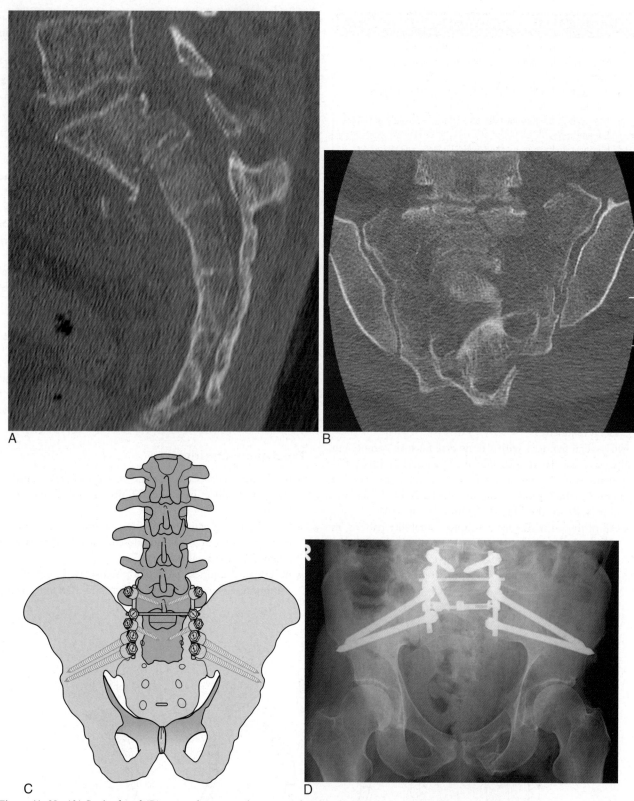

Figure 11–28: **(A)** Sagittal and **(B)** coronal computed tomography images of Denis zone III, Roy-Camille type 3 sacral fracture. **(C)** Schematic illustration and **(D)** anteroposterior radiograph showing fracture stabilization with lumbo-pelvic fixation.

Box 11–17	Gibbons Classification of Cauda Equina Impairment

TYPE	NEUROLOGIC DEFICIT
1	None
2	Paresthesias only
3	Lower extremity motor deficit
4	Bowel or bladder dysfunction

Muscle Grading

0. Total paralysis
1. Palpable or visible contraction
2. Active movement, full range of motion, gravity eliminated
3. Active movement, full range of motion, against gravity
4. Active movement, full range of motion, against gravity and provides some resistance
5. Active movement, full range of motion, against gravity and provides normal resistance
5.* Muscle able to exert, in examiner's judgment, sufficient resistance to be considered normal if identifiable inhibiting factors were not present

NT, not testable. Patient unable to reliably exert effort or muscle unavailable for testing as a result of factors such as immobilization, pain on effort, or contracture.

American Spinal Injury Association Impairment Scale

A = Complete: No motor or sensory function is preserved in the sacral segments S4-S5.
B = Incomplete: Sensory but not motor function is preserved below the neurologic level and includes the sacral segments S4-S5.
C = Incomplete: Motor function is preserved below the neurologic level, and more than half of key muscles below the neurologic level have a muscle grade less than 3.
D = Incomplete: Motor function is preserved below the neurologic level, and at least half of key muscles below the neurologic level have a muscle grade of 3 or more.
E = Normal: Motor and sensory function are normal.
CLINICAL SYNDROMES (OPTIONAL)
Central cord
Brown-Séquard
Anterior cord
Conus medullaris
Cauda equina

Steps in Classification

The following order is recommended in determining the classification of individuals with spinal cord injury.
1. Determine sensory levels for right and left sides.
2. Determine motor levels for right and left sides.
Note: In regions where there is no myotome to test, the motor level is presumed to be the same as the sensory level.
3. Determine the single neurologic level.
This is the lowest segment where motor and sensory function is normal on both sides and is the most cephalad of the sensory and motor levels determined in steps 1 and 2.
4. Determine whether the injury is complete or incomplete (sacral sparing).
If there is no voluntary anal contraction AND all S4-S5 sensory scores are equal to 0 AND if there is no anal sensation, then injury is complete. Otherwise injury is incomplete.
5. Determine ASIA Impairment Scale (AIS) Grade:

Is injury complete? NO ↓	If YES, AIS = A Record ZPP (For ZPP record lowest dermatome or myotome on each side with some (nonzero score) preservation)
Is injury motor incomplete? YES ↓	If NO, AIS = B (Yes, voluntary anal contraction OR motor function more than three levels below the motor level on a given side.)

Are at least half of the key muscles below the (single) neurologic level graded 3 or better?

NO ↓	YES ↓
AIS = C	AIS = D

If sensation and motor function is normal in all segments, AIS = E.
Note: AIS E is used in follow up testing when an individual with a documented SCI has recovered normal function. If at initial testing no deficits are found, the individual is neurologically intact; the ASIA Impairment Scale does not apply.

ASIA, American Spinal Injury Association.

Operative Treatment

- The timing of surgical intervention is dictated by many factors:
    - The patient's physiologic status.
    - The presence of an open fracture or neurologic deficit with sacral root compression.
- Emergent decompression is rarely feasible or safe.
- Effective decompression requires fracture reduction and stabilization and removal of comminuted fracture fragments from within the sacral canal and foramina.
- Percutaneous iliosacral screw fixation is the least invasive of operative stabilization methods, but it does not allow for fracture reduction, is safely feasible only in minimally displaced fractures, and is less biomechanically sound than lumbo-pelvic stabilization methods for fixation of sacral fracture with spino-pelvic dissociation.
    - Patients must wear a HTLSO and restrict weight bearing for 12 weeks postoperatively.
- Sacral alar plates, as described by Roy-Camille, with or without iliosacral screw fixation, offer the ability to stabilize the transverse fracture component but must rely on suboptimal fixation into the frequently comminuted or osteopenic sacral alar to neutralize the loads across the spino-pelvic junction.

unstable lumbo-pelvic junction and decompression of the lumbosacral roots is warranted to:
- Safely mobilize the patient with multiple injuries.
- Provide the best possible environment for recovery of sacral root deficits.
- Protect against the complications of late fracture displacement.

- Weight-bearing must be restricted for 2 to 4 months postoperatively.
- Lumbo-pelvic fixation (Figure 11–28) is a biomechanically validated method that connects solid points of fixation rostral (lumbosacral pedicles) and caudal (iliac wings) to the injury.
- Preliminary results suggest a negligible rate of fixation failure and reliable fracture union without displacement despite immediate, unrestricted weight bearing.
- Wound-related complications approach 20%, without long-term sequelae.

Conclusion

- Approximately 15,000 patients per year sustain SCI in the United States and Canada.
- The prognosis for survival and recovery is improving, with lower mortality rates and less severe cord injuries being seen in rehabilitation centers. However, except in rare cases, a complete cervical cord injury is associated with little chance of functional recovery.
- Prevention of SCI therefore plays a vital role. A lower incidence of SCIs and higher proportion of incomplete rather than complete injuries from vehicular trauma have been observed with improved patient retrieval methods, the use of effective restraint systems, including airbags, and enforcement of drunk driving laws. Diving accident awareness has also played an important role.
- However, further efforts are needed and should focus on fall prevention in the elderly; the use of helmets in bicycling, skiing, and snowboarding; rule enforcement in contact sports, such as football; and additional measures aimed at preventing motor vehicle collisions.
- Once a spinal injury has been sustained, aggressive hemodynamic resuscitation and a thorough understanding of basic spinal injury and stability patterns allow for appropriate treatment and the best possible functional result.

Annotated References
Patient Evaluation

1. Blackmore CC, Mann FA, Wilson AJ: Helical CT in the primary trauma evaluation of the cervical spine: an evidence based approach, *Skel Radiol* 29:632-639, 2000.

This review summarizes the cost-effectiveness and clinical effectiveness of screening helical computed tomography (CT) of the cervical spine (c-spine) for trauma patients. It demonstrates how, when all short-term and long-term costs are considered, CT may cost less than traditional radiographic screening. In addition to having higher sensitivity and specificity for c-spine injury, CT screening may improve clinical efficiency by allowing more rapid radiologic clearance of the c-spine, particularly in patients who are involved in high-energy trauma, who sustain head injury, or who have neurologic deficits.

2. Hoffman JR, Mower WR, Wolfson AB, et al: Validity of a set of clinical criteria to rule out injury to the cervical spine in patients with blunt trauma. National Emergency X-Radiography Utilization Study Group, *N Engl J Med* 343:94-99, 2000.

This prospective, observational study sought to validate a previously published set of clinical criteria (NEXUS low-risk criteria) aimed at identifying patients who did not require radiographic clearance of the cervical spine by evaluating 34,069 patients who underwent radiographic screening of the cervical spine (c-spine) after blunt trauma. Patients were required to meet the following five criteria to be classified as having a low probability of injury: no midline cervical tenderness, no focal neurologic deficit, normal alertness, no intoxication, and no painful, distracting injury. This method identified all but 8 of the 818 patients who had cervical spine injury (99% sensitivity, 99.8% negative predictive value, 12.9% specificity, 2.7% positive predictive value). Only two patients classified as unlikely to have an injury according to the above criteria were noted to have a clinically significant injury (99.6 % sensitivity, 99.9 % negative predictive value, 12.9% specificity, 1.9% positive predictive value). By using the low-risk criteria described above, radiographic imaging could have been avoided in the 4309 (12.6%) of the 34,069 evaluated patients.

3. Steill IG, Wells GA, Vandemheem KL, et al: The Canadian C-spine rule for radiography in alert and stable trauma patients, *J Am Med Assoc* 286:1841-1848, 2001.

The authors describe a clinical decision-making rule that is highly sensitive for detecting acute cervical spine (c-spine) injury and allows the potential for more selective use of screening radiographs in alert and stable trauma patients. The Canadian C-Spine Rule comprises three main questions: (1) Is there any high-risk factor present that mandates radiography (age >65 years, dangerous mechanism, or paresthesias in the extremities)? (2) Is there any low-risk factor present that allows safe assessment of range of motion (simple rear-end motor vehicle collision, sitting position in the emergency department, ambulatory at any time since the injury, delayed onset of neck pain, or absence of midline cervical spine tenderness)? (3) Is the patient able to actively rotate the neck 45 degrees to the left and right? Among the study sample of 8924 patients, 151 (1.7%) had an important c-spine injury. This rule was noted to have 100% sensitivity and 42.5% specificity for identifying the 151 clinically important c-spine injuries. Implementation of these criteria would have resulted in a potential radiography ordering rate of 58.2%. This highly sensitive decision rule for the use of c-spine radiography in alert and stable trauma patients was noted to have the potential to standardize c-spine evaluation in the emergency department and diminish the use of unnecessary c-spine radiography.

4. Steill IG, Clement CM, McKnight RD, et al: The Canadian c-spine rule versus the NEXUS low-risk criteria in patients with trauma, *N Engl J Med* 349:2510-2518, 2003.

This prospective cohort study performed in nine Canadian emergency departments compared the Canadian C-spine Rule (CCR) to the NEXUS low-risk criteria (NLC). The CCR and NLC were interpreted by 394 physicians for 8283 patients before these patients had radiographic evaluation. The authors determined that the CCR was more sensitive (99.4% versus 90.7%, $P < 0.001$) and more specific (45.1% versus 36.8%, $P < 0.001$)

than the NLC for injury, and its use would have resulted in lower radiography rates (55.9% versus 66.6%, $P < 0.001$). The authors concluded that for alert patients with trauma who are in stable condition, the CCR is superior to the NLC.

Upper Cervical

5. Anderson PA, Montesano PX. Morphology and treatment of occipital condyle fractures. *Spine.* 1988 Jul;13(7):731-6.

6. Anderson LD, D'Alonzo RT. Fractures of the odontoid process of the axis. *J Bone Joint Surg Am.* 1974 Dec;56(8):1663-74.

7. Bellabarba C, Mirza SK, West GA, et al: Diagnosis and treatment of craniocervical dissociation: one institution's experience with 17 consecutive survivors over eight years, *J Neurosurg Spine* 4:429-440, 2006.

In this retrospective analysis, the authors describe their clinical experience in treating 17 survivors of craniocervical dissociation. They noted a high rate of delayed diagnosis (76%) despite the consistent (94%) presence of abnormal radiographic screening markers for upper cervical injury. Patients with delayed diagnoses had a higher likelihood of neurologic deterioration before surgical intervention (38%) as compared to patients with a timely diagnosis (0%). Posterior occipitocervical arthrodesis was noted to be neuroprotective. Patients with even severe upper cervical spinal cord injuries (SCIs) showed a high potential for neurologic improvement, as the average American Spinal Injury Association (ASIA) motor score improved from 50 preoperatively to 79, and 6 of the 8 (75%) patients with nonfunctional incomplete (ASIA B, C) SCI regained functional neurologic capacity. The authors recommend careful scrutiny of the cervical spine (c-spine) radiographs, using Harris' lines to evaluate craniocervical alignment. However severe instability was noted to be present even with small amounts of displacement. If a craniocervical dissociation is suspected but not definitively recognized, as in patients in whom only minimal malalignment is appreciated on screening imaging studies, traction testing is advocated to confirm the diagnosis. A classification system based on the degree of craniocervical instability rather than on the direction of displacement has been proposed by the authors: stage 1—minimally displaced on initial imaging studies, stable on traction testing; stage 2—minimally displaced on initial imaging studies, unstable on traction testing; stage 3—highly displaced on initial imaging studies. Posterior occipitocervical arthrodesis is recommended as early as reasonably possible. Even patients with severe neurologic deficits have the potential for substantial functional recovery.

8. Clark CR, White AA 3rd: Fractures of the dens: a multicenter study, *J Bone Joint Surg Am* 67:1340-1348, 1985.

This multicenter survey was conducted by the Cervical Spine Research Society regarding the management of odontoid fractures. Type II fractures were found to be the most problematic. The initial management of these fractures with a halo device was successful in 68% of patients, whereas posterior cervical fusion was successful in 96% of patients, albeit with a higher complication rate. With type II injuries, the degree of angulation (>10 degrees) and amount of displacement (>5 mm) were considered important predictive factors in determining the risk of failed nonoperative treatment as a result of nonunion or malunion. Type III injuries were found to be associated with high rates of malunion after rigid collar immobilization, giving rise

to the recommendation that a halo device or surgery may be indicated for nonimpacted type III fractures.

9. Levine AM, Edwards CC: The management of traumatic spondylolisthesis of the axis, *J Bone Joint Surg Am* 67:217-226, 1985.

In this classic article, the authors analyze a case series of 52 patients with traumatic spondylolisthesis of the axis with respect to injury types, patterns of neurologic injury, associated injuries, injury mechanisms, and results of treatment. They noted the following distribution of injury types: 15 (29%) type I fractures; 29 (56%) type II fractures; 3 (6%) type II-A fractures; and 5 (10%) type III fractures. Associated neurologic deficits were found in only four patients. Closed head injuries were seen in 11 (21%) patients. Thirteen (25%) patients had other fractures of the cervical spine (c-spine). Type I fractures were stable injuries and were treated with a rigid collar. Type II injuries were reduced with the patient in halo traction and then immobilized in a halo vest. Type II-A injuries were reduced manually and placed in a halo vest. Type III injuries were grossly unstable and required surgical stabilization. All of the fractures healed, although the use of early halo-vest immobilization for displaced fractures resulted in significant residual deformity.

10. Traynelis VC, Marano GD, Dunker RO, Kaufman HH. Traumatic atlanto-occipital dislocation. Case report. *J Neurosurg.* 1986 Dec;65(6):863-70.

Lower Cervical

11. Allen BL Jr, Ferguson RL, Lehmann TR, et al: A mechanistic classification of closed, indirect fractures and dislocations of the lower cervical spine, *Spine* 7:1-27, 1982.

This classic article describes a mechanistic classification of subaxial cervical spine injuries, which are categorized as: (1) distractive extension, (2) compressive extension, (3) vertical compression, (4) compressive flexion, (5) distractive flexion, and (6) lateral flexion. Although the classification system is somewhat cumbersome to use on an every day basis, it provides valuable insight into understanding the injury pattern based on the presumed mechanism. The authors also describe the likelihood of neurologic injury for the various injury types. They discuss the value of tailoring treatment based on the injury mechanism, although a strict association between injury mechanism and surgical approach has not been borne out in subsequent literature.

12. Grant GA, Mirza SK, Chapman JR, et al: Risk of early closed reduction in cervical spine subluxation injuries, *J Neurosurg* 90:13-18, 1999.

The authors retrospectively reviewed 121 patients with traumatic cervical spine (c-spine) injuries to determine the risk of neurological deterioration following early closed reduction. They noted that closed reduction using Gardner-Wells tong traction was successful in 97.6% of patients. The incidence of disc herniation and disruption was 22% and 24%, respectively, but the presence of disc herniation or disruption did not affect the degree of neurological recovery. One (1.3%) of 80 patients deteriorated neurologically 6 hours following closed reduction and for reasons not directly related to the reduction maneuver. The authors concluded that, although disc herniation and disruption occur following cervical fracture-subluxations, neurologic deterioration following closed reduction in these patients is rare. They recommended early closed reduction without prior magnetic resonance imaging (MRI) in alert, examinable patients presenting with significant motor deficits.

13. Kwon BK, Vaccaro AR, Grauer JN, et al: Subaxial cervical spine trauma, *J Am Acad Orthop Surg* 14:78-89, 2006.

This article serves as a useful review of current concepts pertaining to subaxial cervical spine (C-spine) trauma, including epidemiology, anatomy, biomechanics, classification, management, and complications.

14. Moore TA, Vaccaro AR, Anderson PA: Classification of lower cervical spine injuries, *Spine* 31:S37-S43, 2006.

The authors introduce the Cervical Spine Injury Severity Score, a new classification system that adds a quantification of stability to the usual morphologic injury descriptions in an attempt to both simplify and standardize the treatment of subaxial cervical spine (c-spine) fractures. This system is based on a four-column model of the c-spine, with the four columns consisting of the anterior column, both lateral pillars, and the posterior osseoligamentous complex. Mechanistic injury descriptions are purposefully avoided in this classification system because they are not felt to have a strong interobserver consensus and do not reliably predict the best treatment approach or prognosis. The authors noted high intraobserver and interobserver agreement using the Cervical Spine Injury Score.

Cervicothoracic Junction

15. Ames CP, Bozkus MH, Chamberlain RH, et al: Biomechanics of stabilization after cervicothoracic compression-flexion injury, *Spine* 30:1505-1512, 2005.

In this cadaveric biomechanical study, the authors sought to determine whether anterior, posterior, or combined anterior and posterior instrumentation provides the best stability for treating cervicothoracic fractures with flexion-distraction injury patterns in which C7 anterior superior endplate compression fractures were combined with compromise of the C6-C7 posterior ligamentous complex. They found that posterior instrumentation alone allowed an 89% smaller range of motion during lateral bending and 64% smaller range of motion during axial rotation than anterior instrumentation alone. Stability was also noted to improve when posterior instrumentation was extended from T1 to T2. In general, they also found that combined anterior and posterior instrumentation outperformed either anterior or posterior instrumentation alone, although the purely biomechanical nature of this study does not allow it to address whether the degree of increased stability justifies the increased morbidity of a combined approach.

16. Bellabarba C, Nemecek AN, Chapman JR: Management of injuries to the cervicothoracic junction, *Techniques in Orthopaedics* 17:355-364, 2003.

The authors review anatomic considerations and diagnostic and treatment challenges pertaining to injuries of the cervicothoracic junction.

17. Chapman J, Anderson PA, Pepin C, et al: Posterior instrumentation of the unstable cervicothoracic spine, *J Neurosurg* 84:552-558, 1996.

In one of the first clinical studies to evaluate posterior instrumentation of the injured cervicothoracic junction, the authors reported on 23 patients with instability of the cervicothoracic region who were treated with posterior instrumented arthrodesis using AO reconstruction plate fixation between the lower cervical and upper thoracic spine, followed by 2 months of external bracing postoperatively. They reported a solid arthrodesis in all patients, without significant loss of alignment. There were no neurovascular or pulmonary complications. One postoperative wound infection required debridement but not hardware removal. The authors conclude that posterior plate fixation provides satisfactory treatment of cervicothoracic instability.

18. Daffner SD, Vaccaro AR: Managing disorders of the cervicothoracic junction, *Am J Orthop* 31:323-327, 2002.

The authors review the anatomy, diagnosis, and treatment of disorders affecting the cervicothoracic junction. The authors review the anatomy, diagnosis, and treatment of disorders affecting the cervicothoracic junction.

19. Vaccaro AR, Conant RF, Hilibrand AS, et al: A plate-rod for treatment of cervico-thoracic disorders: comparison of mechanical testing with established cervical spine in vitro load testing data, *J Spinal Disord* 13:350-355, 2000.

The authors perform a biomechanical analysis of a combination plate rod construct (PRC) that was developed to accommodate the changes in anatomy and larger forces that occur across the transition between the posterior cervical and thoracic spine. The PRC was noted to compare favorably to established maximal load data on posterior cervical fixation systems using lateral mass screws and was noted to have greater strength and resistance to failure than is necessary to sustain maximal in vivo cervical spine (c-spine) loads. The authors concluded that specialized instrumentation for cervicothoracic posterior fixation provide an excellent option for spinal fixation across the cervicothoracic junction because of their potentially superior biomechanical qualities and improved versatility in addressing the complex anatomic features of the cervicothoracic transition zone.

Thoracolumbar

20. Bransford R, Bellabarba C, Thompson JH, et al: The safety of fluoroscopically-assisted thoracic pedicle screw instrumentation for fracture stabilization, *J Trauma* 60:1047-1052, 2006.

The authors sought to determine the perioperative safety of placing thoracic pedicle screws based on anatomic landmarks, intraoperative fluoroscopy, and preoperative computed tomography (CT) imaging for the treatment of thoracic spine fractures. They retrospectively reviewed 245 consecutive patients with spine fractures requiring pedicle screw fixation between T1 and T10. Screws placed at T11 and T12 were not included because it was felt that both the large number of screws placed at these levels and the relative ease of their placement compared to more rostral nontransitional thoracic levels would skew the results in a manner that would underrepresent the true risk of thoracic screw placement. Major complications were defined as a potentially life-threatening vascular injury, neurologic deterioration, pneumothorax or hemothorax, and tracheoesophageal injury. Of the 1533 pedicle screws placed between T1 and T10 in these 245 patients, no patient sustained a major complication related to screw placement. Three patients (1.2%) required a secondary procedure for prophylactic revision of 4 (0.26%) malpositioned screws. The authors concluded that pedicle screws can be safely placed in the thoracic spine for the treatment of spine fractures using preoperative imaging evaluation, standard posterior element landmarks, and intraoperative fluoroscopy.

21. McAfee PC, Yuan HA, Fredrickson BE, et al: The value of computed tomography in thoracolumbar fractures: an analysis of one hundred consecutive cases and a new classification, *J Bone Joint Surg Am* 65:461-473, 1983.

In this classic article, the authors use a computed tomography-based (CT-based) analysis to develop a thoracolumbar classification system that comprises the following injury types: compression fracture, stable burst fracture, unstable burst fracture, Chance fracture, flexion-distraction injury, and fracture-dislocation. In particular, it emphasized the flexion-distraction injury as an unstable variant whereby a seemingly innocuous anterior column fracture was accompanied by tension failure of the posterior osseoligamentous complex.

22. Gertzbein SD, Court-Brown CM, Marks P, et al: The neurological outcome following surgery for spinal fractures, *Spine* 13:641-644, 1983.

The authors sought to establish whether anterior or posterior surgical intervention led to a more favorable neurologic outcome for patients with incomplete neurologic deficits as a result of spinal injuries with greater than 20% encroachment of the spinal canal. Sixty consecutive patients were divided into two groups, those undergoing posterior surgery alone, and those undergoing anterior surgery for formal decompression with or without anterior or posterior instrumentation. In those patients undergoing posterior surgery, neurologic improvement of 83% was achieved in patients with incomplete lesions, whereas 88% improvement was found in those undergoing the anterior procedure. There was no statistical difference in neurologic outcome between these two groups. They concluded that there was no apparent difference between the degree of bony encroachment of the spinal canal and the initial Frankel grade, nor was there a clear difference in neurologic outcome between patients with incomplete spinal cord injury undergoing anterior versus posterior surgery.

23. Vaccaro AR, Lehman RA, Hurlbert RJ, et al: A new classification of thoracolumbar injuries: the importance of injury morphology, the integrity of the posterior ligamentous complex, and neurologic status, *Spine* 30:2325-2333, 2005.

In this study, the authors introduce the Thoracolumbar Injury Classification and Severity Score (TLICS), a new classification system that they propose as practical yet comprehensive. The goal of this system is to assist in deciding the need for operative versus nonoperative care and the surgical treatment approach for unstable injury patterns. The TLICS is based on three injury characteristics: (1) morphology of injury determined by radiographic appearance, (2) integrity of the posterior ligamentous complex, and (3) neurologic status of the patient. These characteristics were used to calculate the injury severity score, with a maximum value of 10 points, which allowed these patients to be stratified into surgical and nonsurgical treatment groups. Patients with a score of 3 or less were considered to be best treated nonoperatively, patients with scores of 5 or greater were deemed to require surgical intervention, and patients with a score of 4 could be treated either operatively or nonoperatively. The authors also propose a methodology for determining the best operative approach for specific surgical injury patterns.

24. Wood K, Butterman G, Mehbod A: Operative compared with nonoperative treatment of a thoracolumbar burst fracture without neurological deficit: a prospective, randomized study, *J Bone Joint Surg Am* 85:773-781, 2003.

This study constitutes the first prospective randomized study examining the outcome of operative versus nonoperative intervention in patients who sustained thoracolumbar burst fractures without neurologic deficit. Forty-seven consecutive patients with stable thoracolumbar burst fractures and no neurologic deficit were randomized to either an operative (posterior or anterior arthrodesis and instrumentation) or nonoperative (application of a body cast or orthosis) treatment group. There was no significant difference in spinal alignment or canal compromise between the two treatment groups at follow-up. In addition, no significant difference was found between the two groups with respect to return to work. The average pain scores at follow-up were similar for both groups. Although preinjury disability scores were similar for both groups, at the time of the final follow-up, patients who were treated nonoperatively reported less disability. Final scores on the SF-36 and Oswestry questionnaires were similar for the two groups, although certain trends favored those treated without surgery. Complications were more frequent in the operative group. The authors concluded that operative intervention did not appear to provide any significant advantage to patients with stable burst fractures and normal neurologic examinations.

Sacrum

25. Bellabarba C, Schildhauer TA, Vaccaro AR: Complications associated with surgical stabilization of high-grade sacral fracture-dislocations with spino-pelvic instability, *Spine* 31: S80-S88, 2006.

This retrospective review examines the complications associated with decompression and spino-pelvic fixation in 19 patients with highly displaced, Denis Zone III U-type sacral fracture-dislocations with spino-pelvic dissociation. The authors found that complications were primarily wound-related or hardware-related. Complications involved the incidental finding of asymptomatic broken rods in 6 out of 19 (31%) patients and wound healing disturbances, including acute infection, seromas, or hematomas requiring surgical debridement, in 5 out of 19 (26%) patients. There were no lasting complications such as chronic osteomyelitis noted. Eight patients in total (42%) required a return to the operating room (OR), including the five patients with wound problems listed previously and three additional patients who requested hardware removal after their fracture had healed as a result of prominence of their iliac screw heads. There were no patients who experienced the loss of alignment or loosening of hardware that has been problematic with other methods of fixation for these injuries. There were no patients who experienced secondary neurologic deterioration. The authors concluded that, despite the high likelihood of secondary procedures, spino-pelvic fixation with pedicle and iliac wing screws is an effective treatment method for these high-energy, highly displaced, unstable and comminuted sacral fractures with spino-pelvic dissociation.

26. Denis F, Davis S, Comfort T: Sacral fractures: an important problem. Retrospective analysis of 236 cases, *Clin Orthop Relat Res* 227:67-81, 1988.

The authors analyzed a large series of sacral fractures and classify these fractures according to anatomic location and likelihood of neurologic injury. Zone I injuries, which are defined as being isolated to the sacral ala, have the lowest likelihood of associated neurologic deficits, which normally occur in the L5 distribution. Zone II injuries, which involve the neuroforamina but not the sacral canal, have a higher likelihood of neurologic deficits and involve primarily sensorimotor dysfunction of the ipsilateral lower extremity. Zone III injuries, which involve the sacral canal, carry the highest likelihood of neurologic deficits, the majority of which are cauda equina syndromes.

27. Gibbons KJ, Soloniuk DS, Razack N: Neurological injury and pattern of sacral fractures, *J Neurosurg* 72:889-893, 1990.

This study examines the type and severity of neurological injuries that occur with sacral fractures and classifies these injuries on a scale of 1 to 4 as follows: Type 1—normal sensorimotor function. Type 2—lower extremity paresthesias. Type 3—motor deficit in the lower extremities. Type 4—cauda equina syndrome with bowel and bladder dysfunction.

28. Isler B. Lumbosacral lesions associated with pelvic ring injuries. *J Orthop Trauma,* 1990;4(1):1-6.

29. Nork SE, Jones CB, Harding SP, et al: Percutaneous stabilization of U-shaped sacral fractures using iliosacral screws: technique and early results, *J Orthop Trauma* 15:238-246, 2001.

This article discusses the technique of iliosacral screw fixation followed by 12 weeks of HTLSO bracing and protected weight bearing for the treatment of minimally displaced Denis zone III, sacral U-type fractures. Displacement that was sufficiently small to allow safe iliosacral screw placement and sufficient integrity of the upper sacral bodies to allow for acceptable iliosacral screw purchase were conditions for the use of this technique. Of the 13 patients who met these criteria, 11 patients had bilateral iliosacral screws placed, 1 had two unilateral screws placed, and 1 had a single unilateral screw placed. Only the patient with a single unilateral screw had loosening of his hardware. Preoperatively, sacral kyphosis averaged 29 degrees, whereas postoperative sacral kyphosis averaged 28 degrees. All fractures healed clinically and radiographically. Of the nine patients with preoperative neurologic deficits, both (22%) patients who had residual deficits had associated multiple level lumbar burst fractures, which required decompression and instrumented stabilization. The authors recommend this technique as a minimally invasive method for treating sacral U-type fractures with a sufficiently low degree of displacement and sacral comminution to allow for effective and safe iliosacral screw placement.

30. Roy-Camille R, Saillant G, Gagna G, et al: Transverse fracture of the upper sacrum: suicidal jumper's fracture, *Spine* 10:838-845, 1985.

The authors further characterize what we now define as zone III sacral fractures according to the displacement and angulation of their transverse fracture component as follows: Type 1—flexion injury with kyphosis but no translation; type 2—flexion injury with kyphosis and retrolisthesis; type 3—extension injury with anterolisthesis. This article does not discuss the type 4 axial loading fracture with comminution of the upper sacrum, which was subsequently added to the classification by Strange-Vognsen and Lebech: *J Ortho Trauma* 5:200-203, 1991.

31. Schildhauer TA, Bellabarba C, Nork SE, et al: Decompression and lumbo-pelvic fixation for high grade sacral fracture-dislocations with spino-pelvic dissociation, *J Orthop Trauma* 20:447-457, 2006.

In this retrospective review, the authors analyze a consecutive series of 19 patients who presented with highly displaced, comminuted zone III sacral U-type fracture-dislocations with spino-pelvic dissociation and cauda equina syndrome. All patients were treated with decompression and spino-pelvic fixation from either the L4 or L5 pedicles to the iliac wings, and the authors provide a description of their surgical technique. Reduction was achieved with a combination of femoral traction, intraoperative traction using the femoral distractor with pins in the L5 pedicle and the ilium and direct intraoperative manipulation of the upper sacral fragment. When possible, iliosacral screws were placed to help maintain the sacral reduction and to add an additional plane of fixation. Sacral fractures healed in all patients, and no patient experienced a loss of reduction. Average sacral kyphosis improved from 43 to 21 degrees. Fifteen patients (83%) had full or partial recovery of bowel and bladder deficits. Average Gibbons score improved from 4 to 2.8 at 31-month average follow-up. Wound infection (16%) was the most common complication. Complete recovery of cauda equina function was more likely in patients with continuity of all sacral roots (86% versus 0%, P = 0.00037) and incomplete deficits (100% versus 20%, P = 0.024). The authors concluded that lumbo-pelvic fixation provided reliable fracture stability and allowed consistent fracture union without loss of alignment. The effect of decompression on neurologic outcome was more difficult to quantify and was influenced, in part, by completeness of the injury and presence of sacral root disruption.

32. Strange-Vognsen and Lebech: An unusual type of fracture in the upper sacrum, *J Ortho Trauma* 5:200-203,1991.

33. Daffner SD, Vaccaro AR: Managing disorders of the cervicothoracic junction, *Am J Orthop* 31:323-327, 2002.

34. Vaccaro AR, Conant RF, Hilibrand AS, et al: A plate-rod for treatment of cervico-thoracic disorders: comparison of mechanical testing with established cervical spine in vitro load testing data, *J Spinal Disord* 13:350-355, 2000.

Thoracolumbar

35. Bransford R, Bellabarba C, Thompson JH, et al: The safety of fluoroscopically-assisted thoracic pedicle screw instrumentation for fracture stabilization, *J Trauma* 60:1047-1052, 2006.

36. McAfee PC, Yuan HA, Fredrickson BE, et al: The value of computed tomography in thoracolumbar fractures: an analysis of one hundred consecutive cases and a new classification, *J Bone Joint Surg Am* 65:461-473, 1983.

37. Gertzbein SD, Court-Brown CM, Marks P, Martin C, et al: The neurological outcome following surgery for spinal fractures, *Spine* 13:641-644, 1988.

38. Vaccaro AR, Lehman RA, Hurlbert RJ, et al: A new classification of thoracolumbar injuries: the importance of injury morphology, the integrity of the posterior ligamentous complex, and neurologic status, *Spine* 30:2325-2333, 2005.

39. Wood K, Butterman G, Mehbod A, et al: Operative compared with nonoperative treatment of a thoracolumbar burst fracture without neurological deficit: a prospective, randomized study, *J Bone Joint Surg Am* 85:773-781, 2003.

Sacrum

40. Bellabarba C, Schildhauer TA, Vaccaro AR: Complications associated with surgical stabilization of high-grade sacral fracture-dislocations with spino-pelvic instability, *Spine* 31: S80-S88, 2006.

41. Denis F, Davis S, Comfort T: Sacral fractures: an important problem. Retrospective analysis of 236 cases, *Clin Orthop Relat Res* 227:67-81, 1988.

42. Gibbons KJ, Soloniuk DS, Razack N: Neurological injury and pattern of sacral fractures, *J Neurosurg* 72:889-893, 1990.

43. Nork SE, Jones CB, Harding SP, et al: Percutaneous stabilization of U-shaped sacral fractures using iliosacral screws: technique and early results, *J Orthop Trauma* 15:238-246, 2001.

44. Roy-Camille R, Saillant G, Gagna G, et al: Transverse fracture of the upper sacrum: suicidal jumper's fracture, *Spine* 10:838-845, 1985.

45. Schildhauer TA, Bellabarba C, Nork SE, et al: Decompression and lumbo-pelvic fixation for high grade sacral fracture-dislocations with spino-pelvic dissociation, *J Orthop Trauma* 20:447-457, 2006.

Pelvic Fractures

H. Claude Sagi, MD

Pelvic Anatomy

- The pelvis is a ring structure composed of the two hemi-pelves and the sacrum.
- Each hemi-pelvis or innominate bone is the result of fusion of three embryonic bones: the ilium, the pubis, and the ischium.
- The pelvic ring is completed anteriorly at the pubic symphysis, which is a symphyseal joint between the two pubic bodies.
- The pelvic ring is completed posteriorly by three structures: the two iliac segments of the innominate bones and the sacrum.
- The sacrum represents the terminal segments of the spinal column and is connected to each innominate bone via the sacro-iliac (SI) joints.
- The sacrum forms a keystone type articulation with the innominate bones by virtue of its wedge shape.
- The SI joints are inherently unstable, and the maintenance of pelvic ring integrity is wholly dependent on ligamentous support for stability (Figure 12–1).
- With weight bearing, the natural tendency is for each hemi-pelvis to externally rotate and shift cephalad and posterior.
- The pelvic ligaments resist these deformations.
- The posterior SI ligaments are the strongest ligaments in the body, and the most important in resisting posterior and cephalad displacement.
- The symphyseal ligaments contribute at most 15% of the total pelvic ring stability.[1]
- The bladder is immediately posterior to the pubic bodies and symphysis.
- The L5 nerve root lies directly on the sacral ala as it courses to join the lumbo-sacral plexus.
- The superior gluteal artery is immediately lateral to the inferior aspect of the SI joint as it arises from the internal iliac artery to exit the greater sciatic notch with the superior gluteal nerve.

- The obturator nerve and artery course along the quadrilateral plate (medial wall) of the acetabulum as they exit the superior and lateral quadrant of the obturator foramen (Figure 12–2).

Epidemiology

- Insufficiency fractures occur in an increasingly large number of patients with the aging population.
- Stress and fatigue fractures occur in high-level athletes or military recruits.
- Traumatic disruptions result from high-energy injuries, such as (in order of decreasing frequency) motorcycle

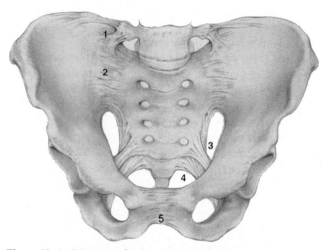

Figure 12–1: Diagram of pelvic bony and ligamentous anatomy. 1. Ilio-lumbar ligaments from the transverse process of L5 to the iliac crest. 2. Sacro-iliac ligaments posteriorly (anterior, posterior, and intraarticular). 3. Sacro-spinous ligaments. 4. Sacro-tuberous ligaments. 5. Symphyseal ligaments anteriorly. (From Fractures of the Pelvis and Acetabulum, ed. GF Zinghi, Thieme Medical Publishers, 2004).

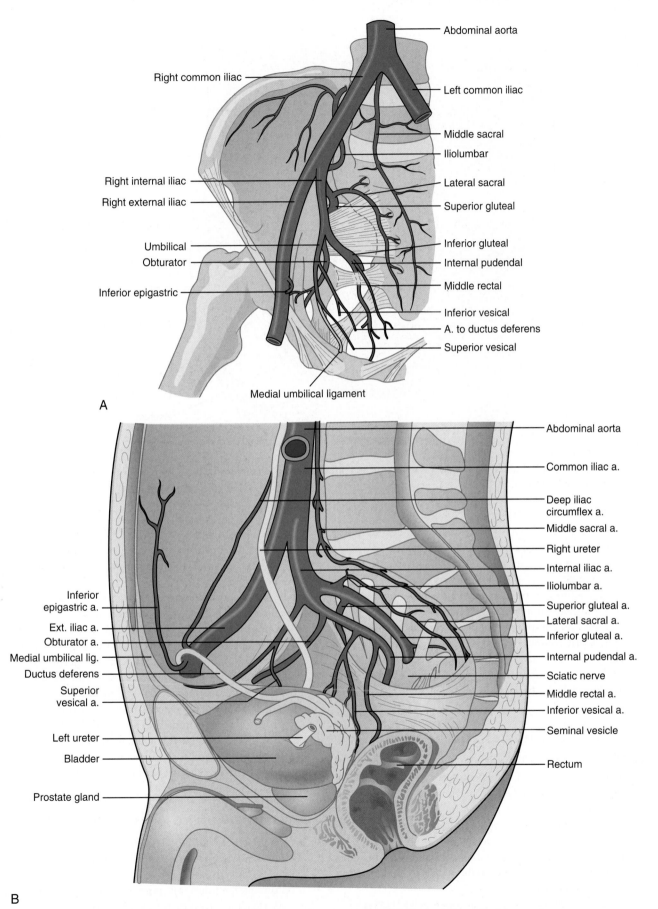

Figure 12–2: **(A)** Anterior view of pelvic arteries with respect to boney anatomy. **(B)** Sagittal view of pelvic arteries and nerves with respect to bony anatomy.

(Continued)

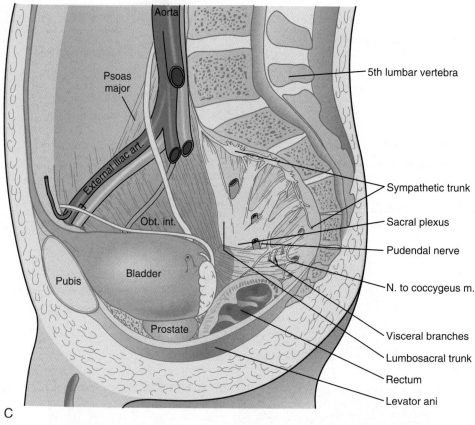

Figure 12–2, cont'd: **(C)** Sagittal view of nerves with arteries removed. (From Clemente H, Gray CD: *Gray's anatomy*, ed 30, Philadelphia, 1985, Lea & Febiger.

crashes, auto-pedestrian collisions, falls from height, motor vehicle accidents, or crush injuries.[2,3]

- Pelvic fractures occur in at least 20% of blunt trauma admissions.[2,4]
- Pelvic fractures occur most frequently in young males.
- They can result in small, insignificant fractures of the pubic rami with no compromise of pelvic ring stability or major injuries that completely disrupt the integrity of the pelvic ring with life-threatening bleeding or visceral injury.
- Pelvic fractures often result in significant chronic pain, permanent disability, and loss of socioeconomic structure.

Associated Injuries and Mortality

- The pelvic ring encloses the true pelvis (organs contained below the pelvic brim, extraperitoneal) and the false pelvis (organs contained above the pelvic brim, peritoneal and retroperitoneal).
- The most commonly associated injuries are to structures contained within the true pelvis:
  - The internal iliac arterial and venous systems and branches
  - The bladder (20%)[5] and urethra (14%)[6]
  - The lumbo-sacral plexus
  - The rectum and vaginal vault (open pelvic fractures)[7]

- Injuries to structures within the false pelvis as a direct result of the pelvic fracture are uncommon, but severe iliac wing fractures with abdominal wall disruption can result in intestinal injury.
- Morbidity and mortality from pelvic fractures is high and results primarily from the associated injuries:
  - Hemorrhage from pelvic bleeding is by far the most common complication and results in more deaths than any other injury directly related to the pelvic fracture.
  - The mortality of a pelvic fracture with an associated bladder rupture approaches 35% in some series.[8,9]
  - The mortality of open pelvic fractures involving the perineum, which was initially as high as 50%,[10] has decreased to as low as 2% with liberal use of diverting colostomy.[11]
  - Injury of the lumbo-sacral plexus can lead to significant permanent disability and pain.

Classification of Pelvic Fractures

- Pelvic fractures can be categorized as:
  - Low-energy injuries in osteoporotic bone (insufficiency fractures).
  - Low-energy injuries in normal bone subjected to cyclic overloading (stress or fatigue fractures).

- High-energy injuries in normal or pathologic bone (traumatic disruptions).
- High-energy traumatic fractures are classified according to the mechanism (Young and Burgess) and injury pattern (Tile and Orthopaedic Trauma Association [OTA]):

Young[12]

- Lateral compression (LC) type: rami fractures plus:
  - LC I: sacral fracture on side of impact (usually impacted fracture).
  - LC II: crescent fracture on side of impact.
  - LC III: type I or II injury on side of impact with contralateral open-book injury.
- Antero-posterior compression (APC) type: symphysis diastasis or rami fractures plus:
  - APC I: minor opening of symphysis and sacro-iliac (SI) joint anteriorly (SI, STL, and SSL intact)
  - APC II: opening of anterior SI (STL and SSL), intact posterior SI ligaments
  - APC III: complete disruption of SI joint and all supporting ligaments.
- Vertical shear (VS) type
  - Vertical displacement of hemi-pelvis with symphysis diastasis or rami fractures anteriorly
  - Iliac wing fracture, sacral facture, or SI dislocation posteriorly
- Combination (CM) type: any combination of above injuries

Tile[13]

- Type A: pelvic ring stable
  - A1: fractures not involving the ring (i.e., avulsions, iliac wing, or crest fractures)
  - A2: stable minimally displaced fractures of the pelvic ring
- Type B: pelvic ring rotationally unstable, vertically stable
  - B1: open book
  - B2: LC, ipsilateral
  - B3: LC, contralateral, or bucket handle type injury
- Type C: pelvic ring rotationally and vertically unstable
  - C1: unilateral
  - C2: bilateral
  - C3: associated with acetabular fracture

Orthopaedic Trauma Association[14]

- 61-A: No disruption of pelvic ring
  - 61-A1: fracture of innominate bone, avulsion
  - 61-A2: fracture of innominate bone, direct blow
  - 61-A3: fracture of sacrum or coccyx, transverse
- 61-B: Partial disruption of posterior ring
  - 61-B1: unilateral APC-type injury
  - 61-B2: unilateral LC-type injury
  - 61-B3: bilateral partial disruption of posterior ring.

- 61 C: Complete disruption of posterior ring
  - 61-C1: through iliac wing
  - 61-C2: through SI joint
  - 61 C3: through sacrum (sacral fracture)
- Sacral fractures can be further categorized depending on the type of injury:
  - Longitudinal fractures that give rise to vertical instability and disruption of the pelvic ring
  - Transverse fractures that result in spinal pelvic dissociation or sacral fracture dislocation but do not disrupt the pelvic ring

Denis (Sacral Fractures)[15]

- Zone 1: alar zone, longitudinal or oblique (risk of neurologic injury ≈6%)
- Zone 2: foraminal zone, longitudinal or oblique (risk of neurologic injury ≈30%)
- Zone 3: sacral spinal canal involvement, transverse (risk of neurologic injury ≈60%)
- Zone 3 transverse fractures can occur either above or below the level of the SI joints and generally do not affect stability of the pelvic ring but can affect stability of the spinal-pelvic junction.
- Fractures below the SI joints usually result from a direct blow to the distal sacrum or coccygeal region.
- Fractures within the region of the SI joints result from a hyperflexion of the pelvis with axial loading ("suicidal jumper's fracture"[16]) and are usually associated with bilateral longitudinal sacral fractures (U-shaped sacral fracture) resulting in spinal-pelvic dissociation. These are unstable injuries with variable degrees of kyphosis and translation, canal compromise, and cauda equina syndrome.[17]

Imaging of Pelvic Fractures
Plain Radiographs

- Anteroposterior (AP) pelvis view as a part of the initial trauma series screening.
- Inlet view (X-ray beam is directed caudally, approximately 60 degrees to the radiographic film):
  - As the plane of the pelvic brim is 45 to 60 degrees to the long axis of the body, this view simulates looking directly into the pelvis from above along its longitudinal axis.
  - The inlet view shows (Figure 12–3):
    - External or internal rotation of the hemi-pelvis.
    - Opening of the SI joint or sacral fracture.
    - AP displacement of the hemi-pelvis.
- Outlet view (X-ray beam is directed cephalad, approximately 45 degrees to the radiographic film):
  - This view simulates looking at the pelvis and sacrum or SI joints directly en-face.
  - The outlet view shows (Figure 12–4):
    - Cephalad or vertical shift of the hemi-pelvis.
    - Sacral fractures relative to the foramina.

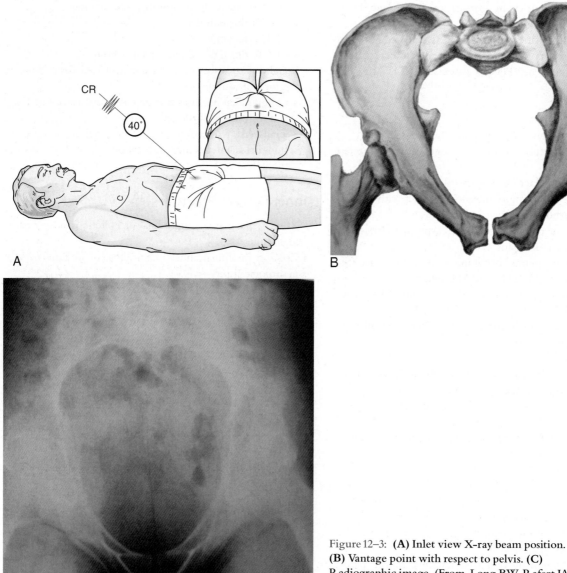

Figure 12–3: **(A)** Inlet view X-ray beam position. **(B)** Vantage point with respect to pelvis. **(C)** Radiographic image. (From Long BW, Rafert JA: *Orthopaedic radiography*, ed 1, Philadelphia, 1995, W. B. Saunders.

- It is important to remember that these radiographs are taken at ≈45 degrees to the long axis of the patient's body.
- Therefore a given amount of shift on the inlet or outlet view is in fact the sum of displacement vectors in both the coronal and axial planes.
- If on the AP radiograph one sees an inlet view of the upper sacrum and an outlet view of the lower sacrum, a lateral X-ray and computed tomography (CT) scan are mandatory to rule out occult sacral fracture-dislocation (U-shaped sacral fracture).

Computed Tomography Scan

- CT scanning is imperative in any suspected pelvic ring injury.
- Three-millimeter (3 mm) axial cuts are the most important.

- Three-dimensional (3D) reconstructions can sometimes help with fracture pattern assessment, but they are not necessary.
- Sagittal plane reconstructions can be helpful in diagnosing occult "U-shaped" sacral fracture or dislocations (see below under sacral fractures), which might be missed with poor quality AP and lateral sacral or lumbo-sacral spine radiographs.
- If any seemingly insignificant fracture is seen on the pelvic radiographs then CT scanning is mandatory to rule out other occult injuries.
- Any ring structure (i.e., the pelvis) that is disrupted in one region must (by virtue of ring mechanics) be disrupted in another region.

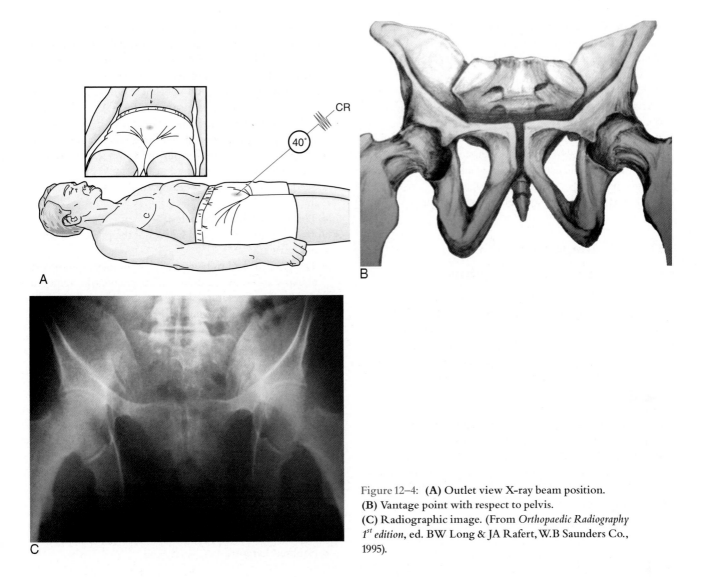

Figure 12–4: **(A)** Outlet view X-ray beam position.
(B) Vantage point with respect to pelvis.
(C) Radiographic image. (From *Orthopaedic Radiography
1st edition*, ed. BW Long & JA Rafert, W.B Saunders Co.,
1995).

Retrograde Urethrography and Cystography

- Mandatory in pelvic fractures with ring disruption to rule out urethral or bladder injury (Box 12–1).
- Foley catheter partially inserted into urethra, balloon inflated with 2 to 3 ml of sterile saline, and then 10 to 15 ml of water-soluble contrast.

Box 12–1	Clues to Urethral or Bladder Injury

- Scrotal or labial ecchymosis
- Blood at the urethral meatus
- Inability to void
- Anteroposterior compression injury or bilateral superior or inferior pubic rami fractures
- High-riding prostate on rectal examination

- Outlet view of the pelvis is taken; if no extravasation is seen, then the catheter is advanced into the bladder with further injection of 300 ml of water-soluble contrast.
- If passage of the catheter is not easily performed, then suprapubic catheterization is performed well above the umbilicus if possible (to avoid contamination of potential future anterior pelvic operations).
- In stable patients who are going to undergo CT scanning, CT cystography is equally as accurate.[18]

Pelvic Angiography

- Indicated if hemodynamic instability persists despite:
  - Adequate volume resuscitation.
  - Other sources of hemorrhage are ruled out (abdomen, thorax, and long-bone fractures).
  - Attempts to "close" the pelvic ring have failed to stop pelvic hemorrhage.

- Vast majority of pelvic hemorrhage arises from venous bleeding (85%).
- Venous bleeding is not amenable to angiographic embolization.
- Arterial bleeding is usually from branches of the internal iliac system (median sacral, superior gluteal, pudendal, or obturator arteries).
- If diagnostic peritoneal lavage (DPL) is being performed to rule out abdominal hemorrhage, then it must be performed above the umbilicus and arcuate line to avoid false-positive results from pelvic hemorrhage.
- See Figure 12–5 example of gluteal artery injury.

Initial Management of the Patient with Pelvic Fracture

- Initial ED and trauma-bay management are governed by the Advanced Trauma Life Support (ATLS)[19] protocol with attention to the airway, breathing, and circulation.
- If hemodynamic instability persists and is deemed to be secondary to pelvic fracture hemorrhage, then temporary stabilization and reduction of the pelvic volume is recommended when the pelvic ring is open (open-book–type injury):
  - Wrapping a sheet around the patient transversely with the force applied at the greater trochanters.
  - Application of a pelvic binder.[20]
  - Application of an external fixator (either in the Emergency Department (ED) or operating room [OR])
- Anterior external fixators (either in the iliac crest or supraacetabular bone) are capable of closing the open-book pelvis provided that the posterior ring is intact and can act as a hinge.

- Pelvic clamps that engage the posterior pelvis in the iliac fossa or groove are able to close and stabilize the posterior ring as well; however, they require expertise in application, and there have been reports of pelvic, spinal canal, and even rectal perforation with these devices.[21–23]
- The pneumatic anti-shock garment (PASG)[24–26] has been used in the past for emergent treatment of pelvic fracture hemorrhage. This device served three potential functions:
  - First, it returned blood from the lower extremities to the central vascular system.
  - Second, it could close, at least partially, open-book–type injuries, and
  - Third, it stabilized the pelvis.
- Potential shortcomings and failures of the pneumatic anti-shock garment:
  - The garment had to be partially or completely removed to allow access to the abdomen in patients who required abdominal exploration.
  - Reports of compartment syndrome and skin necrosis.
- If the pelvic ring is disrupted with vertical displacement but no opening, then longitudinal skeletal traction is applied either through the tibia or the femur if possible.
- Stabilization of the pelvic fracture allows clot formation and cessation or at least slowing of bleeding from the disrupted vessels and bone edges.

Physical Examination (Box 12–2)

- This essentially encompasses the secondary survey of the ATLS protocol.[19]
- The abdominal examination should focus on:
  - Tenderness, fullness, or rigidity.
  - Abdominal wall disruptions, defects, or open wounds.
  - Flank ecchymosis.

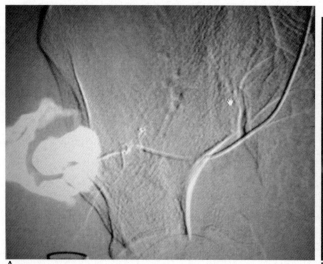
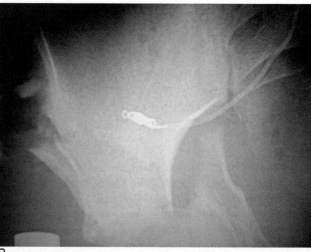

A   B

Figure 12–5: **(A)** Example of injury to superior gluteal artery. Note extravasation of contrast. **(B)** Superior gluteal artery tear treated with interventional angiographic coiling.

1. Flank, perineal, scrotal, or labial ecchymosis
2. Tender abdomen
3. Externally rotated lower extremities
4. Leg length discrepancy
5. Rectal or vaginal bleeding
6. Unilateral lower extremity neurologic deficit

- Presence of internal de-gloving or a Morel-Lavalle lesion (separation of the subcutaneous tissues from the underlying fascia). This can be recognized by extensive ecchymosis and subcutaneous fluctuance or fluid wave.
- The rectal and vaginal examination should focus on:
  - Position of the prostate (high-riding prostate may be a sign of urethral injury).
  - Palpable bone fragments that have penetrated the rectum or vagina.
  - Defects or tears in the wall of the rectum or vagina indicating possible bony penetration.
  - Rectal or vaginal bleeding indicating possible tears or bony penetration.
  - Urethral bleeding indicating possible urethral or bladder disruption.
  - Scrotal or labial swelling and ecchymosis indicating pelvic hemorrhage.
  - Rectal tone, perianal sensation, voluntary sphincter control and bulbo-cavernosus reflex to assess for the presence of cauda equina syndrome or lower sacral nerve root injury.
- The extremity examination should focus on:
  - Leg length discrepancy and presence of external rotation.
  - High incidence of associated acetabulum, hip, and knee injuries.

- The neurologic examination:
  - L1-L2: ilio-psoas (hip flexors) and upper anterior thigh sensation.
  - L3-L4 quadriceps (knee extensors) and lower anterior thigh or medial calf sensation.
  - L5 extensor hallucis and digitorum longus (toe dorsiflexion) and lateral calf or dorsum of foot sensation.
  - S1 gastro-soleus complex (ankle plantar flexion) and posterior calf sensation.
  - S2-S3 flexor hallucis and digitorum longus (toe plantar flexion) and sole of foot sensation.

Assessing for Pelvic Ring Instability

- Instability can exist in three planes:
  - Axial plane instability:
    - Internal rotation of the hemi-pelvis with lateral compression force.
    - External rotation of the hemi-pelvis with anterior compression force.
    - Radiographically greater than 2.5 cm of symphysis diastasis implies disruption of symphysis and sacrotuberous or spinous ligaments.
    - Clinically palpable opening or closing of the pelvis with AP and LC.
    - Fluoroscopic demonstration of opening of the pelvis anteriorly with AP compressive force.
    - See Figure 12–6.
  - Coronal plane instability (VS):
    - Radiographically seen as any vertical (caudal or more commonly cephalad) displacement of the hemi-pelvis or fractured L5 spinous process.
    - Clinically palpable motion or severe pain with longitudinal traction and axial compression of lower extremity.
    - Fluoroscopic demonstration of vertical movement of the hemi-pelvis.

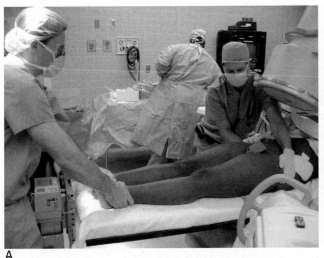
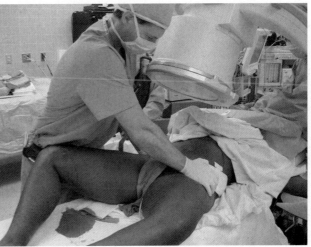

A   B

Figure 12–6: **(A)** Lateral compression assessing internal rotation. Note assistant internally rotating legs.
(B) Anteroposterior compression assessing external rotation.

- See Figure 12–7.
- Sagittal plane instability:
  - Anterior or posterior translation of the hemi-pelvis.
  - Not directly assessable by physical examination (although a bony prominence may be palpable posteriorly with posterior shift).
  - Radiographically best appreciated on the axial CT scan or inlet view X-ray.
  - Note that what appears to be posterior translation on the axial CT is usually a combination of sagittal plane rotation and proximal migration of the hemi-pelvis
  - See Figure 12–8.
- Once the patient has been diagnosed with a pelvic ring injury and the fracture pattern has been characterized, the patient is admitted to the intensive care unit (ICU)

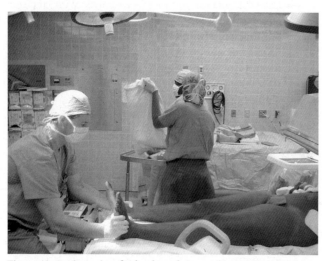

Figure 12–7: **Assessing for leg length inequality with vertical (or caudally directed) force.**

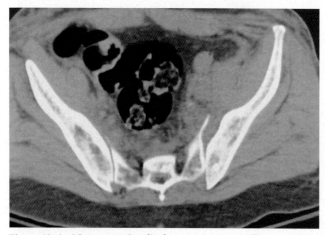

Figure 12–8: **Note posterior displacement at sacro-iliac joint but negligible posterior displacement anteriorly indicating anterior sagittal plane rotation (extension of the hemi-pelvis).**

for volume resuscitation, hemodynamic monitoring, and temporary pelvic stabilizing measures.

- Review of imaging studies and physical examination help to guide definitive treatment and fracture stabilization, which can be pursued once the patient's condition and associated injuries permit.
- Generally speaking, open reduction and internal fixation (ORIF) of pelvic fractures should be delayed for 3 to 5 days to allow for hemodynamic stabilization, volume resuscitation, and clot maturation. This helps to diminish blood loss and allow the surgeon to operate in a more controlled environment.
- If, however, the patient is going to the OR for an exploratory laparotomy, consideration can be made for early anterior fixation of the pelvic ring, and if indicated, percutaneous fixation of the posterior ring. However:
  - Contraindications to open plate fixation of the anterior ring include:
    - Open abdomen that is not amenable to closure secondary to swelling.
    - Bladder rupture not immediately repaired by urologists.
    - Suprapubic catheter communicating directly with anterior wound.

Treatment of Pelvic Fractures and Dislocations

Some Basic Tenets of Pelvic Fixation Biomechanics

- With complete instability of the posterior ring (i.e., the posterior SI ligaments are disrupted), anterior fixation alone is inadequate.
- With complete instability of the posterior ring and VS, any posterior ring fixation should be supplemented with some form of anterior ring stabilization.
- With partial instability of the pelvic ring (i.e., the posterior SI ligaments are intact), anterior ring fixation alone is adequate, and full weight bearing may be permitted.

Anterior Pelvic Ring Injuries

Symphysis Diastasis

- Options include an anterior external fixator or internal fixation with plate and screws (Figure 12–9).
- Available data from biomechanical studies have shown that there is:
  - No significant difference between external or internal fixation of the pelvis for controlling the symphysis or anterior ring.[27]
  - No significant difference between two-hole, multihole, or multiplane symphyseal plates.[28,29]
  - Significant improvement in pelvic stability with some form of anterior fixation in VS injury patterns.[30]

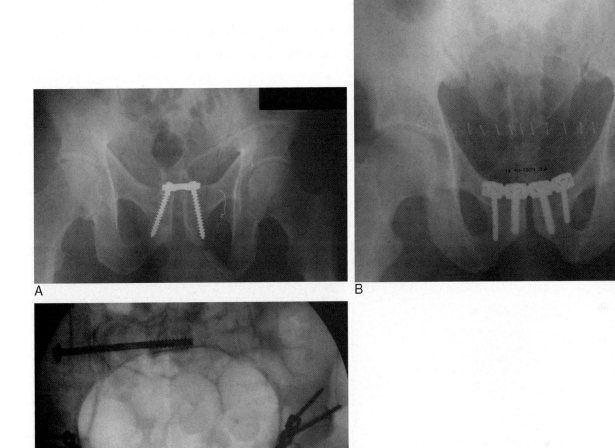

Figure 12–9: **(A)** Two-hole symphyseal plate. **(B)** Multihole symphyseal plate. **(C)** Reconstruction plate for rami fractures.

- Although earlier clinical studies have shown no difference between two-hole plates and multihole plates,[31] newer data suggest that two-hole plates may have a higher reoperation rate and incidence of pelvic malunion.[32]
- Pros of external fixation:
  - Can be used just as easily for both rami fractures and symphysis disruption.
  - Can be applied in the ED, intensive care unit (ICU), or OR.
  - Can be used when contamination from abdominal and genitourinary injuries complicates the clinical picture.
  - Can be removed in the clinic or office setting.
- Cons of external fixation:

- External device that interferes with positioning, sitting, and clothing.
- Pin site care and infection can be problematic, particularly with obese patients.
- More difficult to obtain and maintain an anatomic reduction of the anterior pelvic ring.
- Pros of internal fixation:
  - No interference with positioning, sitting, or clothing.
  - No problems with pin site care.
  - Anatomic reduction of the anterior pelvic ring.
- Cons of internal fixation:
  - Cannot be used with abdominal or pelvic contamination

- Formal operation is required for hardware removal or revision.
- Interferes with relaxation and opening of the pelvis during delivery of a fetus.

Rami Fractures

- Again, the options of external fixation or internal fixation exist.
- Plating rami fractures is more difficult than symphyseal disruptions because the fracture is often lateral, underneath the femoral neurovascular bundle. This requires additional exposure or dissection using the ilio-inguinal or Stoppa approaches.
- Plating in this instance does not have the long-term sequelae of hardware failure or removal and obstetrical concerns.
- Retrograde medullary ramus screws are a novel technique that allows percutaneous application of internal fixation of the ramus fracture.

- This technique does require that near anatomic reduction (at times using a miniopen maneuver to reduce the fracture with a bone hook) of the ramus fracture be obtained before screw insertion because the ramus offers a narrow corridor for safe screw placement.[33]

Posterior Pelvic Ring Injuries

Iliac Wing Fractures

- Iliac wing fractures can be addressed through an anterior approach with the lateral window of the ilio-inguinal or Smith-Peterson exposures, or a posterior approach with an incision along the iliac crest to SI joint and elevation of the gluteal musculature from the outer table of ilium (Figure 12–10).
- Depending on the patient's condition, fracture pattern and associated pelvic or acetabular injuries, one approach may offer advantages over the other.

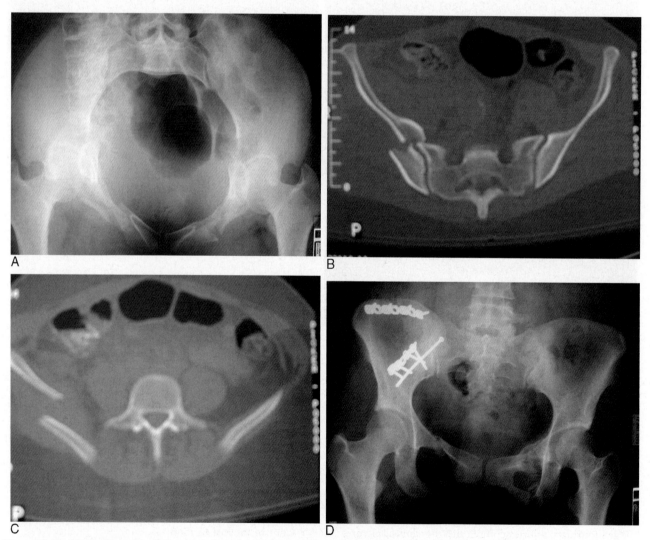

Figure 12–10: **(A)** Radiograph of iliac wing fracture. **(B)** and **(C)** Axial computed tomography scan of iliac wing fracture. **(D)** Iliac wing fracture treated with open reduction and internal fixation.

- As a general rule, the anterior approach is better tolerated by the patient and associated with less blood loss.
- However, if the iliac wing fracture is posterior, then exposure of both sides of the fracture and application of fixation may be difficult through an anterior approach.
- Generally, a single reconstruction plate or lag screw along the crest supplemented with a second reconstruction plate or lag screw at the level of the pelvic brim or sciatic buttress will suffice in neutralizing deforming forces until healing has occurred.[34]
- Bowel injury or herniation is possible with these injuries and should be looked for on CT and at operation.[35,36]

Sacro-Iliac Joint Dislocations

- Again, the SI joint can be approached from either anterior or posterior exposures as described previously (Figure 12–11).

- It is often easier to reduce the SI joint and apply reduction clamps from posterior; however, attention must be paid to closing the anterior aspect of the joint, which can be difficult from posterior. Often the surgeon relies on the ilio-sacral screw or supplemental anterior fixation to close any residual anterior SI diastasis.
- With the patient prone, careful attention must be paid to positioning so that pelvic external rotation and posterior translation is not worsened or that internal rotation and anterior translation are not impeded during reduction maneuvers. To prevent this, the patient should not be resting on the anterior superior iliac spine (ASIS).
- Anterior reduction and fixation is possible but requires dissection out onto the sacral ala. This places the L5 nerve root at risk of injury if care is not taken to stay strictly subperiosteal. Once dissection has progressed medial enough,

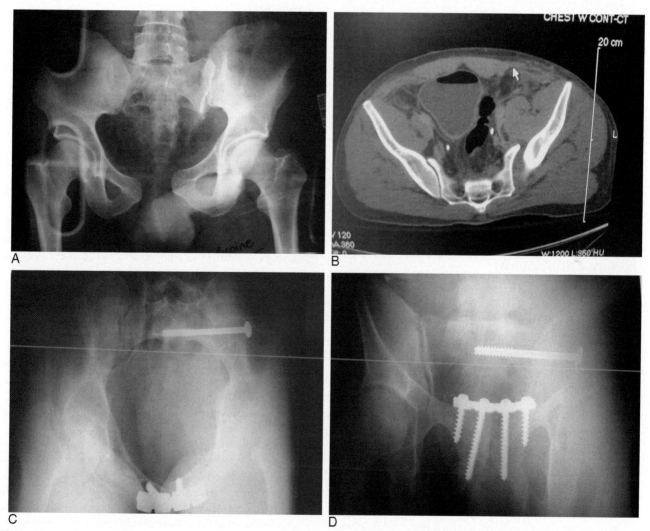

Figure 12–11: **(A)** Anteroposterior radiograph of a sacro–iliac dislocation. **(B)** Axial computed tomography scan showing complete sacro–iliac dislocation **(C)** and **(D)** inlet and outlet radiographs showing stabilization with ilio-sacral screw.

a sharp Homan retractor can be placed into the sacral alar bone to protect the L5 nerve root.[37]

- Fixation options include ilio-sacral screws, anterior SI plating, and posterior transiliac plating or compression rods.
- Biomechanical studies have not shown any significant differences between any of these techniques in terms of strength.[27]
- Biomechanical studies *have not* shown that more than one SI screw (either two into S1 or one into S1 and one into S2) is superior to a single screw into S1.[38]
- Pros and cons of ilio-sacral screw fixation[39–47]:
  - It can be applied percutaneously if closed manipulative reduction is possible.
  - It can be applied in either the prone or supine position.
  - It can be applied in situations of severe soft-tissue damage where open procedure would be compromised.
  - Skilled radiographic interpretation and 3D spatial thinking with good-quality intraoperative fluoroscopic imaging are mandatory.
- Pros and cons of anterior SI plating[37]:
  - It uses anterior approaches as described above for iliac wing fractures.
  - It is particularly useful if additional ipsi-lateral anterior pelvic or acetabular procedures are performed.
  - It requires dissection and placement of fixation onto the sacral ala, which places the L5 nerve root at risk.
  - It does not visualize the lower aspect of the joint.
- Pros and cons of transiliac bars or plates[48]:
  - It crosses the normal contralateral SI joint.
  - In thin patents, fixation can be prominent and bothersome occasionally causing skin breakdown.

Crescent Fractures (Sacro–Iliac Joint Fracture-Dislocations)

- This injury involves a fracture of the iliac wing that starts at the crest and exits into the SI joint (Figure 12–12).[49,50]
- A variable-sized fragment of posterior crest containing the posterior superior iliac spine (PSIS) remains attached to the sacral ala via the posterior SI ligaments.
- This crescentic fragment can be used as an aid to reduction as it is located anatomically with respect to the sacral ala.
- Standard fixation involves a superiorly placed reconstruction plate along the crest with supplemental lag screws from the posterior inferior iliac spine (PIIS) into the sciatic buttress just above the greater notch.
- As the crescentic fragment becomes smaller, this injury approaches and behaves more like an SI dislocation. Consideration must be given to supplemental SI screw fixation for small crescentic fragments.
- There are no data to indicate at which point the fragment is too small, and the surgeon must rely on radiographic appearance at the time of surgery.

Sacral Fractures

- Appropriate treatment of these injuries depends on:
  - Location of the fracture line (as outlined in the classification section).
  - Presence of impaction.
  - Integrity of the L5-S1 facet joint.
  - Presence and type of neurologic deficit (radiculopathy or cauda equina syndrome).
- Any longitudinal sacral fracture that is impacted without vertical shift or leg-length discrepancy can be treated with a trial of nonoperative care as impaction provides some stability to the fracture and pelvic ring.
- Three to 5 days of bedrest then mobilization with protected weight-bearing is safe.
- Repeat inlet, outlet, and AP pelvic radiographs are performed within the first week of mobilization.
- If no shift occurs, then continuation of protected weight-bearing for 12 weeks with close radiographic follow-up is indicated.
- The presentation of the patient in bed is often a good indicator whether or not nonoperative care will be possible in a non-displaced fracture. Those patients that have difficulty rolling over and using a bed pan effectively without severe lower back pain tend to have unstable injuries and may require evaluation of pelvic stability under general anesthetic and fluoroscopy with or without internal fixation.

Zone One Sacral Fractures, Nonimpacted with Displacement

- Treatment consists of reduction and stabilization of both the posterior and anterior pelvic ring.
- SI screws or trans-iliac bars/plates are satisfactory.
- Anterior plating is not applicable since dissection onto the anterior sacrum poses too great a risk to neurovascular structures.

Zone Two Sacral Fractures, Nonimpacted with Displacement

- By definition these fractures traverse the sacral foramina.
- Treatment and fixation of these injuries must therefore take into account the potential for traumatic and iatrogenic injury to the sacral nerve roots.
- Careful neurologic assessment must document function of the sacral nerve roots as outlined previously.
- Carefully scrutinizing the CT scan should rule out compression of the sacral nerve roots by fracture fragments or fracture-dislocation of the L5-S1 facet joint.
- If nerve root compression is observed and the patient exhibits neurologic deficits or symptoms attributable to that lesion, then the patient should have a sacral nerve root decompressive laminectomy in addition to fracture reduction and stabilization.

CHAPTER 12 Pelvic Fractures **223**

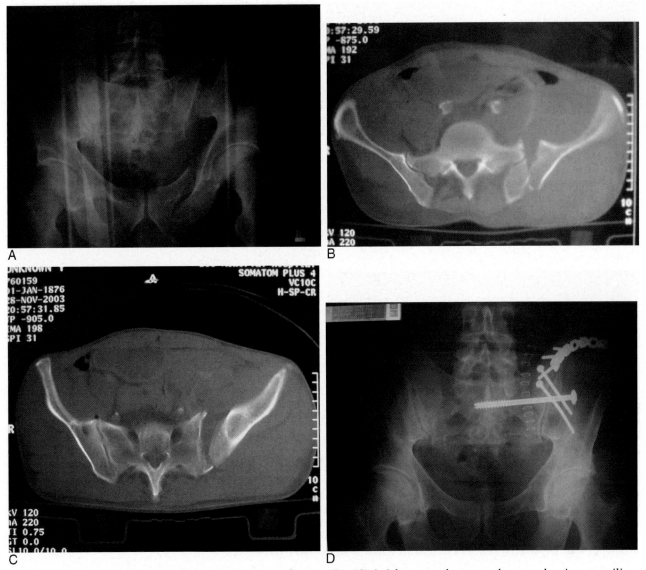

Figure 12–12: **(A)** Anteroposterior radiograph of a crescent fracture **(B)**. **(C)** Axial computed tomography scans showing sacro-iliac joint fracture dislocation. **(D)** Crescent fracture treated with posterior open reduction and internal fixation.

- In zone 2 fractures that have minimal or no comminution with an intact L5-S1 facet joint, SI screw fixation with supplemental anterior stabilization is adequate.
- In fractures where there is significant comminution or the L5-S1 facet joint is disrupted, SI screw or transiliac compression rod, bar, or plate fixation is less reliable with a high reported failure rate both clinically and biomechanically.[51–54]
  - SI screws rely on compression for stability.
  - SI screws are placed at 90 degrees to plane of displacement.
  - SI screws are not a fixed-angle device.
  - As a result, SI screws for this particular injury pattern resist vertical shear deforming forces poorly (see Figure 12–14).
- Spinal-pelvic fixation (also known as lumbo-pelvic fixation or triangular osteosynthesis) has been used to address these concerns for this particular clinical scenario.[55,56]

- A lumbar pedicle screw is connected to an iliac screw positioned at the PSIS.
- This connection uses clamps that are fixed angle and aligns the fixation vertically to resist VS forces.
- The fixation is often used to supplemented a "position" SI screw (not placed under compression). This "triangular" construct resists vertical displacement and rotation around the iliac screw.
- Biomechanical and clinical studies have confirmed the superiority of this fixation technique over SI screws for this particular injury pattern.[57]
- See Figure 12–15.
- Pros and cons of spinal-pelvic fixation:
  - Because spinal-pelvic fixation is rigid and fixed-angle, early (immediate to 4 to 6 weeks) weight bearing is permitted.

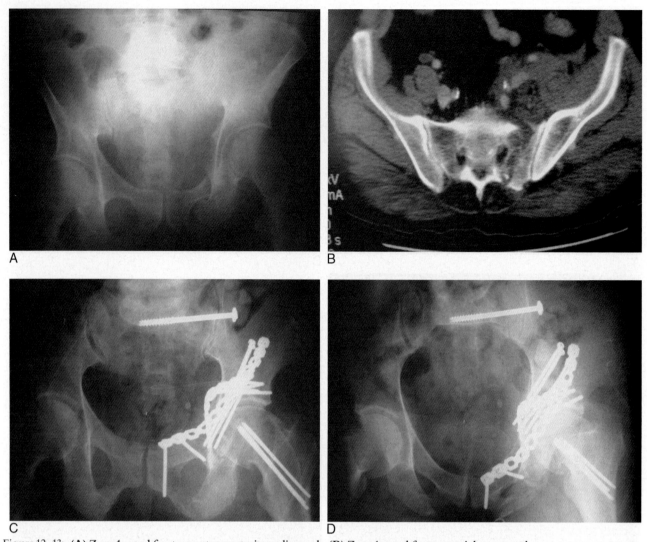

Figure 12–13: **(A)** Zone 1 sacral fracture anteroposterior radiograph. **(B)** Zone 1 sacral fracture axial computed tomography scan. **(C)** and **(D)** Zone I sacral fracture treated with ilio-sacral screw.

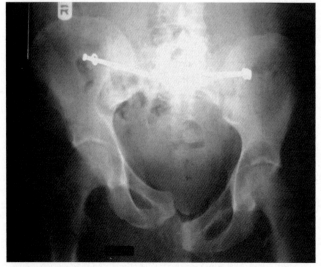

Figure 12–14: Failure of ilio-sacral screw with comminuted zone 2 vertical shear sacral fracture.

- Little to no postoperative loss of reduction is observed compared with traditional ilio-sacral screw fixation.[58]
- The fixation can be quite prominent at the PSIS in thin patients.
- This fixation crosses two potentially normal articulations (the SI joint and L5–S1 joint) and limits the small but normal motion that occurs with normal activities at these articulations. Most patients complain of implant activity-related low-back pain or discomfort that almost invariably necessitates fixation removal once the fracture is healed by CT scan examination at 6 months.

Type Three Sacral Fractures

- These injuries usually present as an open-book–type pattern with diastasis anteriorly and gapping of the sacral fracture posteriorly secondary to external rotation of the hemi-pelvis.[59,60]

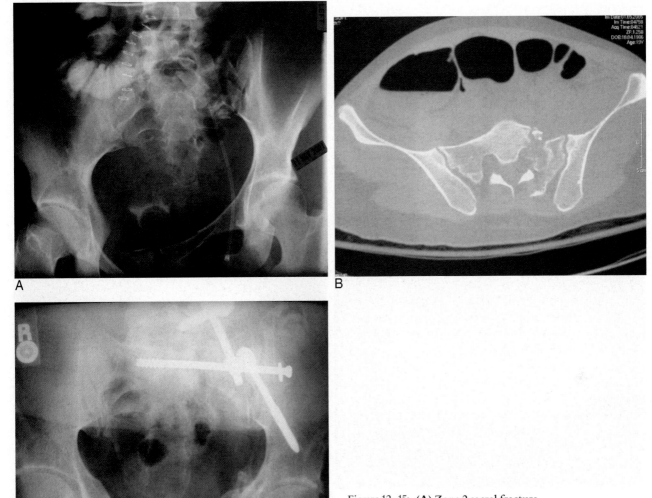

Figure 12–15: **(A)** Zone 2 sacral fracture anteroposterior radiograph. **(B)** Zone 2 sacral fracture axial computed tomography scan. **(C)** Zone 2 sacral fracture treated with spinal-pelvic fixation construct.

- VS or vertical displacement usually does not occur secondary to the buttressing effect of the L5 vertebra and L5-S1 facet joint above. With significant energy and disruption of the L5-S1 facet joint however, VC can occur.[61]
- These injuries can be treated by closing the pelvic ring anteriorly, and if residual fracture gap exists in the sacrum, a long SI screw can be placed across into the contralateral and SI joint ilium to compress the fracture and prevent fibrous nonunion.
- If there is VS with comminution and facet disruption, then consideration should be given to spinal-pelvic fixation.
- See Figure 12–16.

Transverse and U–Shaped Sacral Fractures

- These injuries do not disrupt the integrity of the pelvic ring.
- They can, however, result in discontinuity of the spine and pelvis (spinal-pelvic dissociation) or compression of the sacral spinal canal and cauda equina syndrome.[16,62–66]

- Appropriate neurologic examination is critical. If a rectal examination is not performed, occult cauda equina syndrome will not be diagnosed.
- Transverse fractures below the level of the SI joints do not compromise pelvic ring or spinal-pelvic stability. Consideration of operative treatment therefore is predicated on the presence of cauda-equina syndrome (see Figure 12–17).
- Transverse fractures at the level of the SI joints are associated with bilateral longitudinal fractures, usually of the zone 2 pattern and hence the *u* shape. These are highly unstable at the spinal-pelvic junction with resultant kyphotic or translational deformity. Operative stabilization is required for mobilization or sacral canal decompression if indicated (see Figure 12–18).
- Treatment consists of decompressing the spinal canal, reducing the deformity, and stabilizing the fracture.
- Often, placing the patient prone and extending the hips will affect some reduction and canal decompression.

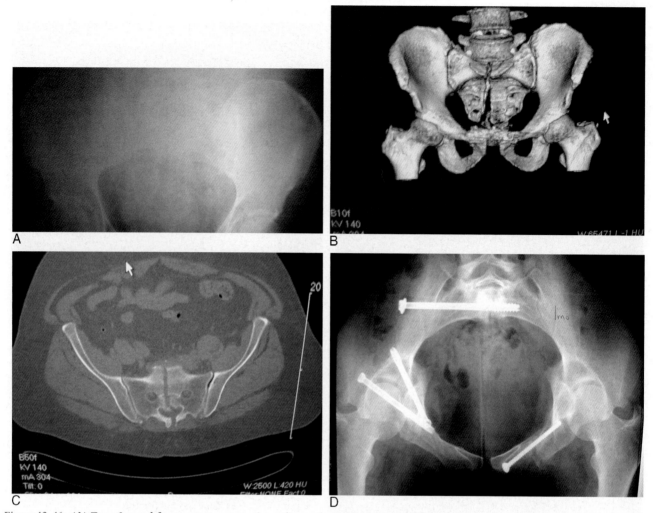

Figure 12–16: **(A)** Zone 3 sacral fracture anteroposterior radiograph. **(B)** Zone 3 sacral fracture three–dimensional reconstruction view. **(C)** Zone 3 sacral fracture axial computed tomography scan. **(D)** Zone 3 sacral fracture treated with ilio-sacral screws.

- If the patient has signs of cauda equina syndrome, then sacral laminectomy should be performed.
- Stabilization involves controlling the sagittal plane deformation (increased kyphosis and anterior translation). To effectively control the sagittal plane deforming forces, the posterior tension band must be restored.
- Spinal-pelvic fixation or standard lumbo-sacral instrumentation has the ability to lock into the lumbar spine and reestablish a stable connection to the pelvis while resisting anterior rotation and translation (see Figure 12-19).
- There are also reports in the literature advocating the application of bilateral SI screws alone for securing stable impacted forms of this injury pattern.[67]

Outcome Studies for Pelvic Fractures

- Stabilization of unstable pelvic injuries has only recently evolved to include early internal fixation and restoration of anatomic relations.

- Before the 1980s, little was understood regarding the biomechanics and contributions to stability of the various pelvic bony and ligamentous structures.
- As recently as the 1970s, many pelvic ring disruptions were treated with nonoperative techniques; generally skeletal traction and pelvic slings to prevent excessive cephalad migration of the hemi-pelvis. However, many clinicians have documented the high incidence of poor functional outcome and chronic pain in patients with vertically unstable pelvic fractures treated nonoperatively.[13,68,69]
- The results of these and other studies provided the impetus to pursue operative means to achieve and maintain anatomic reduction.
- Operative stabilization began with anteriorly placed external fixators alone, which were found to be nearly totally ineffective at controlling vertical and posterior displacement of the posterior aspect of the ring.[70]
- Clinical outcome studies with the use of external fixators subsequently found that results were not improved over nonoperative management, and in fact, traction and pelvic sling alone may have been more successful at treating this unstable injury.[71,72]

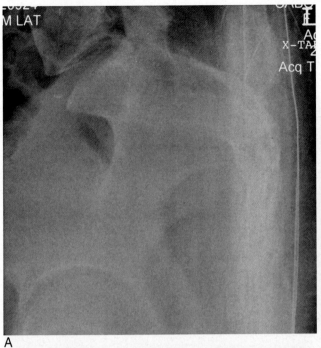

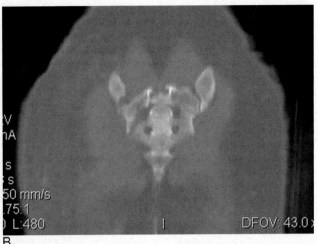

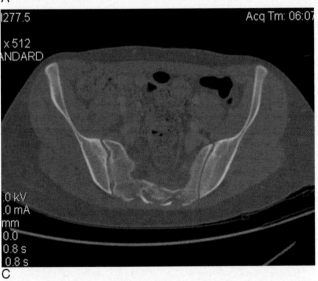

Figure 12–17: **(A)** X-ray and **(B)** and **(C)** computed tomography of infraarticular transverse sacral fracture (no spinal or pelvic ring instability).

- Improved short-term patient outcome with early stabilization of the pelvic fracture and mobilization of the patient and numerous reports citing improved outcome with anatomic reduction of the posterior ring continued to provide the impetus to develop more rigid and stable posterior fixation constructs.[73–76]

- Supplemental fixation of the anterior aspect of the pelvic ring has been shown to provide further biomechanical stability in the case of the vertically unstable hemipelvis.[38]

- Early outcome studies support the position that the long-term functional results are improved if reduction with less than 1 centimeter of combined displacement of the posterior ring is obtained, especially with pure dislocations of the sacro-iliac complex.[77]

- Fractures of the posterior ring tend to do better, presumably because bone healing can restore initial strength and stability, SI dislocations rely purely on ligamentous healing and scar formation and these patients tend to fair worse in terms of short-term and long-term problems with pain and ambulation when compared to patients with other fracture patterns.[78]

- However despite seemingly anatomic reductions (or near anatomic) more recent clinical outcome studies have shown that with modern fixation techniques, a substantial proportion of patients continue to have poor outcomes with chronic posterior pelvic pain.[79–81]

- This is likely related to multiple confounding factors such as:
  - Trauma patients often have a borderline socioeconomic status with poor social and financial support groups.

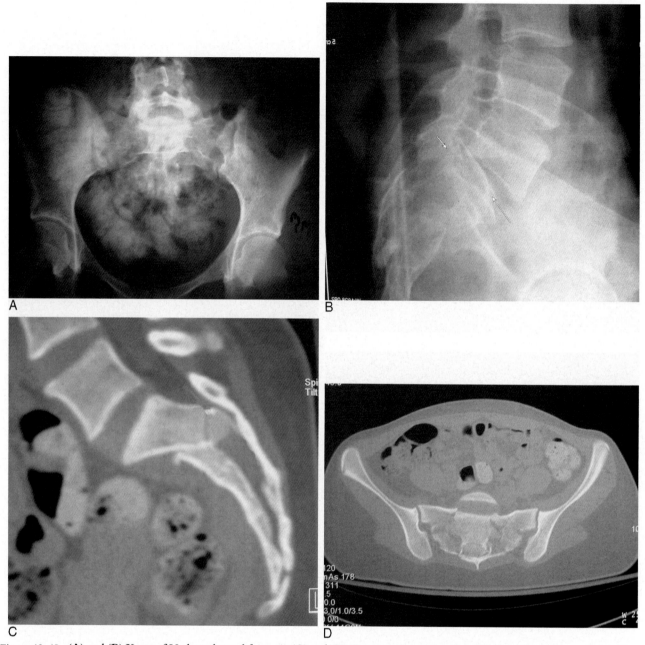

Figure 12–18: **(A)** and **(B)** X-ray of U-shaped sacral fracture. **(C)** and **(D)** Computed tomography of U-shaped sacral fracture (spinal pelvic dissociation). Note that sacro-iliac joints are intact, but the lumbo-sacral spine is not in continuity with the sacro-iliac joints.

- Extensive soft-tissue damage and associated long-bone and extremity fractures.
- Associated neurologic, visceral, and urogenital injuries with dyspareunia, sexual dysfunction, and incontinence.[82]
- Prolonged recovery and rehabilitation time with loss of job, home, and family.
- Outcome studies after fixation of pelvic injuries are difficult to interpret because of poor follow-up, heterogeneity of the injury pattern, associated visceral and neurologic injury, and the lack of a reliable outcome measure for pelvic ring injuries.
- Recent clinical outcome studies have shown that with current fixation techniques, a substantial proportion of patients continue to have poor outcomes with chronic posterior pelvic pain despite seemingly anatomic reductions and healing, with less than 50% returning to previous level of function and work status.

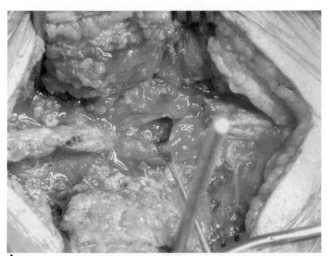

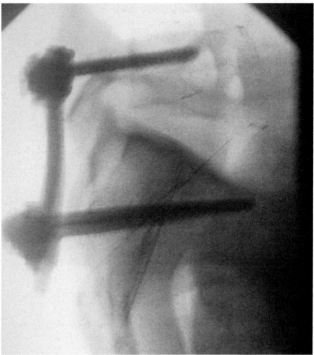

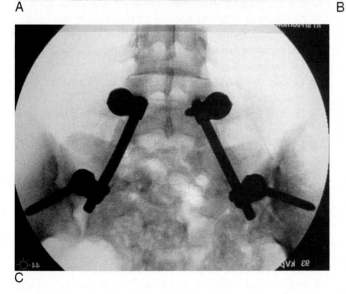

Figure 12–19: **(A)** Decompression of cauda equina.
(B) Reduction of kyphosis. **(C)** Spinal-pelvic fixation.

Other Clinical and Technical Considerations

What about the APC-1 and APC-2 injury with only partial instability of the posterior ring? (i.e., how do you treat the patient with intact posterior SI ligaments and symphyseal diastasis?)

- Because the posterior SI ligaments are intact, symphyseal plating should restore pelvic ring stability and the patient may bear weight immediately.
- In general, if the posterior SI ligaments are intact, then full weight bearing on the affected extremity is permitted.

- If the posterior ring is completely disrupted, then toe-touch weight bearing only is permitted (spinal-pelvic fixation being the only exception).

How much symphysis diastasis is too much?

- The answer lies in the back at the SI joint on CT scan.
- Greater than 2.5 cm implies disruption of the anterior SI, sacrotuberous (ST), and sacrospinous (SS) ligaments.[1]
- If the diastasis is less than 2.5 cm and the anterior SI joint is not open, then examination under anesthetic to assess SI stability is indicated

- If the SI joint opens anteriorly with manual AP or LC then anterior fixation is required.
- If the SI joint remains closed and stable, then full weight bearing is permitted.

Does it matter which of the posterior or anterior ring injuries is fixed first?

- For functional and outcome reasons, the focus is on reducing the posterior ring anatomically.
- Therefore placing anterior fixation that will inhibit or block reduction of the posterior pelvic ring must be avoided.
- If anterior fixation is placed first, then the patient should be positioned such that access to the anterior fixation is possible in the event that its removal or loosening is possible to allow anatomic reduction of the posterior ring. Does posterior fixation that crosses the SI joint need to be removed?
- The long-term effects of SI screws and transiliac bars or plates are not known.
- Certainly, some patients continue to complain of posterior pain long after their injury has healed.
- Whether this is the result of associated neurologic and soft-tissue injury or the effects of retained fixation on normal pelvic biomechanics has yet to be determined.

Appendix 1: Technical Aspects and Technique Tips

Closed reduction of posterior ring injuries:

- Longitudinal traction is the principle maneuver.
- Free-draping the affected extremity to allow internal and external rotation of the limb and hemi-pelvis is also helpful.
- External rotation of the limb will open the pelvis anteriorly but close it posteriorly, particularly if the symphysis is fixed.
- Internal rotation of the limb will close the symphysis and anterior SI joint if the posterior ring is fixed or uninjured. If the anterior ring is fixed, then internal rotation of the limb can help to disimpact or laterally translate the posterior ring.
- Place a bump under the affected PSIS if posterior displacement exists.
- If patient is prone, do not rest the patient on anterior superior iliac spine on the injured side because it will cause posterior translation of the hemi-pelvis.

Ilio-sacral screws:

- Patient may be positioned prone or supine.
- Entry point externally is typically 10 to 20 mm anterior to the crista glutea midway from the iliac crest to the greater sciatic notch.

- Percutaneous procedures must be wary of injury to the superior gluteal neurovascular bundle[83–85].
- "Safe" placement is maximized by careful attention to radiographic boney landmarks[86–90]:
- The screw should have a trajectory tracking posterior to anterior and slightly inferior to superior (i.e., parallel to the joint).
- The screw should be above the S1 foramen on the outlet view.
- The screw should be in the anterior aspect of the sacral body or promontory on the inlet view.
- The screw should be below the iliac-cortical densities or sacral alar slope line on the lateral view.
- All three radiographic projections are important.
- Watch out for sacral dysmorphism (abnormal developmental anatomy at the lumbo sacral junction). There may be incomplete or complete failure to segment or fuse giving "lumbarized S1 vertebrae or "sacralized" L5 vertebrae.

Symphyseal Plating:

- Use of a Pfannenstiel-type of an incision for the skin, with a vertical split in the rectus abdominis along the linea alba facilitates closure and decreases the risk of hernia.
- Dissection along the anterior aspect of the pubic body to allow placement of large reduction tongs into the obturator foramen is not necessary.
- Protect the bladder and bladder neck and urethra with a malleable retractor.
- Have a Foley catheter in place to allow palpation of the urethra and decompression of the bladder.
- Monitor the urine in the Foley bag for new hematuria, which may indicate an iatrogenic bladder injury.
- Use a multihole plate with at least two screws on either side of the symphysis.

Annotated References

1. Vrahas M, Hearn TC, Diangelo D, et al: Ligamentous contributions to pelvic stability, *Orthopedics* 18:271-274, 1995.
A cadaveric biomechanical analysis that determined the respective contributions of the primary pelvic ligaments to pelvic ring stability. Important in that it relates ligamentous stability and importance to loading patterns and combinations of ligamentous disruption. The posterior sacro-iliac and symphyseal ligaments are the most important.

2. Demetriades D, Karaiskakis M, Toutouzas K, et al: Pelvic fractures: epidemiology and predictors of associated abdominal injuries and outcomes, *J Am Coll Surg* 195:1-10, 2002.
Review of over 16,000 patients from Trauma Registry examining risk factors for bleeding and death and associated injuries in patients with traumatic pelvic fractures. The most common visceral injuries in severe pelvic fractures were liver and bladder (about 15%). Motor vehicle crash is the most common mechanism of injury, with the overall mortality at about 1% for those patients succumbing as a direct result of the pelvic fracture.

3. Dalal SA, Burgess AR, Siegel JH, et al: Pelvic fracture in multiple trauma: classification by mechanism is the key to pattern of organ injury, resuscitative requirements, and outcome. *J Trauma* 29:981-1002, 1989.

4. McMurtry R, Walton D, Dickinson D, et al: Pelvic disruptions in the poly-traumatized patient: a management protocol. *Clin Orthop* 151:22-30, 1980.

5. Fallon B, Wendt JC, Hawtrey CE: Urological injury and assessment in patients with fractured pelvis. *J Urol* 131:712-714, 1984.

6. Cass AS, Godec CJ: Urethral injury due to external trauma, *Urology* 11:607-611, 1978.

7. Rothenberger DA, Velasco R, Strate F, et al: Open pelvic fracture: a lethal injury, *J Trauma* 18:184-187, 1978.

8. Flancbaum L, Morgan AS, Fleisher M, et al: Blunt bladder trauma: manifestation of severe injury, *Urology* 31:220-222, 1988.

9. Cass AS: The multiply injured patient with bladder trauma, *J Trauma* 24:731-734, 1984.

10. Raffa J, Christensen NM: Compound fractures of the pelvis, *Am J Surg* 132:282-286, 1976.

11. Richardson JD, Harty J, Amin M, et al: Open pelvic fractures, *J Trauma* 22:533-538, 1982.
Review of staged protocol in treating open pelvic fracture. Stressing the major complications of lethal hemorrhage and infection found in earlier series, the authors demonstrate the efficacy of an aggressive approach using embolization, wound packing, and diverting colostomy.

12. Young JWR, Burgess AR, Brumback RJ, et al: Pelvic fractures: value of plain radiography in early assessment and management, *Radiology* 160:445-451, 1986.
A classic article describing the mechanistic approach to classifying pelvic fractures, which is still the most commonly used today. A must-read and must-know for anyone that may be dealing with pelvic fractures in any way.

13. Tile M: Pelvic fractures: should they be fixed? *J Bone Joint Surg Br* 70:1-12, 1988.

14. OTA classification of fractures, *J Orthop Trauma* 10(Suppl):66-75, 1996.

15. Denis F, Davis S, Comfort T: Sacral fractures, an important problem: retrospective analysis of 236 cases, *Clin Orthop* 227:67-81, 1988.
A classic article that really brought greater understanding to the treatment of sacral fractures. Really more of an epidemiologic retrospective review describing mechanisms of injury and incidence of neurological injury as related to injury pattern, but it remains to this day the article that helps us better understand sacral fractures with regards to pelvic ring stability.

16. Roy-Camille R, Saillant G, Gagna G, et al: Transverse fracture of the upper sacrum: suicidal jumper's fracture, *Spine* 10:838-845, 1984.

17. Strange-Vognsen HH, Lebech A: An unusual type of fracture in the upper sacrum, *J Orthop Trauma* 5:200-203, 1991.

18. Peng MY, Parisky YR, Cornwell EE, et al: CT cystography versus conventional cystography in evaluation of bladder injury, *Am J Roentgenol* 173:1269-1272, 1999.

19. American College of Surgeons Committee on Trauma: *Advanced Trauma Life Support for Doctors*, ed 6, 1997.

20. Bottlang M: Noninvasive reduction of open-book pelvic fractures by circumferential compression, *J Orthop Trauma* 16:367-373, 2002.

21. Pohlemann T: Pelvic emergency clamps: anatomic landmarks for a safe primary application, *J Orthop Trauma* 18:102-105, 2004.

22. Ertel W, Keel M, Eid K, et al: Control of severe hemorrhage using C-clamp and pelvic packing in multiply injured patients with pelvic ring disruption, *J Orthop Trauma* 15:468-474, 2001.

23. Gansslen A, Giannoudis P, Pape HC: Hemorrhage in pelvic fracture: who needs angiography? *Curr Opin Crit Care* 9:515-523, 2003.
An excellent review of pelvic hemorrhage and angiography, with the ultimate supposition that open packing and pelvic clamp application is safer and better for patients, particularly those in extremis.

24. Mattox KL, Bickell W, Pepe PE, et al: Prospective randomized evaluation of antishock MAST in post-traumatic hypotension, *J Trauma* 26:779-786, 1986.

25. Flint LM, Brown A, Richardson JD, et al: Definitive control of hemorrhage in pelvic crush injuries, *Ann Surg* 189:709-716, 1979.

26. Brotman S, Browner BD, Cox EF: MAS trousers improperly applied causing a compartment syndrome in the lower extremity, *J Trauma* 22:598-599, 1982.

27. Hearn TC, Tile M: The effects of ligament sectioning and internal fixation of bending stiffness of the pelvic ring. In: Proceedings of the 13th International Conference on Biomechanics. Perth, Australia, December, 1991.

28. Simonian PT, Schwappach JR, Routt ML, et al: Evaluation of new plate designs for symphysis pubis internal fixation, *J Trauma* 41:498-502, 1996.

29. Stocks GW, Gabel GT, Noble PC, et al: Anterior and posterior internal fixation of vertical shear fractures of the pelvis, *J Orthop Res* 9:237-245, 1991.

30. Sagi HC, Ordway NT, DiPasquale T: Biomechanical analysis of fixation for vertically unstable sacro-iliac dislocations with ilio-sacral screws and symphyseal plating, *J Orthop Trauma* 18:135-139, 2004.
Cadaveric biomechanical study comparing the stability of one versus two ilio-sacral screws with and without a two-hole symphyseal plate. No significant benefit was found with two ilio-sacral screws. However fixation of the anterior aspect of the ring significantly enhanced pelvic ring stability in the vertical shear model.

31. Webb LX, Gristina AG, Wilson JR, et al: Two-hole plate fixation for traumatic symphysis pubis diastasis, *J Trauma* 28:813-817, 1988.

32. Sagi HC, Papp S: Comparative and clinical and radiographic outcome of two-hole and multi-hole symphyseal plating. Presented at the Annual Meeting of the Orthopaedic Trauma Association, Ottawa, Canada, October 2005.

33. Routt ML Jr, Simonian PT, Grujic L: The retrograde medullary superior pubic ramus screw for the treatment of anterior pelvic ring disruptions: a new technique, *J Orthop Trauma* 9:35-44, 1995.

34. Simonian PT, Routt ML Jr, Harrington RM, et al: The unstable iliac fracture: a biomechanical evaluation of internal fixation, *Injury* 28:469-75.

35. Charnley GJ, Dorrell JH: Small bowel entrapment in an iliac wing fracture, *Injury* 24:627-628, 1993.

36. Emery KH: Lap belt iliac wing fracture: a predictor of bowel injury in children, *Pediatr Radiol* 32:892-895, 2002; Epub Jul 26, 2002.

37. Simpson LA, Waddell JP, Leighton RK, et al: Anterior approach and stabilization of the disrupted sacroiliac joint, *J Trauma* 27:1332-1339, 1987.

38. Sagi HC, Ordway N, DiPasquale T: Biomechanical analysis of fixation for vertically unstable sacroiliac dislocations with iliosacral screws and symphyseal plating, *J Orthop Trauma* 18:138-143, 2004.

39. Routt ML, Simonian PT, Mills WJ: Iliosacral screw fixation: early complications of the percutaneous technique, *J Orthop Trauma* 11:584-589, 1997.

40. Routt ML, Simonian PT, Agnew SG, et al: Radiographic recognition of the sacral alar slope for optimal placement of iliosacral screws: a cadaveric and clinical study, *J Orthop Trauma* 10:171-177, 1996.

41. Shuler TE, Boone DC, Gruen GS, et al: Percutaneous iliosacral screw fixation: early treatment for unstable pelvic ring disruptions, *J Trauma* 38:453-458, 1995.

42. Keating JF, Werier J, Blachut P, et al: Early fixation of the vertically unstable pelvis: the role of iliosacral screw fixation of the posterior lesion, *J Orthop Trauma* 13:107-113, 1999.

43. Xu R, Ebraheim NA, Robke J, et al: Radiologic evaluation of iliosacral screw placement, *Spine* 21:582-588, 1996.

44. Templeman D, Schmidt A, Freese J, et al: Proximity of iliosacral screws to neurovascular structures after internal fixation, *Clin Orthop* 329:194-198, 1996.
Another key article on the anatomy in various regions of the sacrum, lending support for the current recommendations for safe placement of ilio-sacral screws.

45. Ebraheim NA, Xu R, Biyani A, et al: Morphologic considerations of the first sacral pedicle for iliosacral screw placement, *Spine* 22:841-846, 1997.

46. Day CS, Prayson MJ, Shuler TE, et al: Trans-sacral versus modified pelvic landmarks for percutaneous iliosacral screw placement: a computed tomographic analysis and cadaveric study, *Am J Orthop* 29:16-21, 2000.

47. Carlson DA, Scheid DK, Maar DC, Baele JR, Kaehr DM. Safe placement of S1 and S2 iliosacral screws: the "vestibule" concept. *J Orthop Trauma* 2000 May; 14:264-269.

48. Shaw JA, Mino DE, Werner FW, et al: Posterior stabilization of pelvic fractures by use of threaded compression rods: case reports and mechanical testing, *Clin Orthop* 192:240-254, 1985.

49. Borrelli J Jr, Koval KJ, Helfet DL: Operative stabilization of fracture dislocations of the sacroiliac joint, *Clin Orthop Rel Res* 329:141-146, 1996.

50. Borrelli J Jr, Koval KJ, Helfet DL: The crescent fracture: a posterior fracture dislocation of the sacroiliac joint, *J Orthop Trauma* 10:165-170, 1996.
A classic article describing the sacro-iliac fracture dislocation injury pattern and the implications thereof associated with ligamentous stability of the pelvic ring. The authors were able to demonstrate an effective extraarticular method of fixation that did not compromise the sacro-iliac joint. This is a retrospective review of only 22 patients.

51. Griffin DR, Starr AJ, Reinert CM, et al: Vertically unstable pelvic fractures fixed with percutaneous ilio-sacral screws: does posterior injury pattern predict fixation failure? *J Orthop Trauma* 17:399-405, 2003.
A great article finally lending support to the anecdotal opinions that ilio-sacral screw fixation applied in the conventional sense was associated with a high failure rate in the fixation of comminuted sacral fractures.

52. Pohlemann T, Angst M, Schneider E, et al: Fixation of transforaminal sacrum fractures: a biomechanical study, *J Orthop Trauma* 7:107-117, 1993.

53. Gorczyca JT, Varga E, Woodside T, et al: The strength of iliosacral lag screws and trans-iliac bars in the fixation of vertically unstable pelvic injuries with sacral fractures, *Injury* 27:561-564, 1996.

54. Simonian PT, Routt ML, Harrington RM, et al: Internal fixation of the transforaminal sacral fracture, *Clin Orthop* 323:202-209, 1996.

55. Schildhauer TA, Josten C, Muhr G: Triangular osteosynthesis of vertically unstable sacrum fractures: a new concept allowing early weight-bearing, *J Orthop Trauma* 12:307-314, 1998.
Clinical series retrospective review introducing the concept of lumbo-pelvic fixation for the treatment of vertically unstable pelvic injuries associated with transforaminal sacral fractures. Demonstrated the strength of the construct with little to no loss of reduction, even in those patients permitted immediate weight-bearing.

56. Kach K, Trentz O: Distraction spondylodesis of the sacrum in "vertical shear lesions" of the pelvis, *Unfallchirurg* 97:28-38, 1994.

57. Schildhauer TA, Ledoux WR, Chapman JR, et al: Triangular osteosynthesis and iliosacral screw fixation for unstable sacral fractures: a cadaveric and biomechanical evaluation under cyclic loads, *J Orthop Trauma* 17:22-31, 2003.

58. Sagi, HC, DiPasquale T, Militano U: Radiographic and functional outcome of vertically unstable transforaminal sacral fractures treated with spinal-pelvic (lumbo-pelvic) fixation, Presented at the 20th Annual Meeting of the Orthopaedic Trauma Association, Fort Lauderdale, FL, October 2004.

59. Moed BR, Morawa LG: Displaced midline longitudinal fracture of the sacrum, *J Trauma* 24:435-437, 1984.

60. Weisel SW, Zeide MS, Terry RL: Longitudinal fractures of the sacrum: case report, *J Trauma* 19:70-71, 1979.

61. Isler B: Lumbosacral lesions associated with pelvic ring injuries, *J Orthop Trauma* 4:1-6, 1990.

62. Savolaine ER, Ebrahim NA, Rusin JJ, et al: Limitations of radiography and computed tomography in the diagnosis of transverse sacral fracture from a high fall, *Clin Orthop* 272:122-126, 1991.

63. LaFollette BF, Levine MI, McNeish LM: Bilateral fracture-dislocation of the sacrum: a case report, *J Bone Joint Surg* 68-A:1099-1101, 1986.

64. Takahara T, Masada K, Goto Y, et al: Isolated fracture-dislocation of the sacrum: a case report, *J Trauma* 34:600-601, 1993.

65. Singh AK, Fleetcroft JP: Bilateral fracture-dislocation of the sacrum, *Injury* 20:301-303, 1989.

66. Marcus RE, Hansen ST: Bilateral fracture-dislocations of the sacrum: a case report, *J Bone Joint Surg* 66-A:1297-1299, 1984.

67. Nork SE, Jones CB, Harding SP, et al: Percutaneous stabilization of U-shaped sacral fractures using iliosacral screws: technique and early results, *J Orthop Trauma* 15:238-246, 2001.
An interesting article presenting the concept of the u-shaped sacral fracture, which in effect is more of a spinal dislocation than a pelvic ring injury. The injury morphology and epidemiology are nicely presented along with reduction maneuvers and fixation techniques using ilio-sacral screws.

68. Routt ML, Nork SE, Mills WJ: High energy pelvic ring disruptions, *Orthop Clin North Am* 33:59-72, 2002.

69. Holdsworth F: Dislocation and fracture dislocation of the pelvis, *J Bone Joint Surg* 30:461-466, 1948.

70. Slatis P, Huittenen V-M: Double vertical fractures of the pelvis: a report on 163 patients, *Acta Chir Scand* 138:799-807, 1972.

71. Semba R, Yasukawa K, Gustilo R: Critical analysis of results of 53 Malgaigne fractures of the pelvis, *J Trauma* 23:535-537, 1983.

72. Kellam J: The role of external fixation in pelvic disruptions, *Clin Orthop* 241:66-82, 1989.

73. Cole JD, Blum DA, Ansel LJ: Outcome after fixation of unstable posterior pelvic ring injuries, *Clin Orthop* 329:160-179, 1996.

74. Kregor PJ, Routt ML: Unstable pelvic ring disruptions in unstable patients, *Injury* 30:SB19-SB28, 1999.

75. Goldstein A, Phillips T, Sclafani SJ, et al: Early open reduction and internal fixation of the disrupted pelvic ring, *J Trauma* 26:325-333, 1986.
One of the early classic articles demonstrating that early pelvic ring stabilization and patient mobilization using a staged protocol had a clear benefit over nonoperative treatment.

76. Latenser BA, Gentilello LM, Tarver AA, et al: Improved outcome with early fixation of skeletally unstable pelvic fractures, *J Trauma* 31:28-31, 1991.

77. Tornetta P III, Matta JM: Outcome of operatively treated unstable posterior pelvic ring disruptions, *Clin Orthop* 329:186-193, 1996.
A classic article looking at a large single surgeon series of unstable pelvic injuries treated operatively. The whole notion of 1 cm combined displacement of the posterior aspect of the ring being related to a poorer functional outcome originated from this analysis.

78. Dujardin FH, Hossenbaccus M, Duparc F, et al: Long-term functional prognosis of posterior injuries in high-energy pelvic disruption, *J Orthop Trauma* 12:145-150, 1998.

79. Nepola JV, Trenhaile SW, Miranda MA, et al: Vertical shear injuries: is there a relationship between residual displacement and functional outcome? *J Trauma* 46:1024-1030, 1999.
An interesting paper with perhaps a more rigid analysis of the functional outcome (using SF-367 and Iowa pelvic scores) of patients with vertical shear fractures and dislocations of the pelvis. It refutes the above findings stating that residual displacement does not affect functional outcome, rather the associated the injuries and socioeconomic impact of the pelvic fracture.

80. Van den Bosch EW, Van der Kleyn, Hogervorst M, et al: Functional outcome of internal fixation for pelvic ring fractures, *J Trauma* 47:365-371, 1999.

81. Pohlemann T, Gansslen A, Schellwald O, et al: Outcome after pelvic ring injuries, *Injury* 27:SB31-SB38, 1996.

82. Copeland CE, Bosse MJ, McCarthy ML, et al: Effect of trauma and pelvic fracture on female genitourinary, sexual, and reproductive function, *J Orthop Trauma* 11:73-81, 1997.
A great article (retrospective review) that identified and categorized concisely for the first time the specific problems that women have subsequent to pelvic fracture. Trauma patients with and without pelvic fractures were compared. Urinary and sexual dysfunction were high and having had a displaced pelvic fracture significantly increased the risk for cesarean section.

83. Collinge C, Coons D, Aschenbrenner J: Risks to the superior gluteal neurovascular bundle during percutaneous iliosacral screw insertion: an anatomical cadaver study, *J Orthop Trauma* 19:96-101, 2005.

84. Matta JM, Saucedo T: Internal fixation of pelvic ring fractures, *Clin Orthop Rel Res* 242:83-97, 1989.

85. Moed BR, Karges DE: Techniques for reduction and fixation of pelvic ring disruptions through the posterior approach, *Clin Orthop Rel Res* 329:102-114, 1996.

86. Carlson DA, Scheid DK, Maar DC, et al: Safe placement of S1 and S2 iliosacral screws: the "vestibule" concept, *J Orthop Trauma* 14:264-269, 2000.

87. Day CS, Prayson MJ, Shuler TE, et al: Transsacral versus modified pelvic landmarks for percutaneous iliosacral screw placement—a computed tomographic analysis and cadaveric study, *Am J Orthop* 29:16-21, 2000.

88. Sagi HC, Lindvall EM: Inadvertent intra-foraminal iliosacral screw placement despite apparent appropriate positioning on intra-operative fluoroscopy, *J Orthop Trauma* 19:130-133, 2005.

89. Xu R, Ebraheim NA, Robke J, et al: Radiologic evaluation of iliosacral screw placement, *Spine* 21:582-588, 1996.

90. Routt ML Jr, Simonian PT, Agnew SG, et al: Radiographic recognition of the sacral alar slope for optimal placement of iliosacral screws: a cadaveric and clinical study, *J Orthop Trauma* 10:171-177, 1996.
A key article that stresses the importance of the lateral X-ray in placing ilio-sacral screws to avoid injury to the L5 nerve root as it passes over the sacral ala. Relying on inlet and outlet views only for placement of screws is inadequate.

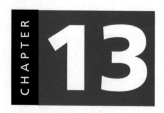

CHAPTER 13

Fractures of the Acetabulum

Thomas G. DiPasquale, DO

- Complex three-dimensional (3D) normal anatomy is altered by multidirectional forces resulting in 10 commonly accepted fracture patterns and occasional variances that do not quite fit.
- Acetabular fractures are typically the result of high-energy blunt trauma forces applied through the greater trochanter, the knee (in a flexed position), the foot (with knee extended), and the posterior aspect of the pelvis often with significant associated injuries requiring coordination of various medical and surgical services
- The acute management of acetabular fractures begins with a detailed clinical evaluation to identify life-threatening injuries, complications associated with the acetabular fracture, and associated skeletal injuries.
- The quality of reduction of the acetabular fractures is the single most important factor in the long-term outcome of these patients followed by the avoidance of commonly known complications of the injury or surgery.
- The acetabular paradox is that the fracture patterns that are more easily approached are the ones with the worse results, and the fracture patterns that are more difficult to approach have the best results.

Clinical Evaluation

- The initial clinical evaluation of acetabular fractures essentially involves resuscitation by Advanced Trauma Life Support (ATLS) guidelines for life-threatening injuries, including aggressive fluid resuscitation and massive transfusion protocols for hypovolemic shock.[1]
- Preoperative angiography and therapeutic embolization may be necessary if the patient is hemodynamically unstable and if the fracture involves the greater sciatic notch, thus injuring the superior gluteal artery.[2,3]
- A thorough preoperative neurologic assessment should always be performed and documented.

- Except for patients with open injuries or irreducible hip dislocations, surgical treatment of the acetabular fracture is usually nonemergent.
- Open fractures need debridement and open reduction and internal fixation (ORIF), and irreducible hip dislocations may require emergent surgical reduction and ORIF if the acetabular fracture is unstable.
- The presence of intraarticular loose bodies is not necessarily an indication for emergency surgery of the acetabulum witen hip subluxations is present and can be addressed during the definitive procedure.
- Balanced skeletal traction by distal femoral, proximal tibial, or calcaneal traction pins provide temporary stabilization when intraarticular fragments are present or acetabular incongruency exists before definitive fixation.
- In approximately 20% of cases, damage to the sciatic nerve can occur by direct compression from posterior wall fractures, the femoral head associated posterior hip dislocations, or by entrapment of the nerve in the fracture site with posterior column and transverse fractures that occur near the greater sciatic notch.[4]
- Subcutaneous soft-tissue degloving injuries over the greater trochanter are termed *Morel-Lavallee lesions*.[5] This lesion develops as a large ecchymotic region with soft fluctuance on palpation possibly requiring aspiration or decompression. Placement of trochanteric traction pins should be avoided through this lesion.
- Disruptions of the pelvic ring are common with acetabular fractures. The most frequent are associated anterior vertical fractures into the obturator foramen.[5]
- The presence of suprapubic catheters and colostomies might necessitate changing the planned surgical approach.[6]
- Noninvasive color venous Doppler ultrasound (US) can be used to screen patients for deep vein thrombosis (DVT) distal to the inguinal ligament, whereas magnetic

resonance venography (MRV) or traditional contrast venography might be necessary to screen for DVTs proximal to the inguinal ligament before surgery.[7,8] Various schemes have been proposed to diminish the risk of DVT and pulmonary embolism (PE).

Radiographic Evaluation

- The radiographic evaluation involves the use of standard radiographs, two-dimensional (2D), and 3D computed tomography (CT) to identify the fracture pattern and assist with preoperative planning.
- The radiographic evaluation of acetabular fractures described by Letournel and Judet[5] begins with the standard anteroposterior (AP) radiograph (Figure 13–1A) and the 45-degree oblique Judet views (iliac and obturator views) (Figure 13–1B and C).
- Inlet and outlet views of the pelvis are required for associated fractures of the pelvic ring (Figure 13–2).

The Anteroposterior Radiograph

- On the AP view, six fundamental radiographic landmarks are (Figure 13–3):
  1. Iliopectineal line: represents the anterior column
  2. Ilioischial line: landmark of the posterior column
  3. Radiographic U or teardrop: created by a confluence of the inner aspect of the acetabular fossa (lateral limb) and the anteroinferior portion of the quadrilateral surface (medial limb)
  4. Roof: represents the superior weight-bearing portion of the acetabulum
  5. Anterior wall: represents the lateral rims of these respective structures
  6. Posterior wall: represent the lateral rims of these respective structures

The Judet Oblique Views

- The iliac oblique view projects the iliac wing on profile and demonstrates the anterior wall, the posterior column

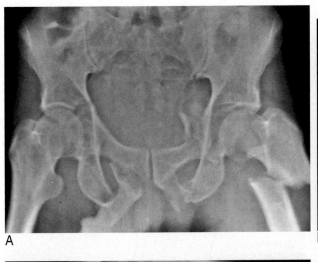

A

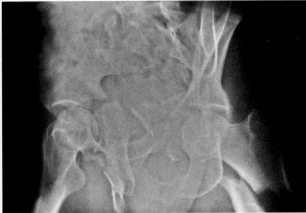

B

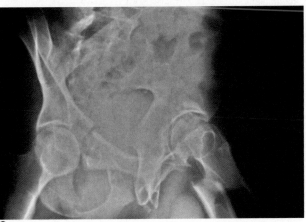

C

Figure 13–1: **A,** Example of anteroposterior radiograph of pelvis. **B,** Example of iliac oblique Judet view of right hip: obturator oblique view of left hip. **C,** Example of obturator oblique Judet view of right hip: iliac view of left hip.

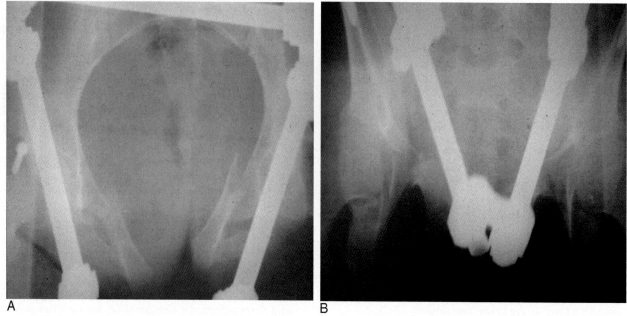

A

B

Figure 13–2: **A,** Pelvic inlet view. **B,** Pelvic outlet view.

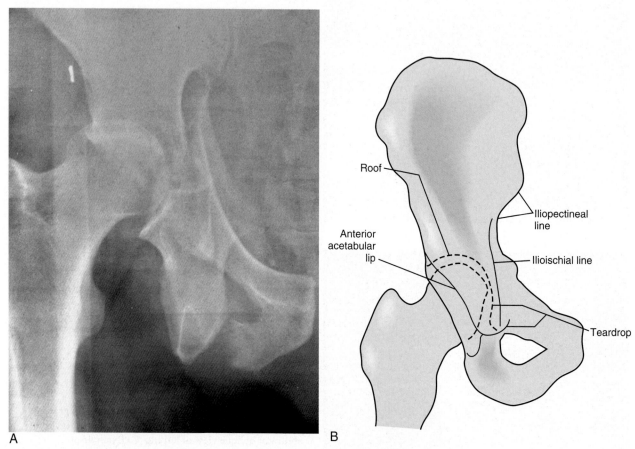

A

B

Figure 13–3: **A,** Example of anteroposterior radiograph. **B,** Diagram of anteroposterior view with the six radiographic landmarks.

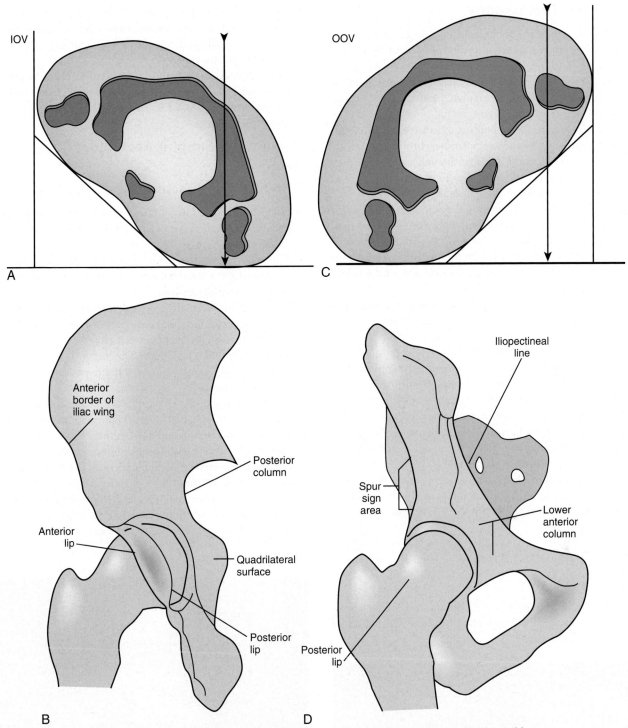

Figure 13–4: **A,** Diagram of patient positioning for iliac oblique Judet view. **B,** Radiographic landmarks visible on iliac oblique Judet view. **C,** Diagram of patient positioning for obturator oblique Judet view. **D,** Radiographic landmarks visible on obturator oblique Judet view. (A and C from Letournel E, Judet R: *Fractures of the acetabulum.* Elson RA, translator and editor. Berlin, 1981, Springer-Verlag.)

(ilioischial line), the quadrilateral surface, and posterior superior roof arc (Figure 13–4).

- The obturator oblique view projects the obturator foramen on profile and demonstrates the posterior wall, the anterior column (iliopectineal line), and the anterior superior roof arc.

- These views are necessary for assessing congruence between the roof of the acetabulum and femoral head.

Computed Tomography

- A 2D CT scan of the abdomen should is often obtained as part of most trauma series protocols. Newer spiral CT scans are 1 to 1.5 mm thick, but older scanners should have 2-mm contiguous bone window sections with no overlap through the acetabulum and 5-mm sections through the remaining pelvis.
- Most new scanners have built-in software that easily converts the data to 3D and multiplanar reconstruction views. These 3D views vastly improve the understanding of the fracture patterns and how the fragments might look through the various surgical exposures.
- The 2D CT defines fracture lines in the sagittal and coronal planes, marginal impaction, intraarticular loose fragments, concentricity of reduction, medial displacement, femoral head impaction or fracture, rotation of articular fragments, and aids in estimation of the size of the posterior wall fragment (Figure 13–5).
- The CT scan also helps define associated pelvic ring injuries, sacral fractures, sacroiliac joint dislocations, and difficult acetabular-pelvic fracture patterns.
- Fracture lines in the sagittal plane represent transverse, oblique, and wall fractures. Fracture lines in the coronal plane represent column fractures and vertical limb of T-shaped fractures. (This takes extensive thought to truly understand).
- 3D imaging aids in the understanding of the complex pathoanatomy, precise plane of the fracture, the degree of disruption of the articular surface, and spatial relationships of the fragments[9] (Figure 13–6).
- The evaluation of late reconstructions that require an osteotomy for surgical correction of acetabular nonunion, or malunion is facilitated with the CT images.

Acetabular Fracture Classification

- The most universally accepted classification of acetabular fractures was originally described by Judet and Letournel in 1964 and modified by Letournel.[5,10]

- This classification system was the first to integrate pelvic anatomy and fracture biomechanics into useful clinical material that allowed the surgeon to correctly approach these difficult fractures.
- The Orthopaedic Trauma Association has modified Letournel's classification to allow computerized coding according to the AO *Comprehensive Classification of Fractures of Long* Bones.[11,12]

Elementary (Simple) Acetabular Fractures

Posterior Wall Fractures

- Posterior wall fractures are the most common acetabular fractures and can occur at any level of the posterior wall (Figure 13–7).
- These fractures involve the posterior acetabular rim, a portion of the retroacetabular surface, and a variable segment of articular cartilage.
- Careful attention of the posterior column during surgery can demonstrate nondisplaced transverse or posterior column fracture lines that might not have been apparent on preoperative radiographs or CT scans.
- Posterior wall fractures can be a single posterior fragment or multifragmented.
- Marginal impactions, or acetabular depression fractures, occur in the presence of single fragment or multifragment posterior wall fracture when the femoral head impacts into the cancellous bone of the intact posterior column, rotating impacting an osteochondral fragment of the acetabulum.
- The CT scan is helpful for evaluation of marginal impaction of the posterior wall fragments, loose fragments in the joint, evaluation of joint concentricity, and estimation of the size of the posterior wall fragment.

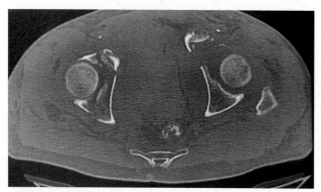

Figure 13–5: **Example of two-dimensional axial computed tomography scan.**

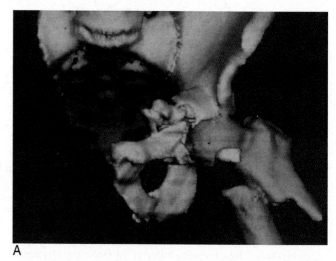

A

Figure 13–6: **A, Example of three-dimensional computed tomography scan.**

(*Continued*)

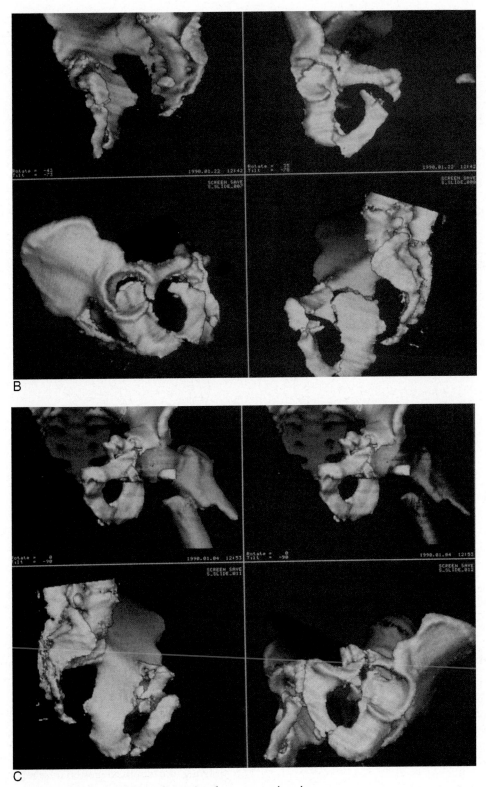

Figure 13–6, cont'd: **B and C,** Example of three-dimensional reconstructive views.

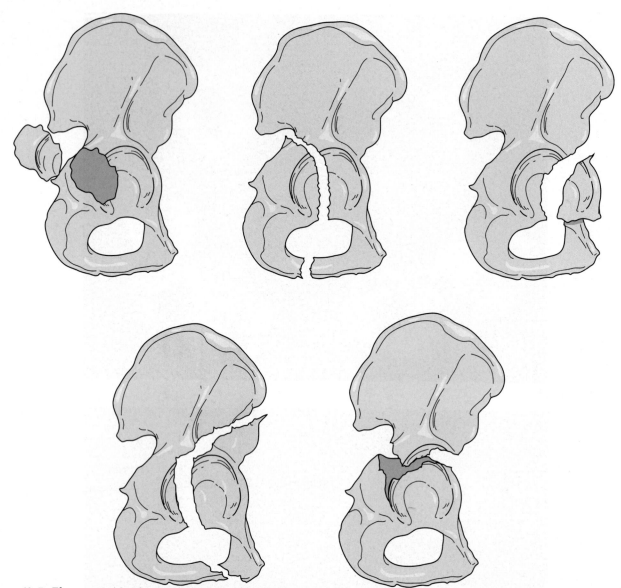

Figure 13–7: Elementary (simple) acetabular fracture patterns. (Modified from Letournel E, Judet R: *Fractures of the acetabulum*, Elson R A, translator and editor. Berlin, 1981, Springer-Verlag.)

Posterior Column Fractures

- The posterior column fracture is characterized by disruption of the ischial portion of the pelvis with wide medial displacement of the retroacetabular surface.
- The vertical fracture line usually originates superiorly at the greater sciatic notch, extends inferiorly through the roof or weight-bearing dome, and exits through the obturator foramen.
- Usually an associated fracture of the inferior pubic ramus also is evident, which exits posteriorly through the ischial tuberosity.
- On the AP view, medial displacement of the femoral head is seen, driving the quadrilateral surface and the sciatic buttress into the true pelvis.

- The iliac oblique view shows the internal and superior boundaries of the displaced fragment and the normal anterior border of the acetabulum.
- The obturator oblique view shows the intact iliopectineal line and the anterior column structures.
- Letournel[5] described the "gull sign" in association with posterior column fractures: The articular cartilage accompanying the displaced posterior segment hinges inward creating an image with the intact portion of the roof that looks like a bird in flight.

Anterior Wall Fractures

- The anterior wall fracture involves the central portion of the acetabulum anteriorly.

- The roof segment has minimal involvement, and the inferior pubic ramus usually is not fractured.
- Radiographs show a fracture and possible displacement through the iliopectineal line that is best seen on the obturator oblique view. This view also demonstrates the degree of involvement of the superior weight-bearing dome.
- The iliac oblique view can show interruption of the anterior rim contour.

Anterior Column Fractures

- These fractures may begin high along the anterior iliac crest and extend distally through the acetabulum or low through the superior pubic ramus and pubic portion of the acetabulum.
- Regardless of the fracture level, the pelvic brim and iliopectineal line are always disrupted.
- The AP radiograph shows an intact posterior column with the ilioischial line unbroken.
- On the obturator oblique view, the iliopectineal line is disrupted and the iliac oblique view reveals the intact posterior elements.
- The CT scan shows displacement of the anterior column and is useful in determining the involvement of the roof segment.
- The roof segment or a portion of it can be displaced medially, as seen in high or intermediate anterior column fractures. However this type of displacement can also be found with anterior column posterior hemi-transverse fractures and both column fractures of the acetabulum.

Transverse Fractures

- Transverse fractures separate the acetabulum into superior and inferior segments and involve both the anterior and posterior columns.
- In a transverse fracture, the fracture line extends obliquely in the transverse place from the anterior to posterior column.
- Judet[10] subdivided transverse fractures according to the levels at which these fractures occur through the acetabulum (Figure 13–8):

1. Transtectal types of fracture occur through the superior weight-bearing dome of the articular surface.
2. Juxtatectal types are seen between the superior acetabular articular surface and the superior margin of the cotyloid fossa.
3. Infratectal types transect the anterior and posterior columns below the junction of the cotyloid fossa and weight-bearing dome.

- The radiographic characteristics of transverse fractures reveal disruption of all vertical lines.
- The iliac oblique view best shows the transverse fracture fragment and level through the posterior column.
- The obturator oblique view best shows the transverse fracture line and level through the anterior column.
- The roof arc is measured from the angle formed between two lines, one drawn vertically through the geometric center of the acetabulum and the other drawn from the fracture line to the geometric center of the acetabulum.

Associated (Complex) Acetabular Fractures

T-Shaped Acetabular Fractures

- The T-shaped acetabular fracture is a transverse fracture with a vertical fracture component splitting the cotyloid fossa and quadrilateral surface, thereby dividing the anterior and posterior columns inferiorly (Figure 13–9).
- Like the simple transverse fracture it can be classified as transtectal, juxtatectal, or infratectal.
- The radiographic key to identifying this fracture pattern is the vertical component. The vertical fracture line usually exits through the obturator foramen with or without an extension of the fracture line through the pubic ramus or ischium.
- The vertical fracture component must be evaluated on the Judet views to distinguish T-shaped fractures from other fractures involving both columns. However, the vertical fracture line can also split into the ischium or superior ramus, leaving the obturartor foramen intact.

Associated Posterior Column or Posterior Wall Fractures

- The fracture line of the posterior column extends from the sciatic notch through the cotyloid fossa and usually enters the obturator ring.
- The AP view shows the intact iliopectineal line along with a disruption of the ilioischial line and central displacement of the femoral head.
- The teardrop might be distorted.
- The obturator oblique view shows a fracture of the ischium or obturator ring with a displaced posterior wall fragment projecting into the soft tissues.
- The iliac oblique view shows the intact anterior column with a displaced ilioischial line.

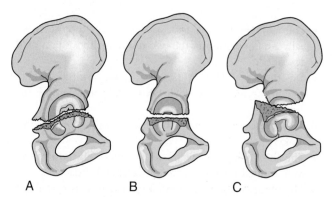

Figure 13–8: Schemes of transverse fractures. **A,** Infratectal type. **B,** Juxtatectal type. **C,** Transtectal type.

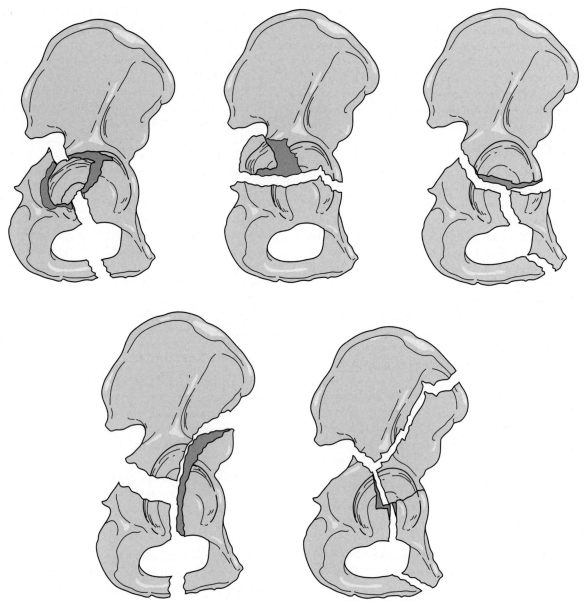

Figure 13–9: Associated (complex) acetabular fracture patterns. (Modified from Letournel E, Judet R: *Fractures of the acetabulum*, Elson RA, translator and editor. Berlin, 1981, Springer-Verlag.)

- The posterior column fracture is often nondisplaced; however, the femoral head is usually dislocated, with the posterior wall fracture being the major component.

Associated Transverse or Posterior Wall Fractures

- The transverse component of this associated injury resembles that previously described, yet the posterior wall fragment rarely reduces when the head is repositioned under the acetabular roof.
- Like the simple transverse pattern, it might also be transtectal juxtatectal, or infratectal.

- The radiographic characteristics of this pattern are essentially a combination of the two distinct patterns previously described.
- On the AP view, a posterior fracture-dislocation of the hip typically is seen with all vertical landmarks disrupted.
- The iliopectineal and ilioischial lines are transversely broken.
- The iliac oblique view shows an intact iliac wing and a well-defined fracture of the quadrilateral surface.
- The obturator oblique view shows the posterior wall deficiency, posterior displacement, and the level of the transverse fracture segment.

- Associated transverse or posterior wall fractures include the rotational component seen with the transverse fracture pattern.
- The obturator foraminal segment can rotate around vertical and horizontal axes. The inferior segment might protrude medially due to the force of the femoral head.
- The 2D CT scan is of little value in the classification or treatment of this fracture pattern; however, 3D reconstructions are easier to interpret and are of help.

Associated Anterior Column or Anterior Wall or Posterior Hemi-Transverse Fractures

- The fracture line routinely detaches from the anterior wall at the anteroinferior spine and passes inferiorly though the cotyloid fossa, usually exiting at the junction of the superior ramus.
- The size of the anterior component varies with the mechanism of injury.
- The posterior hemi-transverse component is a pure transverse fracture of the posterior column only, but this pattern is sometimes referred to as reverse T-shaped.
- Generally, this is a nondisplaced fracture that is located in the lower half on the posterior column and remains intact with the obturator ring.
- Unlike the associated both-column fracture, intact articular acetabular cartilage always remains attached to the iliac wing.
- Radiographically, the AP view demonstrates a nondisplaced fracture of the posterior column.
- The iliopectineal line is always displaced with this fracture pattern.
- The iliac oblique view demonstrates a fracture through the quadrilateral surface.
- The obturator oblique view depicts the size of the anterior wall or column.
- The CT scan might help to distinguish it from a transverse T-shaped or associated both-column patterns.

Associated Both-Column Fractures

- Technically, there are many fracture patterns that involve both anterior and posterior columns (i.e., transverse, transverse or posterior wall, anterior column or posterior hemi-transverse, T-shaped, and both column),but there is only one both column fracture as described by Judet.[10]
- This complex fracture pattern is distinguished from all others in that the articular surface is completely detached from the remainder of the portion of the iliac wing that articulates with the sacroiliac joint.
- The anterior and posterior columns separate from each other.
- The principal posterior column fragment has a fracture line that characteristically begins at the greater sciatic notch and exits inferiorly.

- Secondary fracture lines might be transmitted anywhere in the retroacetabular surface.
- Anterior column involvement can extend though the iliac wing and include anterior wall comminution.
- The obturator ring is frequently disrupted at several locations.
- "Central dislocation" of the femoral head is usually seen on the AP view with the acetabular roof or dome segment demonstrating severe comminution.
- Malrotation frequently obliterates the ilioischial line, but the iliac wing fractures are readily identified on the iliac oblique view.
- This view also demonstrates the loss of all articular relationships of the acetabulum with the iliac wing.
- This type of fracture pattern is most commonly associated with a "spur sign."
- 2D CT demonstrates severe fracture comminution and the size of the fracture fragments, whereas 3D CT scanning can be useful in determining fracture accessibility through a single anterior approach as opposed to an extensile or combined, elective, anterior, or posterior approach.

Treatment Principles
Nonsurgical Management

- The AP and Judet radiographs, taken with traction removed, must first be inspected for congruence between the femoral head and acetabulum. Any degree of incongruence involving the weight-bearing surface of the acetabulum is unacceptable and warrants surgical care.
- Measurements of roof arc angles taken off the AP, iliac oblique, and obturator oblique radiographs can quantify the involvement of the weight-bearing dome of the acetabulum[13] (Figure 13–10).
- The roof arc is measured from the angle formed between two lines, one drawn vertically through the geometric center of the acetabulum and the other drawn from the fracture line to the geometric center of the acetabulum.
- When the angles from the three views are all individually greater than 45 degrees, then the weight-bearing dome is considered to have adequate stable coverage (Figure 13–11).
- Fracture lines that are 10 mm below the CT scan cut through the top of the acetabulum dome also correlates to the 45-degree roof arc angle.[14]
- When the criteria of these roof arc measurements are met and the femoral head is congruent within the acetabulum, nonsurgical treatment is indicated.
- Low transverse fractures not involving the weight-bearing dome and distal anterior column fractures commonly meet these criteria.
- When the roof arc angle is less than 45 degrees and femoral head congruence is maintained, traction might be offered to the appropriate patient in lieu of surgical

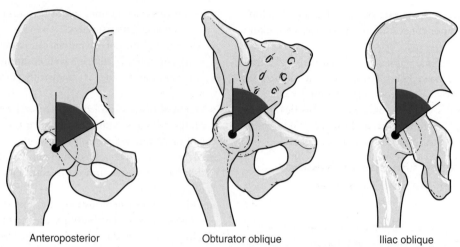

Anteroposterior   Obturator oblique   Iliac oblique

Figure 13–10: Roof arc angle measurements from the anteroposterior, iliac oblique, and obturator oblique views.

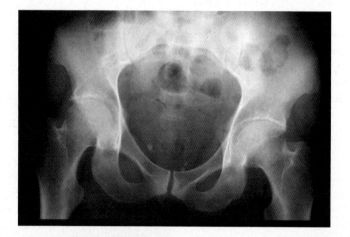

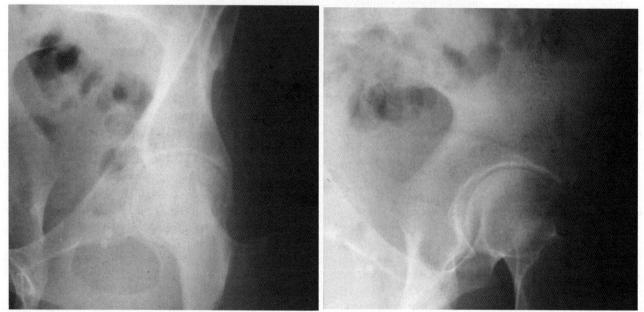

Figure 13–11: Radiographic examples of roof arc angles greater than 45 degrees.

stabilization. However this pattern is considered unstable, and early weight bearing is inadvisable.

- Criteria that might contraindicate nonsurgical care for acetabular fractures, even when the roof arc angle is greater than 45 degrees, are intraarticular fragments and marginal impaction fractures.
- Secondary congruence is seen with some both-column fractures and can be treated with nonsurgical methods. For secondary congruence to occur, the acetabular surface is medially displaced and free floating but remains congruent with the femoral head.
- The results of nonsurgical care for fractures with secondary congruence are not as good as those with anatomic reduction of the joint; however, the results are better than those for displaced fractures of the acetabular roof.
- Total hip arthroplasty might be planned on a delayed basis when symptomatic posttraumatic arthritis develops.
- A rehabilitation protocol must be developed.

Surgical Management

- The goals of surgery are to reduce or delay posttraumatic arthritis, create a foundation on which a salvage procedure, such as total hip arthroplasty or hip arthrodesis, can be performed, and most importantly allow early mobilization of the patient with stable range of motion of the hip.
- Surgical approaches include:
  1. Ilioinguinal: appropriate for anterior wall, anterior column, anterior wall or posterior hemi-transverse, some transverse, both-column, and some T-shaped fractures (Figure 13–12).
  2. Iliofemoral-Extensile: appropriate for both-column fractures with extension into the sacroiliac joint or older than 20 days, and some T-shaped fractures older than 15 days (Figure 13–13).
  3. Posterior Kocher-Langenbeck (KL): appropriate for posterior wall, posterior column, posterior wall or posterior column, some transverse, transverse or posterior wall, and some T-shaped fractures (Figure 13–14).
  4. Suprapubic: mostly for symphysis disruptions but can be easily converted to a modified Stoppa approach[18] for medial buttressing of quadrilateral plate and posterior column reduction.
  5. Modified Stoppa approach[18]: appropriate for displaced anterior column or wall fractures, transverse fractures, T-shaped fractures, both-column fractures, and anterior wall or anterior column fractures associated with posterior hemi-transverse component.[18] This approach is becoming more popular with experienced acetabular surgeons. Direct visualization is limited to the operating surgeon. The modified Stoppa approach allows exposure of the medial fractures of the quadrilateral plate. Buttress plating is more direct to prevent medial femoral head protusion.
  6. Combined or staged approaches may be needed if anterior and posterior reduction and fixation is required.

- The only true emergency in these fractures is the irreducible hip dislocation, which must be reduced immediately to decrease the theoretical incidence of osteonecrosis.
- The primary goal in acetabular fracture surgery is to restore the joint surface; the goal should not be primary total hip replacement.[15,16]
- Best results are usually obtained by addressing the displaced acetabular fracture with ORIF.[17]
- In patients with significant preexisting arthritis, hip arthroplasty might be performed in conjunction with internal fixation, although this is associated with a high rate of acetabular component failure.

Avoidance of Complications

- The incidence of infection is between 3% and 6% in most large series, however, this can be increased by the presence of open wounds, degloving injuries, obesity, and open fractures of the ipsilateral extremity.[5] Prophylactic antibiotics, usually a first-generation cephalosporin, should be started approximately 30 minutes before skin incision is made. Generally, unless there is a breach in sterility, the antibiotics should not be continued after surgery.
- Indwelling urinary catheters can be a source of infection and should be avoided. Intermittent catheterization for urinary retention has been shown to have a lower incidence of urinary infections.[19]
- DVT prophylaxis can be provided with low dose anticoagulation, such as heparin preoperatively and warfarin (Coumadin) postoperatively. Low molecular weight heparins (LMWHs) can be used as antithrombotics both

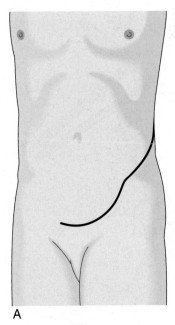

A

Figure 13–12: **A, Ilioinguinal approach according to Letournel. Positioning and incision** (*left side*). (*Continued*)

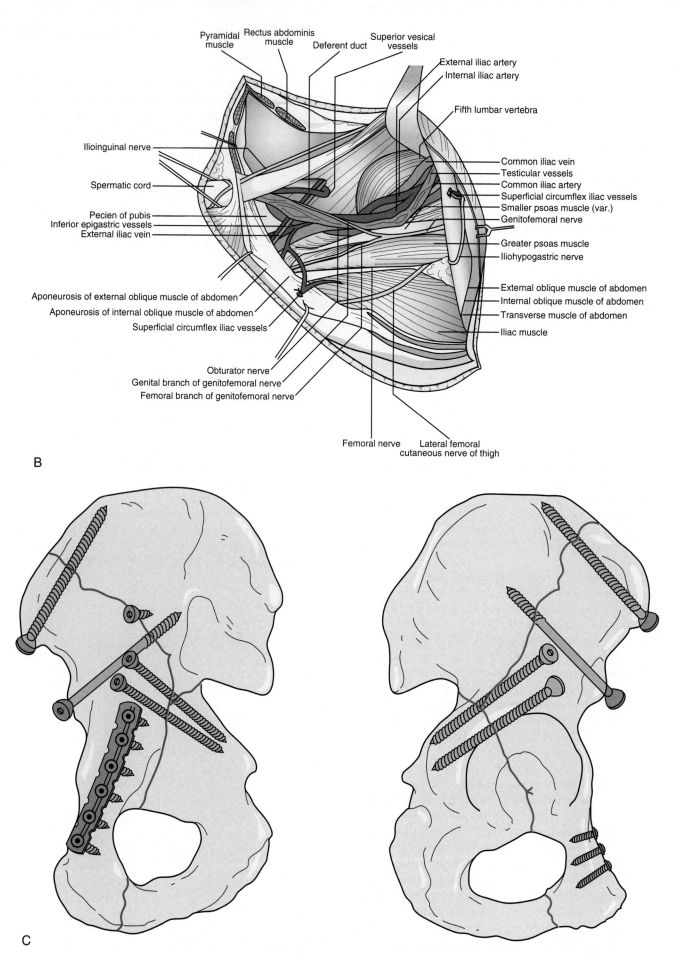

Pyramidal muscle
Rectus abdominis muscle
Deferent duct
Superior vesical vessels
External iliac artery
Internal iliac artery
Fifth lumbar vertebra

Ilioinguinal nerve
Spermatic cord
Pecien of pubis
Inferior epigastric vessels
External iliac vein

Common iliac vein
Testicular vessels
Common iliac artery
Superficial circumflex iliac vessels
Smaller psoas muscle (var.)
Genitofemoral nerve
Greater psoas muscle
Iliohypogastric nerve

External oblique muscle of abdomen
Internal oblique muscle of abdomen
Transverse muscle of abdomen
Iliac muscle

Aponeurosis of external oblique muscle of abdomen
Aponeurosis of internal oblique muscle of abdomen
Superficial circumflex iliac vessels

Obturator nerve
Genital branch of genitofemoral nerve
Femoral branch of genitofemoral nerve

Femoral nerve
Lateral femoral cutaneous nerve of thigh

B

C

Figure 13–12, cont'd: **B,** Anatomic exposure for ilioinguinal approach. **C,** Internal fixation of a combined anterior column and posterior hemi-transverse fracture using the ilioinguinal approach.

(*Continued*)

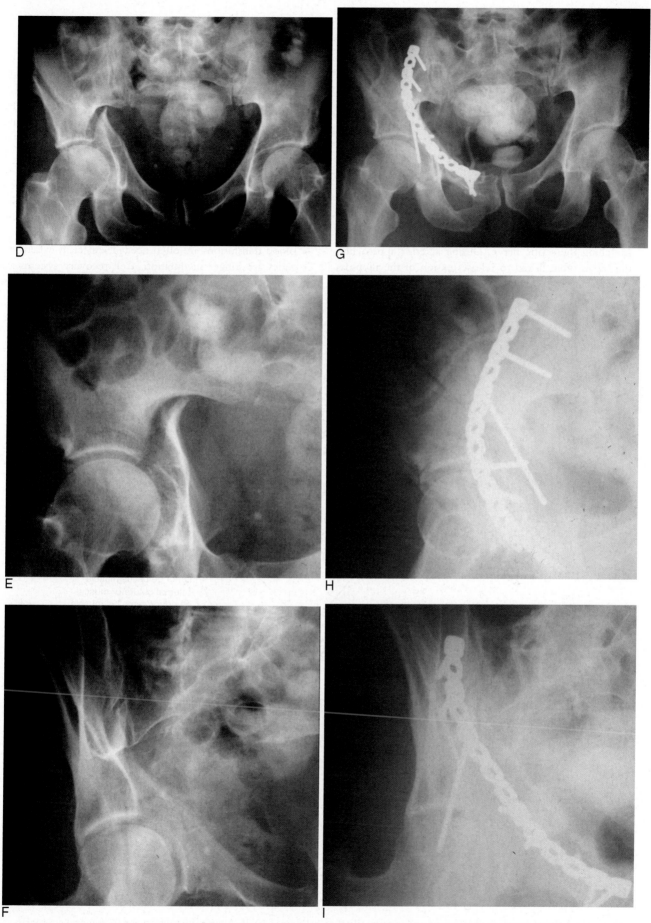

Figure 13–12, cont'd: **D, E, F,** Anteroposterior and Judet radiographs of anterior column posterior hemi-transverse fracture. **G, H, I,** Postoperative radiographs of ilioinguinal approach. (**A and B** from Bauer R, Kershbaumer F, Poisel S: *Operative approaches in orthopedic sugery and traumatology,* New York, 1987, Thieme Medical Publishers. **C** from Muller ME, Allgower M, Schneider R, Willenegger H: *Manual of internal fixation: techniques recommended by the AO-ASIF Group.* Berlin, 1991, Springer-Verlag.)

preoperatively and postoperatively. Although the LMWHs are more expensive, they can be given easily without the need to perform and monitor expensive lab tests. Mechanical compression devices can be used in combination or in the event of a contraindication to the use of anticoagulant therapy. If preoperative Dopplers suggests a thrombus, then inferior vena cava filtration is indicated.

- Iatrogenic nerve injury can be avoided by careful attention to the leg position during surgery. During a posterior K-L approach, the hip is extended and the knee flexed to avoid stretching the sciatic nerve. During anterior approaches, the hip is often flexed to release tension of the iliopsoas muscle but this tensions the sciatic nerve in the greater sciatic notch. This approach has been shown to have higher iatrogenic nerve injury than was once thought.[20] Intraoperative somatosensory evoked potential (SSEPs) and electromyographys (EMGs) are expensive and have not shown to be any better than careful attention to technique.

- The lateral femoral cutaneous nerve is intentionally cut or stretched during the ilioinguinal approach but rarely causes significant disability. It is most important to forewarn patients so they are not surprised by postoperative numbness of the anterior thigh.

- Blood transfusions are often needed, especially when surgeries are longer in duration. Cell recovery systems are available and can capture up to 50% of the blood lost

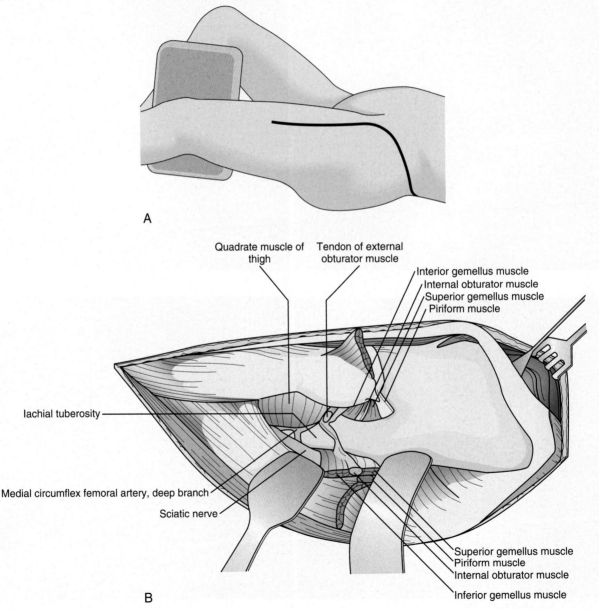

Figure 13–13: **A,** Judet approach. Positioning and incision (iliofemoral approach). **B,** Anatomic exposure for iliofemoral approach.

(Continued)

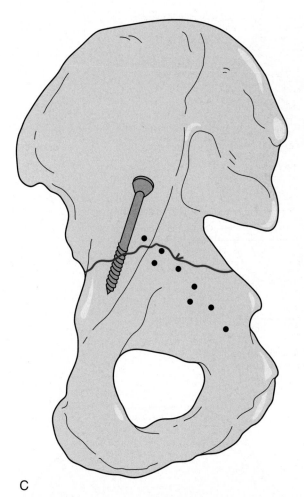
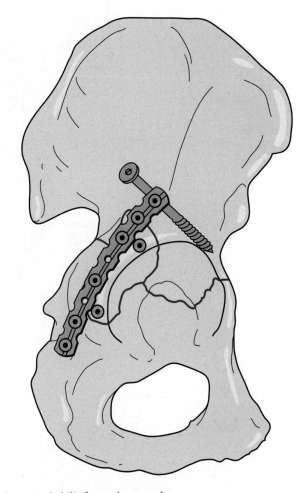

C

Figure 13–13, cont'd: **C,** Internal fixation of a both column fracture using the extended iliofemoral approach.
(**A** and **B** from Bauer R, Kershbaumer F, Poisel S: *Operative approaches in orthopedic sugery and traumatology,* New York, 1987, Thieme Medical Publishers. **C** from Muller ME, Allgower M, Schneider R, Willenegger H: *Manual of internal fixation: techniques recommended by the AO-ASIF Group.* Berlin, 1991, Springer-Verlag.)

during the operation for retransfusion. Postoperative blood recovery systems are also available. Cross-matched blood must be planned for and available.

- Heterotopic ossification (HO) can occur, especially with posterior and extended ilioinguinal approaches. Indomethacin alone or in combination with low-dose radiation has been routinely used in the postoperative period for 6 to 12 weeks.[21] Late resection may be needed for the most severe cases.

- Intraarticular hardware placement can ruin an excellent reduction. Intraoperative C-arm fluoroscopy can show the extraarticular placement of all screws. If the views are suboptimal, such as in obese patients, than intraoperative auscultation with a sterile esophageal stethoscope can be used accurately to detect inadvertent intraarticular hardware.

- Posttraumatic arthritis occurs in 20% to 30% of cases. If limited to mild aching with weather change or excessive activity, over-the-counter antiinflammatory medication may be used. Severe arthritis can occur despite anatomic reduction and may require total hip arthroplasty.

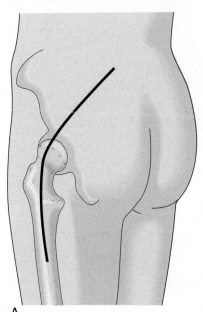

A

Figure 13–14: **A,** Posterior (Kocher-Langenbeck) approach to the hip joint. Positioning and incision.

(Continued)

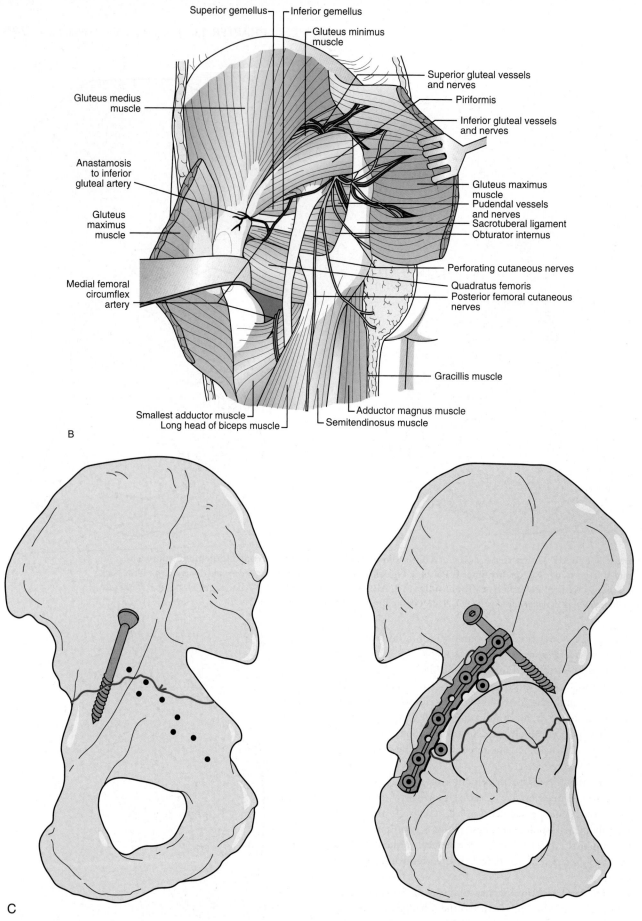

Figure 13–14, cont'd: **B,** Anatomic exposure for Kocher–Langenbeck approach. **C,** Internal fixation of a combined transverse and posterior wall fracture using the Kocher–Langenbeck approach. (**A** and **B** from Bauer R, Kershbaumer F, Poisel S: *Operative approaches in orthopedic sugery and traumatology,* New York, 1987, Thieme Medical Publishers. **C** from Muller ME, Allgower M, Schneider R, Willenegger: *Manual of internal fixation: techniques recommended by the AO-ASIF Group.* Berlin, 1991, Springer-Verlag.)

Postoperative Care and Expectations

- Patients are usually discharged from the hospital 3 to 4 days postoperatively with isolated injuries and no complications.
- Patients will usually ambulate with crutches or a walker for 12 weeks. Weight bearing is restricted on the affected extremity to 10 to 20 kg or the weight of the leg. Cane-assisted ambulation is begun at 3 months and continued as long as the patient has a limp. Patients usually limp when they first get up from the bed or chair. This "start-up limp" is usually the result of scar tissue that needs to be stretched before resolving. Patients often limp at the end of a long day. This "lack of endurance limp" is usually the result of muscle fatigue and will resolve after reconditioning.
- Patients are routinely seen postoperatively at 2 weeks for a wound check and suture removal.
- AP and Judet view radiographs are obtained at 6 weeks, 3 months, 6 months, and 1 year.
- DVT prophylaxis is discontinued as soon as the patient is ambulatory. Bedridden patients are continued on their DVT prophylaxis regimen until ambulatory.
- HO prophylaxis is discontinued if no radiographic findings of HO formation is seen at 6 weeks. Otherwise it is continued for an additional 6 weeks.

Annotated References

1. American College of Surgeons Committee on Trauma: *Advanced Trauma Life Support Program for Physicians*, Chicago, IL, 1993, American College of Surgeons.

2. Bossee MJ, Poka A, Reinert CM, et al: Preoperative angiographic assessment of the superior gluteal artery in acetabular fractures requiring extensile surgical exposures, *J Orthop Trauma* 2:303-307, 1988.

3. Juliano PJ, Bosse MJ, Edwards KJ: The superior gluteal artery in complex acetabular procedures: a cadaveric angiographic study, *J Bone Joint Surg Am* 76:244-248, 1994.

A study of fresh cadavers was performed to assess the collateral circulation to the abductor muscle flap created by the various pelvic exposures in the presence of an occlusive injury to the ipsilateral superior gluteal artery. Preoperative assessment of the superior gluteal artery is recommended for a patient who is a candidate for an extensile exposure for an acetabular procedure. If the superior gluteal artery is occluded, a combined ilioinguinal and posterior operative approach should be considered.

4. Fassler PR, Swiontkowski MF, Kilroy AW, et al: Injury of the sciatic nerve associated with acetabular fractures, *J Bone Joint Surg Am* 75:1157-1166, 1993.

The patients who had isolated, mild involvement of the peroneal nerve had a favorable prognosis, but those who had a severe injury of the peroneal component, whether it was isolated or associated with an injury of the tibial component, did not recover good function.

5. Letournel E, Judet R, editors *Fractures of the acetabulum*, ed 2. Berlin, 1993, Springer-Verlag.

Detailed comparison of acetabular care.

6. Matta JM, Letournel E, Browner BD: Surgical management of acetabular fractures. In Anderson LD editor: *American Academy of Orthopaedic Surgeons Instructional Course Lectures XXXV*, St. Louis, MO, 1996, Mosby.

We have each experienced a significant learning phase for surgical treatment of these fractures. However problems of articular reduction remain significant, particularly for complex fractures. It is our opinion that a certain degree of centralization of acetabulum fracture treatment—especially for the associated types—can lead to an improved standard of care overall.

7. Montgomery KD, Potter HG, Helfet DL: Magnetic resonance venography to evaluate the deep venous system of the pelvis in patients who have an acetabular fracture, *J Bone Joint Surg Am* 77:1639-1649, 1995.

The authors performed a prospective, blinded study to assess and compare the values of preoperative contrast venography and magnetic resonance venography (MRV) in the detection of deep venous thrombosis (DVT) in the thigh and pelvis of 45 consecutive patients who had a displaced acetabular fracture. The MRV and contrast venography were performed an average of 7 days (range, 1 to 29 days) after the injury. MRV is noninvasive, does not require the use of contrast medium, images the proximal aspects of both lower extremities simultaneously, and most importantly, allows for the identification of DVT in the pelvis.

8. Montgomery KD, Potter HG, Helfet DL: The detection and management of proximal deep venous thrombosis in patients with acute acetabular fractures: a follow up report, *J Orthop Trauma* 11:330-336, 1997.

Magnetic resonance venography (MRV) is a sensitive screening examination that allows the placement of inferior vena cava filters based on documented proximal thrombosis. The authors anticipate that preoperative deep venous thrombosis (DVT) screening with MRV will significantly decrease the incidence of fatal pulmonary embolism in this high-risk population.

9. Martinez CR, DiPasquale TG, Helfet DL, et al: Evaluation of acetabular fractures with two- and three-dimensional CT, *Radiographics* 12:227-242, 1992.

10. Judet R, Judet J, Letournel E: Fractures of the acetabulum: classification and surgical approaches for open reduction. Preliminary report. *J Bone Joint Surg Am* 46:1615-1646, 1964.

11. Orthopaedic Trauma Association Committee for Coding and Classification: Fracture and dislocation compendium, *J Orthop Trauma* 10:73, 1996.

12. Muller ME, Nazarian S, Kock P, Schatzker J: *The comprehensive classification of fractures of long bones*, New York, 1996, Springer-Verlag.

13. Matta J: Operative indications and choice of surgical approach for fractures of the acetabulum, *Tech Orthop* 1:13-22, 1986.

14. Tornetta P 3rd: Non-operative management of acetabular fractures: the use of dynamic stress views, *J Bone Joint Surg Br* 81:67-70, 1999.

To assess the stability of the hip after acetabular fracture, dynamic fluoroscopic stress views were taken of 41 acetabular fractures that met the criteria for nonoperative management. These included roof arcs of 45 degrees, a subchondral computed tomography (CT) arc of 10 mm, displacement of less than 50% of the posterior wall, and congruence on the anteroposterior (AP) and Judet views of the hip. There were three unstable hips that were treated by open reduction and internal fixation. The remaining 38 fractures were treated nonoperatively with early mobilization and delayed weight bearing. At a mean follow-up of 2.7 years, the results were good or excellent in 91% of the cases. Three fair results were ascribed to the patients' other injuries. Dynamic stress views can identify subtle instability in patients who would normally be considered for nonoperative treatment.

15. Romness CR, Lowell JD: Prognosis of fractures of the acetabulum, *J Bone Joint Surg Am* 43:30-59, 1961.

16. Jimenez ML, Tile M, Schenk RS: Total hip replacement after acetabular fracture, *Orthop Clin North Am* 28:435-446, 1997.

The controversies surrounding total hip arthroplasty after acetabular fracture are presented in this article. Hip arthroplasty for acute treatment of acetabular fractures is rarely indicated. In general, total hip arthroplasty should be reserved for the late salvage of hips in which symptomatic, posttraumatic arthritis has developed after acetabular fracture. Preoperative, intraoperative, and postoperative management are discussed. Modern surgical techniques may improve the long-term survival of total hip arthroplasty after acetabular fracture, particularly the acetabular component.

17. Helfet DL, Borrelli J, DiPasquale T, et al: Stabilization of acetabular fractures in elderly patients, *J Bone Joint Surg Am* 74:753-765, 1992.

Eighteen patients who were 60 years or older and had an acute displaced fracture of the acetabulum were managed with open reduction and internal fixation (ORIF). All of the patients had ORIF with either the ilioinguinal approach (13 patients) or the Kocher-Langenbeck approach (5 patients). ORIF of selected displaced acetabular fractures in the elderly can yield good results and may obviate the need for early and often difficult total hip arthroplasty.

18. Cole JD, Bolhofner BR: Description of operative technique and preliminary operative results, *Clin Orthop* 305:112-123, 1994.

Between March 1991 and December 1992 the authors surgically treated 55 acetabular fractures using a modified Stoppa anterior intrapelvic extensile approach. Indications for utilization of this approach included displaced anterior column or wall fractures, transverse fractures, T-shaped fractures, both column fractures and anterior column or wall fractures associated with a posterior hemi-transverse component. Clinical results were excellent (47%), good (42%), fair (9%), and poor (2%). The modified STOPPA incision offers the experienced trauma surgeon a new approach for fixation of displaced acetabular fractures. The approach offers improved reduction and fixation possibilities and may decrease the rate of complications associated with extrapelvic or extensile approaches.

19. Turi MH, Hanif S, Fasih O, Shaikh MA: Proportion of complications in patients practicing clean intermittent self catheterization (CISC) vs indwelling catheter, *J Pak Med Assoc* 56:401-404, 2006.

The authors compared the complications especially for infection in two groups; in group A, those performing clean intermittent self-catheterization (CISC) and in groupB, patients with indwelling catheters. CISC is much safer practice with less complications and infection rate than indwelling catheters.

20. Haidukewych GJ, Scaduto J, Herscovici D Jr, et al: Iatrogenic nerve injury in acetabular fracture surgery: a comparison of monitored and unmonitored procedures, *J Orthop Trauma* 16:297-301, 2002.

The authors review experience with iatrogenic nerve injuries and evaluate the efficacy of intraoperative monitoring in a large consecutive series of operatively treated acetabular fractures. The use of intraoperative monitoring did not decrease the rate of iatrogenic sciatic palsy. Further study involving larger prospective, randomized methodology appears warranted. Sciatic nerve injury was more common in ilioinguinal approaches in both groups, likely resulting from reduction techniques for the posterior column performed with the hip flexed, placing the sciatic nerve under tension.

21. Moed BR, Letournel E: Low dose irradiation and indomethacin prevent heterotopic ossification after acetabular fracture surgery, *J Bone Joint Surg Br* 76:895-900, 1994.

From 1987 to 1991, the authors treated 53 patients with 54 fractures of the acetabulum by reconstruction through a posterior or an extended iliofemoral surgical approach. For prophylaxis against heterotopic ossification they used perioperative irradiation and indomethacin. The combination therapy proved effective; 44 fractures showed no heterotopic ossification and 10 showed Brooker class I. The functional results were good, and there were no complications of this therapy. Irradiation with 1200 cGy did not appear to offer any therapeutic advantage over the 700 cGy dose.

CHAPTER 14

Proximal Femur Fractures

George J. Haidukewych, MD

- Fractures and dislocations around the hip remain among the most common and challenging injuries encountered.
- With the ever-growing elderly population with osteopenic bone, the number of fractures continues to proportionately increase.
- Additionally, younger patients may sustain various fractures and dislocations around the hip as a result of high-energy trauma, many of which can threaten the vascularity of the femoral head and the long-term prognosis of the hip joint.

Hip Dislocations

- Hip dislocations typically result from high-energy trauma, usually a motor vehicle accident.
- Associated injuries are common and have been reported in over 70% of patients.
- Hip dislocations are generally classified as either anterior or posterior. Regardless of the type of dislocation, it should be emphasized that post-reduction 3-mm cut computed tomography (CT) scanning is mandatory, even if the plain films appear completely normal. Small osteochondral intraarticular fragments, acetabular, and proximal femoral fractures must be excluded by CT scanning after closed reduction.
- If closed reduction is unobtainable, a CT scan should be obtained before surgery. This may guide the surgeon when selecting operative approach and evaluating appropriate treatment of associated fractures.

Anterior Hip Dislocations

- Anterior hip dislocations are extremely rare and account for the minority of all hip dislocations. They have been subdivided into those that are superior or inferior in relationship to the pubic ramus; however, their treatment is the same.
- The patient may present with the extremity held in an abducted externally rotated "figure four" position after

a high-energy injury. Femoral head fractures are commonly associated with anterior hip dislocations and can involve impaction or osteochondral injury of the femoral head on the acetabular rim.

- Closed reduction requires complete muscle relaxation, traction, extension, and gentle internal rotation. If closed reduction is unsuccessful, then open reduction should be performed usually through an anterior approach.
- Forceful closed reduction attempts are not recommended as a result of possibility of iatrogenic femoral neck or acetabular fracture.

Posterior Hip Dislocations

- Posterior hip dislocations account for the vast majority of all hip dislocations (approximately 90%). These are typically caused by an axial force to the flexed hip, such as one would sustain in a dashboard injury.
- Bone quality and the position of the limb at the time of impact determines whether an associated acetabular fracture or a simple dislocation occurs. Traumatic posterior hip subluxations without dislocation have also been reported with the pathognomonic magnetic resonance imaging (MRI) findings of iliofemoral ligament rupture, hemarthrosis, and marginal posterior acetabular wall avulsion fracture.
- The treatment of isolated posterior dislocations involves emergent closed reduction or if necessary, open reduction. Open reduction of irreducible posterior dislocations usually proceeds through the Kocher-Langenbeck approach. Identification and careful protection of the sciatic nerve is recommended because it may be tented by the displaced femoral head.
- Dislocations with associated posterior wall fractures are treated as indicated based on fragment size, displacement, and hip stability. Postreduction treatment of a simple hip dislocation, regardless of direction, involves early mobilization with gait aids as needed for patient comfort.

- Patients should be instructed to avoid hyperflexion of the hip for posterior dislocations and extension and external rotation for anterior dislocations.

Complications

- A substantial subset of patients will remain persistently symptomatic after sustaining a hip dislocation. Good-to-excellent results have been reported in about 70% of patients.
- Posttraumatic arthritis has been reported in over 15% of patients in several long-term studies.
- Osteonecrosis of the femoral head can occur in approximately 10% of hip dislocations. The risk of osteonecrosis increases with the presence of an associated fracture of the acetabulum, likely as a result the more extensive soft tissue injury. Osteonecrosis has also been reported after traumatic hip subluxations as well.
- Early reduction of simple dislocations and fracture dislocations has been suggested to lower the rate of osteonecrosis.
- Sciatic nerve injuries have been documented in as many as 8% to 19% of patients. These are most commonly associated with posterior dislocations.

Femoral Head Fractures

- Femoral head fractures have been categorized by Pipkin into four types based on location of the fracture fragment in relation to the fovea centralis and presence of associated fractures.
- Type 1 fractures are inferior to the fovea, type 2 fractures are superior to the fovea, type 3 also involves a femoral neck fracture, and type 4 also involve a fracture of the acetabulum.
- Patients with types 1, 2, and 4 femoral head fractures should undergo emergent closed reduction of the hip dislocation with postreduction CT scanning to evaluate fracture displacement. In general, femoral head fractures are treated based on fragment location, size, displacement, and hip stability.
- A nondisplaced or minimally displaced Pipkin type 1 fracture can be managed nonoperatively. A small or comminuted displaced Pipkin type 1 fracture can usually be simply excised resulting from the fact that this fracture is below the weight-bearing dome of the femoral head while larger fragments may require surgical fixation.
- Pipkin type 2 fractures mandate accurate anatomic reduction and stable internal fixation. Titanium countersunk screw fixation is preferred to allow MRI imaging in the future, if needed.
- The anterior Smith-Peterson approach is generally preferred as a result of improved visualization for reduction and internal fixation and a lower complication rate as compared to a posterior approach. A trochanteric flip may be added.
- Pipkin type 3 fractures are extremely rare and usually occur in younger patients. These should be treated with internal fixation of both the femoral neck and femoral head fracture. In older patients with poor bone quality and low functional demands, prosthetic replacement is probably more predictable and is generally preferred.
- Pipkin type 4 fractures are treated based on the location of the femoral head fracture and the type of associated acetabular fracture. The most common clinical scenario is a posterior wall acetabular fracture associated with a small, displaced, inferior (infra-foveal) femoral head fracture. This combination of injuries may be treated through a Kocher-Langenbeck approach with excision of the inferior femoral head fragment and simultaneous internal fixation of the posterior acetabular wall fracture.
- A larger (suprafoveal) femoral head fracture in this situation may require an anterior exposure for femoral head fracture fixation and a posterior exposure for posterior acetabular wall fixation or the use of an extensile approach.

Hip Fractures

General Considerations and Risk Factors

- Although hip fractures typically occur in elderly, osteopenic patients after low-energy falls, these injuries also occur in younger active patients, usually as a result of high-energy trauma.
- With increasing longevity, the number of hip fractures sustained on an annual basis continues to increase.
- Decision making regarding treatment is based on fracture pattern, patient age, associated injuries, and medical comorbidities.

Clinical and Radiographic Evaluation

- Most hip fractures occur after low-energy falls in elderly patients. Attention to associated injuries, frequently involving the ipsilateral upper extremity, is important.
- In the elderly, frail population with multiple medical comorbidities, preoperative medical evaluation and optimization is important. The orthopedic surgeon is frequently the first physician to recognize osteopenia in these patient and appropriate evaluation and treatment is recommended.
- Elderly patients with hip fractures should be brought to surgery as soon as medical optimization is obtained. The benefits of early mobilization in this cohort should not be underestimated.
- In the younger patient population life-threatening injuries, if present, should be managed first, and then the hip fracture should be treated in an urgent fashion.

- The majority of hip fractures will be evident on antero-posterior and lateral radiographs. However, occult or stress fractures of the femoral neck may require additional imaging modalities for diagnosis.

- MRI can be extremely helpful in not only rapidly determining whether a fracture is present but also ruling out other potential causes of hip pain, such as pubic ramus fractures or osteonecrosis. MRI can also provide information on fracture location (femoral neck or intertrochanteric) and fracture verticality.

- Radionucleotide bone scanning can also be useful in this setting, especially if symptoms have been present for several days; however, it cannot provide as much rapid information as can be obtained from an MRI scan.

Femoral Neck Fractures
Classification

- Multiple classification schemes for femoral neck fractures exist; however, the most commonly used is that of Garden. Although four types are described, most surgeons group these fractures into those that are displaced (types III and IV) or nondisplaced (types I and II) because treatment decisions and prognosis are grouped in this manner as well.

- The Pauwels' classification has divided femoral neck fractures based on increasing amounts of fracture verticality measured from the horizontal as type 1, 30 degrees; type 2, 50 degrees; and type 3, 70 degrees. These fractures have been thought to behave in biomechanically distinct ways based on the increase in shear forces imparted at the fracture site by increasing degrees of fracture verticality.

- Some authors have recommended the use of a fixed-angle internal fixation device for higher shear angle (more vertical) transcervical and basicervical fractures, and cancellous screws alone for fractures with lower shear angle (more horizontal) transcervical fractures based on this theoretical concern.

Treatment Options
Nondisplaced Femoral Neck Fractures

- Nondisplaced fractures are treated similarly regardless of patient age, with internal fixation typically involving multiple parallel cannulated cancellous screws. Nonoperative treatment is reserved for only the most frail, essentially nonambulatory patients with prohibitive medical comorbidity and minimal discomfort from the injury.

- Subsequent displacement of nondisplaced or valgus impacted fractures treated nonoperatively has been demonstrated in nearly 40% of patients in a recent series with increased rates of osteonecrosis and nonunion.

- Recent cadaveric data demonstrated superiority of three screws over two screws when used to stabilize subcapital fractures in an inverted triangular configuration.

- It is important to place the screws near the cortex of the femoral neck to allow host bone to support the shafts of the screws and avoid varus, shortening, and external rotation displacement (Figures 14–1 and 14–2).

- Rates of nonunion of less than 5% and osteonecrosis of less than 10% have been reported with this technique. Early patient mobilization postoperatively is encouraged.

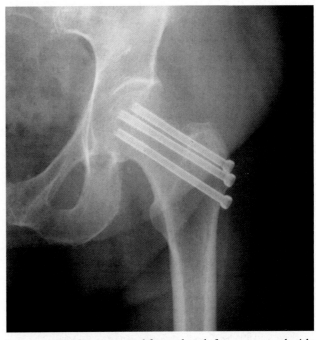

Figure 14–1: **Valgus impacted femoral neck fracture treated with three cannulated cancellous screws, anteroposterior view.**

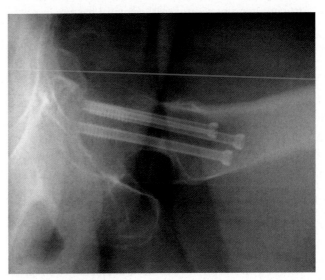

Figure 14–2: **Lateral view.**

Displaced Femoral Neck Fractures in Young Patients

- A displaced femoral neck fracture in the young patient should be treated expeditiously. In theory, fracture displacement can kink any vessels that have not been disrupted by the injury. Additionally, intracapsular tamponade can occur as a result of fracture hematoma, which may impede blood flow to the femoral head.

- Clinical data had documented lower rates of osteonecrosis with early treatment.

- A gentle closed reduction attempt is reasonable; however, multiple aggressive attempts at closed reduction are not indicated as a result of potential damage to the remaining femoral head vascularity or potential fracture comminution. If closed reduction is excellent, internal fixation should be performed as fracture pattern (verticality) dictates.

- If closed reduction is not obtainable, then open reduction is indicated. There are no generally accepted guidelines on what constitutes an acceptable femoral neck fracture reduction.

- In general, anatomic reduction is recommended. A slight valgus reduction is acceptable; however, any varus should be avoided. Review of a radiograph of the contralateral hip can assist the surgeon in determining the neck-shaft angle that is anatomic for the patient.

- Typically the Watson-Jones or Hardinge approaches are used allowing direct visualization of the fracture fragments, anatomic reduction, and internal fixation, usually with multiple parallel cannulated cancellous screws.

- If the fracture exhibits high verticality and a tendency to shear intraoperatively, screws alone are not recommended, and a fixed-angle device should be used. In one series, transcervical shear fractures exhibited a high failure rate when treated with screws alone.

- The role of capsulotomy in the treatment of femoral neck fractures remains controversial. Original fracture displacement probably determines the fate of the femoral head. Capsulotomy is recommended because it is relatively simple to perform, exposes the patient to minimal additional risk, and may reduce the intracapsular tamponade effect. In the young patient efforts are focused on preservation of the femoral head and avoiding arthroplasty at a young age.

- More data are needed to clearly determine if capsulotomy significantly alters the prognosis for young patients with displaced femoral neck fractures.

Displaced Fractures in Older Patients

- Resulting from the challenges of achieving stable proximal fragment fixation in osteopenic bone, the need for a predictable operation with a low fixation failure rate and the need for early, full weight-bearing mobilization, prosthetic replacement has been favored in the United States for the treatment of displaced femoral neck fractures in older patients.

- A failure rate of nearly 40% has been recently reported in ambulatory elderly patients with displaced femoral neck fractures treated with internal fixation. Fixation failure rates of 30% to 40% have been consistently reported over multiple series over the past few decades.

- In sharp contrast, multiple series evaluating the outcome of prosthetic replacement in this setting have consistently demonstrated predictable pain relief, functional improvement, and importantly, a low reoperation rate for a patient population that cannot tolerate the prolonged convalescence and multiple surgeries associated with fixation failure.

- Once prosthetic arthroplasty has been chosen, further controversy surrounds the selection of the type of arthroplasty, unipolar or bipolar, hemiarthroplasty, total hip arthroplasty, and the type of fixation, cemented or uncemented.

- Good-to-excellent results can be expected with either cemented or uncemented newer generation arthroplasties.

- Risks of uncemented arthroplasty include femoral fracture, prosthesis subsidence, and anterior thigh pain. Careful attention to accurate prosthetic sizing and appropriate seating on the calcar is essential.

- Cementation of the prosthesis has the risk of intraoperative death or embolization of marrow content during cementation. This may be reduced by canal venting and gentle cement pressurization.

- It should be noted, however, that the available literature suggests generally better outcomes with cemented arthroplasties. In the nonambulatory patient when the procedure is performed predominantly for pain control, first-generation uncemented (Austin-Moore type) prostheses can be used.

- Considerable data exist comparing unipolar to bipolar bearings for elderly patients with displaced femoral neck fractures. Short-term to midterm follow-up studies demonstrate no clear difference in morbidity, mortality, or functional outcome. Longer term follow-up suggests a lower reoperation rate for bipolar bearings (Figure 14–3). This is not surprising because patients who live longer are probably more active, and acetabular erosion is a time-dependent phenomenon.

- Total hip arthroplasty has been classically recommended for patients with displaced fractures and symptomatic ipsilateral degenerative change of the hip. This combination of pathology, however, is rare. Recent studies have expanded the indications to include active elderly patients with displaced femoral neck fractures and otherwise normal hip joints resulting from the more predictable pain relief and better function total hip arthroplasty provides, as compared to hemiarthroplasty.

- The main complication of hip arthroplasty performed in this setting is dislocation, with rates averaging 10% across

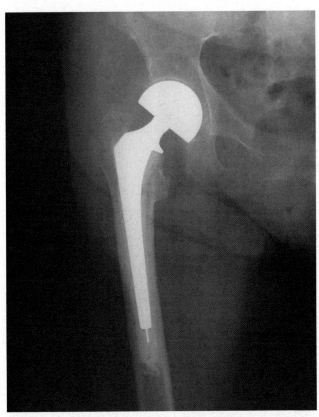

Figure 14–3: Cemented bipolar hemiarthroplasty.

multiple series. Of those that dislocate, approximately 25% become recurrent dislocators.

- A recent metaanalysis demonstrated a mean dislocation rate approximately seven times greater for total hip arthroplasty compared to hemiarthroplasty in this setting. Considering the enormous number of patients with displaced femoral neck fractures treated annually, the potential societal and economic impact of such dislocations can be substantial.
- Use of the anterolateral approach decreases the dislocation rates as does the selective use of larger diameter femoral heads, which should be considered when performing total hip arthroplasty in this setting.

Complications

- Nonunion is rare in the younger patient, with most series reporting rates of less than 10%. Secondary surgeries such as valgus-producing osteotomies are successful in ultimately achieving union, likely as a result of the excellent bone stock and healing potential in a young patient.
- Valgus intertrochanteric osteotomies convert the shear forces of a vertical fracture line to compressive forces by increasing fracture horizontality. Nonunion is more common in the older patient, with rates averaging less than 5% for

nondisplaced fractures and to over 30% for displaced fractures. Nonunion in the older patient is typically treated with hip arthroplasty.

- Rates of posttraumatic osteonecrosis have averaged 10% for nondisplaced fractures and 25% for displaced fractures.
- Not all patients with osteonecrosis will be symptomatic and require further treatment. The treatment of symptomatic posttraumatic osteonecrosis varies by patient age and osteonecrosis grade.

Intertrochanteric Hip Fractures
Classification

- Various classifications for intertrochanteric fractures have been proposed, but none has been widely accepted. Commonly, fractures are described by the number of "parts" and the presence of certain fracture characteristics that indicate greater instability.
- For example, a large posteromedial fragment, a reverse obliquity configuration, or subtrochanteric extension are commonly considered features that result in more "unstable" fractures. Intertrochanteric fractures are treated similarly regardless of patient age. Choice of internal fixation device should be based on fracture pattern.

Sliding Hip Screw

- The most important variables under a surgeon's control when treating an intertrochanteric hip fracture include correct device selection based on fracture pattern, accurate reduction, and placement of the lag screw into the center of the femoral head.
- Most intertrochanteric fractures can be treated successfully with the sliding hip screw device. This device offers the advantages of a simple, predictable operative technique, and a long clinical history of successful results. An increasing rate of failure and hardware cutout with poor implant placement or poor reduction has been documented.
- The "tip to apex distance" has been described as a guide to accurate screw placement and should be less than 25 mm. Ideally, a "center-center" position with the lag screw within 1 cm of the subchondral bone on both anteroposterior and lateral views is preferred (Figure 14–4).
- It should be emphasized that the sliding hip screw should never be used for fractures with reverse obliquity because in this situation this device does not allow controlled collapse and fracture compression but allows shear across the fracture site with medial displacement of the distal fragment, excessive sliding, and eventual lag screw cut-out (Figure 14–5).
- In one series, a 56% failure rate was noted for reverse obliquity fractures treated with a sliding hip screw. For intertrochanteric fractures with reverse obliquity either a 95-degree fixed-angle device (such as the 95-degree

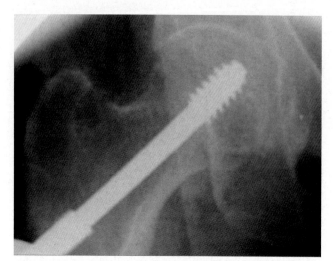

Figure 14–4: A well-placed sliding hip screw with deep and central position of the lag screw into the femoral head.

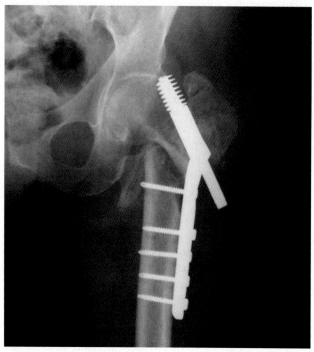

Figure 14–5: Failed fixation and cutout of a reverse obliquity fracture treated with a sliding hip screw.

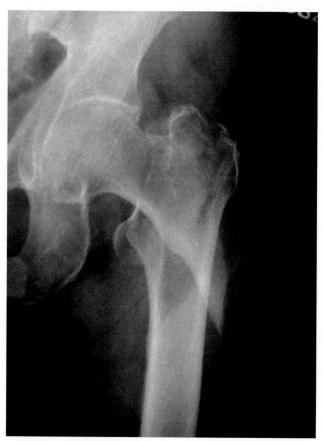

Figure 14–6: A four-part comminuted intertrochanteric fracture with reverse obliquity.

Intramedullary Devices

- Multiple studies, both randomized and nonrandomized, prospective and retrospective, comparing intramedullary (IM) devices to sliding hip screws for the fixation of intertrochanteric fractures exist. Although the concept of managing these fractures through small incisions and avoiding the usually bloody dissection of the vastus lateralis necessary for side plate placement is appealing, the literature has not demonstrated the clear advantage of IM devices to justify their routine use.

- In earlier series that evaluated outdated nail designs, higher complication rates, including iatrogenic femur fractures were reported. Contemporary IM implant designs have addressed many of these concerns and may allow more minimally invasive fracture management techniques.

- A recent prospective, randomized series of 400 patients comparing the redesigned Gamma nail to a sliding hip screw demonstrated a higher (but not statistically significant) rate of complications with the Gamma nail. The authors concluded that the routine use of the Gamma nail cannot be recommended.

- Currently, IM devices may be most suitable for fractures with reverse obliquity, high subtrochanteric, or intertrochanteric fractures with subtrochanteric extension. More

dynamic condylar screw, the condylar blade plate) or an cephalomedullary device is recommended.

- A recent prospective randomized series documented superior outcomes of intramedullary techniques over a 95-degree dynamic condylar screw (Figures 14–6 and 14–7).

- Recent studies have compared the results of sliding hip screws with two-hole side plates to conventional four-hole side plates for both stable and unstable fractures. No difference in clinical outcomes was noted. The shorter side plates offer the advantage of less soft-tissue dissection.

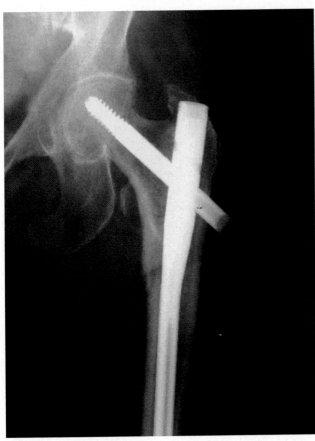

Figure 14–7: **Postoperative view after treatment with an intramedullary hip screw.**

data are needed to define which fractures benefit the most from IM fixation and whether further design refinements will decrease the complications noted in earlier series, thereby making intramedullary fixation more widely applicable.

Primary Prosthetic Replacement

- The role of primary prosthetic replacement for intertrochanteric fractures remains controversial. The potential advantages of primary prosthetic replacement in the face of an unstable intertrochanteric fracture in a patient with severely osteopenic bone include relatively predictable pain relief, early mobilization, and the fact that reoperation rates may be lower.
- The disadvantages include the more extensive nature of the surgical procedure, the frequent necessity to use calcar replacing, long-stem cemented implants in medically frail patients, and the fact that often comminuted, osteopenic trochanteric fragments need to be stabilized with some form of internal fixation.
- It should be noted from the literature that the overwhelming majority of well-reduced intertrochanteric hip fractures treated with properly selected, and accurately implanted internal fixation devices will heal predictably without complication.

- Additionally, should failure occur, prosthetic replacement for salvage of failed internal fixation has demonstrated excellent durability and predictable pain relief. Prosthetic replacement as the acute treatment for intertrochanteric fractures should be reserved for patients with pathologic fractures resulting from neoplasm, neglected fractures with deformity and poor bone stock precluding internal fixation or those that have failed internal fixation attempts.
- Additionally, prosthetic replacement may be a reasonable therapeutic option for patients with severe ipsilateral symptomatic degenerative joint disease or certain unfavorable fracture patterns associated with poor bone quality.

Subtrochanteric Fractures

- The subtrochanteric area of the femur experiences some of the highest biomechanical stresses in the human body. In general, the subtrochanteric region is considered the anatomic region immediately below the lesser trochanter to the proximal aspect of the femoral isthmus.
- Various classification systems, including the Russell-Taylor classification, have been proposed based on the location of the fracture relative to the lesser trochanter and the presence of fracture line extension into the piriformis fossa.
- More proximal subtrochanteric fractures often involve extension of the fracture line into the piriformis fossa which influences internal fixation device selection. Multiple fixation methods have been described, including the use of the sliding hip screw, dynamic condylar screw, or angled blade plate for more proximal ("high") subtrochanteric fractures, and interlocking cephalomedullary nailing for more distal ("low") subtrochanteric fractures.
- In general, if the piriformis fossa is intact, a nailing technique is preferred. If the lesser trochanter is intact and the proximal fragment is of sufficient length, then fixation into the femoral head is usually not necessary and a standard antegrade nail with locking into the lesser trochanter is adequate.
- With shorter proximal fragments without piriformis fossa involvement, cephalomedullary so-called "reconstruction" nailing with interlocking screw fixation into the femoral head and neck is preferred. A preoperative CT scan may be helpful to evaluate the integrity of the proximal fragment when plain radiographs are difficult to interpret as a result of patient size, proximal fragment rotation, and so on.
- If plating techniques are chosen for comminuted fractures, the vascularity of the medial bony fragments should be carefully preserved by avoiding dissection and periosteal stripping in this region. Areas of comminution should be "bridged," and stable proximal and distal fixation should be obtained while maintaining correct limb alignment, length, and rotation. Such "indirect" reduction techniques

have demonstrated high union rates but are technically demanding. Although plating techniques are associated with potentially lower rates of malalignment, dissection and blood loss can be substantial.

- Biomechanically, IM fixation of subtrochanteric fractures is generally preferred. Nails provide load sharing stability that allows early postoperative weight bearing that plated fractures typically cannot tolerate. This may be advantageous in patients with multiple injuries with other extremity injuries.

- Nailing short subtrochanteric fractures can be challenging as a result of the flexed, abducted, and externally rotated position of the proximal fragment. Great care should be taken to avoid varus proximal fragment malalignment, which can occur with conventional antegrade nails placed through a starting point that is too lateral.

- The use of newer nails designed for entry through the tip of the greater trochanter may facilitate access to the IM canal and results in less potential malalignment for these challenging fractures, however, there is little data to substantiate this speculation.

Pathologic Fractures of the Proximal Femur

- Metastatic disease commonly involves the proximal femur, affecting the femoral neck in 50%, subtrochanteric region in 30%, and intertrochanteric region in 20%.

- Decision making regarding whether some form of prophylactic internal fixation or hip arthroplasty is appropriate is based on the anatomic location of the lesion, size of the lesion, the extent of bony destruction, and anticipated life expectancy.

- In general it has been recommended that lesions that cause more than 50% destruction of a cortex or those that present with functional pain be stabilized. Complete fractures should be treated surgically in all but the most infirm patients. High-quality preoperative radiographs of the acetabulum and entire length of the femur are mandatory to evaluate for ipsilateral lesions.

- Other sites of bony pain should also be evaluated by plain films and bone scintigraphy. Appropriate preoperative workup in consultation with an oncologist is recommended.

- A fracture resulting from a solitary pathologic lesion of the proximal femur requires a pathologic tissue diagnosis before internal fixation or prosthetic replacement even in a patient with a prior cancer history. This will help avoid the rare but potentially disastrous complication of internal fixation of a primary malignancy. If necessary, a CT scan can be obtained of the proximal femur and the acetabulum to further evaluate for proximal lesions.

- The entire femur should be protected by the internal fixation device, typically a third-generation cephalomedullary nail. Lesion debulking and methacrylate augmentation of the fixation construct may be necessary for larger lesions.

- If extensive involvement of the proximal femur precludes predictable and durable internal fixation, then prosthetic replacement can provide functional improvement and pain relief in this cohort. Modular, so-called "tumor" prostheses are available to manage bony deficiency and restore leg length and hip stability. Pathologic fractures of the femoral neck, head, and intertrochanteric region often require treatment with prosthetic replacement.

- Medical comorbidities are extremely common and multidisciplinary management with a medical oncologist, radiation oncologist, nutritionist, and such is recommended.

- Postoperative radiation to the entire construct and surgical bed, after the surgical wound has healed, is recommended to minimize the chance of tumor progression and implant failure. Should fixation failure occur, conversion to hip arthroplasty has been shown to predictably improve function and relieve pain, however, these reconstructions are plagued by a high rate of postoperative infection.

Annotated References

Hip Dislocations and Femoral Head Fractures

Ganz R, Gill TJ, Gautier E, et al: Surgical dislocation of the adult hip a technique with full access to the femoral head and acetabulum without the risk of avascular necrosis, *J Bone Joint Surg Br* 83:1119-1124, 2001.
The authors describe a safe operative approach for hip dislocation in 213 hips with no cases of avascular necrosis (AVN). This approach, known as the "trochanteric flip" is useful for multiple degenerative and traumatic disorders of the hip joint.

Moorman CT, Warren RF, Hershman EB, et al: Traumatic posterior hip subluxation in American football, *J Bone Joint Surg Am* 85:1190-1196, 2003.
The authors discuss the clinical presentation, magnetic resonance imaging (MRI) findings, suggested treatment, and outcomes of eight football players with traumatic hip subluxation. Two of eight developed osteonecrosis and required total hip arthroplasty.

Sahin V, Karakas ES, Aksu S, et al: Traumatic dislocation and fracture-dislocation of the hip: a long term follow-up study, *J Trauma* 54:520-529, 2003.
Forty-seven patients with hip dislocation and fracture-dislocation were followed a mean of 9.6 years. Seventy-one percent had medium-to-very-good results. Sixteen percent developed posttraumatic degenerative joint disease, and 9.6% developed osteonecrosis. Early reduction improved outcomes.

Stannard JP, Harris HW, Volgas DA, et al: Functional outcome of patients with femoral head fractures associated with hip dislocations, *Clin Orthop* 377:44-56, 2000.
The authors provide a thorough review of the principles of treatment and confirm the need for early reduction, anatomic reduction, and stable internal fixation for good results. The Kocher-Langenbeck

approach was associated with a 3.2 times higher incidence of avascular necrosis (AVN) compared to the Smith-Peterson approach.

Femoral Neck Fractures

Bhandari M, Devereax PJ, Swiontkowski MF, et al: Internal fixation compared with arthroplasty for displaced fractures of the femoral neck: a meta-analysis, *J Bone Joint Surg Am* 85:1673-1688, 2003.

The authors evaluated published trials between 1969 and 2002 on the treatment of displaced femoral neck fractures in patients age 65 or older. Arthroplasty provided a significantly lower rate of revision surgery ($p = 0.0003$) but was associated with greater blood loss, longer operative time, and a trend toward higher mortality in the first 4 months (NS).

Haidukewych GJ, Israel TA, Berry DJ: Long-term survivorship of cemented bipolar hemiarthroplasty for fracture of the femoral neck, *Clin Orthop* 403:118-126, 2002.

The results of 212 patients over the age of 60 treated with cemented bipolar hemiarthroplasty are reported. Overall 10-year survivorship free of reoperation for any reason was 94%. Only one patient was revised for acetabular cartilage wear. Over 90% of patients had no or minimal pain at follow-up, and the dislocation rate was less than 2%.

Jain R, Koo M, Kreder HJ, Schemitsch EH, et al: Comparison of early and delayed fixation of subcapital hip fractures in patients sixty years of age or less, *J Bone Joint Surg Am* 84:1605-1612, 2002.

Delayed treatment of subcapital fractures was associated with a higher rate of osteonecrosis; however, this complication did not significantly affect functional outcome at follow-up.

Keating JF, Mzasson M, Scott N, et al: Randomized trial of reduction and fixation versus bipolar hemiarthroplasty versus total hip arthroplasty for displaced subcapital fractures in the fit older patient, Presented at the American Academy of Orthopaedic Surgeons 70th Annual Meeting, New Orleans, LA,

The authors demonstrate superior functional outcomes for fractures treated with total hip arthroplasty when compared to open reduction and internal fixation (ORIF) or hemiarthroplasty.

Maurer SG, Wright KE, Kummer FJ, et al: Two or three screws for fixation of femoral neck fractures? *Am J Orthop* 32:438-442, 2003.

Three screws demonstrated less fracture displacement than two screws in axial loading in embalmed cadaveric specimens with subcapital osteotomies.

McKinley JC, Robinson CM: Treatment of displaced intracapsular hip fractures with total hip arthroplasty: comparison of primary arthroplasty with early salvage arthroplasty after failed internal fixation, *J Bone Joint Surg Am* 84:2010-2015, 2002.

The authors demonstrate better outcomes and fewer complications with primary arthroplasty than when arthroplasty is performed after internal fixation fails in a matched pair case controlled study.

Ong BC, Maurer SG, Aharonoff GB, et al: Unipolar versus bipolar hemiarthroplasty: functional outcome after femoral neck fracture at a minimum of thirty-six months of follow-up, *J Orthop Trauma* 16:317-322, 2002.

No difference in functional outcome at midterm follow-up is noted between unipolar and bipolar cemented hemiarthroplasties.

Robinson CM, Saran D, Annan IH: Intracapsular hip fractures: results of management adopting a treatment protocol, *Clin Orthop* 302:83-91, 1994.

One hundred sixty-six fractures were managed by a protocol involving open reduction and internal fixation (ORIF) for fractures in patients younger than 65 or for those patients with non-displaced fractures, arthroplasty for those older than 85, and based on a physiologic status score in those between 65 and 85. Only 5% of the total group required reoperation.

Rogmark C, Carlsson Å, Johnell O, et al: Primary hemiarthroplasty in old patients with displaced femoral neck fracture: a 1-year follow-up of 103 patients aged 80 years or more, *Acta Orthop Scand* 73:605-610, 2002.

Primary hemiarthroplasty demonstrated a lower failure rate than those treated with internal fixation. There was no difference in hospital stay or mortality.

Sharif KM, Parker MJ: Austin Moore hemiarthroplasty: technical aspects and their effects on outcome, in patients with fractures of the neck of femur, *Injury* 33:419-422, 2002.

This retrospective study evaluates radiographic findings with outcomes and revision rates for 243 patients with a mean age of 81 years treated with Austin-Moore hemiarthroplasty. Undersizing of the prosthetic head and poor seating of the prosthesis on the calcar were associated with loosening and residual pain.

Tanaka J, Seki N, Tokimura F, et al: Conservative treatment of Garden stage I femoral neck fracture in elderly patients, *Arch Orthop Trauma Surg* 122:24-28, 2002.

Nonoperative treatment of Garden 1 femoral neck fractures demonstrated a 39% nonunion rate.

Intertrochanteric Hip Fractures

Adams CI, Robinson CM, Court-Brown CM, et al: Prospective randomized controlled trial of an intramedullary nail versus dynamic screw and plate for intertrochanteric fractures of the femur, *J Orthop Trauma* 15:394-400, 2001.

Four hundred patients were randomized for either a sliding hip screw or a Gamma nail. The nailed group had a higher rate of reoperations and complications (NS). The authors conclude that the routine use of an intramedullary device is not recommended.

Haidukewych GJ, Berry DJ: Hip arthroplasty for salvage of failed treatment of intertrochanteric hip fractures, *J Bone Joint Surg Am* 85:899-905, 2003.

The durability and predictable functional improvement of hip arthroplasty for failed treatment of intertrochanteric fractures is documented in 60 patients. Long-stem, calcar replacing prostheses are commonly required. The greater trochanter was a persistent source of discomfort in a substantial subset of patients.

Haidukewych GJ, Israel TA, Berry DJ: Reverse obliquity of fractures of the intertrochanteric region of the femur, *J Bone Joint Surg Am* 83:643-650, 2001.

The authors demonstrate a 56% failure rate when the sliding hip screw was used for a reverse obliquity fracture. The 95-degree blade plate had the lowest failure rate. Few patients were treated with intramedullary fixation during the study period. The authors conclude that the sliding hip screw is contraindicated for reverse obliquity fractures.

Janzig HM, Howben BJ, Brandt SE, et al: The Gotfried percutaneous compression plate versus the dynamic hip screw in the treatment of peritrochanteric hip fractures: minimal invasive treatment reduces operative time and postoperative pain, *J Trauma* 52:293-298, 2002.
One hundred fifteen patients randomized to either the percutaneous compression plate or sliding hip screw are reviewed. The percutaneous plate demonstrated lower operative time and less pain, but more mechanical complications.

Kosygan KP, Mohan R, Newman RJ: The Gotfried percutaneous compression plate compared with the conventional classic hip screw for the fixation of intertrochanteric fractures of the hip, *J Bone Joint Surg Br* 84:19-22, 2002.
One hundred eleven prospectively randomized to the percutaneous compression plate or sliding hip screw are reported. The percutaneous plate was associated with less blood loss and fewer transfusions but longer operative time. There was no difference in complications or fracture healing.

Sadowski C, Lubbeke A, Saudan M, et al: Treatment of reverse oblique and transverse intertrochanteric fractures with use of an intramedullary nail or a 95 degrees screw-plate: a prospective, randomized study, *J Bone Joint Surg Am* 84:372-381, 2002.
Intramedullary fixation demonstrated a lower rate of fixation failure than the 95-degree dynamic condylar screw.

Subtrochanteric Fractures

Barquet A, Francescoli L, Rienzi D, et al: Intertrochanteric-subtrochanteric fractures: treatment with the long Gamma nail, *J Orthop Trauma* 14:324-328, 2000.
Fifty-two fractures with a mean follow-up of 16 months are reviewed.
A 100% union rate is reported with few complications.

Vaidya SV, Dholakia DB, Chatterjee A: The use of a dynamic condylar screw and biologic reduction techniques for subtrochanteric femur fractures, *Injury* 34:123-128, 2003.
Thirty-one patients were treated with indirect reduction techniques.
The authors report a 100% union rate; 6.4% had a malunion.

van Doorn R, Stopert JW: The long Gamma nail in the treatment of 329 subtrochanteric fractures with major extension into the femoral shaft, *Eur J Surg* 166:240-246, 2000.
Retrospective review of 304 fractures. Seven patients (2%) developed nonunion. Results were generally good.

Classic Bibliography
Hip Dislocations and Femoral Head Fractures

Dreinhofer KE, Schwarzkopf SR, Haas NP, et al: Isolated traumatic dislocation of the hip: long-term results in 50 patients, *J Bone Joint Surg Br* 76:6-12, 1994.

Marchetti ME, Steinberg GG, Coumas JM: Intermediate-term experience of Pipkin fracture-dislocations of the hip, *J Orthop Trauma* 10:455-461, 1996.

Pipkin G: Treatment of grade IV fracture-dislocation of the hip: a review, *J Bone Joint Surg Am* 39:1027-1042, 1957.

Stewart MJ, Milford LW: Fracture-dislocation of the hip: an end-result study, *J Bone Joint Surg Am* 36:315-342, 1954.

Thompson VP, Epstein HC: Traumatic dislocation of the hip: a survey of two hundred and four cases covering a period of twenty-one years, *J Bone Joint Surg Am* 33:746-778, 1951.

Upadhyay SS, Moulton A, Srikrishnamurthy K: An analysis of the late effects of traumatic posterior dislocation of the hip without fractures, *J Bone Joint Surg Br* 65:150-157, 1983.

Femoral Neck Fractures

Alho A, Benterud JG, Solovieva S: Internally fixed femoral neck fractures: early prediction of failure in 203 elderly patients with displaced fractures, *Acta Orthop Scand* 70:141-144, 1999.

Asnis SE, Wanek-Sgaglione L: Intracapsular fractures of the femoral neck: results of cannulated screw fixation, *J Bone Joint Surg Am* 76:1793-1803, 1994.

Booth KC, Donaldson TK, Dai QG: Femoral neck fracture fixation: a biomechanical study of two cannulated screw placement techniques, *Orthopedics* 21:1173-1176, 1998.

Calder SJ, Anderson GH, Jagger C, et al: Unipolar or bipolar prosthesis for displaced intracapsular hip fracture in octogenarians: a randomized prospective study, *J Bone Joint Surg Br* 78:391-394, 1996.

Chua D, Jaglal SB, Schatzker J: Predictors of early failure of fixation in the treatment of displaced subcapital hip fractures, *J Orthop Trauma* 12:230-234, 1998.

Garden RS: Malreduction and avascular necrosis in subcapital fractures of the femur, *J Bone Joint Surg Br* 53:183-197, 1971.

Hammer AJ: Nonunion of the subcapital femoral neck fracture, *J Orthop Trauma* 6:73-77, 1992.

Lee BP, Berry DJ, Harmsen WS, et al: Total hip arthroplasty for the treatment of an acute fracture of the femoral neck: long term results, *J Bone Joint Surg Am* 80:70-75, 1998.

Lu-Yao GL, Keller RB, Littenberg B, et al: Outcomes after displaced fractures of the femoral neck: a meta-analysis of one hundred and six published reports, *J Bone Joint Surg Am* 76:15-25, 1994.

Maruenda JI, Barrios C, Gomar-Sancho F: Intracapsular hip pressure after femoral neck fracture, *Clin Orthop* 340:172-180, 1997.

Parker MJ, Blundell C: Choice of implant for internal fixation of femoral neck fractures: meta-analysis of 25 randomized trials including 4,925 patients, *Acta Orthop Scand* 69:138-143, 1998.

Swiontkowski MF, Thorpe M, Seiler JG, et al: Operative management of displaced femoral head fractures: case-matched comparison of anterior versus posterior approaches for Pipkin I and Pipkin II fractures, *J Orthop Trauma* 6:437-442, 1992.

Intertrochanteric Hip Fractures

Baumgaertner MR, Curtin SL, Lindskog DM, et al: The value of the tip-apex distance in predicting failure of fixation of peritrochanteric fractures of the hip, *J Bone Joint Surg Am* 77:1058-1064, 1995.

Koval KJ, Sala DA, Kummer FJ, et al: Postoperative weight-bearing after a fracture of the femoral neck or an intertrochanteric fracture, *J Bone Joint Surg Am* 80:352-356, 1998.

Kyle RF, Gustilo RB, Premer RF: Analysis of six hundred and twenty-two intertrochanteric hip fractures, *J Bone Joint Surg Am* 61:216-221, 1979.

Parker MJ, Pryor GA: Gamma versus DHS nailing for extracapsular femoral fractures: meta-analysis of ten randomized trials, *Int Orthop* 20:163-168, 1996.

Subtrochanteric Fractures

Kinast C, Bolhofner BR, Mast JW, et al: Subtrochanteric fractures of the femur: results of treatment with the 95 degree condylar blade plate, *Clin Orthop* 238:122-130, 1989.

Russell TA, Taylor JC: Subtrochanteric fractures of the femur. In Browner BD, Jupiter JB, Levine AM, et al editors: *Skeletal trauma*, ed 2, Philadelphia, 1997, W. B. Saunders.

Sanders R, Regazzoni P: Treatment of subtrochanteric femur fractures using the dynamic condylar screw, *J Orthop Trauma* 3:206-213, 1989.

Siebenrock KA, Muller U, Ganz R: Indirect reduction with a condylar blade plate for osteosynthesis of subtrochanteric femoral fractures, *Injury* 29:7-15, 1998.

Wiss DA, Brien WW: Subtrochanteric fractures of the femur: results of treatment by interlocking nailing, *Clin Orthop* 283:231-236, 1992.

CHAPTER 15

Femoral Shaft Fractures

William M. Ricci, MD

Fractures of the femoral shaft are among the most common operatively treated fractures. Although seemingly associated with a simple treatment algorithm (as the vast majority are treated operatively) and a consensus treatment modality of intramedullary (IM) nailing that is one of the most common and familiar procedures performed for fracture in orthopaedics, femoral shaft fracture is associated with significant patient morbidity and potential challenges for the surgeon. As the femur is the largest bone in the human body, high-energy trauma is required to cause fracture. For this reason, associated musculoskeletal and other system injuries are common. The optimal timing of surgical intervention and the proper surgical technique continue to be refined. The challenge for the orthopaedic surgeon is to synthesize all of the factors that contribute to choosing the proper treatment modality, choose the most appropriate timing for treatment, and execute the procedure with precision.

Classification

The Winquist classification describes the degree of comminution of femoral shaft fractures.[1] Because fracture comminution involves more of the diameter of the bone, the Winquist Type increases (Figure 15–1).

- Type 0 fractures have no comminution.
- Type I fractures have a small area of comminution with greater than 75% of the diameter of the bone remaining in continuity.
- Type II fractures have increased comminution but with at least 50% of the diameter intact.
- Type III fractures have less than 50% cortical contact.
- Type IV fractures, have no abutment of the cortices at the level of the fracture to prevent shortening.

The AO/OTA Classification

According to the Orthopaedic Truama Association (OTA) classification,[2] fractures of the femoral shaft are designated as "32." The tens place indicates the bone (femur = 3), the ones place indicates the location (1 = proximal end segment, 2 = middle [shaft], 3 = distal end segment.)

- Type 32A fractures are simple (without comminution; equivalent to Winquist Type 0 fractures).
- Type 32B are comminuted but maintain some degree of cortical continuity between the proximal and distal shaft fragments (can be equivalent to Winquist Types I, II, or III fractures).
- Type 32C fractures have loss of continuity between the proximal and distal fragments (equivalent to Winquist Type IV fractures).
- Further subtypes represent increasing fracture complexity.

Evaluation

Routine evaluation of femur fractures includes anteroposterior (AP) and lateral plain film radiographs of the entire femur (including the hip and knee joints).

- Associated femoral neck fractures, although estimated to be present in only 1% to 8% of femoral shaft fractures, have a high incidence of being misdiagnosed (>30%). All patients with femoral shaft fractures should have, in addition to the AP and lateral views of the entire femur, separate preoperative AP and lateral radiographic views of the femoral neck. Computed tomography (CT) scans have proven useful to diagnose occult femoral neck fractures. Recent studies have advocated routine preoperative CT scans in patients with high-energy injury mechanisms.[3]
- Careful postoperative evaluation of the femoral neck is also indicated because of the risk for creating an iatrogenic femoral neck fracture or displacement of previously occult femoral neck fracture during nailing of the femoral shaft.
- Fractures of the femur are usually associated with relatively high-energy trauma. Accordingly, patients should be

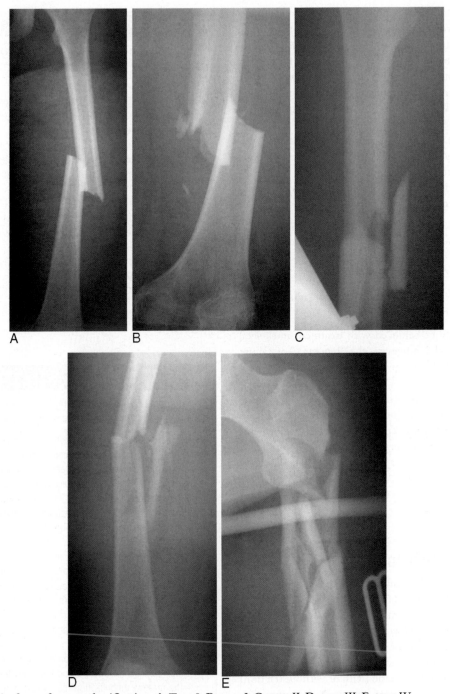

Figure 15–1: **Winquist femur fracture classification. A,** Type 0; **B,** type I; **C,** type II; **D,** type III; **E,** type IV.

carefully and systematically evaluated for associated injuries. The mechanism of injury can help heighten the suspension for other particular injuries.

• Knee injuries are commonly associated with femur fractures, especially those resulting from motor vehicle accidents in which there is direct impact of the knee into the dashboard.

   • Associated knee injury occurs in approximately 40% of patients and can include ligamentous injuries, meniscal injuries, and bone contusion.[4]

• Knee stability should be evaluated with careful examination under anesthesia immediately after femur fracture stabilization.

• Patients with persistent knee pain should be evaluated for occult internal derangement and bone contusion usually with magnetic resonance imaging (MRI) scanning.

• Falls from a height can be associated with other injuries that are commonly associated with axial loading, such as calcaneus fractures and spinal compression fractures.

- Visceral, chest, and head trauma should always be ruled out in patients with high-energy femoral shaft fractures.
- Bleeding at the site of femoral shaft fracture is usually self-limited but can be several hundred milliliters. In patients with bilateral femoral shaft fractures or those with other long-bone fractures, the cumulative bleeding can be clinically significant. These patients should be monitored closely for anemia and hemodynamic changes.
- Associated vascular injury is uncommon, but patients with diminished or asymmetric pulses should be carefully evaluated for associated vascular injury.
- Neurologic deficit associated with penetrating trauma may require acute surgical exploration.

Treatment Options
Nonsurgical Treatment

Nonsurgical treatment has a limited role for adult patients with femoral shaft fractures.

- Union can usually be achieved with treatment in skeletal traction (Box 15-1); however, the frequency of failure resulting from malalignment and shortening can be as high as 66%.
- Severely debilitated, nonambulatory patients or those patients with contraindications to anesthesia are candidates for nonoperative treatment with skeletal traction for 6 weeks followed by cast-brace application.
- Patients with paraplegia can be treated nonoperatively with pillow splints. However those that rely on an intact femur for independent transfers should be considered for operative treatment.

Intramedullary Nailing

Locked intramedullary (IM) nailing remains the gold standard treatment for patients with femoral shaft fractures.[1] Reported healing rates have been remarkably consistent as being between 90% and 95% (and as high as 99%) with low associated complication rates.[1] Nails can be inserted with or without reaming and can be locked in static or dynamic mode. Patients can be placed either supine (with or without traction) or in the lateral decubitus position. The optimal combination of reaming (Box 15-2), locking, and position are dependant on factors related to the patient (Box 15-3), fracture stability (Box 15-4), fracture location (Box 15-5), soft tissue injury, and surgeon. Various insertion techniques, such as antegrade though the piriformis fossa, antegrade through the greater trochanter, or retrograde through an intraarticular intercondylar starting point, may be used (Box 15-6). Healing and infection rates can be expected to be similar regardless of the selected starting point. Functional outcome and other complications after IM nailing can be specific to the particular technique that is used and will be discussed later in this chapter.

Box 15–1 | Skeletal Traction

Skeletal traction is most often used for temporary stabilization if a delay in operative treatment is expected to be greater than 12 to 24 hours.

- Traction through the distal femur is most common. Traction through the proximal tibia may be used provided there are no ligamentous knee injuries.
- Skeletal traction applied to the distal femur provides improved stability and comfort compared to traction applied through the tibia by avoiding traction across the knee joint and allowing for knee flexion.
- Balanced suspension traction configuration (Figure 15–2) should provide approximately 20 to 30 degrees of hip flexion, 20 to 30 degrees of knee flexion, support for the posterior thigh, and support for the posterior calf.
- A traction force of approximately 20 to 40 pounds should be used depending on the size of the patient.

Box 15–2 | Reaming

Reamed intramedullary (IM) nailing for treatment of femoral shaft fractures remains the gold standard with regard to fracture healing.

- Theoretic local and systemic detrimental affects associated with reaming have made reaming controversial.
- Animal studies have demonstrated that reaming damages the IM blood supply. However, this vascularity returns quickly.
- Despite the destruction of the endosteal blood supply, prospective randomized trials have demonstrated reamed nail insertion provides lower nonunion healing rates (1.7%) than nonreamed insertion (7.5%).[33]
  - Reaming is associated with increased IM pressures that theoretically increases fat embolization compared to nonreamed nailing. However the correlation between raised IM pressure and fat embolization has not been shown in humans.
  - Fat embolization has been shown to be similar with reamed nailing, unreamed nailing, and plating of femoral shaft fractures.
  - Marrow content embolization during the reaming process is less than that during fracture and less than that for nail insertion. The marrow embolization that occurs during reaming is usually subclinical. The risks associated with reaming are therefore outweighed by the benefits of reaming on the healing process.
  - The benefits of reaming for the healing process are thought to be deposition of bone graft material at the fracture site and stimulation of a favorable inflammatory response.
- No difference in pulmonary complications has been demonstrated between reamed nailing and unreamed nailing in multiple prospective randomized studies and in retrospective reviews.
- Sharp reamers, proper reamer design, and slow passage of the reamer can decrease IM pressures and fat embolization and should be used especially for patients with associated chest or lung injury.

Box 15–3	Indications of Borderline Patient Status

1. Pulmonary dysfunction
2. Hypothermic
3. Coagulopathy
4. Shock

Box 15–4	Fracture Stability

- Axially stable fractures: Winquist type I and type II fractures are considered to be axially stable.
  - They are more amenable to earlier (usually immediate) weight bearing after intramedullary (IM) nailing.
  - Dynamic interlocking can be used for axially stable fracture patterns, but occult fracture lines can lead to undesired shortening.
- Axially unstable fractures: Winquist type III and type IV fractures are considered to be axially unstable.
  - Weight bearing after IM nailing of axially unstable injuries should only be considered if treated with a statically locked construct.
  - Fatigue fracture of interlocking screws can lead to a large degree of shortening in comminuted fractures. Such "autodynamization" can be beneficial to the healing process but is at the expense of limb shortening.
  - Shortening as a result of interlocking screw fracture can lead to undesirable nail protrusion. This is especially problematic after retrograde nailing when nail protrusion is into the knee (Figure 15–5).
- Rotationally stability is determined by the amount of comminution and obliquity of the fracture.
  - Oblique fractures are more rotationally stable.
  - Transverse fracture patterns are less rotationally stable.
  - Severely comminuted fractures are least rotationally stable.

Box 15–5	Fracture Location

- The location of the fracture along the length of the shaft is usually described as being of the proximal, middle, or distal one third.
- There is overlap between subtrochanteric and proximal one-third shaft fractures and between supracondylar and distal one-third fractures.
- Fractures within the zone 5 cm below the lesser trochanter are usually considered to be in the subtrochanteric region but can also be classified as proximal third shaft fractures.
- Fractures within the zone of the distal metaphyseal flare are usually considered in the supracondylar region but can also be classified as distal third shaft fractures.

Insertion Technique and Starting Points

Piriformis Fossa Starting Point

Relative Advantages of Piriformis Fossa Starting Point

The piriformis fossa starting point is the gold standard for IM nailing of femur fractures.

- The major advantage of the piriformis fossa compared to the greater trochanter or retrograde intercondylar starting points are its colinear axis with the shaft of the femur and its extraarticular location, respectively.
- Because it is colinear with the long axis of femur, the piriformis fossa is optimal for obtaining satisfactory fracture reduction.

Relative Disadvantages of Piriformis Fossa Starting Point

- The required dissection through the gluteal muscles and disruption of the external rotator tendons can contribute to functional disability.
- The piriformis fossa is technically more difficult to instrument particularly in muscular and obese patients.

Box 15–6	Nailing Technique

Antegrade Nailing

Positioning

- Supine positioning on a fracture table with skin traction through the distal limb is the most common position for antegrade nailing.
- Skeletal traction can also be applied through either the femur or tibia (in the absence of knee ligament injury).
- Traction is applied against a padded peroneal post that is usually positioned against the ipsilateral ischium. Placement of the post against the contralateral ischium allows more adduction of the proximal fragment. This can facilitate access to the entry portal and is particularly useful during antegrade nailing of patients with obesity and those with proximal fractures.
- The opposite leg is usually placed in the hemi-lithotomy position to facilitate lateral fluoroscopic radiography. The peroneal nerve passes across the fibula, should be free of pressure, and well padded to avoid iatrogenic peroneal nerve injury.
- The limb that is elevated into the hemi-lithotomy position is subject to elevated compartment pressures and should be monitored carefully especially when injured or when surgery is prolonged.
- Placement of the opposite leg in skin traction with the two limbs scissored relative to one another is another technique that helps improve access to the starting portal. Traction applied to the contralateral limb prevents the pelvis from rotating toward the effected limb and therefore provides relative adduction of the operative hip relative to the pelvis.
- Antegrade nailing without traction on a radiolucent table with or without the use of a femoral distractor can reduce operative time and because of better assessment of the contralateral limb, can facilitate obtaining proper rotational alignment.

- The lateral decubitus position provides hip flexion and adduction and therefore offers improved ease of access to the piriformis fossa. However, it is more difficult to control and evaluate femoral rotation and to control the distal fragment that tends to drift into valgus.

Starting Point

- Instrumentation of the starting point, piriformis fossa or greater trochanter, can be performed either open or percutaneously with a skin entry site that is several centimeters proximal to the greater trochanter. Fluoroscopic imaging is used to confirm proper placement of the starting point instrument (Figure 15–7A, B, and C).
- The local soft tissues should be protected during instrumentation of the femur to minimize damage and development of heterotopic bone (Figure 15–7D and E).
- The starting point is confirmed with anteroposterior (AP) and lateral radiographs and should be colinear with the long axis of the femur in both views for antegrade piriformis and retrograde nailing. When performing antegrade trochanteric nailing, the starting point should be colinear with the long axis on the lateral view (Figure 15–7C) and can be slightly off axis on the AP view (Figure 15–7B).
  - The off-axis angulation that can be accepted with trochanteric nailing is dependent on the proximal lateral bend of the nail system being used but is generally approximately five degrees.
  - The most common mistake during trochanteric nailing is to start too lateral (lateral to the tip of the trochanter) and to aim too medial (toward the lesser trochanter). This risks creation of a varus deformity and iatrogenic fracture comminution of the medial cortex.
  - The proper starting point for trochanteric nailing is usually at or just medial to the tip of the trochanter with a trajectory nearly central to the canal (Figure 15–7B).

Reduction, Canal Preparation, and Nail Insertion

- Once the proximal fragment is opened, the fracture is reduced then a guidewire is passed across the fracture site. The maneuvers used to obtain fracture reduction for passage of the guidewire should be recreated during reaming to avoid asymmetric reaming of a malaligned fracture that invariably results in similar malalignment after passage of the nail. In general, the fracture alignment at the time of guidewire placement and reaming is the alignment that should be expected after nailing.
- Reaming is usually to a size approximately 1 to 2 mm larger than the diameter that causes "chatter." Extensive reaming of the endosteal cortex was previously performed to provide for insertion of large-diameter nails that were required to provide adequate strength. Modern titanium nails are of sufficient strength that such overreaming is unnecessary and to avoid thermal injury should be avoided.
- Less overreaming is acceptable when using a relatively flexible nail or when the femur is relatively straight (and the nail has a similar bow). More overreaming is indicated when using a relatively rigid nail, when the femur has a large bow, or when there is significant mismatch between the bow of the femur and that of the nail. The nail diameter should be 1 to 2 mm smaller than the largest used reamer.
- The nail's anterior bow can be taken advantage of during trochanteric nailing of proximal fractures to avoid iatrogenic comminution of the medial cortex. The nail is rotated 90 degrees (apex medial) on insertion. Once the nail is across the fracture, it is gradually derotated (Figure 15–2C, D, and E).
- The optimal anterior or posterior position for the piriformis fossa starting point depends on the relative curvature of the native femur and the selected nail
  - Biomechanical studies have demonstrated that an anterior piriformis fossa starting point must be avoided because increased hoop stresses at this location can lead to iatrogenic fracture of the proximal fragment.[34]
  - The greater the anterior bow (decreased radius of curvature) of the selected nail, the more posterior the starting point should be.

Retrograde Nailing

Positioning

- Retrograde nailing is most often performed with the patient in the supine position on a radiolucent table. This allows unencumbered access to the starting point from the foot of the table.

Starting Point

- The initial starting point for retrograde nailing was the medial femoral condyle. This entry portal was not ideal as a result of its off-axis location and a lack of implants designed for this starting point.
- The proper insertion site for retrograde nailing is intraarticular and centered or slightly medial in the intracondylar notch in the coronal plane (AP view) and centered at the apex of Blumensaat's line in the saggital plane (lateral view; Figure 15–8).

Reduction, Canal Preparation, and Nail Insertion

- The principles for fracture reduction, canal preparation, and nail insertion are the same for retrograde nailing as for antegrade nailing.
- Insertion of the nail beneath the articular surface is critical to avoid damaging the patella articular cartilage.
- Multiple distal interlocking screws should be used (especially in patients with axially unstable fractures) to minimize the risk of distal screw fracture and subsequent migration of the nail into the knee (Figure 15–4).

- Patients with obesity are prone to complications with nailing through the piriformis fossa, such as fracture of the greater trochanter and difficulty in obtaining a proper starting point.[5] In this group of patients, nailing through the greater trochanter or retrograde nailing should be considered.

- The lateral femoral circumflex artery is at high risk of injury,[6] but such injury does not appear to be clinically relevant in adults. However, as a result of the association of avascular necrosis (AVN) with the piriformis fossa starting point, this entry portal is contraindicated in children and in adolescents with open physes.

- Use of the piriformis fossa starting point should be avoided when fractures extend into the piriformis fossa.

Greater Trochanter Starting Point

Gerhard, generally thought of as the father of intramedullary nailing, used the tip of the grater trochanter as his entry portal with the patient in the supine position. In Europe, this remains the entry site of choice for antegrade femoral nailing. In the United States, the greater trochanteric starting point lost favor to the piriformis starting point (initially popularized with the patient in the lateral position to facilitate access to the piriformis fossa) resulting from problems associated with the greater trochanter entry portal being off axis from the femoral canal.

Relative Advantages of Greater Trochanter Starting Point

- The greater trochanteric starting point offers advantages as a result of its more subcutaneous position than the piriformis fossa. This facilitates ease of insertion, especially in muscular and obese patients.

- The improved technical ease of the greater trochanter starting point is evidenced by reduced operative times and reduced radiation exposure compared to nailing through the piriformis fossa.[7]

- Nailing through the greater trochanter reduces damage to the short external rotators compared to nailing through the piriformis fossa.[6] Conversely, there is more disruption of the gluteus medius tendon with the greater trochanteric starting point.[6] A 17-mm trochanteric entry hole encompasses 27% of the gluteus medius tendon.[8] The functional significance of these differences remains uncertain, however, clinical experience and preliminary data suggests that any differences are subtle.

Relative Disadvantages of Greater Trochanter Starting Point

- Iatrogenic fracture comminution of the medial cortex, especially when the femoral fracture is located within the proximal third of the diaphysis, can be associated with trochanteric nailing (Figure 15–2A and B). Refined insertion techniques that exploit the anterior bow of the nail can help reduce this complication (Figure 15–2C, D, and E).

- Varus malalignment can result when using the trochanteric starting point with nails designed without a proximal trochanteric bend (Figure 15–3A, B, and C). New implants designed specifically for use with a greater trochanteric starting point with a proximal lateral bend reduce the risk of varus malalignment (Figure 15–3D and E).

- Contraindications for use of the trochanteric starting point are relative and include situations where proximal exposure is undesirable.

Results of Antegrade Nailing

- Early results of trochanteric nailing using nails specifically designed for this starting portal (with a proximal lateral bend) have reduced the complications previously seem with this starting point and straight nails (without a proximal lateral bend).

- Healing and complication rates have been similar to those seen with antegrade nailing using the piriformis fossa.

- Functional outcome, based on early reports, also appear to be similar to those with piriformis fossa nailing.

Retrograde Nailing

Retrograde nailing of femoral shaft fractures was developed to address situations in which antegrade nailing was either difficult or undesirable. The patient with ipsilateral femoral neck and femoral shaft fractures was one of the first such indications for retrograde nailing technique. This combination of fractures was difficult to treat with first-generation and second-generation femoral nails. Retrograde nailing of femoral shaft fractures has since evolved to be a viable alternative to antegrade nailing (Box 15-7).[9]

Relative Advantages of Retrograde Nailing

- The advantages of retrograde nailing relate to ease of access to the starting point and to ease of simultaneous access to other anatomic areas in the patient with multiple injuries.

Box 15–7 | **Current Indications for Retrograde Intramedullary Nailing**

- Clinical situations in which proximal access to the femur for antegrade nailing is either impossible or not desired are indications for retrograde nailing. These include patients with obesity, ipsilateral acetabular fracture, pregnancy, ipsilateral femoral shaft and proximal femur fractures, ipsilateral femoral shaft and tibial shaft fractures, traumatic thorough knee amputation, polytrauma, and those with spine trauma.

- Routine use of retrograde nailing for treatment of isolated femoral shaft fractures is limited by the unknown long-term effects on the knee.

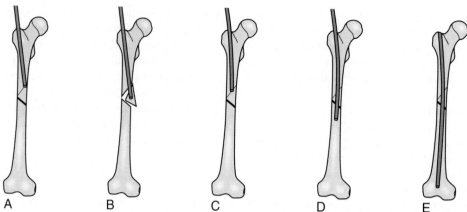

Figure 15–2: Avoiding iatrogenic comminution during trochanteric femoral nailing. An off-axis starting point (**A**) can force nail to aim medially and can lead to (**B**) iatrogenic fracture comminution. This complication can be avoided by using taking advantage of the nails anterior bow. **C**, The nail is rotated 90 degrees on insertion such that the anterior bow is apex medial such that the tip of the nail does not aim medially. It is passed beyond the fracture site without causing iatrogenic comminution (**D**) then gradually derotated during final seating (**E**).

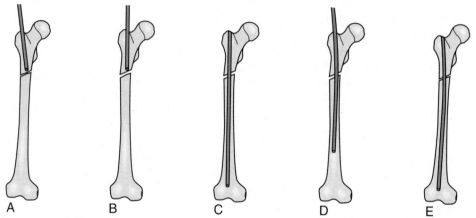

Figure 15–3: Avoiding varus malalignment during trochanteric nailing. **A**, The off-axis trochanteric starting point causes the nail to aim eccentrically. **B**, Varus deformity is created when aligning the nail with the distal fragment and is maintained after final seating of the nail (**C**). A nail with a proximal lateral bend temporarily creates varus (**D**) that is corrected as the bent proximal portion of the nail engages the proximal fracture fragment (**E**).

- Retrograde nailing does not compromise surgical approaches about the hip in patients with acetabular or pelvic fractures.
- Retrograde nailing may provide improved ease of obtaining proper fracture alignment of distal shaft fractures, decreased operating room (OR) time, and decreased blood loss compared to antegrade nailing.[9]
- Facilitates treatment of patients with ipsilateral femoral neck or intratrochanteric fractures.

Relative Disadvantages of Retrograde Nailing

- The greatest disadvantage of retrograde nailing through the currently standard intraarticular starting point is the requirement for a knee arthrotomy, drilling through the articular cartilage of the trochlea, and risk for damage to the under surface of the patella (Figure 15–4). All of which may contribute to knee problems.

- When proper technique is used (see Box 15–6), there is not an increase in patella-femoral contact pressures associated with retrograde nailing. The region of the hole made for the starting point contacts the patella only during terminal flexion.

Results of Retrograde Nailing

- The results of retrograde nailing when reamed interlocked nails are used can be expected to be similar to other nailing techniques with regard to healing, infection, and malalignment (although retrograde nailing may facilitate reduction of distal fractures resulting from improved control of this fragment).
- Complications specific to retrograde nailing technique are related knee problems. The incidence of knee pain after retrograde nailing has been reported as 7% to 60%. The knee pain is usually mild but occasionally effects normal function. It can be difficult to discern if knee symptoms

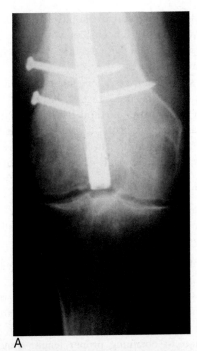

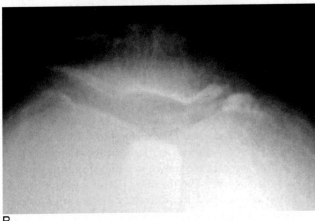

B

Figure 15–4: Complication of retrograde nailing. Destruction of the articular surface of the patella can occur when a retrograde nail protrudes into the knee joint. **A,** Fracture of the distal interlocking screws lead to shortening and backing of this retrograde nail into the knee resulting in severe destruction of the patella seen on the merchant view radiograph **(B).**

are attributable to the initial injury mechanism or resulting from the nailing procedure. When patients with known traumatic knee injury are excluded, knee problems are more common after retrograde nailing (36%) than after antegrade nailing (9%).[9]

- Knee stiffness and septic arthritis have not been shown to be significant problems after retrograde nailing.[10,11]
- Contraindications to retrograde nailing occur when access to the knee is compromised or is ill advised. Knee contracture such that 45 degrees of flexion cannot be achieved can prevent adequate access to the starting point.

- Active or prior knee infection is another contraindication to retrograde nailing.

Plating

Plate fixation of acute femoral shaft fractures is reserved for the pediatric population and for adults in situations in which IM nailing is either impossible or undesirable.

- Plate fixation is indicated for patients with ipsilateral femoral neck and shaft fractures, extremely small intramedullary canals, associated vascular injury, and those with periprosthetic fractures about IM implants.
- When plating femoral shaft fractures, minimally invasive methods, such as indirect reduction techniques and submuscular plating, should be used to reduce soft-tissue disruption and maximize healing potential.
- Plates with locking screws have theoretic advantages in osteoporotic bone, but the specific benefits and indications of such devices for femoral shaft fractures are yet to be proven.

External Fixation

External fixation as definitive treatment of acute femoral shaft fractures is limited to the pediatric population.

- In adults, external fixation can be useful as temporary fixation when acute IM nailing is ill advised, such as for application of damage control principles or for severely contaminated open wounds, especially when repeated access to a contaminated IM canal is indicated.
- External fixation can be useful to provide provisional stabilization in patients with associated vascular injury where time constraints preclude IM nailing.

Timing of Surgical Treatment

Recommendations for the timing of surgical treatment for patients with femoral shaft fractures have changed over the past three decades. Delayed stabilization, as advocated in the 1950s, was associated with increased incidence of systemic complications, such as pulmonary failure and multisystem organ failure, that are related to sustained fat embolization from the nonstabilized femur. This lead to a trend toward early (within 24 hours of injury) femur fracture stabilization especially for patients with multiple injuries. Compared with delayed stabilization early stabilization has been associated with decreased mortality and decreased pulmonary complications, such as adult respiratory distress syndrome (ARDS), fat embolism syndrome (FES), pneumonia, and pulmonary failure.

Damage Control Orthopaedics

The practice of immediate stabilization of femoral shaft fractures in patients with multiple injuries has recently come into question. It has been theorized that the systemic stress of orthopaedic procedures, the associated blood loss and the potential for hypothermia and systemic cytokine release may be detrimental to the patient with multiple injuries. Based on these theories the concept of "damage control orthopaedics" has emerged. The principals of which include early, rapid, and temporary stabilization of long-bone fractures usually with external fixation. This is followed by definitive management after intensive care unit (ICU) optimization of the patient.

- Conversion of external fixation to IM nailing can usually be performed up to 2 weeks after external fixation application without increased risk of infection so long as the pin sites are clean.
- The data to support damage control orthopaedics remains theoretical without good level I clinical evidence.
- It has been suggested that the ideal group of patients that would benefit from damage control principles are the so called borderline or at-risk patient as defined in Box 15–7.

Special Situations

Open Fractures

Open fractures of the femur, which is surrounded and protected by a large envelope of muscle, are much less common than with the tibia, which is largely subcutaneous. Because of the presence of this large protective soft-tissue envelope, open fractures are often associated with significant soft-tissue trauma.

- Small skin wounds can disguise more significant deep muscle and periosteal injury.
- All open fractures of the femoral shaft (except gunshot wounds) should be emergently treated.
- Wounds should be extended for evaluation of the deep soft tissues.
- All nonviable soft tissues and bone should be debrided.
- Serial debridements at 24- to 48-hour intervals are indicated with higher grade open injuries until all nonviable soft tissues and bone are removed.
- Although closure of contaminated wounds should be avoided, whether clean wounds should be left open or closed between serial debridements is controversial.
- Immediate IM nailing of open femoral shaft fractures is indicated except when repeat access to a contaminated IM canal is required, in which case provisional external fixation is useful. IM nailing can be performed once the canal has been sufficiently cleansed.
- Intravenous (IV) antibiotics should be initiated on arrival at a care center and continued until definitive would closure.
- Routine wound culture is not indicated.

Gun Shot Fractures

Fractures of the femur as a result of gun shot wounds are technically open fractures, however, they can usually be treated as closed injuries.

- The entry and exit wounds should be debrided locally at the level of skin and subcutaneous tissue.
- The deeper tissues do not require formal irrigation and debridement.
- Fracture stabilization can thereafter follow standard treatment for closed fractures.
- The exception to this method is high-velocity gun shot wounds and shotgun blasts at close range that have severe soft-tissue compromise. In these instances, treatment should be as for other high-grade open injuries.

Vascular and Nerve Injuries

Femoral shaft fractures associated with either vascular or nerve injury are relatively uncommon (<1%) and are usually associated with penetrating trauma.

- Timing of fracture stabilization relative to vascular repair is controversial.
- Skeletal stabilization before vascular repair theoretically reduces risk of disruption of the repair compared to when stabilization is performed after vascular repair.
  - Attention to obtaining proper length should be performed before neurovascular repair.
  - The most expeditious stabilization method is usually external fixation. In the absence of pin-tract infection, conversion to IM nailing within 2 weeks can be performed safely. Great care should be taken to avoid disruption of the soft-tissue repair during the secondary nailing procedure.
  - Another expeditious alternative is retrograde nailing with interlocking deferred until after neurovascular repair.
- Vascular repair before skeletal stabilization decreases ischemic time and has been shown to reduce the need for associated fasciotomy. The theoretic risk of repair disruption during subsequent fracture fixation has not been evident based on results of small case series.[12,13]

Compartment Syndrome

Compartment syndrome associated with femoral shaft fracture is uncommon. However, a heightened index of suspension for compartment syndrome should accompany injuries with a crushing mechanism, prolonged compression, vascular injury, systemic hypotension, and coagulopathy.

- When a clinical diagnosis of compartment syndrome is made, fasciotomy should be preformed emergently.
- Compartment pressure measurements can be used as an adjunct to clinical diagnosis, especially in obtunded patients.

Obese Patients

It is estimated that approximately 30% to 40% of adults in the United States will soon be considered obese. Difficulty in obtaining a proper starting point for antegrade femoral nailing in obese patients is responsible for increased number of complications when nailing with an entry site through the piriformis fossa in this patient population.

- Better results have been obtained with nailing through the tip of the greater trochanter[14] especially with newer implants that have a proximal lateral bend designed for this insertion site.[15]
- Obesity is a relative indication for retrograde nailing.

Floating Knee (Ipsilateral Associated Tibia Fracture)

This combination of fractures is usually associated with high-energy trauma.

- Good results, similar to those found after high-energy isolated injury, have been obtained with retrograde nailing of the femur followed by antegrade nailing of the tibia through a single anterior knee approach.[16]

Ipsilateral Proximal and Shaft Fractures

Ipsilateral proximal femur fracture and femoral shaft fracture are uncommon, with the association occurring in approximately 5% of all femoral shaft fractures (Figure 15–5A). However when present they have been shown to be missed in up to 30% of cases.

- All patients with femoral shaft fracture should be evaluated for ipsilateral proximal femur fracture. Missed proximal components can lead to complications especially when displacement of an initially nondisplaced femoral neck fracture occurs. Nonunion, malunion, or AVN can be disastrous when occurring in young patients. These complications can be avoided with timely recognition and operative stabilization of both fractures.
- A femoral neck component of such injuries is of the highest priority for optimal but not necessarily initial, stabilization.
- Separate treatment with retrograde nailing or plating of the shaft combined with standard fixation of the proximal fracture is associated with the best results.[17]
- Reduction of the femoral neck fracture can be difficult without an intact shaft component.
- Provisional fixation of the femoral neck before retrograde nailing, such as with guidewires for cannulated screws, can help avoid further displacement during the retrograde nailing portion of the procedure (Figure 15–5B).
- Control of the shaft component, obtained after locked retrograde nailing (Figure 15–5C, D, E, F, and G), facilitates reduction of the proximal fracture either with manual traction or subsequent placement of the limb in traction on a fracture table.
- Simultaneous treatment of the proximal and shaft fractures using a single IM device in reconstruction mode is another alternative but is technically difficult and is associated with a higher complication rate especially when applied for an associated femoral neck fracture.

- Femoral neck fractures, when associated with shaft fractures, are most often vertically oriented. This fracture pattern is subject to high shear forces and has little inherent stability. A sliding hip screw construct with a derotation screw may provide improved biomechanics over cannulated lag screws for these vertical fractures.

Periprosthetic Femoral Shaft Fracture

The incidence of periprosthetic femoral fractures has risen over the last decade concurrent with the aging population and the increasing number of arthroplasties being performed.

- The optimal management strategies remain unclear as an array of treatment options are described in the literature without a clear consensus emerging on the most appropriate method.[18,19] Most recently, treatment has focused on open reduction with internal fixation (ORIF) or revision arthroplasty procedures with or without supplementary autologous or allogeneic bone grafting.[20–22]
- A successful approach to the management of periprosthetic femur fractures must consider the fracture location relative to the femoral component, the implant stability, the quality of the surrounding bone, and the medical and functional status of the patient.[23]
- Fractures about well-fixed femoral implants do not require revision arthroplasty. Stabilization with ORIF using lateral plates secured with screws through native bone and cables in the zone of the IM implant (Figure15-6) is the preferred method.[24–27] Screws in the trochanteric region and unicortical locked screws in the region of the IM implant may be used as adjuncts to cables.
- Plate osteosynthesis combined with a cortical strut allograft placed subperiosteally 90 degrees from the plate requires extensive disruption of periosteal soft tissues, which can adversely effect fracture healing.
- Contemporary fracture fixation techniques, which minimize soft-tissue disruption and periosteal stripping, using a single lateral plate without structural allograft have been successfully applied to the treatment of periprosthetic femoral shaft fractures about stable IM implants.[28]
- Fracture about a loose hip arthroplasty stem usually requires revision arthroplasty. Long noncemented stems provide IM stabilization. Adjuvant structural allografting is indicated to treat associated cortical bone defects. Lateral plate fixation is indicated when adequate stabilization can not be obtained by IM means.

Complications
Malalignment

Malalignment of femoral shaft fractures is usually related to lapses in surgical technique. Careful preoperative planning, execution, and postoperative evaluation are necessary to provide optimal fracture alignment. Whenever possible,

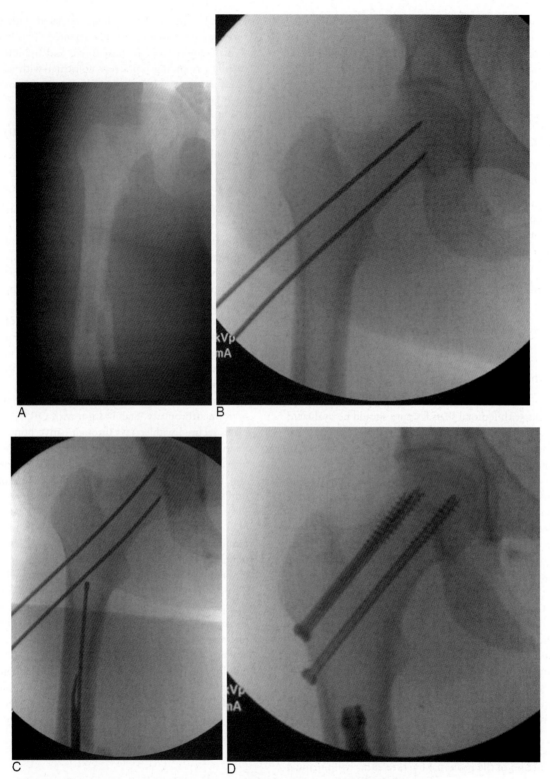

Figure 15–5: Ipsilateral femoral shaft and femoral neck fractures. **A,** Anteroposterior radiograph depicting ipsilateral femoral neck and shaft fractures. **B,** Provisional stabilization of the neck component with terminally treaded 2.7-mm wires. **C,** Retrograde nailing being performed after provisional stabilization of the neck component. **D, E,** Anteroposterior and lateral fluoroscopic views showing definitive fixation of the femoral neck.

(Continued)

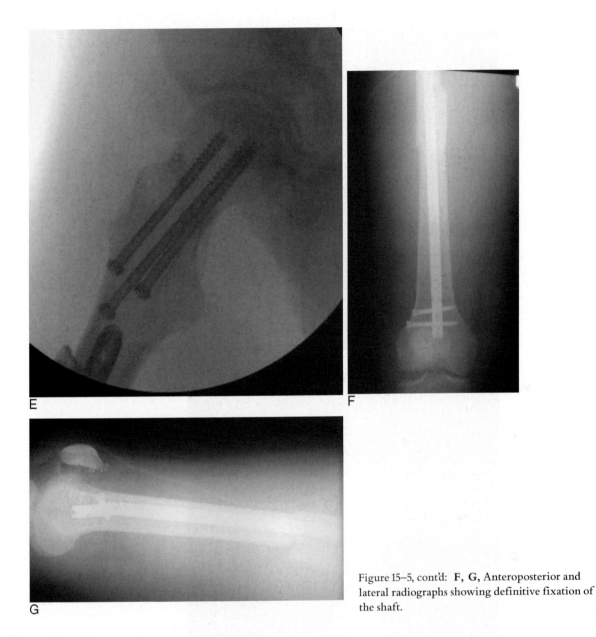

E

F

G

Figure 15–5, cont'd: **F, G,** Anteroposterior and lateral radiographs showing definitive fixation of the shaft.

malalignment should be identified and treated before leaving the operative suite after the index procedure to avoid a secondary surgical procedure.

- Limb length can be difficult to properly determine in patients with comminuted fractures. In such instances, careful clinical or radiographic comparison to the uninjured limb is indicated.
- Rotational symmetry compared to the uninjured limb should be performed immediately after definitive fracture stabilization before leaving the operating suite. When rotational malalignment is identified, immediate correction should be performed.
- Coronal and sagittal plane alignment is closely related to surgical precision, the location of the fracture, the relative location of the fracture, and the starting point for nailing.[29] During IM nailing of any long-bone fracture,

proper sagittal and coronal plane alignment can be obtained when the nail is aligned with the central axis of both the proximal and distal fracture fragments.

- With IM nailing, fractures of the middle third of the shaft are the easiest to reduce and have a low incidence of angular malalignment (2%). The narrow isthmus, which is located at the proximal portion of the middle third of the shaft, serves to align the proximal and distal fracture fragments.
- Fractures of the proximal third are the most difficult to reduce and are at highest risk of malalignment usually consisting of flexion or varus deformity in up to 30% of cases.
- Distal-third fractures are associated with an intermediate risk of malalignment up to 10%.
- Antegrade nailing can facilitate improved reduction for proximal fractures and retrograde nailing for distal fractures.

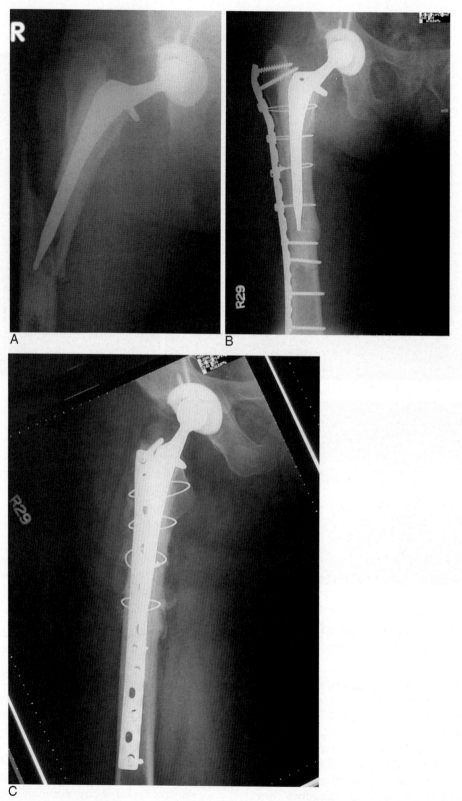

Figure 15–6: Periprosthetic femoral shaft fracture. **A,** Injury radiographs shows fracture involving the tip of the well fixed femoral stem. **B, C,** Anteroposterior and lateral radiographs show the healed fracture after treatment with a lateral plate without structural allograft.

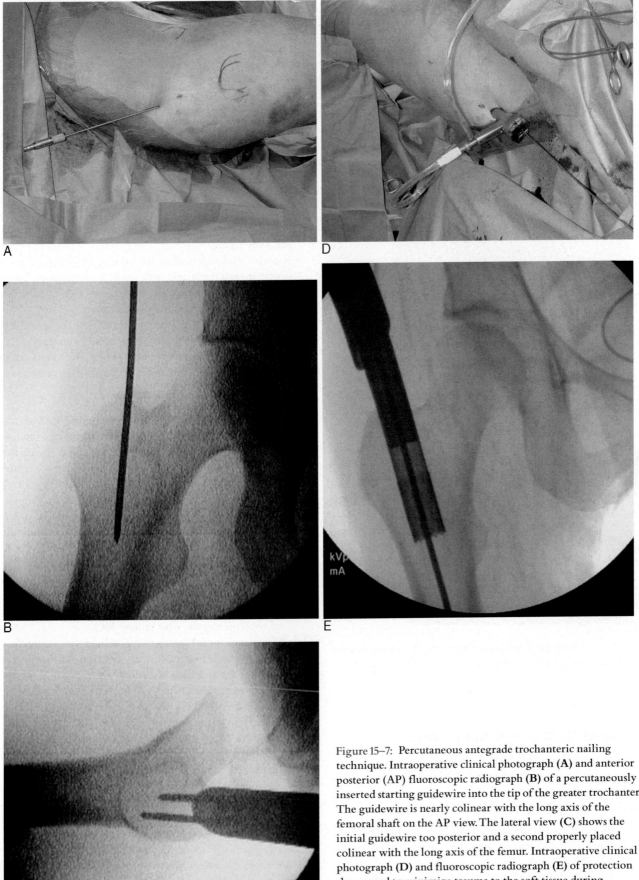

Figure 15–7: Percutaneous antegrade trochanteric nailing technique. Intraoperative clinical photograph (**A**) and anterior posterior (AP) fluoroscopic radiograph (**B**) of a percutaneously inserted starting guidewire into the tip of the greater trochanter. The guidewire is nearly colinear with the long axis of the femoral shaft on the AP view. The lateral view (**C**) shows the initial guidewire too posterior and a second properly placed colinear with the long axis of the femur. Intraoperative clinical photograph (**D**) and fluoroscopic radiograph (**E**) of protection sleeve used to minimize trauma to the soft tissue during instrumentation of the femoral canal. **E,** Lateral radiograph shows one guidewire too posterior and one properly placed colinear with the long axis of the femur.

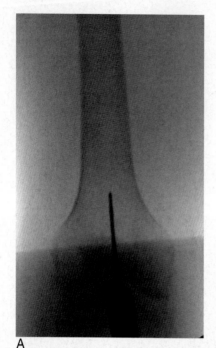

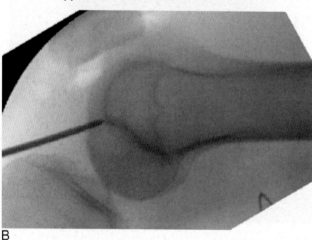

Figure 15–8: Retrograde nailing technique. **A, B,** Anteroposterior and lateral radiographs depicting the proper starting point for retrograde nailing.

Delayed Unions and Nonunions

Healing complications, such as delayed unions and nonunions, can be expected in 5% to 10% of patients with femoral shaft fracture. It is incumbent on the surgeon to take steps to avoid such complications.

- Gaps between fracture ends, especially for transverse and oblique fracture patterns, should be avoided. This can be accomplished with "back or forward slapping" during IM nailing. Failure to achieve close abutment of fracture ends can be the result of improper rotational alignment.

In such cases, adjustment of rotation often leads to anatomic abutment of the fracture ends. Anatomic alignment of the endosteal and periosteal cortical lines helps to confirm proper rotation.

- Dynamization can be employed for the treatment of delayed unions treated with IM nails. However its effectiveness remains unproven. It should be reserved for axially stable fracture patterns to avoid undesirable shortening. Dynamization of a retrograde femoral nail should be performed by removing proximal rather than distal interlocking screws so that the nail will not back into the knee joint.
- Reamed exchange nailing has been successful in achieving union in approximately 40% to 80% of cases of femoral nonunion and is one of the treatments of choice, particularly in the absence of angular deformity.
- Compression plating with judicious use of autologous bone graft is also an effective treatment modality.[30] It is a particularly attractive option when exchange nailing has failed or when deformity correction is necessary.

Functional Disability

- Pain and functional disability after femoral shaft fracture can occur regardless of the mode of treatment. Soft-tissue injury associated with the initial fracture, particularly injury to the quadriceps muscles, can lead to persistent pain and knee contracture. Pain and disability can also be related to the surgical procedure. Although nailing is considered the gold standard method of treatment of femoral shaft fractures, it is not without associated morbidity.
- Antegrade femoral nailing can be associated with hip disfunction and hip pain in up to 40% of patients.[31,32]
  - Heterotopic ossification (HO) and prominent implants increase the incidence of these complications.
  - Thorough irrigation of the surgical wound and the use of tissue protectors may reduce HO.
  - Whenever possible, the nail should be countersunk beneath bone to minimize soft-tissue irritation and related pain and muscle dysfunction.
- Retrograde femoral nailing is associated with more problems related to the knee and less related to the hip as compared to antegrade nailing.
  - Injury to the patella-femoral articulation can be avoided with retrograde nailing by countersinking the nail beneath the articular surface.
  - Retrograde nails should be locked with at least two distal interlocking bolts, especially for axially unstable fractures, to avoid migration of the nail into the knee joint.
- Interlocking screws should not be left protruding through bone, especially about the medial side of the knee.
- Adequate rehabilitation with attention to abductor, quadriceps, and hamstring strengthening can reduce muscle dysfunction.

Other Complications

Other complications associated with treatment of femoral shaft fractures are unusual but can be serious.

- Femoral neck fracture is perhaps the most serious complication relating to femoral nailing. A proper starting point for antegrade nailing (avoiding an anterior piriformis fossa starting point) and careful preoperative evaluation for occult fractures should help reduce the risk of this complication.
- Use of the hemi-lithotomy position for antegrade femoral nailing increases compartment pressures in the well leg. Prolonged use of this position should be used with caution to avoid contralateral leg compartment syndrome, especially in patients with injury to the contralateral limb.
- Excessive and prolonged traction against a peroneal post should be avoided to minimize the risk of pudendal and sciatic nerve injury from compression and stretch, respectively

Annotated References

1. Winquist RA, Hansen ST, Clawson DK: Closed intramedullary nailing of femoral fractures, *J Bone Joint Surg Am* 66:529-539, 1984.
Classic study of 520 femoral shaft fractures treated with antegrade nailing. Results that included a union rate of 99.1% and an infection rate of 0.9% established intramedullary (IM) femoral nailing as the treatment of choice for this injury.

2. Orthopaedic Trauma Association: Fracture and dislocation compendium, *J Orthop Trauma* 10:1-55, 1996.
Supplement to the *Journal of Orthopaedic Trauma* that describes and illustrates the official fracture classification system adopted by the Orthopaedic Trauma Association.

3. Yang KH, Han DY, Park HW, et al: Fracture of the ipsilateral neck of the femur in shaft nailing: the role of CT in diagnosis, *J Bone Joint Surg B* 80:673-678, 1998.
A combined retrospective and prospective analysis of 152 femoral shaft nailings. Fourteen ipsilateral neck fractures were ultimately identified. Eight were initially missed. Six of these eight undisplaced fractures were shown to have been present before operation by retrospective review of abdominal computed tomography (CT) scans. The other two were thought to be iatrogenic from the intramedullary (IM) nailing procedure. Routine CT scans were advocated for high-risk patients.

4. Blacksin MF, Zurlo JV, Levy AS: Internal derangement of the knee after ipsilateral femoral shaft fracture: MR imaging findings. *Skeletal Radiol* 27:434-439, 1998.
Magnetic resonance imaging (MRI) of the ipsilateral knee was performed on 34 patients with closed femoral shaft fractures who also had knee pain at the time of fracture, soft-tissue swelling or an effusion of the knee, or a positive knee examination under anesthesia. Twenty-seven percent of patients demonstrated meniscal tears, 38% medial collateral ligament injury, 21% posterior cruciate ligament injury, and 32% bone bruises.

5. McKee MD, Waddell JP: Intramedullary nailing of femoral fractures in morbidly obese patients, *J Trauma* 36:208-210, 1994.
Intraoperative and postoperative complications were found to be numerous in seven patients who underwent reamed femoral nailing and met the criteria for morbid obesity. Problems included difficulty in establishing a start point that resulted in two fractures of the greater trochanter, and one partial trochanteric osteotomy was necessary for access in a third patient.

6. Dora C, Leunig M, Beck M, et al: Entry point soft tissue damage in antegrade femoral nailing: a cadaver study, *J Orthop Trauma* 15:488-493, 2001.
A cadaver evaluation that compared soft-tissue injury for different starting portals during antegrade femoral nailing. The piriformis fossa, although geometrically ideal and most recommended, caused the most significant damage to muscle and tendons and to the blood supply to the femoral head.

7. Ricci WM, Schwappach J, Coupe K, et al: Trochanteric vs. piriformis entry portal for the treatment of femoral shaft fractures. Annual Meeting of the Orthopaedic Trauma Association, 2004.
A prospective analysis of 108 patients treated with antegrade femoral nailing with either a piriformis or trochanteric nail entry portal. A femoral nail specially designed for trochanteric insertion resulted in equally high union rates, equally low complication rates, and functional results similar to conventional antegrade femoral nailing through the piriformis fossa. As a result of increased ease of insertion, decreased operative time, and decreased fluoroscopy time, the greater trochanter entry portal coupled with an appropriately designed nail represents a rational alternative for antegrade femoral nailing.

8. McConnell T, Tornetta P III, Benson E, et al: Gluteus medius tendon injury during reaming for gamma nail insertion, *Clin Orthop Relat Res* 199-202, 2003.
A cadaveric study that quantified damage to the gluteus medius tendon secondary to reaming of the greater trochanter necessary for safe Gamma nail insertion. In 27 of 34 specimens, the portal was contained completely within the tendinous insertion of the gluteus medius. The percentage of the tendon insertion disrupted by the reamer ranged from 14.8% to 52.5% with an average of 27%. During appropriate placement of the Gamma nail, damage to the gluteus medius tendon is unavoidable and should be recognized as a potential cause of postoperative morbidity.

9. Ricci WM, Bellabarba C, Evanoff B, et al: Retrograde versus antegrade nailing of femoral shaft fractures, *J Orthop Trauma* 15:161-169, 2001.
Two hundred eighty-three consecutive adult patients with 293 fractures of the femoral shaft who underwent stabilization with antegrade (153 cases) or retrograde (140 cases) inserted femoral nails were studied. Retrograde and antegrade nailing techniques provided similar results for union (88% to 89%) and malunion (11% to 13%) rates. There were more complications related to the knee after retrograde nailing and more complications related to the hip after antegrade nailing.

10. Moed BR, Watson JT: Retrograde intramedullary nailing, without reaming, of fractures of the femoral shaft in multiply injured patients, *J Bone Joint Surg Am* 77:1520-1527, 1995.
Twenty patients with multiple injuries who had a total of 22 fractures of the femoral shaft were managed with retrograde intramedullary (IM) nailing without reaming. Normal motion of

the knee was regained by all patients, except one who had had an ipsilateral dislocation of the knee.

11. Ostrum RF, DiCicco J, Lakatos R, et al: Retrograde intramedullary nailing of femoral diaphyseal fractures, *J Orthop Trauma* 12:464-468, 1998.

A prospective, consecutive series of 61 femur fractures treated with reamed retrograde nailing. There was a 95% union rate after nailing and dynamization as necessary. No knee problems were associated with the retrograde femoral intramedullary (IM) nailing technique.

12. McHenry TP, Holcomb JB, Aoki N, et al: Fractures with major vascular injuries from gunshot wounds: implications of surgical sequence, *J Trauma* 53:717-721, 2002.

A retrospective review was performed of 27 patients over a 10-year period requiring acute revascularization and fracture fixation for isolated gunshot wound injuries (17 lower and 10 upper extremity). Fracture fixation preceded vascular repair in 5 cases, whereas revascularization preceded bone fixation in 22 cases. There were no cases of vascular repair, shunt disruption, or amputation after fracture fixation. Four of five (80%) patients with orthopedic fixation before revascularization required fasciotomies, whereas 8 of 22 (36%) patients with revascularization before fixation required fasciotomies.

13. Braten M, Helland P, Myhre HO, et al: 11 femoral fractures with vascular injury: good outcome with early vascular repair and internal fixation, *Acta Orthop Scand* 67:161-164, 1996.

A review of 11 consecutive cases with combined femoral fracture and vascular injury presenting with acute ischemia. Vascular repair preceded fracture stabilization in five cases; there were no vascular complications during the subsequent fracture stabilization.

14. Ostrum RF: A greater trochanteric insertion site for femoral intramedullary nailing in lipomatous patients, *Orthopedics* 19:337-340, 1996.

A review of the treatment of 12 femoral shaft fractures and three nonunions in lipomatous patients who had a greater trochanteric insertion point for intramedullary (IM) nailing. Combined with a small proximal extension of the incision, maximal limb adduction, and a slotted IM nail, the greater trochanteric insertion point was effective, and no complications directly related to this procedure were encountered.

15. Ricci W, Devinney S, Haidukewych G, et al: Trochanteric nail insertion for the treatment of femoral shaft fractures, *J Orthop Trauma* 19:511-517, 2005.

A study of 61 consecutive patients with femoral shaft fractures treated with antegrade nailing using a nail specifically designed for trochanteric insertion. Union occurred in all but one fracture after the index procedure. No patient sustained iatrogenic fracture comminution, and there were no angular malunions. Pain was reported as slight in six patients and moderate in two.

16. Gregory P, DiCicco J, Karpik K, et al: Ipsilateral fractures of the femur and tibia: treatment with retrograde femoral nailing and unreamed tibial nailing, *J Orthop Trauma* 10:309-316, 1996.

Twenty-six fractures treated with intramedullary (IM) fixation of both a femoral and tibial shaft fractures using a technique of retrograde insertion of a femoral nail and unreamed insertion of an interlocking tibial nail. The femoral nails were placed either through the medial femoral condyle (*n* = 14) or the

intercondylar notch of the distal femur (*n* = 12). No significant knee problem related to the femoral nailing technique was identified. Thirteen additional operative procedures were required in five complicated tibiae (one nail dynamization, six debridement procedures, five bone grafts, and one muscle flap) after the initial hospitalization. Five additional operative procedures were required in the three complicated femora (two nail dynamizations, one bone graft, and two exchange nailing procedures).

17. Watson JT, Moed BR: Ipsilateral femoral neck and shaft fractures: complications and their treatment, *Clin Orthop* 78-86, 2002.

A retrospective review of 13 patients who had healing complications develop after surgical treatment of ipsilateral femoral neck and shaft fractures. Lag screw fixation of the neck with reamed intramedullary (IM) nailing of the shaft were associated with the fewest complications.

18. Lewallen DG, Berry DJ: Periprosthetic fracture of the femur after total hip arthroplasty: treatment and results to date, *Instr Course Lect* 47:243-249, 1998.

19. Kolstad K: Revision THR after periprosthetic femoral fractures: an analysis of 23 cases. *Acta Orthop Scand* 65:505-508, 1994.

20. Haddad FS, Marston RA, Muirhead-Allwood SK: The Dall-Miles cable and plate system for periprosthetic femoral fractures, *Injury* 28:445-447, 1997.

21. Radcliffe SN, Smith DN: The Mennen plate in periprosthetic hip fractures, *Injury* 27:27-30, 1996.

22. Chandler HP, Tigges RG: The role of allografts in the treatment of periprosthetic femoral fractures, *Instr Course Lect* 47:257-264, 1998.

23. Duncan CP, Masri BA: Fractures of the femur after hip replacement, *Instr Course Lect* 44:293-304, 1995.

24. Wong P, Gross AE: The use of structural allografts for treating periprosthetic fractures about the hip and knee, *Orthop Clin North Am* 30:259-264, 1999.

25. Brady OH, Garbuz DS, Masri BA, et al: The treatment of periprosthetic fractures of the femur using cortical onlay allograft struts, *Orthop Clin North Am* 30:249-257, 1999.

26. Tower SS, Beals RK: Fractures of the femur after hip replacement: the Oregon experience. *Orthop Clin North Am* 30:235-247, 1999.

27. Haddad FS, Duncan CP, Berry DJ, et al: Periprosthetic femoral fractures around well-fixed implants: use of cortical onlay allografts with or without a plate, *J Bone Joint Surg Am* 84:945-950, 2002.

28. Ricci WM, Bolhofner BR, Loftus T, et al: Indirect reduction and plate fixation, without grafting, for periprosthetic femoral shaft fractures about a stable intramedullary implant, *J Bone Joint Surg Am* 87:2240-2245, 2005.

Fifty consecutive patients with periprosthetic femoral shaft fractures about a stable intramedullary (IM) implant were treated with a protocol that included open reduction and internal fixation (ORIF) using indirect reduction techniques and fixation with a single lateral plate without structural allograft. All fractures healed in satisfactory alignment after the index procedure at an average of 12 weeks. Thirty of the 41 patients returned to their baseline ambulatory status. The results of this study support the use of ORIF of periprosthetic femoral shaft fractures about a stable IM implant using indirect reduction methods and a single extraperiosteal lateral fixation plate, without the use of allograft struts.

29. Ricci WM, Bellabarba C, Lewis R, et al: Angular malalignment after intramedullary nailing of femoral shaft fractures, *J Orthop Trauma* 15:90-95, 2001.

A review of femoral shaft fractures treated with antegrade (183 cases) or retrograde (174 cases) intramedullary (IM) femoral nailing. A multiple linear regression statistical analysis determined that proximal fracture location, distal fracture location, and unstable fracture pattern were associated with increasing fracture angulation, whereas fracture location in the middle third, stable fracture pattern, method of treatment (i.e., antegrade or retrograde), and nail diameter were not. The incidence of malalignment was 9% for the entire group of patients, 30% when the fracture was of the proximal third of the femoral shaft, 2% when the fracture was of the middle third, and 10% when the fracture was of the distal third.

30. Bellabarba C, Ricci WM, Bolhofner BR: Results of indirect reduction and plating of femoral shaft nonunions after intramedullary nailing, *J Orthop Trauma* 15:254-263, 2001.

A consecutive series of 23 patients with femoral shaft nonunion after intramedullary (IM) nailing. All were treated with indirect plating techniques and judicious use of autologous bone graft. Twenty-one of the 23 nonunions healed without further intervention at an average of 12 weeks.

31. Bain GI, Zacest AC, Paterson DC, et al: Abduction strength following intramedullary nailing of the femur, *J Orthop Trauma* 11:93-97, 1997.

Hip abductor function, strength, and complaints following insertion of a femoral intramedullary nail were studied in 32 patients who had an intramedullary (IM) nail inserted for an isolated femoral shaft fracture and compared to normal controls. Complaints included trochanteric pain (40%), thigh pain (10%), and limp (13%). There was significant difference in the abduction strength ($P < 0.01$) and abduction ratio ($P < 0.01$) between the control and the treatment group.

32. Biyani A, Jones DA, Daniel CL, et al: Assessment of hip abductor function in relation to peritrochanteric heterotopic ossification after closed femoral nailing, *Injury* 24:97-100, 1993.

The power of hip abduction and the presence or absence of heterotopic ossification was assessed in 25 patients who had undergone antegrade femoral nailing. Clinically important abductor weakness was more likely to be the result of ipsilateral fractures or a long nail rather than heterotopic ossification.

33. The Canadian Orthopaedic Trauma Society: Nonunion following intramedullary nailing of the femur with and without reaming: results of a multicenter randomized clinical trial, *J Bone Joint Surg Am* 85:2093-2096, 2003.

A multicenter, prospective, randomized trial of 224 patients to compare reamed and nonreamed femoral nailing. Nonunion occurred in 7.5% of the nonreamed group and only 1.7% of the reamed group.

34. Johnson KD, Tencer AF, Sherman MC: Biomechanical factors affecting fracture stability and femoral bursting in closed intramedullary nailing of femoral shaft fractures, with illustrative case presentations, *J Orthop Trauma* 1:1-11, 1987.

A study that defined the effect of starting hole position, fracture component length, reamed diameter, and nail type on the potential for femoral bursting and fracture instability. The most significant factor in the proximal femoral component was found to be the position of the starting hole. Anterior displacement by greater than 6 mm from the neutral axis of the medullary canal consistently caused high hoop stresses at the level of the fracture, which resulted in bursting of the proximal femoral component by lifting off the anterior cortex. Hoop stresses at the level of the fracture were less sensitive to lateral or medial placement of the starting hole

CHAPTER 16

Distal Femur Fractures

Brett R. Bolhofner, MD

- Distal femur fractures involve the distal 15 cm of the femur, which includes the epiphyseal or articular segment and the distal femoral metaphysis.
- These fractures account for approximately 6% of femur fractures.

Anatomy

- The condyles are trapezoidal in shape and are narrower anteriorly and wider posteriorly.
- The popliteal artery passes from medial to posterior about 10 cm above the knee joint and so is posterior in most distal femoral fractures.
- The quadriceps produce shortening across the fracture site, and the gastrocnemius muscles produce posterior angulation of the articular segment.
- The knee joint axis is parallel to the ground, and the axis of the distal femur is about 7 degrees compared to the vertical axis.
- The sciatic nerve is directly posterior in the distal femur.

Etiology

- Generally, there is a bimodal distribution between younger patients with high-energy injuries and older patients with low-energy injuries.[1]
- Older patients are predominantly women[1] who sustain ground-level falls.
- Periprosthetic injuries around and above total knee prostheses are becoming more common and are generally low energy.
- High-energy injuries are usually the result of direct trauma to the flexed knee.

Associated Problems

- High-energy injuries may be associated with ligament and tibial plateau injuries.
- High-energy injuries may be associated with a vascular injury.

Classification

- The most commonly used current classification is the Arbeitsgemeinschaft für Osteosynthesfragen (AO) classification[2] (Figure 16–1).

Diagnosis

- Clinical examination in distal femur fractures typically will be remarkable for tenderness, swelling, deformity, and crepitus.
- High-energy injuries may exhibit contusion, abrasion, laceration and vascular compromise.
- Standard anteroposterior (AP) and lateral plain radiographs are often sufficient.
- Computed tomography (CT) scan may be helpful to diagnose or more accurately define intraarticular pathology.
- Magnetic resonance imaging (MRI) may be helpful for delineating some ligamentous associated injuries.

Treatment

- Nonoperative treatment is currently primarily reserved for nondisplaced fractures and in people who are not surgical candidates as a result of medical conditions because of poorer results.[3] Nonoperative treatment includes traction, casting, and cast bracing.[4]
- Operative treatment is generally carried out with either a combination of plates and screws or intramedullary (IM) nails inserted in a retrograde fashion.

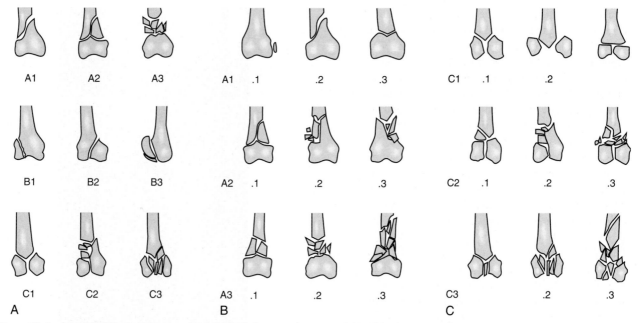

Figure 16–1: **A,** AO/OTA classification. **B,** AO/OTA A type subgroups. **C,** AO/OTA C type subgroups.

- The more difficult the fracture pattern, the more expertise is required for optimal results.
- Open fractures require standard irrigation and debridement protocols and antibiotic coverage. Fixation may be carried out primarily or secondarily depending on wound and patient conditions. A temporary spanning external fixator is a satisfactory temporizing measure in these situations.
- The goal of treatment is restoration of limb axis, knee joint, length, and full function.

Intramedullary Devices

- Satisfactory results of retrograde nailing of distal femur fractures have been reported.[5–7]
- Condylar involvement, that is AO/OTA C3-type and B-type fractures, are relative contraindications in most surgeons' hands.
- Advantages of IM devices are considered to be decreased blood loss, decreased operative times, and less periosteal stripping. The reamings may also serve as bone graft[8] (Box 16–1).
- Nonunion, delayed union, and hardware failure have been reported and may be lessened by bone grafting, larger nails, and locking screws.[7]
- Reduction must be achieved before nail insertion because the nail will not reduce the fracture. Articular fractures will need to be reduced and fixed before nail insertion. Fixation must not interfere with nail entry site.
- Possible drawbacks are difficulty changing a faulty entry site, less secure distal fixation than plate and screw devices, difficult revision in face of nonunion[9] and potential propagation of metaphyseal or diaphyseal infection into the knee joint. The consequences of retrograde entry sites are not completely known.

Box 16–1	**Retrograde Nail**

Advantages

- Decreased blood loss
- Decreased time in the operating room
- Decreased periosteum stripping
- Can be done through smaller incision
- Can load share in the right fracture pattern

Disadvantages

- Does not reduce fracture
- Difficult to use in face of intraarticular fracture patterns
- Less secure fixation of distal segment
- Increased nonunion incidence
- Salvage can be difficult
- Potential intramedullary infection propagation

Retrograde Nail Technique

- Preoperative planning using a tracing of the opposite femur, when available, is helpful. The fracture lines are drawn on the tracing in their reduced position. This is helpful for determining entry site and nail diameter and length.
- The patient is positioned supine on a radiolucent table the entire limb is draped free. A bump or triangle is used to assist in reduction and alignment. Schanz screws may be used to assist reduction.
- In fractures without joint involvement, a small distal incision, large enough to accommodate the nail and insertion instruments, is made.
- If intraarticular fractures are present and nailing is chosen, a medial parapatellar incision is necessary for exposure,

reduction, and fixation of the condyles. The condyles are secured with clamps and fixed with screws, which are typically placed percutaneously. It is critical that the anterior screws not block the nail entry site.

- The entry site for the nail is then established with a guidewire specific to the particular manufacturers nail. Position of the guidewire is verified on AP and lateral imaging. Once again, the fracture must be reduced before the guidewire and subsequent nail insertion.

- Reaming is then carried out in incremental fashion with periodic fluoroimaging. Reaming is carried out past the diaphysis into the proximal metaphysis and over reaming by 1 to 1.5 mm will be helpful for easy nail insertion and any fine tuning of length and rotation, which may ultimately be required.

- The nail is inserted over the guidewire and countersunk below the articular surface. The nail is then locked distally. The distal locking screws are generally not parallel to the joint axis as a result of the valgus orientation of the distal femur.

- The length and rotation are then verified using the opposite leg, clinical examination, and radiograph parameters.[22] The nail is then locked proximally by free hand or lucent drive technique and reexamined. Drill sleeves or trocars are helpful to protect the soft tissues.

- If length or rotation is off, the proximal locking bolts may be removed, reduction adjusted, and nail relocked. If varus or valgus are off, the entire nail must be backed out and blocking screws may be necessary to redirect the nail on reinsertion.

- Range of motion may be initiated early, but weight bearing should probably be protected initially, particularly if intraarticular fractures are present (Figure 16–2).

Plating Options and Treatment

- Plating of distal femur fractures is carried out through two basic approaches. Formal open surgery (Figure 16–3), usually via a lateral approach or alternatively, a minimally invasive approach. There are variations of the open approach including a Tarpo approach,[22] which involves a 15- to 20-cm lateral parapatellar incision for joint exposure and submuscular plate insertion. Tibial tubercle osteotomies and medial approaches are used less frequently. The minimally invasive approach involves a small lateral incision large enough for retrograde insertion of a plate and primarily used in extraarticular fracture patterns.

- Plating options are basically two-conventional and locked. Ninety-five-degree condylar blade plate dynamic, condylar compression screw, and condylar buttress plate are all conventional options. Locked plate options include less invasive stabilization system (LISS; from Synthes, Paoli, Penn.) and similar devices and locking condylar plate (from Synthes, Paoli, Penn) and similar devices. Each has its advantages and disadvantages.

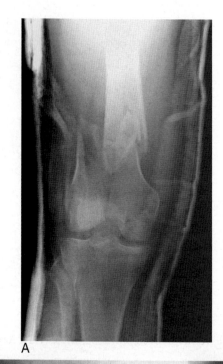

A

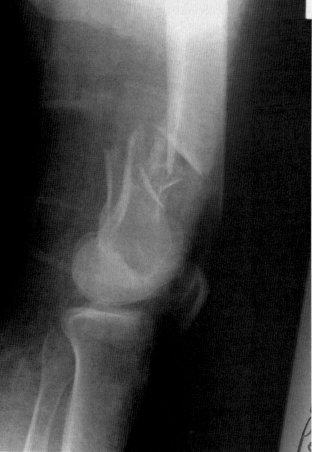

B

Figure 16–2: **A, B,** Anteroposterior and lateral X-rays of C2 **fracture.**

(Continued)

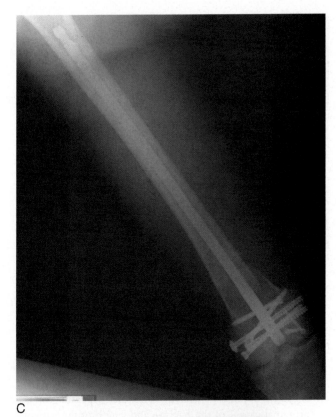

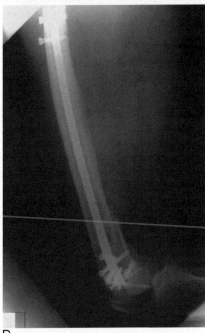

Figure 16–2, cont'd: **C, D,** Anteroposterior and lateral X-rays showing treatment with retrograde nail and lag screws. An advanced application. (Case courtesy of Dolfi Herscovici.)

Ninety-Five-Degree Condylar Plate

- Excellent results have been reported with this device used in conjunction with an open, indirect reduction technique.[10,11]
- Advantages for 95-degree plate are that it is a fixed-angle device, lends itself to preoperative planning and indirect reduction (implant used to reduce the fracture), and is bone sparing (no reaming). This implant is relatively inexpensive and easy to salvage in the case of treatment failure (Box 16–2).
- The disadvantages are that it may be difficult to use in multi-fragmentary intraarticular fracture patterns, and it requires a fairly large (4 cm) distal segment. The insertion can be considered somewhat technically demanding. (Figure 16–4).

Condylar Screw

- Good and excellent results have been reported with this device in supracondylar femur fractures.[12] This is a fixed-angle device.
- The advantages of this device include a guidewire and the ability to adjust the sagittal plane intraoperatively. It is a relatively strong implant and lends itself to preoperative planning and indirect reduction technique. It may be used with a percutaneous technique.[13] It is relatively inexpensive.
- Possible disadvantages include difficulty with use in multi-fragmentary intraarticular fractures and sagittal instability. This implant also requires a large distal segment of at least 4 cm. This implant requires the reaming away of valuable condylar bone, which may be a problem acutely and in cases of failure (Box 16–3).

Condylar Buttress Plate

- Good results have been reported in the literature[10]; however, some authors have recommended adding an adjunctive medial plate. This is not a fixed-angle device.
- The advantages of this plate are ease of use, low cost, and applicability in multifragmentary intraarticular fractures, particularly those with a coronal or Hoffa extension. It does not require a large distal segment.
- The major disadvantage of this plate is varus or valgus instability because the screws do not have a fixed relationship to the condylar head of the plate. Double plating or temporary medial or spanning external fixation may be needed to avoid early collapse[10] (Figure 16–5; Box 16–4).

Locked Plating Options

- Two basic concepts exist—systems such as LISS are applied as internal fixators and hold a reduction stationary that has been achieved by open or closed means (Box 16–5). Systems such as locking condylar plate may be used similarly or in a more conventional technique to assist in achieving

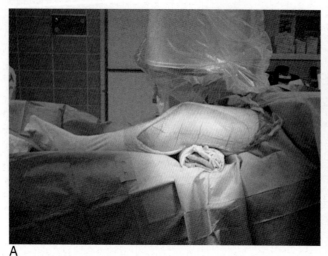
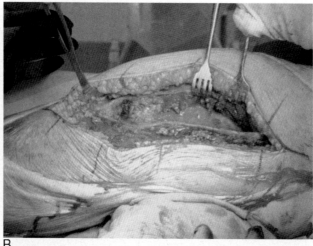

A   B

Figure 16–3: **A,** Set up showing planned incision, C-arm, limb draped free, and bump. The table is radiolucent. **B,** The vastus is retracted anteriorly, and the bone exposure is extraperiosteal.

reduction. All screws in the LISS system are locking screws, whereas locking condylar plate-type implants have combination holes, which may be locked or used with standard screws (Box 16–6).

- Locking screws in these implants allow them to become fixed-angle devices, avoiding dual plating and allowing more distal fixation and fixation in porotic bone[14] (Box 16–7).
- Ninety-three percent union without loss of distal fixation has recently been reported using the LISS system.[15] A significant learning curve is expected with this technique (Box 16–5).

Essence of Plating Technique: Indirect Reduction

- Patient is positioned supine on a radiolucent table. The entire extremity is draped out and a bump under the knee is helpful (Figure 16–3A).
- The recommended equipment includes lucent table, modern C-arm, sterile tourniquet, bone forceps including swivel-footed Verbrugge, and at least four pointed reduction clamps. A distraction or compression device, assorted

retractors including Hohman's, and the instruments for the plate of choice.

- A preoperative drawing using a tracing (reversed) of the contralateral distal femur with the fracture pattern is helpful (Figure 16–4E and F).
- A tourniquet may be used in some cases depending on the proximal extent of the fracture and length of the patient's leg. A sterile tourniquet may be a good option.
- A lateral incision and approach is developed and by elevating the vastus lateralis and the joint is subsequently exposed. (Figure 16–3B).
- The articular surface is reduced and is secured with Kirschner wires (K-wires) and small fragment screws with consideration for the location of the eventual distal plate fixation. It may be helpful to leave some bone clamps in place until the plate is applied to the distal segment.
- The plate of choice is then applied to the distal fragment in its known anatomic position according to the implant selected.
- The plate or condyle construct is then reduced to the shaft. If the plate has been applied correctly, axial alignment should be restored. Rotation and length can then be fine tuned manually or by push and pull screws.
- If the fracture pattern is conducive, the construct may then be axially loaded off a proximal push and pull screw using a clamp or compression device. This will increase stability and allow the plate to load share with the bone (Figure 16–4).

Box 16–2 Plating Options

Angle Blade Plate

Advantages

- Strong
- Useful as reduction tool
- Removes no significant bone

Disadvantages

- Requires relatively large (4 cm) distal fragment
- Difficult to use with multiple intraarticular fragments
- Technically difficult

Essence of Plating Technique: Minimally Invasive

- Patient is positioned supine on a radiolucent table. The entire extremity is draped out and a bump under the knee is helpful and additional bumps may also be helpful.

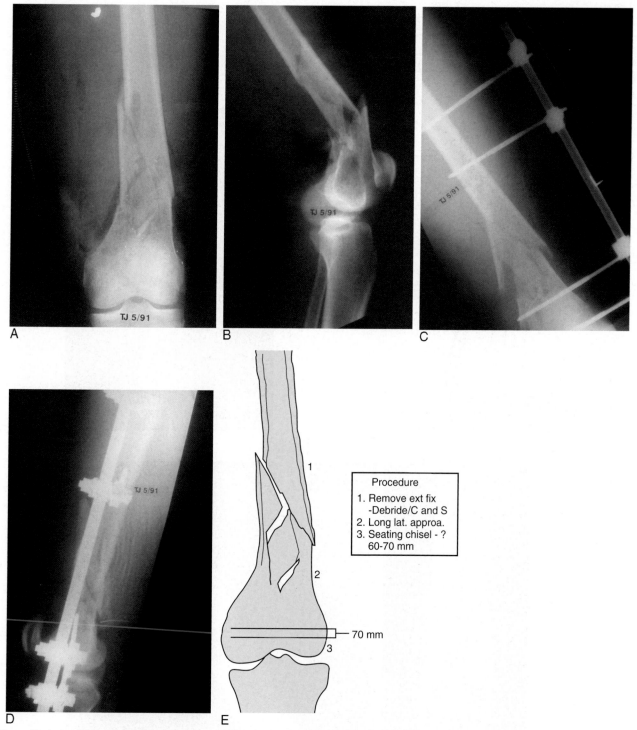

Figure 16–4, cont'd: **A, B,** A-type fracture secondary to gunshot wound. **C, D,** Same fracture with spanning external fixation. **E, F,** Preoperative plan.

- Equipment is the same as with the indirect technique except distraction and compression devices and Verbrugge will not be needed. Shantz pins and external fixation devices may be helpful to achieve and hold reduction. Instruments for the selected plating system should be well known.

- Preoperative planning is the same as with the open technique. Planning is particularly helpful for selection of implant of appropriate length.
- A small lateral or parapatellar incision is made, large enough to allow visualization of the articular surface and insertion of the plate shaft, head, and possible aiming arm.

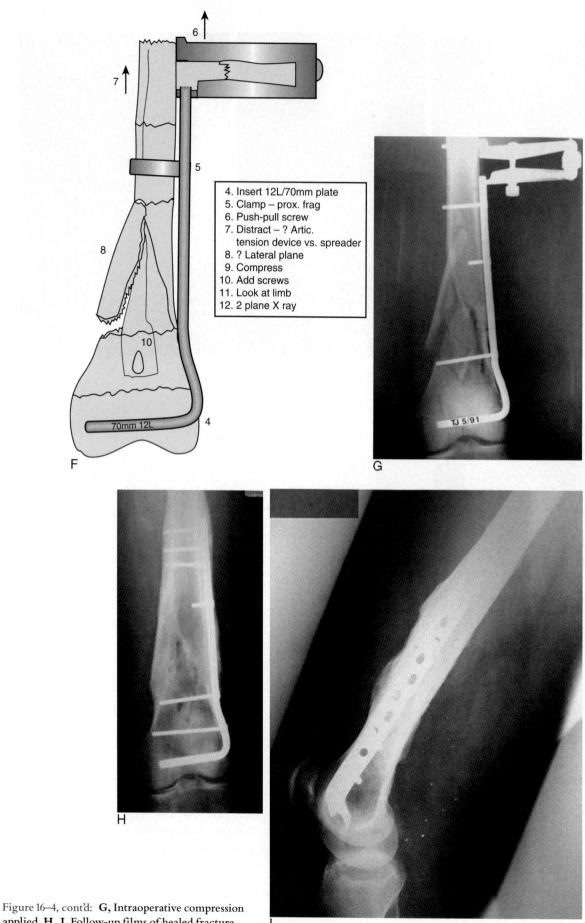

4. Insert 12L/70mm plate
5. Clamp – prox. frag
6. Push-pull screw
7. Distract – ? Artic.
   tension device vs. spreader
8. ? Lateral plane
9. Compress
10. Add screws
11. Look at limb
12. 2 plane X ray

Figure 16–4, cont'd: **G,** Intraoperative compression applied. **H, I,** Follow-up films of healed fracture.

Box 16–3 Condylar Screw

Advantages

- Strong
- Adjustable in sagittal plane
- Can be used as a reduction tool
- Uses guidewire

Disadvantages

- Removes valuable bone
- Difficult to use with multiple intraarticular fragments
- Difficult salvage
- Requires large distal segment
- Some fracture patterns may be sagittally unstable

Box 16–4 Condylar Buttress Plate

Advantages

- Inexpensive and easy to use
- Can be used with multiple intraarticular fractures

Disadvantages

- No axial or angular stability
- May need additional supporting fixation (medial plate, ex fix)

Box 16–5 Less Invasive Stabilization System or Similar Device

Advantages

- Improved fixation in porotic bone and distal fractures
- Bone and soft tissue sparing
- Can be used in any distal fracture pattern
- Minimally invasive

Disadvantages

- Learning curve may be long
- Cannot be used as a reduction tool
- Removal may be problematic
- Cannot be load sharing
- Cost

Box 16–6 Locking Condylar Type Implant

Advantages

- Can be used as a reduction tool
- Can be used with minimal invasive or standard technique
- Guidewire driven
- Can be used in any fracture pattern
- Improved fixation in porotic bone and distal fractures

Disadvantages

- Cost
- Some learning curve involved when switching from conventional plates

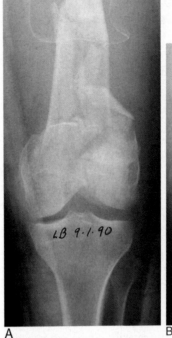
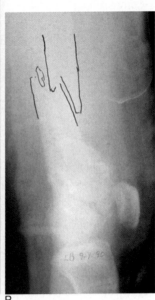
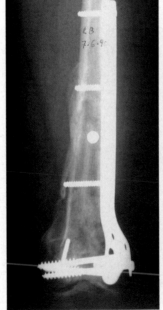
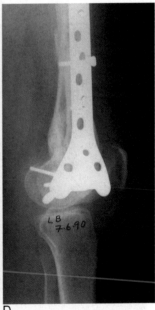

A B C D

Figure 16–5: **A, B,** Anteroposterior and lateral X-rays of C3 fracture. **C, D,** Follow-up films with condylar buttress plate.

- The condyles and articular surface are reduced and secured as in the indirect technique with attention to the eventual distal plate fixation.
- The articular or condylar segment must then be reduced to the shaft by closed or percutaneous means. The plate will generally not assist in the reduction. Rotation, length, and axial alignment must also be confirmed.

Box 16–7	Conventional versus Locked Plates

Conventional

- Cost less
- Long known history and experience
- Familiar technique
- Can be used on many fracture patterns
- Dependent on bone quality
- Difficult to use in more severe fracture patterns, small distal segments

Locked

- Cost more
- Recent history only
- New learning curve for locking screws
- Can be used in nearly all distal fracture patterns
- Independent of bone quality
- Especially useful with difficult fracture patterns, small distal segments

- The selected plate is then slid up the lateral aspect of the distal femur under the vastus lateralis. Some systems may have a handle, which can be helpful, but is not mandatory.

Reduction may be adjusted manually, with bumps or with percutaneous pins and wires (Figure 16–6).

- The plate is then secured to the bone using the specific anatomic landmarks and fluoroscopic views. Specific aiming arms or targeting devices may be available from manufacturers for specific systems. These may be helpful, but the plate may also be applied freehand (Figure 16–5).
- Some systems (e.g., locking condylar plate) may have standard screw options, which may allow the bone to be pulled to the plate, which can be helpful. A locked screw will not pull the bone to the plate and so it cannot be used as a reduction tool (Figure 16–7).

Postoperatively

- Patients are mobilized as soon as possible.
- Initial weight bearing is weight of limb for usually 4 to 8 weeks depending on clinical and radiographic healing. At this time, full weight bearing on locked plates immediately postoperatively has not been recommended.
- Active, active-assisted, and passive range-of-motion exercises are encouraged. A continuous passive motion (CPM) machine may be of some benefit.

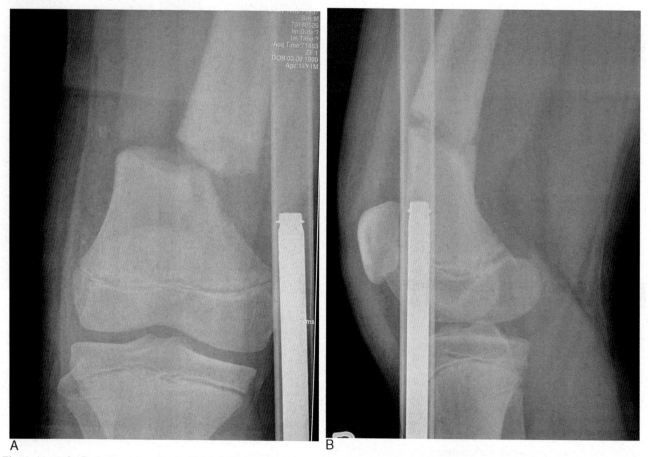

A   B

Figure 16–6: **A, B,** Anteroposterior and lateral X-rays of supracondylar fracture in a skeletally immature patient (14 years old).

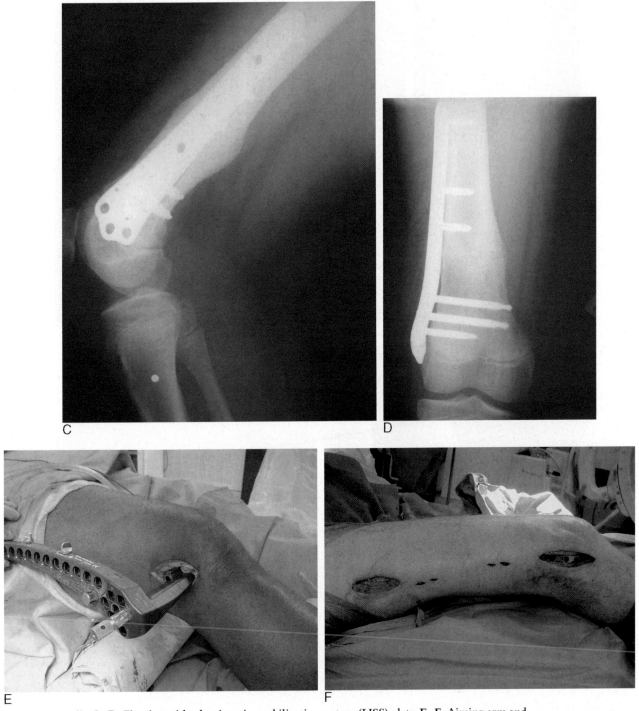

Figure 16–6, cont'd: **C, D,** Fixation with a less invasive stabilization system (LISS) plate. **E, F,** Aiming arm and limited incisions.

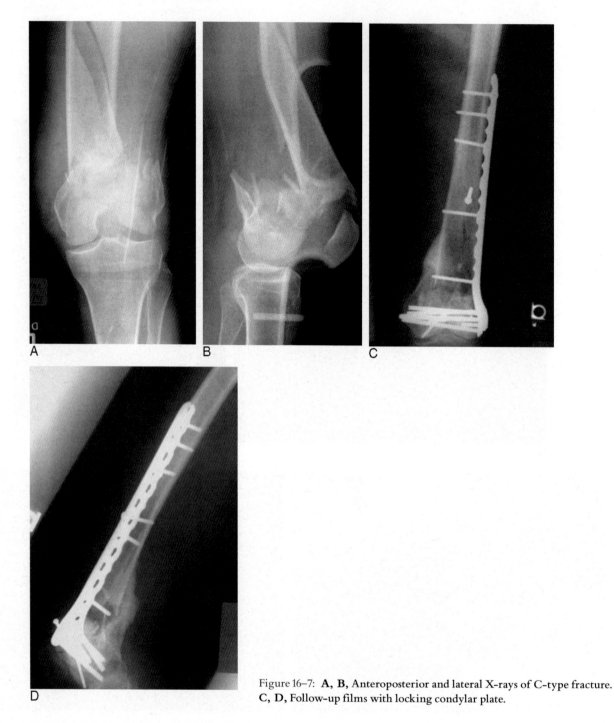

Figure 16–7: **A, B,** Anteroposterior and lateral X-rays of C-type fracture. **C, D,** Follow-up films with locking condylar plate.

- Patients should be followed at least monthly with clinical and radiographic examinations.
- Bracing may be indicated for additional ligament or soft-tissue injury or when fixation is felt to be tenuous.

Periprosthetic Fracture (above a Total Knee)

- These fractures are becoming more common and the ideal treatment has not been defined.

- Nondisplaced and minimally displaced fractures may be treated nonoperatively[16] with good results.
- Surgical problems stem from limited bone available for distal fixation.
- In displaced fractures, if the component is loose then revision surgery is indicated.[17]
- In displaced fractures with solidly fixed components, locked plating has been successful[18] (Figure 16–8).
- Retrograde nailing may be successful if allowed by prosthesis geometry,[19] but distal fixation may be tenuous.

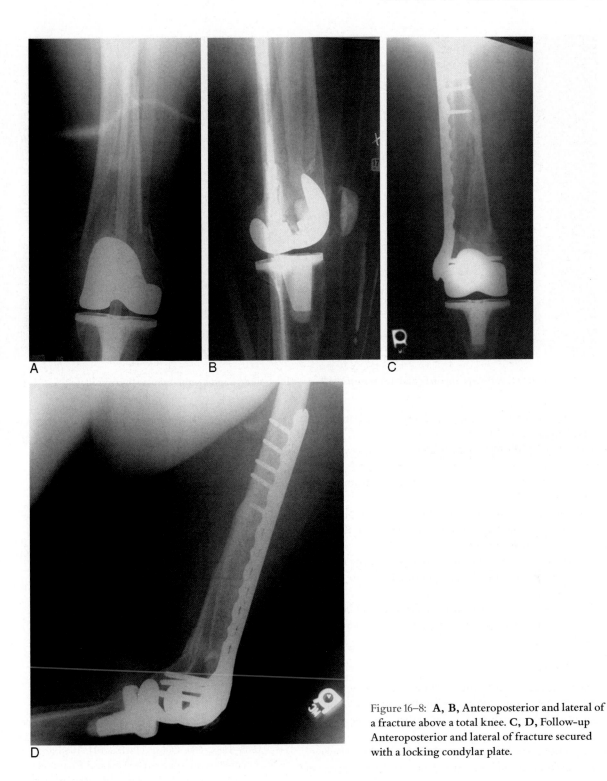

Figure 16–8: **A, B,** Anteroposterior and lateral of a fracture above a total knee. **C, D,** Follow-up Anteroposterior and lateral of fracture secured with a locking condylar plate.

Isolated Condyle (B-Type) Fractures

- These fractures are amendable to lag screw fixation or percutaneous or with open arthrotomy.
- Buttressing the lag screw fixation may be helpful to avoid secondary displacement as a result of axial shearing forces and the

relatively vertical nature of many of these fractures. (Figure 16–9)

Complications

- Infection may occur in 5% to 7% of cases with modern techniques and antibiotic prophylaxis.[10,12] Aggressive

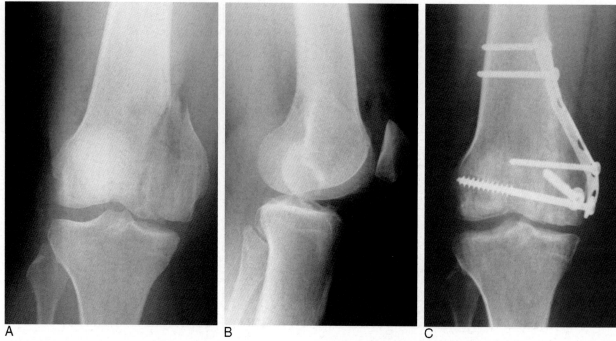

Figure 16–9: **A, B, C,** A B-type medial condyle fracture treated with lag screws and a semi-tubular buttress plate.

management with antibiotics and surgical irrigation and debridement is mandatory.

- Nonunion is probably currently about 5% to 6% with current operative techniques.[10,11,15]
- Malunion has about the same incidence and treatment has been described.[20]
- With current plating and surgical technique, implant failure is probably between 5% to 8% or roughly the same as nonunion or malunion.
- Decreased knee range of motion tends to occur in more severe fracture patterns and may ultimately require surgical intervention.
- The incidence of posttraumatic arthritis of the knee following supracondylar femur fracture is not known.

Summary

- Supracondylar femur fractures, although relatively uncommon, present some treatment challenges as a result of articular and metaphyseal comminution and poor bone quality in many cases.
- Several treatment options are available, each with advantages and disadvantages and are dependent, to a large degree, on the fracture pattern and surgical experience (Box 16–8).
- Because these injuries are relatively uncommon, a treatment technique and implant that can be used for most, if not all fractures, should be considered.
- Good results are possible with traditional and minimally invasive techniques.
- Locking plates appear to offer some advantages for these cases, and early results are promising.

Box 16–8 **Fracture Type**

- A
- B
- C1 and C2
- C3

Fixation Options

- Conventional plate, retrograde nail, and locking plate (the shorter the distal segment the more treatment leans toward locking plate)
- Lag screws or buttress plates
- Conventional plates, retrograde nail, or possible locking plates
- Locking plates

Annotated References

1. Arneson TJ, Melton LJ, Lewallen DG, et al: Epidemiology of diaphyseal and distal femur fractures in Rochester, Minnesota 1965–1984, *Clin Orthop* 234:188-194, 1988.
One hundred twenty-three of 402 femoral fractures exclusive of the hip were noted. The bimodal age and mechanism of supracondylar fractures is reported.

2. Muller ME, Nazarian S, Kuch P, et al: *The comprehensive classification of fractures of long bones*, New York, 1990, Springer-Verlag.
Comprehensive fracture classification scheme. A, B, and C type distal femur fracture classification is generally accepted.

3. Healy WL, Brooker AF: Distal femoral fractures: comparison of open and closed methods of treatment, *Clin Orthop* 166-171, 1983.

Closed treatment is compared to open treatment in 98 distal femur fractures. Patients treated with open method spent less time in the hospital, had better functional results with lower nonunion rates, and had fewer complications.

4. Connolly JF: Closed management of distal femur fractures, *Instr Course Lect* 36:428-437, 1987.

Probably the last good description and argument for closed treatment. Technique for traction, closed reduction, and casting and brace treatment are detailed.

5. Leung KS, Sher W, So WS, et al: Interlocking intramedullary nailing for supracondylar and intercondylar fractures of the distal part of the femu, *J Bone Joint Surg Am* 73:332-340, 1991.

The authors report 95% good-to-excellent results in 37 A, C1 and C2 fractures. One patient had delayed union, and three cases required distal screw removal for irritation. A knee scoring system was used.

6. Butler MS, Brumback RU, Ellison TS, et al: Interlocking intramedullary nailing for ipsilateral fractures of the femoral shaft and distal part of the femur, *J Bone Joint Surg Am* 73:1492-1502, 1991.

The authors report the technique and results of locked nails combined with supplement condylar fixation in patients with shaft and distal fractures occurring ipsilaterally. They consider a coronal extension distally to be a contraindication.

7. Iannacone WM, Bennett FS, DeLong WG Jr, et al: Initial experience with treatment of supracondylar femoral fractures using the supracondylar intramedullary nail: a preliminary report, *J Orthop Trauma* 8:322-327, 1994.

This paper discussed preliminary results in 41 fractures, more than half were open. There were four nonunion and no infections. Nail size of 12 to 13 mm were recommended.

8. Danziger M, Caucci D, Zechner B, et al: Treatment of intercondylar and supracondylar distal femur fractures using the GSH supracondylar nail, *Am J Orthop* 8:684-690, 1995.

The authors describe the technique of retrograde nailing in fractures with intraarticular components. They used 6.5-mm cannulated lag screws to reconstruct the condyles prior to nailing. In 23 fractures, there was one nonunion, one delayed union, one hardware failure, and one nail impingement. No functional score was used.

9. Koval KJ, Seligson D, Roser H, et al: Distal femoral non-union and treatment with a retrograde inserted locked intramedullary nail, *J Orthop Trauma* 9:285-292, 1995.

The authors report failure of union in 9 out of 16 patients treated for nonunion with a retrograde nail. Hardware failure was common.

10. Krettek C, Tscherne H: Distal femur fractures. In FH Fu, CD Harner, KG Vince, editors: *Knee surgery*, Baltimore, 1994, Williams & Wilkins.

11. Bolhofner BR, Carmen B, Clifford P: The results of open reduction and internal fixation of distal femur fractures using a biologic (indirect) reduction technique, *J Orthop Trauma* 10:372-377, 1996.

Using a scoring system, 84% good-to-excellent results were reported in 57 fractures. More severe fracture patterns did worse. Over half of the cases were done with a condylar buttress plate. All were treated with indirect reduction.

12. Ostrum R, Geel C: Indirect reduction and internal fixation of supracondylar femur fractures without bone graft, *J Orthop Trauma* 9:278-284, 1995.

Using an indirect reduction technique 86.6% good-to-excellent results using a scoring system are reported. No cases were bone grafted primarily. There were three failures.

13. Sanders R, Regazzoni P, Reudi T: Treatment of supracondylar-intraarticular fractures of the femur using a dynamic condylar screw, *J Orthop Trauma* 3:214-222, 1989.

This paper describes 71% good-to-excellent results and uses a functional knee scale. More comminuted fractures did worse. Ease of insertion and revision are listed as advantages.

14. Krettek C, Schadelmaier P, Miccau T, et al: Transarticular joint reconstruction and indirect plate osteosynthesis for complex distal femoral fractures, *Injury* 28:A31-A41, 1997.

The authors report a small series of L2 to L3 fractures treated with open reduction and internal fixation (ORIF) of the articular segment followed by sub muscular insertion of a lateral plate. The plate screws were then placed percutaneously.

15. Koval KJ, Hoehl JJ, Kummer FJ, et al: Distal femoral fixation: a biomechanical comparison of the standard condylar buttress plate, a locked buttress plate and the 95-degree blade plate, *J Orthop Trauma* 11:521-524, 1997.

The locked buttress plate was shown to have greater stability in fixation than either of the comparison plates.

16. Kregor PJ, Stannard JA, Zlowodski M, et al: Treatment of distal femur fractures using the less invasive stabilization system, *J Orthop Trauma* 18:509-520, 2004.

Ninety-three percent of fractures healed without bone grafting. Fixation failed proximally five times. Varus collapse was not a problem. There was a 6% malreduction rate. A knee score was not used.

17. Chen F, Munz MA, Bachner BS: Management of ipsilateral supracondylar femur fractures following total knee arthroplasty, *J Arthroplasty* 9:521-526, 1994.

The authors review 12 previously reported studies of 195 periprosthetic distal femur fractures. Patients with displaced fractures had poor results compared with nondisplaced cases. The authors present a treatment algorithm.

18. Henry SL: Management of supracondylar fractures proximal to total knee arthroplasty with GSH supracondylar nail, *Contemp Orthop* 31:231-238, 1995.

Five patients treated with a retrograde GSH nail for periprosthetic distal femur fractures showed improved union rates and less complications compared to previous series treated with plates and screws.

19. Ricci WM, Loftus T, Cox C, Borelli J: Locked plates combined with minimally invasive insertion technique for the treatment of periprosthetic supracondylar femur fractures above a total knee arthroplasty. *J Orthop Trauma*, 20:190-196, 2006.

20. Rolston LR, Christ DJ, Halpern A, et al: Treatment of supracondylar fractures of the femur proximal to a total knee arthroplasty, *J Bone Joint Surg Am* 77:924-931, 1955.

The authors report successful treatment of a distal periprosthetic fracture in four patients. Common prostheses are listed with their intercondylar distances.

21. Bellabarba C, Ricci W, Bolhofner B: Indirect reduction and plating of distal femoral non-unions, *J Orthop Trauma* 16:287-296, 2002.

The authors describe treatment technique and results in 20 nonunions in distal femur fractures. All cases healed and knee scores improved after treatment.

Further Reading

22. Krettek C, Micau T, Grun O, et al: Techniques for assessing limb alignment during closed reduction and internal fixation of lower extremity fractures, *Tech Orthop* 14:247-256, 1999.

The authors describe technical tricks for assessing angular length and rotational alignment during surgery. The cable technique, hyperextension test, meter stick, and hip rotation tests are illustrated.

CHAPTER 17

Knee Dislocations

Seth I. Gasser, MD

- Traumatic knee dislocations are rare, accounting for only 0.02% of all orthopaedic injuries.[1]
- The true number of knee dislocations may be grossly underestimated because this does not take into account those injuries that spontaneously reduce. Recent literature would indicate knee dislocations are much more prevalent.[2]
- A knee dislocation should be considered an orthopaedic emergency as a result of the high incidence of associated vascular injury.
- Historically, traumatic knee dislocations were treated with closed reduction and immobilization. Unfortunately, this often led to unsatisfactory clinical results.
- Today, the preferred treatment for traumatic knee dislocations includes emergent closed reduction, assessment of the neurovascular status, and surgical reconstruction or repair of the injured structures. This approach, although technically challenging, has led to a significant improvement in functional outcomes.

Definition

- A knee dislocation can be defined as a loss of articulation between the tibia and femur.
- Although knee dislocations may occur with an isolated injury to the anterior cruciate ligament (ACL) or posterior cruciate ligament (PCL),[3–5] in the vast majority of cases both cruciate ligaments and one collateral ligament are ruptured. Associated injuries are common, including damage to the posteromedial or posterolateral corner, menisci, articular cartilage, and neurovascular structures.
- Any knee with injury to three major ligaments is assumed to have sustained a dislocation.

Classification

- The anatomic position of the tibia in relation to the femur, the velocity of injury, and the length of time since injury can be used to classify traumatic knee dislocations.

Anatomic Classification

- The anatomic classification of traumatic knee dislocations is based on the position of the tibia in relation to the femur. The majority can be classified as anterior, posterior, medial, lateral, or rotatory.
- Anterior dislocations are the most common and account for approximately 40% of all traumatic knee dislocations.[1,2] The most common mechanism is a posterior directed force to the thigh with the foot fixed on the ground causing a hyperextension type injury.
- Posterior dislocations are the second most common and account for approximately 33% of all traumatic knee dislocations.[1,2] The most common mechanism of injury is a posterior directed force on the proximal tibia with the knee flexed (dashboard injury).
- Lateral dislocations account for approximately 18% of all traumatic knee dislocations and result from a valgus load.
- Medial dislocations account for approximately 4% of all traumatic knee dislocations and result from a varus load.
- Rotatory dislocations are the least common type of traumatic knee dislocation. They often occur via a twisting mechanism and result from a combination of loads described previously. There are several types of rotatory dislocations; however, posterolateral rotatory dislocations are the most common.
  - Posterolateral dislocations may be irreducible by closed means. This occurs when the medial femoral condyle buttonholes through the medial soft-tissue structures.[6–8] In addition, the torn medial collateral ligament (MCL) may be incarcerated in the joint. A "dimple sign" along the medial aspect of the knee should alert the examiner to the possibility of an irreducible rotatory dislocation.

Injury Velocity

- Knee dislocations can be divided into low-velocity and high-velocity injuries.[9]

- Low-velocity injuries are associated with sporting events whereas high-velocity injuries are often secondary to a motor vehicle accident or a fall from a height.
- High-velocity injuries are more likely to be associated with neurovascular damage, associated orthopaedic injuries, and multisystem trauma.
- Recently, a third category of ultra low-velocity knee dislocations has been described in the morbidly obese secondary to a simple fall.

Time since Injury

- Knee dislocations are classified as either acute or chronic.
- Acute dislocations are less than 3 weeks old.
- Chronic dislocations have been present for more than 3 weeks.
  - Primary repair of injured structures (such as collateral ligaments or the posterolateral corner) may not be possible after 3 weeks.
  - An open reduction may be required if the knee is left unreduced for a prolonged period of time.

Associated Injuries

- There are a multitude of associated injures that can occur with a knee dislocation.
- Vascular lesions include injury to the popliteal artery or vein and represent a true orthopaedic emergency.
  - The incidence of popliteal artery injury ranges from 32% to 45%.[10]
  - Early recognition is the key to successful treatment of vascular lesions. A delay in revascularization of 6 to 8 hours may lead to an amputation rate as high as 86%.
  - An intimal tear may result in delayed vascular compromise several days after injury and can occur with normal distal pulses.[11]
  - I recommend an arteriogram in all cases of a suspected knee dislocation.
- Neurologic injury usually involves damage to the peroneal nerve and less commonly the tibial nerve.[12]
  - Nerve injury occurs in 16% to 40% of all knee dislocations.
  - Nerve injuries range from neuropraxia (stretching of the nerve) to neurotmesis (complete transection of the nerve).
  - Peroneal nerve injuries are more common than tibial nerve injuries and are most commonly seen in association with lateral collateral ligament (LCL) and posterolateral corner (PLC) injuries.
  - A careful neurologic evaluation is mandatory for all patients with knee ligament injuries.
- Bony lesions include tibial plateau fractures, distal femoral condyle fractures, femoral and tibial shaft fractures, and avulsion fractures of the ACL, PCL, MCL, or LCL.

- Cartilage lesions include injury to the articular cartilage or menisci.
- Open knee dislocations are rare and require emergent irrigation and debridement to prevent infection.

Anatomy

- Knee stability relies on both the bony anatomy and the soft-tissue structures.
- Dynamic stabilizers include the various muscles that cross the knee joint. Static stabilizers include the bony articulation between the femoral condyles and tibial plateau, ligaments, capsule, and menisci.
- There are four major ligaments:
  - ACL
    - The ACL primarily prevents anterior translation of the tibia relative to the femur. It also functions to limit internal and external rotation with the knee in full extension. The ACL is a secondary stabilizer for varus and valgus stress in the face of a collateral ligament injury. The average size of the ACL is 33 mm × 11 mm. The ACL consists of two bundles: an anteromedial bundle, which is tight in flexion, and a posterolateral bundle, which is tight in extension. Its major blood supply comes from the middle geniculate artery.
  - PCL
    - The PCL prevents posterior translation of the tibia relative to the femur and is considered the primary static stabilizer of the knee. The average size of the PCL is 38 mm × 13 mm. The PCL consists of two bundles: an anterolateral bundle, which is tight in flexion, and a posteromedial bundle, which is tight in extension. Its major blood supply, like the ACL, comes from the middle geniculate artery.
  - MCL
    - The MCL is the primary stabilizer to valgus stress with the knee in 30 degrees of flexion. It secondarily resists anterior and posterior translation and rotation of the tibia on the femur.
  - LCL
    - The LCL is the primary stabilizer to varus stress with the knee in 30 degrees of flexion. It secondarily resists anterior and posterior translation and rotation of the tibia on the femur.
  - PLC
    - The posterolateral corner consists of the LCL, arcuate complex, the popliteus tendon, and the popliteofibular ligament. Together these structures work to prevent excessive external (posterolateral) rotation of the tibia relative to the femur. They also assist the PCL in preventing posterior tibial translation on the femur (Figure 17–1).

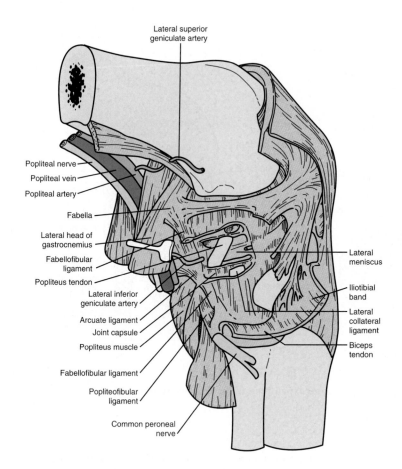

Lateral superior geniculate artery

Popliteal nerve
Popliteal vein
Popliteal artery
Fabella
Lateral head of gastrocnemius
Fabellofibular ligament
Popliteus tendon
Lateral inferior geniculate artery
Arcuate ligament
Joint capsule
Popliteus muscle
Fabellofibular ligament
Popliteofibular ligament
Common peroneal nerve

Lateral meniscus
Iliotibial band
Lateral collateral ligament
Biceps tendon

Figure 17–1: **Anatomy of the posterolateral corner of the knee.** (Davies H, Unwin A, Aichroth P: *Injury* 35, 68-75, 2004).

- Posteromedial corner
  - The posteromedial corner consists of the posterior oblique ligament and the associated posteromedial joint capsule. Together they prevent excessive internal (posteromedial) rotation of the tibia relative to the femur and assist the PCL in resisting posterior tibial translation (Figure 17–2).
- Medial and lateral menisci
  - Functions of the menisci include:
    - Load transmission
    - Shock absorption
    - Joint stability
    - Joint congruity
    - Proprioception
- Neurovascular structures
- The major neurovascular structures at risk from a knee dislocation are the popliteal artery and vein and the tibial and peroneal divisions of the sciatic nerve.
- The neurovascular structures are located within the popliteal fossa, a diamond-shaped area on the posterior aspect of the knee. The fossa is bounded superiorly and laterally by the biceps femoris and superiorly and medially by the semitendinosus, semimembranosus, gracilis, sartorius, and adductor magnus. The medial and lateral heads of the gastrocnemius closes the space distally.

- The popliteal artery is the structure most at risk. Proximally it is tethered at Hunter's canal by the adductor hiatus and distally by the soleus arch. The popliteal artery is considered an "end artery" of the lower extremity. Collateral circulation via the geniculate arteries is not sufficient to maintain viability of the leg.
- The popliteal artery is at risk for iatrogenic injury during reaming of the PCL tibial tunnel as a result of its close proximity to the back of the tibia.
- The popliteal vein is closely associated with the artery but less commonly injured.
- The sciatic nerve divides within the popliteal fossa into the peroneal and tibial divisions. These structures are less likely to be injured than the popliteal artery because they are not tethered.
- The peroneal nerve is most at risk where is crosses the fibular head. Damage to the peroneal nerve is usually associated with varus instability, which causes a traction injury. Care must be taken to avoid iatrogenic damage during dissection for repair of the LCL or PLC.

Evaluation

- Patients are often in a considerable amount of pain or have associated injuries, which makes history and physical examination difficult.[13]

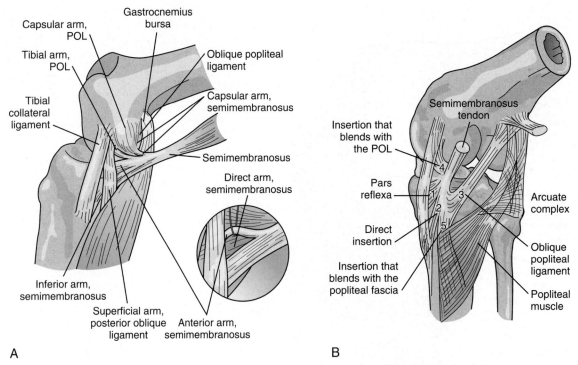

Figure 17–2: **A,** The posterior oblique ligament. **B,** The semimembranosus expansions. (Sims WF, Jacobson, K: *Am J Sports Med* 32, 337-345, 2004).

- The mechanism of injury may provide a clue to the possibility of a severe knee injury.
- Knee dislocations may spontaneously reduce and initially appear benign. A large effusion may be absent as a result of capsular disruption. A careful history and physical examination are crucial to the successful diagnosis and treatment of this injury. A high index of suspicion must be maintained.
- The neurovascular examination is the most important part of the initial assessment. The dorsalis pedis and posterior tibial pulses should be compared with the opposite leg. Doppler examinations and measurement of an ankle brachial index (ABI) compared with the other side are valuable tools in assessing the vascular status of the extremity. A normal examination, however, does not rule out a vascular injury.
- A vascular consultant should be called when there is any suspicion of a vascular injury.
- I currently recommend an arteriogram for all suspected knee dislocations, unless this would delay transport to the operating room (OR) in a patient with obvious vascular compromise. However, obtaining an arteriogram for all knee dislocations is controversial. There is literature to support close observation and serial examinations as acceptable treatment for patients with normal pulses and normal ABIs.[14]
- A venogram may be useful to rule out a popliteal vein injury, if the clinical picture warrants.

- Compartments should be palpated and compartment pressures measured, if any clinical index of suspicion for compartment syndrome exists.

Ligamentous Examination

- Knowledge of the normal tibial step off will prevent misdiagnosing a cruciate ligament injury. With the knee flexed 90 degrees, the medial tibial plateau should be 1 cm anterior to the medial femoral condyle. This normal step off should be established before performing the Lachman and posterior drawer tests.
- The ACL is best examined with a Lachman test. With the knee in 30 degrees of flexion, the distal femur is stabilized with one hand while the other directs an anterior force on the proximal tibia. In the presence of an ACL tear, there will be an excessive amount of anterior translation with a soft endpoint. This should always be compared to the contralateral extremity. The sensitivity of the examination can be increased by flexing and abducting the hip while externally rotating the leg.
- The PCL is best evaluated with the posterior drawer test. This can be accomplished by placing a posterior directed force on the proximal tibia with the knee in 90 degrees of flexion. With a PCL injury an excessive amount of posterior translation will be felt, with a soft endpoint (Figure 17–3). Posterior translation of the proximal medial tibia beyond the medial femoral condyle indicates a grade 3 injury. Again, comparison to the opposite extremity is helpful.

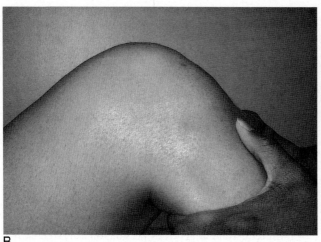
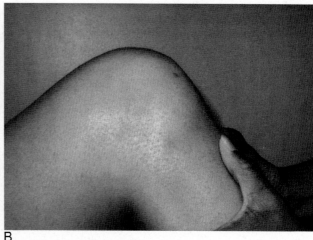

Figure 17–3: **A,** Normal position of the tibia in relation to the femur with knee flexed 90 degrees. **B,** Posterior displacement of the tibia in relation to the femur with knee flexed 90 degrees.

- Loss of the normal prominence of the tibial tubercle on visual inspection, known as the "posterior sag" sign, indicates a PCL disruption.
- The MCL is best assessed by applying a valgus stress with the knee in full extension and 30 degrees of flexion. Laxity at only 30 degrees suggests an isolated MCL injury. Laxity at both 0 degrees and 30 degrees suggests a combination of injuries to both the MCL, posteromedial capsule, and one or both cruciate ligaments.
- The LCL is best assessed by applying a varus stress with the knee in full extension and 30 degrees of flexion. Laxity at only 30 degrees suggests an isolated LCL injury. Laxity at both 0 degrees and 30 degrees suggests a combination of injuries.
- PLC injuries are often missed on initial examination. Evaluating for excessive external rotation in comparison with the opposite extremity best assesses the posterolateral corner. Increased external rotation of the tibia at 30 degrees indicates only an isolated PLC injury. Increased external rotation at both 30 degrees and 90 degrees indicates a combined PLC-PCL injury. The external rotation recurvatum test is performed by lifting the extremity off the examination table by the great toe. Increased external rotation, tibia vara, and recurvatum compared with the opposite extremity indicate an injury to the PLC (Figure 17–4).

Diagnostic Studies
Radiographs

- All suspected knee dislocations should have routine anteroposterior (AP), lateral, and oblique radiographs of the knee. In addition, AP and lateral views of the entire tibia and femur, including the hip and ankle joints, should be obtained to rule out associated fractures. Postreduction films must document a concentric reduction (Figure 17–5).

Magnetic Resonance Imaging

- Once the patient is stabilized, magnetic resonance imaging (MRI) should be obtained. This is helpful in further evaluating the ligaments, tendons, menisci, articular cartilage, and bony structures[15] (Figure 17–6).

Arteriogram

- Vascular injuries can lead to devastating outcomes. The reported incidence of popliteal artery injury is between 32% and 45%. Injuries to the popliteal artery can range from spasm, to an intimal tear, to complete transection. I recommend an angiogram for all suspected knee dislocations. The minimal risk in obtaining this valuable study far outweighs the potential catastrophic complications of missing a vascular injury (Figure 17–7).

Initial Management

- The initial management of all suspected knee dislocations begins with an evaluation of the vascular status and assessment of joint congruity.

Ischemic Limb

- If the knee is found dislocated on examination and there are gross signs of ischemia, an emergent gentle reduction should be performed. After reduction, the neurovascular status should be reevaluated and the extremity placed in a long leg splint.
- If pulses return post-reduction, radiographs should be obtained to ensure concentric reduction, and an arteriogram along with a vascular consult ordered.
- If pulses do not return following reduction, a vascular surgery consultant should be called and an emergent surgical exploration and revascularization performed. Surgery should not be delayed for an arteriogram

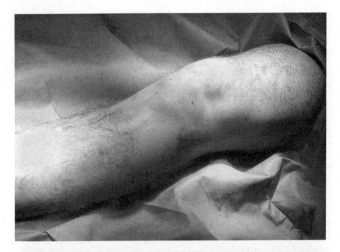

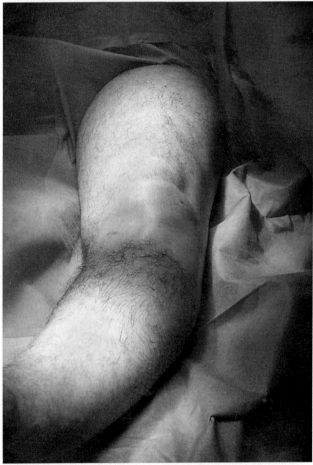

Figure 17–4: **Extremity prepped and draped; the external rotation recurvatum test is performed by lifting the great toe off the examining table. Increased external rotation and recurvatum are indicative of a posterolateral corner injury.**

because one can be performed intraoperatively. It is often helpful for the orthopaedic surgeon to be present during the procedure to discuss future incision sites and to apply a spanning external fixator across the knee

joint if gross instability exists. Simple soft-tissue repairs may also be performed if they are readily exposed through the vascular repair incision, can be done in a timely fashion, and are permitted by the patients overall status. Intraoperative radiographs must be obtained to document a concentric reduction.

Nonischemic Limb

- The first step in treatment of a suspected knee dislocation without vascular compromise is to obtain appropriate radiographs of the extremity.
- After X-rays are obtained and the direction of the dislocation determined, a gentle reduction can be performed under intravenous (IV) sedation. It is important to perform reductions as gently as possible on a relaxed extremity to prevent possible iatrogenic neurovascular injury or worsening of an existing neurovascular injury. Longitudinal traction with manipulation of the proximal tibia in the appropriate direction will usually effect a reduction.
- Following reduction, a repeat neurovascular examination is performed followed by application of a long leg splint. It is important to obtain postreduction radiographs to ensure a concentric reduction.
- An arteriogram can then be obtained to rule out occult vascular damage. Alternatively, serial examination and measurement of ABIs is considered acceptable.
- Intimal damage can be associated with thrombus formation hours or days later, making serial examinations essential.

Indications for Emergency Surgery

Vascular Compromise

- All cases of vascular compromise require a vascular surgery consultation and emergent revascularization.

Compartment Syndrome

- Fasciotomies should be performed on all compartments with elevated compartment pressures and following all revascularization procedures.

Open Dislocation

- The principles of open fracture management can be applied to the open knee dislocation. This includes a thorough irrigation and debridement, IV antibiotics, serial debridements, and wound closure with soft-tissue coverage if needed.
- An external fixator may be necessary to both maintain reduction and provide easy access to the wound.

Irreducible Dislocation

- Irreducible dislocations (typically posterolateral) require open reduction.

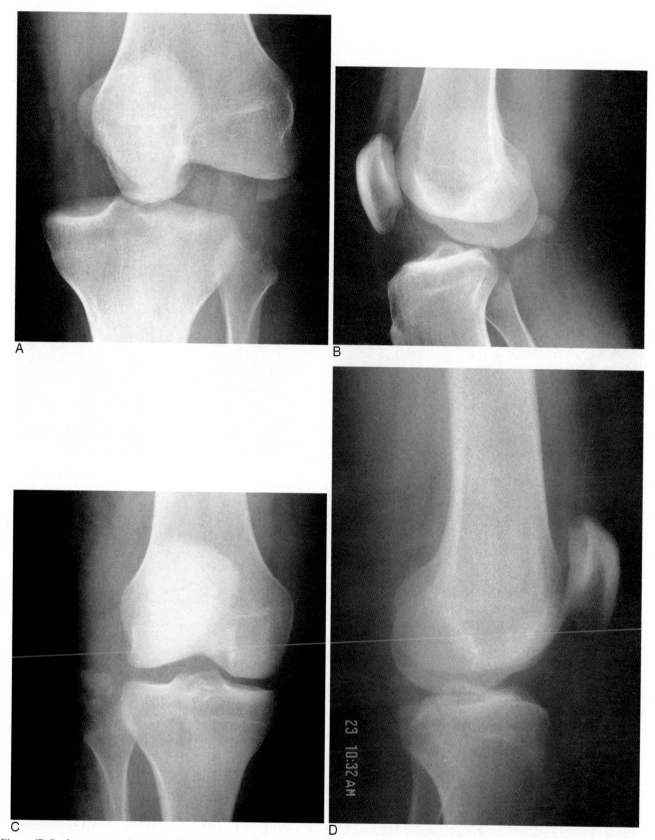

Figure 17–5: Anteroposterior (**A**) and lateral (**B**) radiographs of an uncommon anteromedial dislocation. Postreduction anteroposterior (**C**) and lateral (**D**) radiographs of the same knee.

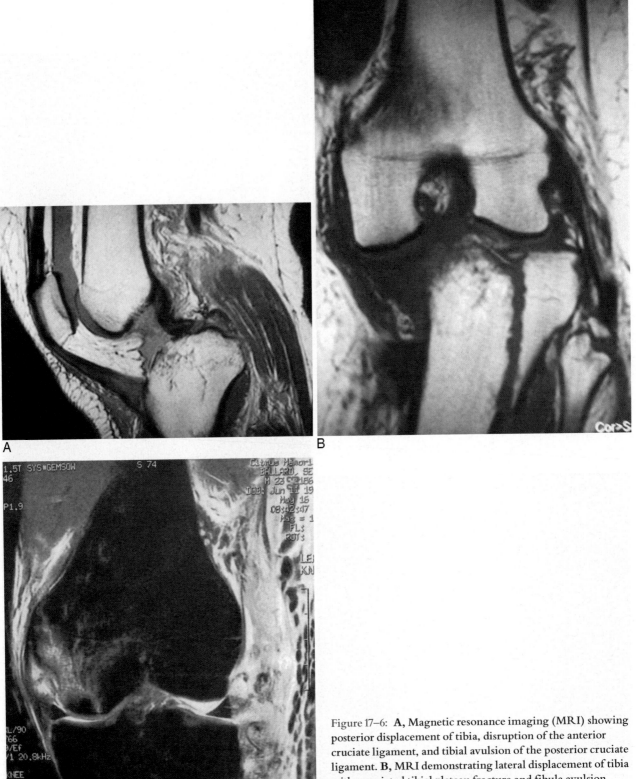

Figure 17–6: **A,** Magnetic resonance imaging (MRI) showing posterior displacement of tibia, disruption of the anterior cruciate ligament, and tibial avulsion of the posterior cruciate ligament. **B,** MRI demonstrating lateral displacement of tibia with associated tibial plateau fracture and fibula avulsion fracture with attached lateral collateral ligament. **C,** MRI reveals significant edema associated with complete disruption of the lateral ligament complex.

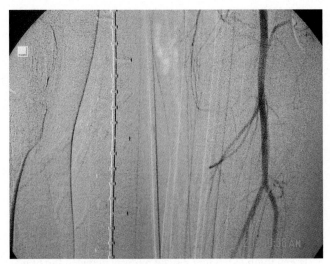

Figure 17–7: **Normal arteriogram.**

- Simple repairs should be performed at the time of open reduction through the same surgical incision. This typically would include the medial or posteromedial capsule and MCL. Definitive ligamentous reconstruction is delayed for several days to weeks. This allows for swelling to decrease and a complete work up with MRI to be performed.

Definitive Management
Background

- Historically, traumatic knee dislocations were treated with closed reduction and immobilization, with variable results.
- Prolonged immobilization has led to unacceptable stiffness, whereas an inadequate length of immobilization may result in excessive instability.
- There have been no prospective randomized studies comparing surgery to immobilization.
- Today, the trend in treatment of traumatic knee dislocations includes emergent closed reduction, assessment of the neurovascular structures, and surgical reconstruction or repair of the injured structures. This approach has led to a significant improvement in functional outcomes.[16,17]

Nonoperative Treatment

- Although the current trend is to treat knee dislocations surgically, there are indications for nonoperative treatment.
- The indications for nonoperative treatment are:
  - An elderly or sedentary patient with low functional demands.
  - A medically debilitated patient or one with posttraumatic comorbidities that would preclude surgical treatment.
  - An active infection.
  - Significant preexisting or posttraumatic arthritis.
  - Certain periarticular and intraarticular fractures.

- Nonoperative treatment protocol:
  - After concentric reduction has been confirmed, the extremity can be immobilized in a number of ways including an external fixator, hinged knee brace, or long leg splint.
  - External fixators are excellent choices for patients who are morbidly obese, have soft-tissue injuries that require observation and treatment, or have undergone vascular repairs.
  - The position to best immobilize the extremity has been widely debated. It varies anywhere from full extension to 45 degrees of flexion. The most important thing to ensure, however, is that a concentric reduction is maintained and documented on serial radiographs.
  - Immobilization is typically continued for 6 to 8 weeks, followed by physical therapy to regain motion.

Surgical Management
General Principals

- The goal of surgical management is to repair or reconstruct cruciate ligament, collateral ligament, capsular, and meniscal injuries.[18] However, not all ligaments have the same intrinsic healing ability. Understanding the following principles greatly helps with surgical planning:
  - ACL tears, LCL tears, and PLC injuries have no potential for intrinsic healing.
  - PCL tears and MCL tears have potential for intrinsic healing.
  - Bony avulsions of the cruciate ligaments are amenable to primary repair if associated with minimal intrasubstance ligament damage.
  - Medial-sided injuries associated with ACL or PCL tears may heal without surgery.
  - PCL tears with grade II laxity can heal with similar long-term results as grade I laxity and do not necessarily require surgery.
  - Grade III PCL tears should be treated with surgical reconstruction.
  - ACL tears associated with grade I or II PCL or MCL tears can initially be treated nonoperatively and reconstructed later as dictated by the patient's symptoms and activity level.
  - LCL and PLC tears are best treated with early repair. Delayed reconstruction leads to less predictable outcomes and poorer functional results.
- As a result, I have developed the following general guidelines for the two most common combination of ligament injuries:
  - ACL-PCL-LCL-PLC injuries are best treated with early primary LCL and PLC repair at 10 days to 3 weeks post-injury and simultaneous or staged ACL and PCL reconstruction.

- ACL-PCL-MCL injuries can be treated with protected range of motion to allow the medial-sided injuries to heal. The extremity can then be reevaluated for residual laxity. Typically, an ACL-PCL reconstruction can be performed electively (6 to 8 weeks) once strength and motion have been restored. In cases with grade II PCL laxity or less, a PCL reconstruction may not be necessary.

Surgical Timing

- When considering the timing of surgical intervention one should consider:
  - Whether the patient has been medically optimized.
  - If an adequate workup, including radiographs and MRI scan, has been performed.
  - If the vascular status been stabilized and confirmed with an arteriogram.
- Typically, surgery is delayed for 10 days to 3 weeks following the initial injury. This delay is important for several reasons:
  - It allows for resolution of acute inflammation and soft-tissue swelling.
  - This "cooling off" period decreases the risk of arthrofibrosis.
  - It allows for the capsular structures to heal, making it easier to perform an arthroscopic procedure without the risk of fluid extravasation (and possible development of a compartment syndrome).
- In contrast, a delay of greater than 3 weeks may result in excessive scarring that precludes the primary repair of structures such as the LCL and PLC.
  - If a delay greater than 3 to 4 weeks is anticipated, nonoperative treatment may be considered initially. After concentric reduction is obtained, the extremity is immobilized for 6 to 8 weeks. Rehabilitation is started following this initial period of immobilization in an attempt to restore motion and strength. The extremity is then reevaluated for stability. If the knee continues to be functionally unstable, surgical reconstruction is planned.

Surgical Procedure: General Principles

- The patient is placed supine on a standard operating room table with a lateral post.
- Perioperative antibiotics are routinely administered.
- A tourniquet may be applied but is not inflated (I do not apply a tourniquet).
- A sandbag is taped to the table in a position that stabilizes the foot with the knee flexed 80 degrees to 90 degrees.
- Pulses are evaluated via palpation and with a Doppler ultrasound before and after the procedure.
- A fluoroscope is available in the room.
- The extremity is carefully examined under anesthesia and compared with the opposite side.

- Planned surgical incisions are marked.
- If greater than 10 days from the initial injury, an arthroscopy is performed first. Meniscal and chondral pathology are addressed and cruciate injury confirmed. Debridement and notchplasty can be performed at this time as well.
- I use an inflow pump with a relatively low pressure setting (50 mm Hg). If excessive fluid extravasation is noted, it may be necessary to complete the arthroscopic portion of the surgery "dry" or convert to an open procedure.
- The calf is intermittently palpated throughout the procedure to be sure a compartment syndrome is not developing.

Open Lateral Collateral Ligament and Posterolateral Corner Repair

- A 10 to 12-cm "hockey stick" incision is made from the lateral thigh extending distally midway between the fibular head and Gerdy's tubercle over the lateral epicondyle.
- Minimal dissection is often required once the skin is incised. The trauma from the injury will typically detach and strip the lateral and posterolateral structures, allowing direct visualization into the lateral compartment of the knee if the capsule has not yet completely healed.
- The peroneal nerve is identified, isolated, and protected throughout the procedure. The nerve is easier to identify proximally posterior to the biceps femoris tendon.
- The following structures (from deep to superficial) are identified and repaired anatomically (Figure 17–8):
  - Lateral meniscus
  - Posterolateral capsule
  - Popliteus tendon
  - Popliteofibular ligament
  - LCL
  - Biceps femoris
  - Iliotibial (IT) band
- The capsule and meniscal attachments are fixed with suture anchors placed just below the joint line (Figure 17–9).
- The popliteus tendon, LCL, and popliteofibular ligament may require augmentation or reconstruction if inadequate tissue is available for primary repair.
- Except for the capsular sutures, the remaining sutures are placed but not tied until after the cruciate ligaments are reconstructed. Tying the capsular sutures allows the joint to remain distended for arthroscopic ACL or PCL reconstruction. By leaving the rest of the incision open, any fluid extravasating during the arthroscopy will drain out the wound and not into the compartments of the lower extremity.

Lateral Collateral Ligament and Posterolateral Corner Reconstruction

- If more than 3 weeks has elapsed since the injury, the LCL or PLC may require augmentation or reconstruction.
- I prefer allografts for LCL or PLC reconstruction. A variety of tendon grafts may be used based on surgeon preference.

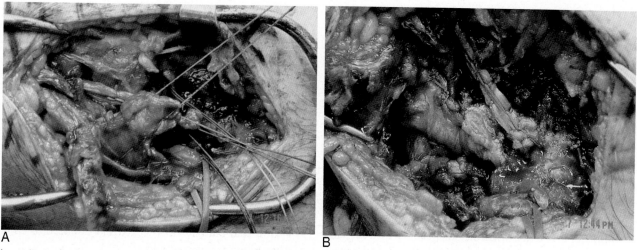

Figure 17–8: **A,** Operative photo showing the lateral structures of the knee: lateral collateral ligament, biceps femoris, peroneal nerve, and sutures in proximal tibia and posterolateral capsule avulsion. **B,** Repair of lateral structures: fibular head, lateral collateral ligament, and biceps femoris.

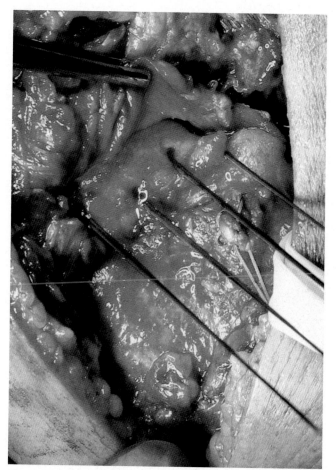

Figure 17–9: Intraoperative photo that shows the posterolateral capsule with four suture anchors placed in the proximal tibia, in preparation for repair.

These include: Achilles, tibialis anterior, semitendinosus, and quadriceps.

- An Achilles tendon allograft is preferred for an isolated LCL reconstruction (Figure 17–10).
  - A 7-mm bone block is fixed to a longitudinal tunnel drilled in the fibular head with an interference screw.
  - The tendon is secured to the anatomic LCL femoral insertion site with suture anchors, or a screw and ligament washer. Alternative fixation involves drilling a 30-mm closed end tunnel obliquely and tensioning the graft by passing the sutures out the medial femoral condyle with a set of Beath pins. The graft is then secured in the tunnel with an interference screw while

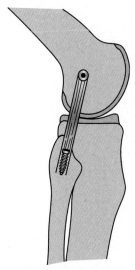

Figure 17–10: Lateral collateral ligament reconstruction.

tensioning the sutures. This is done with the knee in 30 degrees of flexion and a valgus stress applied. The sutures are then tied over a bony bridge on the medial femoral cortex for backup fixation.

- Popliteus complex reconstruction recreates the popliteofibular ligament and is performed with a tibialis anterior or Achilles tendon allograft (Figure 17–11A).
    - A tunnel is created in the proximal aspect of the fibular head at its widest point. This tunnel parallels the oblique slope of the fibular head from proximal posterior to distal anterior. The tunnel is created from anterior to posterior by carefully reaming over a guidewire while protecting the peroneal nerve.
    - One end of the graft is passed through the fibular head from posterior to anterior, while the other end is passed deep to the LCL and placed in a closed end tunnel made at the anatomic femoral insertion site of the popliteus tendon.
    - Fixation is similar to that used for LCL reconstruction. A valgus and internal rotation stress is applied during graft tensioning and fixation with the knee in 30 degrees of flexion.
    - In patients requiring both LCL and popliteofibular reconstruction, a tibialis anterior allograft is used. The procedure mimics that described above for the popliteofibular ligament, except the distal end of the graft is passed through the fibular head from posterior to anterior and then brought back up and attached to the femoral attachment site of the LCL. This recreates both the LCL and the popliteofibular ligament (Figure 17–11B).
- The posterolateral capsule should be advanced anteriorly and imbricated to the LCL.

Medial Collateral Ligament and Posteromedial Corner Repair

- In my experience, MCL and posteromedial corner injuries rarely require surgery.

- If significant valgus laxity (grade III) in full extension persists despite bracing and cruciate ligament reconstruction, the MCL may be primarily repaired, recessed at its femoral attachment, advanced at its distal attachment, or reefed.
- The posteromedial capsule, including the posterior oblique ligament, should be advanced anteriorly and imbricated to the MCL.
- A medial curvilinear incision that incorporates the tibial incision for the ACL or PCL tibial tunnels and extends proximally over the medial epicondyle and lateral thigh is used. The femoral PCL tunnel can also be made through this incision. Care is taken to avoid injury to the infrapatellar branch of the saphenous nerve.
- The repair is tensioned with the knee in 30 degrees of flexion, and the knee then flexed and extended to ensure that motion is not constrained.
- MCL allograft reconstruction may be performed similar to lateral sided injuries but is rarely necessary.

Anterior Cruciate Ligament and Posterior Cruciate Ligament Reconstruction

- Graft selection
    - We recommend allografts for the knee with multiple ligaments injured.[19,20] A bone-patellar tendon-bone allograft is used for ACL reconstruction (Figure 17–12), and an Achilles tendon allograft for PCL reconstruction (Figure 17–13).
- Benefits of allografts:
    - Graft availability.
    - Decreased operative time.
    - Decreased donor site morbidity.
- General rules of thumb for all allografts:
    - Donor age less than 50.

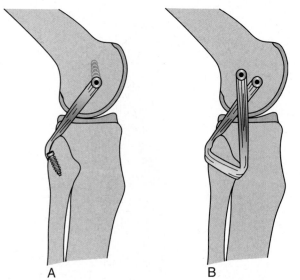

Figure 17–11: **A,** Popliteofibular reconstruction, **B,** Lateral collateral ligament and popliteofibular reconstruction.

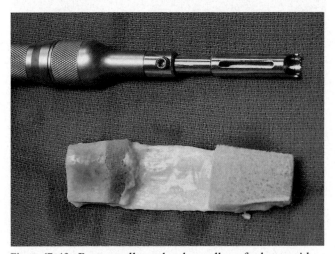

Figure 17–12: **Bone-patella tendon-bone allograft, shown with bone plug harvester. The posterolateral capsule should be advanced anteriorly and imbricated to the LCL. (Courtesy of Stryker Corporation, San Jose, CA)**

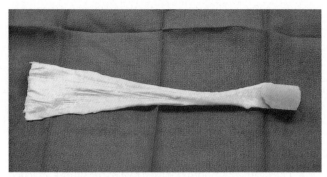

Figure 17–13: **Achilles tendon allograft.**

- Fresh frozen nonirradiated grafts.
- Reputable tissue bank.
- Technical pearls for single bundle arthroscopic PCL reconstruction
  - I prefer a single bundle (anterolateral bundle) technique for the knee with multiple injured ligaments.
  - Graft preparation
    - An Achilles allograft is fashioned to mimic a standard bone-patellar tendon-bone allograft.
    - The bone block of the Achilles allograft is cut with a 9-mm circular oscillating saw (Stryker Corporation; San Jose, Calif.) to a length of 25 mm (Figure 17–14). A second 9-mm bone plug is cut from the remaining calcaneal bone block to a length of 30 mm (Figure 17–15). This free bone plug is then sutured to the tendon end of the graft using #1 nonabsorbable sutures placed through drill holes in the bone plug (Figure 17–16). It is helpful to thin this region of the tendon before attaching the free bone plug to decrease bulk. The tendon length between the plugs is approximately 60 mm (Figure 17–17). This basically creates a bone-tendon-bone construct that can be customized to the desired length and allows interference fixation on both sides of the joint. The femoral plug is sized to fit through

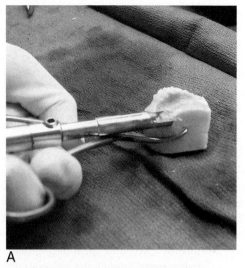

A

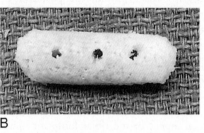

B

Figure 17–15: **A, Harvesting free bone plug. B, Free bone plug with drill holes for suturing.**

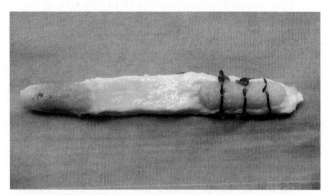

Figure 17–16: **Achilles' tendon allograft with free bone plug attached.**

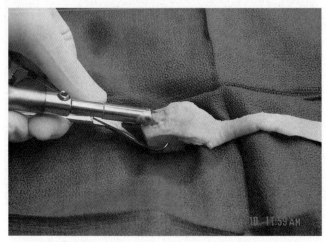

Figure 17–14: **Harvesting tendon with bone plug from Achilles' tendon allograft.**

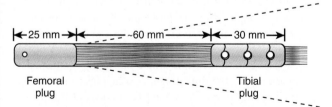

Figure 17–17: **Diagram of complete bone-Achilles tendon-bone allograft. The femoral plug is sized for a 10-mm tunnel. The tibial plug is sized for an 11-mm tunnel. The tibial plug is secured to the graft with three sets of #1 nonabsorbable sutures placed through drill holes. The tendon width is 11 mm. It is not necessary to tabularize the tendon. Simply cut off the excess and secure the plug at the desired length.**

a 10-mm tunnel, whereas the tibial plug is sized for an 11-mm tunnel.

- Advantages of using an Achilles allograft:
  - A free bone block can be attached to the tendon to allow interference screw fixation on both sides of the joint.
  - The tendon length can be adjusted to accommodate each patient.
  - The Achilles tendon has a larger cross-sectional area than the patellar tendon.
- A specially designed angled curette and rasp, inserted through the anteromedial portal and placed through the notch, are used to elevate the posterior capsule off the back of the tibia and debride the PCL tibial footprint. Care is taken to stay directly on bone with these instruments. Extra time spent during this step will facilitate graft passage around the posterior tibia later in the procedure. A radiofrequency probe is helpful in debriding the soft tissue from the notch and maintaining hemostasis.
- The PCL tibial tunnel angle guide is set at approximately 60 degrees and inserted through the anteromedial portal over the back of the tibia so the guide tip is placed 1 cm below the joint line posteriorly and in the distal lateral aspect of the tibial footprint. The starting point on the anterior tibia should be midway between the tibial tubercle and the posteromedial border of the tibia and slightly distal to the tibial tubercle. A 3- to 4-cm longitudinal skin incision is made and will be used for placement of the ACL tibial tunnel as well.
- Using image, the guide pin is drilled into but not through the posterior cortex. A common error is to place this pin too proximal on the posterior tibia. The pin should parallel the proximal tibia-fibula joint on lateral imaging. The tibial tunnel is reamed with an 11-mm reamer under image intensification. Great care is taken to avoid plunging through the posterior cortex. A knee roll placed under the distal thigh facilitates knee flexion to 90 degrees, allowing the neurovascular bundle to fall posteriorly. An accessory posteromedial incision, or a lateral incision if previously made, may be used to allow finger palpation and retractor placement posteriorly to protect the neurovascular bundle. Additionally, a posteromedial portal may be created for direct arthroscopic visualization during this step.
- A two-incision technique is used for placement of the femoral tunnel, which is drilled through a small medial incision over the distal thigh. It is helpful to retract the leading edge of the vastus medalis oblique (VMO) proximally during this step. A femoral guide is used to place a pin 7 mm off the articular cartilage at the 1:00 or 11:00 position for a right or left knee, respectively, in the anterior portion of the PCL footprint. Care is taken to start proximally enough on the anteromedial cortex to avoid "blowing out" the distal femur. A 10-mm reamer is used to create the femoral tunnel.

- A ligament smoother (W. L. Gore & Associates Inc.; Flagstaff, Ariz.) is passed retrograde up the tibial tunnel and retrieved from the posterior compartment using a grasper through the anteromedial portal. This is then pulled into the femoral tunnel and out the medial incision. At this time the position of the gore smoother simulates the PCL, and it can be used to rasp the tunnel edges and subsequently to pass the graft.
- The ligament smoother is used to pass the sutures attached to the femoral plug of the PCL graft up the tibial tunnel, through the joint, and out the femoral tunnel. An arthroscopic suture manipulator placed through the anteromedial portal and into the posterior compartment can be used as a pulley for the sutures to help pass the femoral bone plug around the "killer turn" at the posterior aspect of the tibia (Figure 17–18). Drilling the tibial tunnel 1 mm larger than the femoral tunnel also helps the bone plug pass easier into the joint. The bone plug is then guided into the femoral tunnel under arthroscopic visualization.
- Interference screws are used for graft fixation. The femoral plug is secured with a 7-by-25-mm absorbable screw, whereas the tibial plug is fixed with a 9-by-25-mm absorbable screw. All interference screws are placed over a flexible guidewire to avoid screw plug divergence. I usually back up the tibial fixation by tying the sutures over a post (screw and washer).
- Technical pearls for endoscopic ACL reconstruction
  - Graft preparation
  - Use a bone-patellar tendon-bone allograft with a tendon length less than 50 mm to avoid graft tunnel mismatch (Figure 17–19).

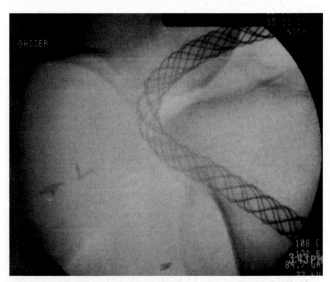

Figure 17–18: **Intraoperative radiograph demonstrating the "Killer corner" with ligament smoother.**

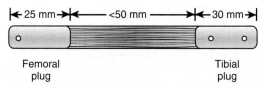

Figure 17–19: **Diagram of complete bone-patella tendon-bone allograft.** The femoral and tibial plugs are sized to fit through a 10-mm tunnel. The tendon width equals 10 mm.

- Both bone plugs are fashioned with a 9-mm circular oscillating saw to allow passage through a 10-mm tunnel and cut to a length of 25 mm (Figure 17–20).
- Anatomic landmarks used for locating the center of the tibial tunnel include:
  - The base of the medial tibial spine.
  - A line projecting from the inner edge of the anterior horn of the lateral meniscus.
  - The posterior half of the ACL tibial footprint.
  - Seven mm in front of the PCL (the smoother may be used to simulate the PCL).
- The tibial tunnel angle guide is typically set between 50 degrees and 55 degrees. I use the $n + 7$ degrees rule to set the tibial tunnel angle guide, in which n represents the tendon length of the graft.
- Start the tibial tunnel at a point midway between the tibial tubercle and the posteromedial border of the tibia. A 1- to 2-cm bony bridge should be present between the ACL and PCL tunnel openings on the anterior tibia, with the PCL tunnel more distal.
- An adequate notchplasty that allows visualization of the periosteum on the posterior aspect of the femur will help avoid anterior femoral tunnel placement, which is the most common technical error in ACL reconstructions.
- Place a knee roll under the distal thigh to allow 90 degrees of knee flexion when locating and drilling the femoral tunnel. This helps avoid posterior wall "blowout."
- Use a 6- or 7-mm over-the-top guide placed through the tibial tunnel to locate the femoral tunnel, at the 10:30 or 1:30 position for a right and left knee, respectively. Ream the tunnel to a depth of 30 mm. It is helpful to ream a 3- to 4-mm footprint to confirm correct placement before committing to drilling the entire tunnel depth.
- Both femoral and tibial tunnels are drilled with a 10-mm reamer.
- Interference screws are used for graft fixation. The femoral plug is fixed with a 7-by-25-mm absorbable screw, whereas the tibial plug is fixed with a 9-by-25-mm absorbable screw. The screws are inserted over a flexible guide wire to ensure proper placement.

Order of Bicruciate Ligament Reconstruction

- Drill the PCL tunnels: tibial, then femoral.
- Drill the ACL tunnels: tibial, then femoral.

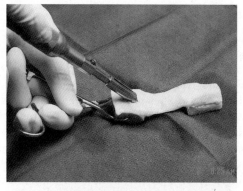

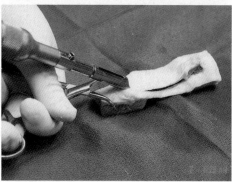

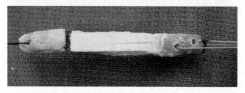

Figure 17–20: **Harvesting graft from bone-patellar tendon-bone allograft.**

- Pass the PCL graft and fix the femoral plug.
- Pass the ACL graft and fix the femoral plug.
- Cycle the knee through a range of motion while applying tension to the tibial sutures of both the ACL and PCL.
- Secure the PCL tibial plug with the knee in 80 degrees to 90 degrees of flexion and moderate tension on the sutures. Be sure the normal medial tibial step, with the medial tibial plateau 1 cm anterior to the medial femoral condyle, is recreated. If the tunnels have been correctly placed, tensioning both sets of sutures should automatically "set" the tibia in the correct position. Back-up tibial fixation of the PCL may be performed if deemed necessary.
- Secure the ACL tibial plug with the knee near full extension and moderate tension on the ACL tibial sutures.
- Tie the previously placed sutures for the medial or lateral or posterolateral repair. For the lateral-sided repair, the knee is placed in 30 degrees of flexion with a valgus and internal rotation stress applied to the tibia. For the medial sided repair, the knee is placed in 30 degrees of flexion with a varus stress applied.

Rehabilitation

- Each patient's rehabilitation will need to be individualized based on the ligaments involved, the quality of the repair, and any associated injuries.
- Patients are typically placed in a knee immobilizer for 3 weeks with a soft support under the proximal third of the tibia to prevent posterior sagging. Toe touch weight bearing with crutches is allowed.
- Isometric quad sets may begin immediately. Active hamstring flexion is avoided for 6 weeks.
- A hinged brace is fit at 3 weeks, and home continuous passive motion (CPM) started for progressive range of motion.[21] The patient is given a referral to begin formal structured physical therapy. Patients may be partial weight bearing with crutches. Full weight bearing is delayed until 6 to 8 weeks postoperatively. Crutches are discontinued when the patient demonstrates good motion, strength, and ambulatory ability.
- Flexion is limited to 90 degrees for the first 8 weeks postoperatively, with the goal of regaining full range of motion by 12 to 16 weeks.
- A functional ACL/PCL brace is fit at approximately 2 months.
- Open chain exercises start at 3 months postoperatively.
- Full recovery generally takes 8 to 12 months.

Complications

- Failure to recognize and treat vascular injuries.
- Iatrogenic neurovascular damage.
- Technical errors in tunnel placement.
- Failure to recognize and appropriately treat all components of instability.
- Osteonecrosis of the medial femoral condyle.
- Persistent loss of knee motion.

Conclusions

- Knee dislocations represent a serious injury, with significant risk for vascular compromise, and should be treated as an orthopaedic emergency.
- Prompt recognition and surgical repair of popliteal artery injuries is required to prevent prolonged ischemia and possible amputation.
- Appropriate surgical intervention results in better outcomes than traditional nonoperative treatment. The goals of surgery are to restore functional stability and motion with early repair and reconstruction of the injured ligaments.
- Surgical treatment is complex and fraught with potential complications and should be performed by those physicians experienced in treating complicated knee ligament injuries.

Annotated References

1. Brautigan B, Johnson D: The epidemiology of knee dislocations, *Clin Sports Med* 19:387-397, 2000.
This article discusses the definition, classification, and epidemiologic patterns of knee dislocation. Mechanisms of injury and injury patterns are described according to a classification system.

2. Rihn JA, Groff YJ, Harner CD: The acutely dislocated knee: evaluation and management, *J Am Acad Ortho Surg.* 12:334-346, 2004.
This is an excellent review article on the acutely dislocated knee. It discusses the entire gamut of the evaluation and management of the dislocated knee.

3. Shelbourne KD, Pritchard J, Rettig AC, et al: Knee dislocations with intact PCL, *Orthop Review* 21:607-609, 610-611, 1992.
This article presents three cases of documented knee dislocation where the posterior cruciate ligament (PCL) is preserved. The authors suggest an intact PCL provides a better prognosis.

4. Bratt HD, Newman AD: Complete dislocation of the knee without disruption of both cruciate, *J Trauma* 34:383-389, 1993.
This article presents four cases of complete knee dislocation without disruption of both cruciate ligaments. It also discusses the biomechanics of the soft-tissue restraints about the knee and analyzes how sufficient laxity can occur, with only one cruciate ligament disruption.

5. Palmer I: On the injuries to the ligaments of the knee joint: a clinical study, *Acta Chir Scand* 53:1-28, 1938.
A historical review of ligament injuries about the knee.

6. Quinlan AG: Irreducible posterolateral dislocation of the knee with buttonholing of the medial femoral condyle, *J Bone Joint Surg Am* 48:1619-1621, 1966.
In this historical paper the authors discuss five case reports of the medial femoral condyle "button-holing" through the medial joint capsule and preventing reduction.

7. Kontakis GM, Christoforakis JJ, Katonis PG, et al: Irreducible knee dislocation due to interposition of the vastus medialis associated with neurovascular injury, *Orthopaedics* 26:645-646, 2003.
This article discusses the soft tissues that can block reduction after a knee dislocation.

8. Huang FS, Simonion PT, Chonsky HA: Irreducible posterolateral dislocation of the knee, *Arthroscopy* 16:323-327, 2000.
This article reviews the literature for cases of irreducible knee dislocations. It also presents an interesting case of posterolateral knee dislocation and many of the associated signs and symptoms of an irreducible knee dislocation (i.e., the dimple sign).

9. Shelbourne KD, Porter DA, Clingman JA, et al: Low-velocity knee dislocation, *Orthop Rev* 20:995-1004, 1991.
This article discusses the evaluation and management of low-velocity knee dislocations.

10. Green NE, Allen BL: Vascular injuries associated with dislocation of the knee, *J Bone Joint Surg Am* 59:236-239, 1977.
This excellent article emphasizes the frequency and the nature of vascular lesions and their treatment and the risk and rate of amputation. The article retrospectively evaluated 245 knee dislocations. Out of the 245 knee dislocations 75 (32%) had a disruption in flow of the popliteal artery. They also found that

there was 86% amputation rate if an ischemic limb is not revascularized within 6 to 8 hours.

11. Barnes CJ, Pietrobon R, Higgins LD: Does the pulse examination in patients with traumatic knee dislocation predict a surgical arterial injury? A meta-analysis, *J Trauma* 53:1109-1114, 2002.

An excellent metaanalysis of the plethora of literature on this subject. The article concludes that the isolated presence of abnormal pulses is not sensitive enough to detect a surgical vascular injury in the presence of a knee dislocation.

12. Goitz RJ, Tomaino MM: Management of peroneal nerve injuries associated with knee dislocations, *Am J Orthop* 32:14-16, 2003.

This article is an excellent discussion of the evaluation of peroneal nerve palsy and provides recommendations of surgical treatment after knee dislocations.

13. Swenson TM: Physical diagnosis of multiple-ligament injured knee, *Clin Sports Med* 19:415-423, 2000.

This article provides an excellent review of the assessment of an acutely dislocated knee. It goes through the physical examination, including ligamentous and vascular examination and radiographic assessment.

14. Standard J, Sheils T, Lopez-Ben R, et al: Vascular injuries in knee dislocation: the role of physical examination in determining the need for arteriography, *J Bone Joint Surg Am* 86:910-915, 2004.

This is a prospective evaluation of 126 patients with an acute multiligamentous knee dislocation at a level one trauma center. Ten patients had abnormal physical examination findings. Nine patients (7% prevalence) had arteriography findings of a flow limiting popliteal artery injury (one false positive physical examination). The authors conclude that serial physical examinations can be used to determine the need for arteriography.

15. Yu JS, Goodwin D, Salonen D, et al: Complete dislocation of the knee: spectrum of associated soft-tissue injuries depicted by MR imaging, *Am J Roentgenol* 64:135-139, 1995.

This article discusses the spectrum of injuries that can be depicted by magnetic resonance imaging (MRI) in patients with a knee dislocation. It also proposes that evidence of injury to the popliteal tendon on MRI is a good prognostic indicator of possible peroneal nerve injury or vascular compromise.

16. Almekinders LC, Dedmond BT: Outcomes of the operatively treated knee dislocation, *Clin Sports Med* 19:503-518, 2000.

This article is a comprehensive review of the outcomes of surgical treatment for acute knee dislocations from 1990 to 2000. The authors noted stiffness and pain were the major postoperative problems as opposed to instability. Return to work and athletic activities were variable.

17. Richter M, Bosch U, Wippermann R, et al: Comparison of surgical repair or reconstruction of the cruciate ligaments versus nonsurgical treatment in patients with traumatic knee dislocations, *Am J Sports Med* 30:718-727, 2002.

This article retrospectively evaluates 89 patients with an 8-year follow-up. The authors conclude surgical repair is better than nonsurgical. Patients younger than 40 and sports injuries versus motor vehicle accidents have a better prognosis. An adequate functional rehabilitation program is also essential in outcome.

18. Harner CD, Waltrip RL, Bennett CH, et al: Surgical management of knee dislocations, *J Bone Joint Surg Am* 86:262-273, 2004.

This is article is an excellent discussion of the authors preferred surgical techniques in the treatment of knee dislocations.

19. Fanelli G: Treatment of combined anterior cruciate ligament-posterior cruciate ligament-lateral side injuries of the knee, *Clin Sports Med* 19:493-502, 2000.

This article discusses arthroscopically assisted combined anterior cruciate ligament-posterior cruciate ligament (ACL-PCL) reconstruction with primary repair of the posterolateral corner. The authors recommend the use of allograft tissue because of the strength of the larger grafts, and absence of donor-site morbidity.

20. Shapiro MS, Freedman EL: Allograft reconstruction of anterior and posterior cruciate ligaments after traumatic knee dislocation, *Am J Sports Med* 23:580-587, 1995.

This study, although limited because it is a retrospective evaluation of only seven patients, serves to reinforce the point that arthrofibrosis can be a complication after surgical reconstruction of multiligamentous injured knee.

21. Noyes FR, Barber-Westin SD: Reconstruction of the anterior and posterior cruciate ligaments after knee dislocation: use of early protected postoperative motion to decrease arthrofibrosis, *Am J Sports Med* 25:769-778, 1997.

This article provides objective data of operative treatment using allogenic tissues and immediate protected knee motion for combined anterior cruciate ligament (ACL) and posterior cruciate ligament (PCL) ruptures. It shows good restoration of function in the majority of cases.

Tibial Plateau and Proximal Tibia Fractures

Eric M. Lindvall, DO

Anatomy

Bone

- Tibia proximally supports body weight through medial and lateral condyles (plateaus).
- Fibula provides strut for muscle attachments in leg; distally important as part of ankle joint and proximally articulates with tibia below knee joint.
- Tibial articular surface slopes 10 degrees to 12 degrees inferiorly from anterior to posterior.
- Medial and lateral eminences provide attachment for medial and lateral menisci and anterior and posterior cruciate ligaments, respectively.
- Tibial tubercle provides attachment site for patellar tendon— approximately 3 cm distal to joint line.
- Lateral tibial plateau convex (Figure 18–1).
- Medial tibial plateau concave (see Figure 18–1).

Soft Tissue

- Lateral meniscus more mobile than medial meniscus.
- Medial collateral ligament (MCL) and lateral collateral ligament (LCL) act as stabilizers against valgus and varus stress, respectively.
- Anterior cruciate ligament (ACL) and posterior cruciate ligament (PCL) act as stabilizers against anterior and posterior tibial translation, respectively.
- Quadriceps and patellar tendons are important structures allowing active knee extension and contain largest sesamoid bone (patella).
- Popliteal fossa contains sciatic nerve (tibial nerve and common peroneal nerve) and popliteal artery before it trifurcates into posterior tibial artery, anterior interosseous artery (dorsal pedis), and peroneal artery.

Tibial Plateau Fractures

Incidence

- Lateral are more common than medial plateau fractures; bimodal distribution, in young adults high-energy fractures are usual, and in the elderly low-energy fractures are usual.[1]

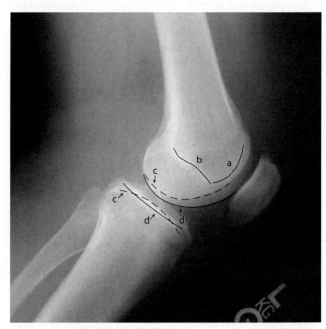

Figure 18–1: **Lateral radiograph demonstrating relationship between femoral and tibial condyles.** *a,* Trochlear groove, *b,* Intercondylar notch, *c,* Lateral tibial plateau and matching lateral femoral condyle, *d,* Medial tibial plateau and matching medial femoral condyle. Note convex lateral tibial plateau and concave medial tibial plateau.

Mechanism of Injury

- Lateral plateau: valgus injury with or without axial loading.
- Medial plateau: varus injury with or without axial loading.
- Bicondylar plateau: axial loading; position of knee (flexion or extension) during load determines location of fracture.
- Direct blow to lateral or medial aspect of knee can also produce appropriate force to cause fracture

Associated Knee Injuries

- Lateral plateau: lateral meniscus, MCL, ACL, and fibular neck or head fracture (peroneal nerve).[2]
- Medial plateau: LCL, medial meniscus, cruciate ligaments, peroneal nerve, or popliteal vessel (Figure 18–2).[2]
- Bicondylar plateau: peroneal nerve, arterial injury, menisci, cruciates (often avulsions), patellar tendon avulsion, fibular neck or head fractures, and tibial tubercle fractures.

Classification

- Schatzker[3]
  - Type I: split lateral plateau
  - Type II: split depression lateral plateau
  - Type III: depression lateral plateau
  - Type IV: medial plateau
  - Type V: bicondylar
  - Type VI: bicondylar with metaphyseal-diaphyseal dissociation
- Moore (fracture or dislocation)[4]
  - Type I: split
  - Type II: entire condyle
  - Type III: rim avulsion
  - Type IV: rim compression
  - Type V: four part

Diagnosis

- History of axial load or valgus or varus stress.
- Physical examination.
  - Knee effusion if truly intraarticular fracture, it is seen within few hours after injury.
  - Decreased range of motion and it is painful.
  - Possible knee instability.
  - Edema or ecchymosis is more commonly seen many hours or days following injury.
  - Must assess for patellar and quadriceps function to rule out injury to extensor mechanism.
  - Must assess neurovascular status; ankle brachial index (ABI) less than 0.9 indicates vascular injury and warrants arteriogram. Assess peroneal nerve function
  - Must assess for signs of compartment syndrome; most commonly seen in proximal tibia fractures in region of greatest muscle mass.
- Radiographs: anteroposterior (AP) and lateral of knee (oblique views if not found on routine orthogonal views); AP and lateral tibia or fibular views to rule out segmental fracture.
- Computerized tomography (CT) helps define entire fracture and all fracture planes to assist with surgical planning.[5] Critical for correct lag screw placement.
- Magnetic resonance imaging (MRI) superior to CT scan in depicting soft-tissue injuries; some authors also prefer over CT for fracture definition.[6]

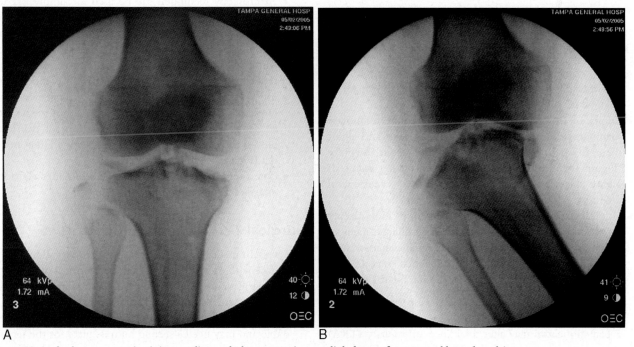

A   B

Figure 18–2: **A,** Anteroposterior injury radiograph demonstrating medial plateau fracture and lateral avulsion fractures. **B,** Varus stress applied while under general anesthetic showing gross instability.

(Continued)

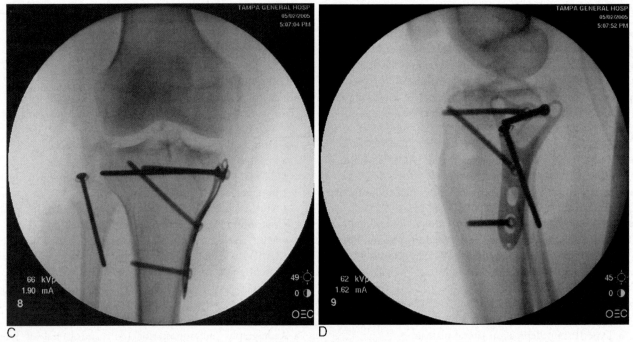

C   D

Figure 18–2, cont'd: **C and D, Medial buttress plating and reattachment of lateral collateral ligament avulsion from fibula with spiked washer. Stability was restored, especially to varus stress.**

Nonoperative Treatment

- It is recommended for nondisplaced, minimally displaced fractures.
- Patients medically incapable of withstanding an operation.
- Patients that would not functionally benefit from restoring knee motion or alignment.
- Nonweight bearing 8 to 10 weeks. Cast or brace.
- Usually can begin motion at 6 weeks in minimally or non-displaced fractures.

Operative Treatment

- Goals remain to restore[1] joint fragments anatomically and metaphyseal or diaphyseal fragments into anatomic alignment.[7]
- Displaced, comminuted patterns often require temporary spanning external fixation to maintain length and alignment through ligamentotaxis while soft tissues stabilize (Figure 18–3); provides traveling traction rather than sedentary skeletal traction; can delay over 3 weeks until definitive surgery if length has been maintained.[8]
- Surgical approaches mainly vary with skin incision; deeper dissection similar. Options include lateral oblique incision, lateral "hockey stick" incision, straight midline incision with deeper fascial lateral oblique or "hockey stick" incision, and medial oblique incision for access to posteromedial tibia.[9]

  - Must *not* strip both medial and lateral aspects of proximal tibia.
  - Lateral incision may alter total knee arthroplasty (TKA) approach if ample time not allowed for skin bridges to revascularize

- Midline approach can be detrimental to patellar tendon if wound dehisces or becomes infected
- If tibial tubercle is fractured, may remain midline and elevate patellar tendon with tubercle and menisci to access both plateaus.[10]
- Must assess for and repair meniscal tears; frequently trapped in fracture when significant lateral depression is noted.
- Arthroscopy technique can be used for simply fracture patterns but must avoid iatrogenic compartment syndrome because fluid can extravasate into proximal tibia through fracture site.[11]
- Minimally displaced or simple depression patterns can reduce percutaneously through cortical window and use of image intensification (lateral depressions will often elevate better when approached from medial side and visa versa as a result of orientation of depressed piece); back fill trough created by tamp with graft material (Figure 18–4).
- One should bone graft the void created after elevation of articular the fragments.[12]

Surgical Techniques and Implants

- Lateral or medial plateau fractures require restoration of joint surface with or without graft, meniscal repair if needed, and buttress plating. "Raft" screws act as scaffolding beneath the joint line, whereas lag screws compress condyles.[13]
- Bicondylar fractures require same principles but are less stable and may need a second buttress plate for the second condyle.[9] One side must involve only limited dissection to avoid "dead bone sandwich."

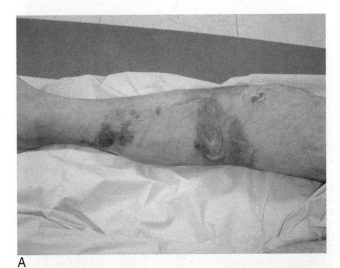

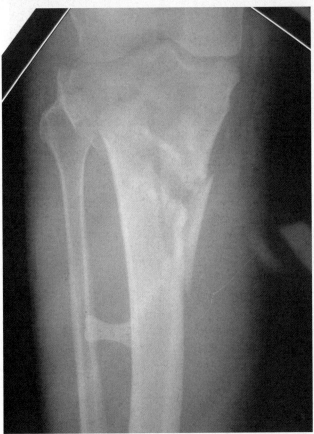

Figure 18–3: **A,** Early fracture blisters and ecchymosis noted after short intensive care unit stay. **B,** Radiograph of same patient depicting comminution of proximal tibia and shortening through fracture.

- Thin wire fixators can be used to avoid large surgical incisions. Wires should be extracapsular to avoid pin tract infection tracking into knee joint.[14]
- Locked plating can provide additional construct stability and often eliminate the second plate (Figure 18–5). Must confirm that orientation of locked screws will actually enter fragment (Figure 18–6) Careful technique must be used because locked plating does not provide traditional buttressing unless traditional unlocked screws are first used to compress the plate to the bone. The unlocked screws can then be exchanged for locked screws after other plate holes have been secured. Primary advantage remains in osteoporotic bone and in bicondylar fractures.
- Reduction techniques include use of large periarticular clamps, bone tamps or elevators to elevate joint fragments, and femoral distractor to help restore alignment and length and gain visualization into joint.[15]
- Bioabsorbable pins allow the assembly of multiple articular fragments without obstructing further reduction as is seen with Kirschner wires (K-wires). Also allow preservation of small articular fragments that would otherwise be too small for screw fixation and likely discarded.
- Some synthetic graft materials (tricalcium phosphates) that harden during surgical repair may soon allow earlier weight bearing.[16]

Postoperative Course

- Goal is to restore knee motion during nonweight-bearing phase.
- Nonweight bearing usually 10 to 12 weeks.
- Once fully weight bearing, focus should shift to strengthening.

Complications

- Malunion—varus malunions seen in bicondylar fractures lead to treatment with dual plating.[17] Wound problems returned focus toward careful soft-tissue handling and maintaining bone vascularity. Locked plating has provided additional stability that can help avoid loss of reduction and varus collapse. Percutaneous medial buttress plating or mini-incision techniques can also be successfully used to prevent varus collapse. Articular malunions eventually lead to arthritic changes, especially in the face of knee instability.
- Infection—almost always adds to knee stiffness. Can also cause loss of joint reduction if graft material is involved and needs to be removed. Midline incision can be problematic if infection develops due to exposed and involved patellar tendon.
- Posttraumatic osteoarthritis—directly related to articular reduction, severity of injury, and residual knee instability. Joint malreduction leads to localized increase in joint reactive forces and therefore accelerated articular wear. It is unknown the amount of articular cell death that will occur as a result of initial trauma. Residual knee instability major cause for poor outcome.[3,17,18] Additional meniscal pathology also leads to poorer outcome.[19]

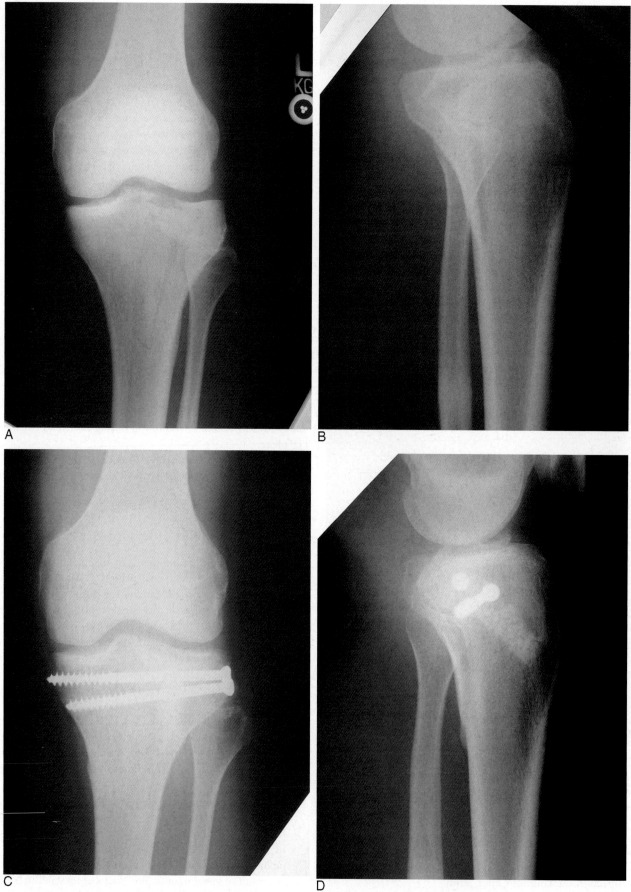

Figure 18–4: Anteroposterior (**A**) and lateral (**B**) radiographs showing posterolateral articular depression with minimally displaced metaphyseal split. **C** and **D**, Radiographs 10 months postoperatively with well-maintained joint reduction and still visible cancellous allograft chips backfilled with tamp into trough created through a cortical window using percutaneous technique.

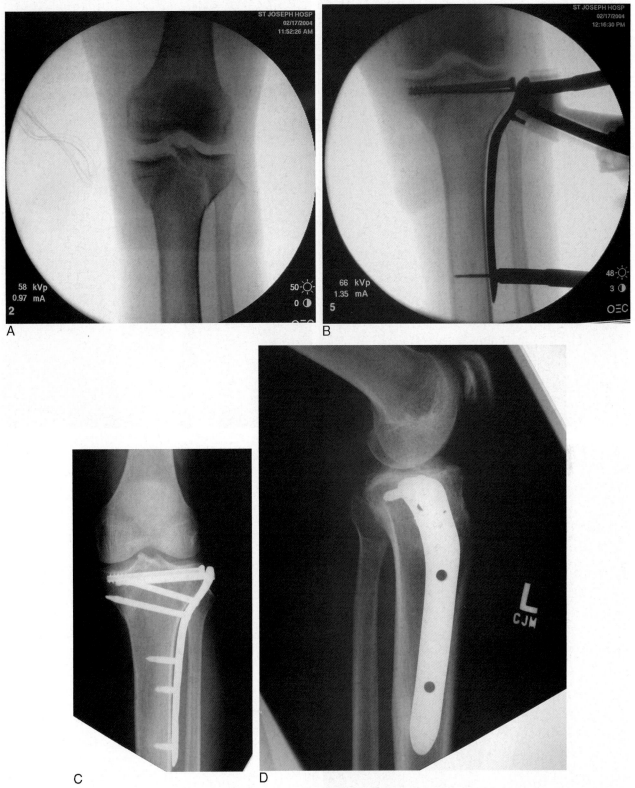

Figure 18–5: **A,** Bicondylar fracture. **B,** Lag screw fixation of condyles followed by percutaneous locked plate insertion. **C** and **D,** Radiographs 18 months after surgery demonstrating healed fracture without collapse.

- Joint stiffness—infection, excessive dissection, open fractures, patient apprehension, and prolonged immobilization can all lead to increased stiffness. Must strive to achieve functional range of motion before full weight bearing. Immobilization better tolerated in nonoperative cases because less scarring occurs.[20]
- Greater malalignment appears to be better tolerated in nonoperative cases.[21]

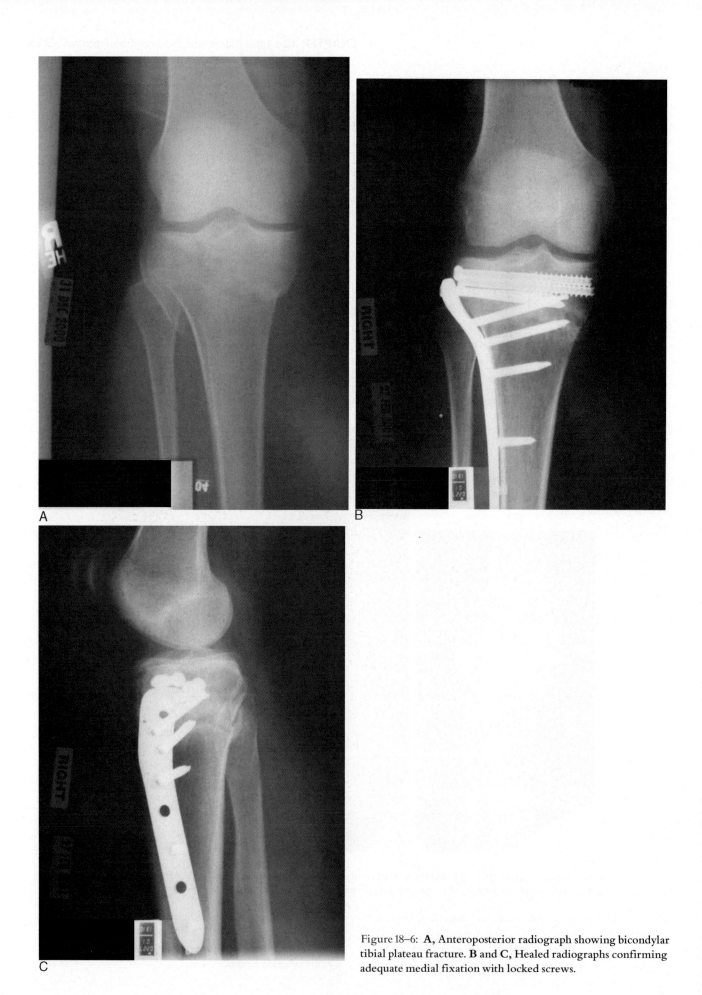

Figure 18–6: **A,** Anteroposterior radiograph showing bicondylar tibial plateau fracture. **B** and **C,** Healed radiographs confirming adequate medial fixation with locked screws.

Extraarticular Proximal Tibia Fractures

Definition

- There is no accepted definition, usually a fracture in metaphyseal zone proximal to diaphysis.
- Usually a result of higher energy injury.
- Frequently are open fractures resulting from crushing mechanism (i.e., car bumper)

Associated Conditions

- High frequency of compartment syndrome—muscle mass resides in the proximal leg and therefore significant muscle injury can occur.
- Vascular injury resulting from proximity to popliteal fossa.
- Knee ligamentous injuries.
- Peroneal nerve injuries because fibular head or neck also typically fractured.
- Often will have fracture extending proximally along the posterior cortex of the proximal fragment, may or may not be displaced (Figure 18–7).
- Unsolved fracture—can be plated, nailed, or treated with external fixation. No accepted standard.

Treatment

- Nonoperative—reserved for nondisplaced or minimally displaced fractures. Must still monitor for compartment syndrome. Also individuals who would not benefit from early knee range of motion or normal limb alignment. Hinged knee brace or cast or splint for 6 to 8 weeks with protected weight bearing.
- Operative treatment—displaced fractures and those benefiting from earlier restoration of knee and limb function.

  - Intramedullary (IM) nailing—must obtain reduction before nail insertion and maintain reduction during nail

insertion. Must be aware of frontal and sagittal plane deformities during nail insertion because nail will *not* reduce fracture but can malreduce fracture. Lateral starting point generally preferred for proximal tibia fractures,[22,23] although others authors disagree.[24] Valgus and apex anterior deformities most common malreduction seen with IM nailing[22,25] (Figure 18–8). Some authors attribute difficulty in fracture reduction to the location of the proximal bend in the nail.[26] The use of

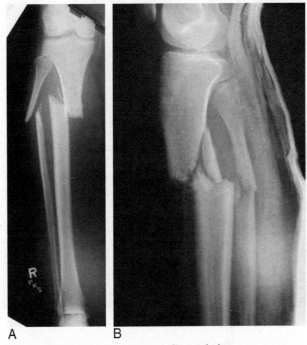

Figure 18–7: **A,** Anteroposterior radiograph demonstrates near diaphyseal location of fracture. **B,** Lateral radiograph reveals more proximal extension in region. This fragment may initially be without displacement.

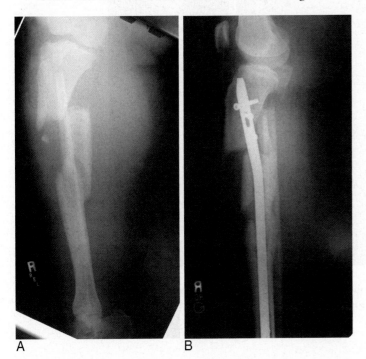

Figure 18–8: **A,** Lateral view of segmental fracture with intact-appearing posterior cortex of proximal fragment. **B,** Extension and translation of proximal fragment with nail inserted (note displacement of posterior cortex of proximal fragment).

blocking screws may also be used to maintain reduction during nail insertion[27] (Figure 18–9)

- Plating—may be more stable construct and does allow for easier reduction with through an open approach.[25] Should avoid significant soft-tissue stripping because this can add to soft-tissue complications. Percutaneous techniques and plating systems have increased popularity of plating as an indirect technique (Figure 18–10)

- External fixation—allows for protection of the soft tissues and early knee motion when compared to cast treatment. Proximal pin sites can lead to septic arthritis with pin tract infection.[14]

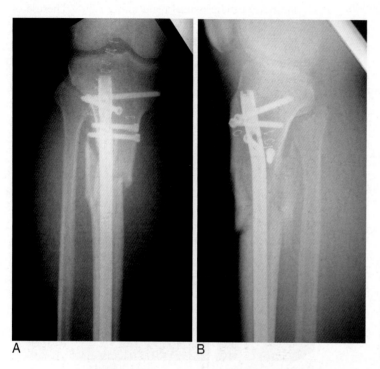

Figure 18–9: **A,** Anteroposterior view demonstrates alignment maintained with intramedullary nail in place (note lateral insertion point of nail). **B,** Lateral view depicting posterior blocking screw to avoid nail deflection off of posterior cortex of proximal fragment; alignment well-maintained without extension of proximal fragment.

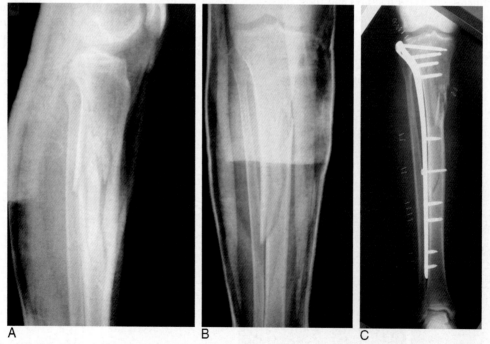

Figure 18–10: Lateral **(A)** and anteroposterior **(B)** radiographs showing proximal extension of fracture posteriorly. **C and D,** Immediate postoperative radiographs after percutaneous locked plating.

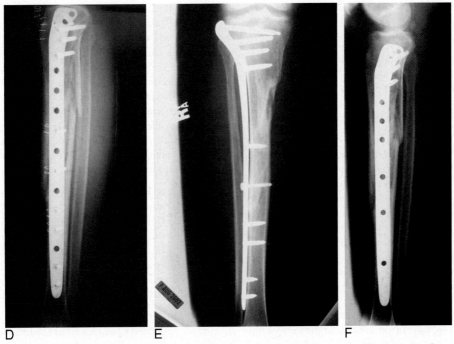

Figure 18–10, cont'd: **E and F,** 1-year follow-up radiographs demonstrating healed fracture with maintained alignment.

Annotated References

1. Honkonen SE: Indications for surgical treatment of tibial condyle fractures, *Clin Orthop* 302:199-205, 1994.
One hundred thirty patients with average follow-up of 6 years. Authors reported incidence of tibial plateau fractures to increase with age in women, resembling any osteoporotic fracture. In men, peak incidence was in third decade of life. Also described radiographic criteria for open reduction internal fixation: lateral plateau-tilt greater than 5 degrees step off greater than 3 mm, widening greater than 5 mm; medial plateau—all fractures except fissures.

2. Delamarter RB, Hohl M, Hopp EJr: Ligament injuries associated with tibial plateau fractures, *Clin Orthop* 250:226-233, 1990.
Thirty-nine patients with tibial plateau and ligament injuries were reviewed with follow-up of more than 1 year. Most common ligament injury (24/39) was medial collateral ligament (MCL), followed by lateral collateral ligament (LCL; 15/39). MCL injuries predominantly in lateral plateau fractures, isolated LCL injuries found equally among medial and lateral plateau fractures. Greater than 10 degrees of instability correlated with poorer results.

3. Schatzker J, McBroom R, Bruce D: The tibial plateau fracture, *Clin Orthop* 138:94-104, 1979.
Ninety-four patients, 70 with average follow-up of 28 months are detailed. Described fracture classification and concluded that a comprehensive approach to tibial plateau fractures is misleading because different fracture patterns behave differently. Confirmed that instability will lead to increased posttraumatic arthritis.

4. Moore TM: Fracture-dislocation of the knee, *Clin Orthop* 156:128-140, 1981.
Moore described a classification for fracture and subluxation or dislocation of the proximal tibia to differentiate these injuries from traditional tibial plateau fractures and true knee dislocations. Significant instability was demonstrated with all five described patterns and was seen in 60% of type I cases and 100% of type 5 cases. These injuries do better than traditional tibial plateau fractures but worse than true knee dislocations.

5. Chan PS, Klimkiewicz JJ, Luchetti WT, et al: Impact of CT scan on treatment plan and fracture classification of tibial plateau fractures, *J Orthop Trauma* 11:484-489, 1997.
Computed tomography scans decreased intraobserver and interobserver variability and increased agreement when added to plain radiographs during fracture classification and surgical planning.

6. Yacoubian SV, Nevins RT, Sallis JG, et al: Impact of MRI on treatment plan and fracture classification of tibial plateau fractures, *J Orthop Trauma* 16:632-637, 2002.
Magnetic resonance imaging (MRI) and plain radiographs were compared to computed tomography (CT) scan and plain radiographs and the authors found MRI superior to CT scan with greater interobserver agreement amongst MRI cases.

7. Stevens DG, Beharry R, McKee MD, et al: The long-term functional outcome of operatively treated tibial plateau fractures, *J Orthop Trauma* 15:312-320, 2001.
Forty-seven patients with tibial plateau fixation and minimum 5-year follow-up, average 8.3-year follow-up. Noted good results with open treatment and recommended surgical treatment for displaced

tibial plateau fractures. Age at time of injury did influence outcome—patients younger than 40 years old did better and those older than 40 years old faired worse.

8. Tscherne H, Lobenhoffer P: Tibial plateau fractures: management and expected results, *Clin Orthop* 292:87-100, 1993.

Proposed soft-tissue classification for open tibia and fibula fractures based on depth of soft-tissue damage not on wound size. Authors suggested initial external fixation for more severe injuries followed by internal fixation.

9. Barei DP, Nork SE, Mills WJ, et al: Complications associated with internal fixation of high-energy bicondylar tibial plateau fractures utilizing a two-incision technique, *J Orthop Trauma* 18:649-657, 2004.

Eighty-three patients with complex tibial plateau fractures (AO/OTA 41-C3) underwent plate fixation through two mini incisions—anterolateral and posteromedial with average follow-up of 36 months. Fifty percent of cases had initial spanning external fixation followed by open reduction and internal fixation (ORIF) with average delay of 9.2 days. Nineteen percent had need for reoperation with 8.4% deep infection rate. Authors noted that locked plating technology may have prevented a second incision but that this technology was not yet available at the time of this study.

10. Fernandez DL: Anterior approach to the knee with osteotomy of the tibial tubercle for bicondylar tibial plateau fractures, *J Bone Joint Surg Am* 70:208-219, 1988.

Osteotomy of tibial tubercle through anterior midline approach—elevation of both menisci allowing exposure of entire joint is described for complex bicondylar tibial fractures.

11. Fowble CD, Zimmer JW, Schepsis AA: The role of arthroscopy in the assessment and treatment of tibial plateau fractures, *Arthroscopy* 9:584-590, 1993.

Authors compared standard open reduction and internal fixation (ORIF) to arthroscopic reduction and percutaneous fixation in split and depression or depression tibial plateau fractures and reported better results with arthroscopic technique as a result of more anatomic reductions, shorter hospital stay, and less complications. They also were able to address associated knee pathology arthroscopically.

12. Lachiewicz PF, Funcik T: Factors influencing the results of open reduction and internal fixation of tibial plateau fractures, *Clin Orthop* 259:210-215, 1990.

Open reduction and internal fixation (ORIF) of 43 patients with average follow-up of 2.7 years. The absence of bone grafting was associated with less than excellent results. Bicondylar fractures resulted in average range of motion of 110 degrees, 18 degrees less than other fracture types.

13. Karunakar MA, Egol KA, Peindl R, et al: Split depression tibial plateau fractures: a biomechanical study, *J Orthop Trauma* 16:172-177, 2002.

Biomechanical cadaveric study showing raft screws to be an effective form of fixation either through a plate or free standing with separate antiglide plate.

14. Marsh JL, Smith ST: External fixation and limited internal fixation for complex fractures of the tibial plateau, *J Bone Joint Surg Am* 77:661-673, 1995.

Twenty-one complex tibial plateau fractures; 7 open and 14 closed fractures with average follow-up 38 months. Closed reduction with interfragmentary fixation of articular fragments and external fixation of metaphyseal and diaphyseal fracture. Bone graft performed in only one patient. Thirty-three percent had pin site infection and 10% developed septic arthritis from intracapsular pin sites. All fractures healed. Authors stated poorer results are more likely from severity of articular injury rather than quality of reduction.

15. Sirkin MS, Bono CM, Reilly MC, et al: Percutaneous methods of tibial plateau fixation, *Clin Orthop* 375:60-68, 2000.

Authors stated unicondylar fractures are most amenable to percutaneous techniques and recommended preoperative computed tomography (CT) scan to accurately define fracture planes. Techniques described include femoral distractor for ligamentotaxis, percutaneous large clamps, cortical windows and tamps to elevate depressed fragments, and raft screws with washers at fracture apex.

16. Lobenhoffer P, Gerich T, Witte F, et al: Use of an injectable calcium phosphate bone cement in the treatment of tibial plateau fractures: A prospective study of twenty-six cases with twenty-month mean follow-up, *J Orthop Trauma* 16:143-149, 2002.

Twenty-six patients that required bone graft underwent injection of a "bone cement" (hardening calcium phosphate). All fractures healed with displacement. Early weight bearing was allowed at mean postoperative follow-up of 4.5 weeks. Concluded that initial mechanical strength of hardening calcium phosphate can allow earlier weight bearing.

17. Rasmussen PS: Tibial condyle fractures, *J Bone Joint Surg Am* 55:1331-1350, 1973.

Two hundred sixty fractures and indication for surgery was instability of knee in extended position. Minimal fixation techniques and instrumentation were available. Authors concluded that medial plateau fractures are important and should undergo repair. They also noted that worse results were found in patients with residual instability and malalignment.

18. Jensen DB, Rude C, Duus B, et al: Tibial plateau fractures: a comparison of conservative and surgical treatment, *J Bone Joint Surg Br* 72:49-52, 1990.

One hundred nine tibial plateau fractures were reviewed; 61 treated with skeletal traction and 48 with surgery with average follow-up of 70 months. Equal comparison was not possible because those in the surgery group had worse injuries. Hospital stay and bed rest were longer in the nonsurgical group, but osteoarthritis was higher in the surgical group. Meniscotomy at time of surgery showed a trend toward greater osteoarthritis.

19. Honkonen SE: Degenerative arthritis after tibial plateau fractures, *J Orthop Trauma* 9:273-277, 1995.

One hundred thirty tibial plateau fractures with average follow-up of 7.6 years. Seventy-six fractures were treated with surgery and 55 treated nonoperatively. Bone grafting was performed in 52 of 76 fractures. Arthritis was related to poor reductions, instability, and especially meniscotomy. Authors also concluded that posttraumatic arthritis seems to almost be an avoidable consequence of tibial plateau fractures.

20. Gausewitz S, Hohl M: The significance of early motion in the treatment of tibial plateau fractures, *Clin Orthop* 202:135-138, 1986.

One hundred twelve fractures with average follow-up of 1.8 years were reviewed for knee range of motion based on treatment. Three groups—those with minimal or no displacement, those with displacement treated nonoperatively, and those with displacement treated operatively. Authors reported that final knee range of motion was affected greatest in those treated operatively and immobilized longer than 6 weeks. Concluded that knee immobilization is tolerated well up to 6 weeks when treated non-operatively but may result in some stiffness when treated operatively and therefore recommended earlier knee motion following operative treatment.

21. Duwelius PJ, Connolly JF: Closed reduction of tibial plateau fractures: a comparison of functional and roentgenographic end results, *Clin Orthop* 230:116-126, 1988.

One hundred tibial plateau fractures with average follow-up of 5.1 years; 73 treated nonoperatively. Good-to-excellent results were reported despite less than satisfactory radiographic results. Authors concluded that most of these fractures can be treated nonoperatively if evaluation of the knee in extension does not demonstrate instability. Instability in extension or medial plateau fractures should receive operative treatment.

22. Freedman E, Johnson E: Radiographic analysis of tibial fracture malalignment following intramedullary nailing, *Clin Orthop* 315:25-33, 1995.

One hundred thirty-three tibial fractures undergoing intramedullary nailing were radiographically reviewed. Proximal third fractures had the greatest rate of malalignment at 58%, compared to 7% for central third, and 8% for distal third fractures. Average valgus was 9.5 degrees and average extension of the proximal fragment was 7.5 degrees in the proximal third fracture group. Authors recommended careful technique and a more lateral insertion site for proximal third fractures.

23. Lang GJ, Cohen BE, Bosse MJ, et al: Proximal third tibial shaft fractures: Should they be nailed? *Clin Orthop* 315:64-74, 1995.

Thirty-two fractures of the proximal third of the tibia that underwent intramedullary (IM) nailing were reviewed. Eighty-four percent had greater than 5 degrees of frontal or sagittal plane angulation. More than 25% had loss of initial reduction noted on follow-up radiographs. Most common deformities were valgus and apex anterior angulation. Authors recommended consideration of others forms of fixation for these fractures or initial plate fixation of the fracture followed by IM nailing for segmental fractures.

24. Buehler KC, Green J, Wall TS, et al: A technique for intramedullary nailing of proximal third tibia fractures, *J Orthop Trauma* 11:218-223, 1997.

Fourteen cases of proximal tibia fractures underwent intramedullary (IM) nailing through a lateral insertion site and the use of a medial femoral distractor. Hypothesis was based on cadaveric transverse cross-sectional data supporting the concept of a wider IM canal laterally. The authors noted that the effective canal width is decreased medially and therefore can cause a valgus malreduction. Twelve of the 14 were treated successfully with this technique.

25. Henley MB, Meier M, Tencer AF: Influences of some design parameters on the biomechanics of the unreamed tibial intramedullary nail, *J Orthop Trauma* 7:311-319, 1993.

Fourteen fresh cadaveric specimens were obtained and underwent intramedullary (IM) nailing with the Synthes (Paoli, Penn.) tibial nail. Authors concluded that the location of the bend in the nail can cause the fracture to result in a malreduction. A nail with a more proximal bend is recommended when treating proximal tibia fractures with an IM nail.

26. Sameulson MA, McPherson EJ, Norris L: Anatomic assessment of the proper insertion site for a tibial intramedullary nail, *J Orthop Trauma* 16:23-25, 2002.

Sixty-one cadaveric legs, with an average age 87 years old, were nailed in a retrograde fashion, and the exit point proximally was mapped. Average canal size was 11 mm and nail used was 7 mm. Authors concluded that starting point should be the medial third of tibial tubercle and that lateral starting points should be avoided.

27. Ricci WM, O'Boyle MO, Borrelli J, et al: Fractures of the proximal third of the tibial shaft treated with intramedullary nails and blocking screws, *J Orthop Trauma* 15:264-270, 2001.

Twelve patients with proximal third tibia fractures underwent intramedullary (IM) nailing and blocking screw placement to help control fracture alignment during nail insertion. Blocking screws proved to be an effective technique to control alignment during nail insertion and avoid valgus malreductions.

Tibial Shaft Fractures

Jeffrey Anglen, MD, FACS

Etiology

- The tibia is the most commonly fractured long bone in the human body.
- Tibia fractures occur in a wide spectrum of ages and from a variety of mechanisms.
- Low-energy mechanisms, such as most sports-related fractures and standing level falls, occur in two age-group peaks. Sporting injuries occur in the second and third decades of life, and fractures through poor quality bone from falls occur in the elderly.
- High-energy fractures, such as pedestrians struck by vehicles, motorcycle accidents, agricultural machines, or gunshots, can occur to patients of any age. In general, high-energy fractures are the most difficult to treat and have the highest risk of complications.

Anatomy

- The tibia is approximately straight, although there may be various degrees of curvature in a normal tibia. The cross section is not circular but roughly triangular. In healthy adults the cortex is quite thick and dense.
- The proximal and distal metaphyses expand and the cortex thins. The expansion of the bone is not symmetrical because it flares more laterally on the proximal end and medially on the distal end.
- As a result the intramedullary (IM) axis of the tibial shaft does not pass exactly through the midpoint of the proximal metaphyseal width, a fact that has important implications for the starting point of a tibial nail (Figure 19–1).
- In the sagittal plane, the proximal metaphysis flares posteriorly much more than anteriorly, placing the tibial shaft axis quite anterior to the midpoint of the metaphyseal anteroposterior (AP) dimension (see Figure 19–1).

- The tibial shaft and tibial joint line angle is approximately 3 degrees of varus in the coronal plane and 10 degrees sloping posterior in the sagittal plane.
- The anterior portion of the proximal tibia includes the tibial tubercle, the attachment of the patellar tendon.
- The anterior medial surface of the tibia is flat and covered only with periosteum and skin. The lateral and posterior surfaces are covered by the muscles of the calf.

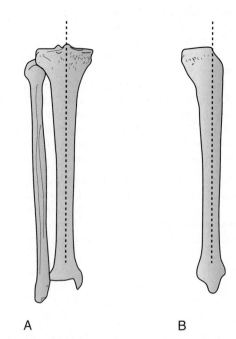

A   B

Figure 19–1: **A,** This diagram shows the frontal projection of the tibia. Notice that the proximal projection of the shaft axis does not line up exactly with the midpoint of the epiphysis. **B,** This diagram showing a lateral projection of the tibia shows that the intra-medullary axis lies anterior to the majority of the epiphysis. The star marks the position for placement of the proximal femoral distractor pin.

- The muscles of the calf are partitioned into four fascial compartments, a common site of compartment syndrome (Figure 19–2).
- The fibula is posterior and lateral to the tibia and surrounded by muscle.
- The popliteal artery and vein and the tibial and peroneal nerves are posterior to the proximal tibia and are close to the bone. The peroneal nerve continues laterally around the neck of the fibula and divides into deep and superficial branches.
- The nutrient artery of the tibia enters posteriorly in the proximal third.

Classification

- Tibia fractures are commonly associated with soft-tissue injury, which can be graded to identify injuries at risk for complications and poor outcome. Open fractures are commonly classified by the Gustilo-Anderson system,[1] whereas the soft-tissue injury in a closed fracture can be graded using the method of Tscherne.[2] Although the Gustilo-Anderson system is widely used, it should be noted that the interobserver reliability is no better than 65% to 70%.
- A Gustilo-Anderson grade I open fracture is one associated with a minor (=1 cm) skin laceration and no significant degloving or excessive contamination. A grade II open fracture demonstrates a skin disruption between 1 and 10 cm in length, again without periosteal stripping or severe contamination. The grade III fractures are the most severe and are subdivided further. Grade III-A denotes a clean laceration greater than 10 cm in total length and may include degloving or skin loss without periosteal stripping. A smaller soft-tissue wound with excessive or exceptional contamination would be graded as III-A by most surgeons. A grade III-B open fracture's defining characteristic is periosteal stripping—exposed, devitalized bone. In some cases and situations, this may require a soft-tissue flap for coverage but not always. With newer wound treatments, the need for flaps is decreasing, and in any event, the wound classification should determine the treatment rather than the other way around. A grade III-C open fracture is a fracture with any size or amount of soft-tissue injury associated with a vascular disruption that requires repair (i.e., producing limb ischemia).
- The Tscherne classification of closed soft-tissue injury is less commonly used and probably has even less interobserver reliability but is useful to read and understand. There are four grades of soft-tissue injury, 0 to 3.[2]
  - Grade 0 indicates a simple fracture configuration, with little or no soft-tissue injury.
  - In grade 1, there is a mild- to moderate-energy severe fracture pattern, associated with a superficial abrasion or contusion. The soft-tissue damage is mild to moderate and may be the result of fragment pressure from within.
  - In grade 2, there is a moderate-energy fracture pattern with a deep contaminated abrasion with local damage to skin or muscle. This type includes impending compartment syndrome.
  - In grade 3, there is a high-energy fracture pattern with extensive contusion or crushing of skin or subcutaneous tissue. There may be avulsion of skin (closed degloving) and damaged muscle.
- Tibial fractures can be described by location (metaphyseal, diaphyseal, proximal, distal, or segmental), comminution, displacement (shortening, rotation, angulation, or translation), and fracture pattern (transverse, spiral, oblique, or butterfly).
- The Orthopaedic Trauma Association (OTA) classification system is useful to categorize groups of fractures for comparison of series, particularly in research communications. Tibial fractures are type 42, and the next level of description is A (simple), B (wedge), or C (complex) (Figure 19–3).

Patient Evaluation

- Although a high-energy open tibia fracture can be a dramatic and arresting injury, the orthopaedic consultant should remember to do a full evaluation of the patient, as in any multiple trauma situation. The ABCs of trauma evaluation must not be forgotten. During the secondary evaluation of the musculoskeletal system, every body surface should be inspected, looking for laceration, contusion, swelling, abrasion, ecchymosis, or deformity. Every bone and joint should be palpated for stability, crepitus, tenderness, and range of motion.

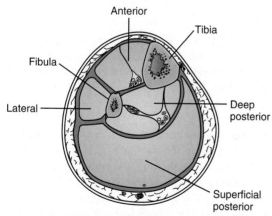

Figure 19–2: This cross-sectional diagram of the leg shows the four fascial compartments: anterior, lateral, deep posterior, and superficial posterior. The anterior compartment contains the anterior tibialis, the extensor hallucis longus, and the extensor digitorum. The lateral compartment contains the peroneus longus and brevis. The deep posterior compartment contains the flexor hallucis longus, the flexor digitorum, and the posterior tibialis. The superficial posterior compartment contains the soleus and gastrocnemius.

Groups:

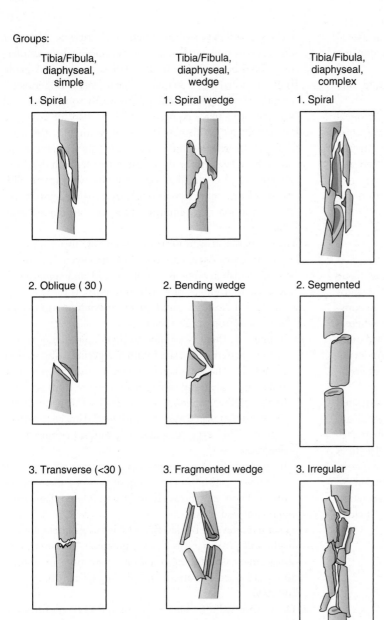

Tibia/Fibula, diaphyseal, simple

1. Spiral

2. Oblique (30)

3. Transverse (<30)

Tibia/Fibula, diaphyseal, wedge

1. Spiral wedge

2. Bending wedge

3. Fragmented wedge

Tibia/Fibula, diaphyseal, complex

1. Spiral

2. Segmented

3. Irregular

Figure 19–3: **The Orthopaedic Trauma Association and Arbeitsgemeinschaft für Osteosynthesefragen (AO) classification system for fractures of the tibial shaft.** *J Orthop Trauma* 10:52, 1996.

- Neurovascular examination of the limb should include palpation of the soft-tissue compartments, dorsalis pedis and posterior tibial pulse, evaluation of capillary refill, sharp and touch sensation in all nerve root distributions of the foot, and active and passive motion of the toes and ankles. "Wiggles toes" is not adequate. Beware the passive recoil after toe plantar flexion that simulates active dorsiflexion. Gently judge strength against resistance if possible. Remember that the examination may change over time and should be repeated at intervals in patients at risk. Document carefully and completely, particularly any deficits found or suspected.

- Compare to the uninjured side, particularly for swelling in the soft tissues (compartment syndrome). Missed compartment

syndrome is a common cause of lawsuits, so have a low index of suspicion for this condition. Initial signs include pain on passive motion of the toes and tense swelling. In obtunded patients, palpation may be the only clue, other than history. Compartment syndrome can happen in open fractures. The diagnosis is primarily made clinically, but direct measurement can be used to rule it out. The compartment pressure should be measured at multiple sites, including particularly the level of the fracture. Elevated pressures in the correct clinical setting confirm the diagnosis and indicate fasciotomy. Various pressure level thresholds have been advocated in the literature, but compartment pressures within 30 mm Hg of the diastolic blood pressure or within 40 mm Hg of the mean arterial pressure can be considered to represent compartment syndrome. Examination should be repeated at intervals.

- Open wounds should be examined and described in the chart, perhaps with a drawing. Note the location, size, and character of soft-tissue wounds and the presence of contamination or devitalized tissue. Severely contaminated wounds can be irrigated with a liter of saline. Wounds should not be repeatedly probed but should be covered with a sterile, compressive dressing after the initial examination and protected from further contamination in the hospital. Initial cultures are not useful.

- Regardless of the ultimate treatment selected, a fractures tibia should be gently realigned in the emergency department (ED) with adequate analgesia and a splint placed to protect the limb. A posterior long leg plaster slab or a U-shaped sugar tong splint can be used. Access to the soft tissues for repeat evaluation should not be impaired by the splint.

- Ice and elevation are helpful to control pain and swelling. If compartment syndrome is not suspected, elevation should be above the heart. If extremity perfusion ("impending compartment syndrome") is a concern, elevation to the level of the heart may be more prudent.

Definitive Treatment
Nonsurgical Treatment

- Many if not most tibial shaft fractures can be treated successfully without surgery.

- Traditionally, nonoperative treatment consisted of immobilization of the limb in a long leg cast and protection from weight bearing from several weeks or months. Although tedious and inconvenient, this method resulted in a high rate of union and ultimate return to satisfactory function. Rehabilitation required to address stiffness and weakness was often prolonged.

- Sarmiento[3] have developed and advocated the concept of functional fracture bracing, in which the patient is placed in a premolded, somewhat pliable, removable fracture brace after about 4 weeks of casting. This method encourages early motion of adjacent joints and earlier weight bearing. It facilitates quicker healing and return to function.

- Malalignment is the most frequent complication of closed treatment. Although minor degrees of shortening and deformity are common with this treatment, they are of no functional significance. The amount of deformity that will be functionally significant is unknown and probably varies among patients with different expectations and activity levels. The relationship between tibial deformity and arthritis of the knee or ankle remains unclear.

- Analysis of radiographs reveals that the deformity seen on the original film does not increase over time with functional brace treatment. In other words, the first radiograph shows the maximum deformity possible for the fracture;

if it is acceptable, the fracture can be treated without surgery.

- There has not been a direct comparison between functional brace treatment and IM nailing. Comparisons between IM nailing and cast immobilization (with some patients having screws or wiring before the cast) suggest a higher rate of nonunion, delayed union, decreased mobility, and more time off work with casting but a much higher rate of anterior knee pain with nailing.[4,5]

- Certain fractures can be predicted to do poorly without surgical treatment.
  - Open fractures require surgical treatment of the wound, and many will require continued access to the soft tissues, which might be obstructed by casts or braces.
  - Highly comminuted (= 50% of circumferential cortical continuity) or otherwise unstable fractures, such as those with greater than 2 to 3 cm shortening, greater than 50% translation, or segmental patterns. Significant instability is the fracture characteristic most apt to indicate the need for early operative intervention.[6]
  - Reduction is difficult to maintain in spiral fractures of the tibia with similar factures of the fibula at another level.
  - Tibial shaft fractures with intact fibulae have a high risk of varus nonunion or malunion when treated closed.
  - Fractures with associated ipsilateral femur fractures or intraarticular fractures of the knee or ankle.
  - Fractures that cannot be maintained in "acceptable" alignment by casting or bracing. The limits of acceptable deformity are controversial. Various authors have suggested acceptable limits of 5 degrees to 10 degrees of varus, 4 degrees to 10 degrees of valgus, 5 degrees to 20 degrees of AP angulation, 5 degrees to 20 degrees of rotation, and 10 to 20 mm of shortening.[6]

External Fixation

- External fixators can be of several types. Half-pin fixators use larger pins with threaded tips, and the pins extend through the skin on one side of the bone. The pins are coupled to external rods. Circular (wire or ring) fixators use thin wires (1.5 to 2 mm) that are placed all the way through the limb and are held under high tension by complete or partial rings around the limb. The rings are then connected together into a frame by coupling to rods. The Ilizarov fixator was the first of this type. Hybrid fixators use both rings and independent half pins, usually consisting of a ring near the epiphysis and half pins in the diaphysis.

- External fixation is useful with open fractures or other soft-tissue injuries, such as burns, compartment syndrome, and contaminated abrasions.

- Compared to IM nailing, external fixation in open tibial fractures leads to more problems with malalignment and "surgical interface" (incision, pin site, or percutaneous screw site) infection.[7]

- Although a full discussion of external fixation technique is beyond the scope of this text, a few points may be helpful.
  - Plan pin placement to avoid potential incisions and to minimize the amount of soft tissue penetrated. In the tibial shaft, that usually means anterior or anteromedial placement of half pins.
  - Maximum stability is achieved by spreading the pins as widely as possible in the segment. Generally, two pins per bone segment is adequate fixation. For temporary fixators as described in this chapter, one centrally threaded transfixion pin in each segment is enough.
  - Pins should be placed through small skin incisions to avoid tethering skin or other structures. The soft tissues are gently spread to periosteum, a small elevator is used, and drill guides with a trocar allow the drill to be positioned directly on the bone.
  - Predrilling and hand insertion of pins is preferable to self-drilling pins as a result of reduced heat of insertion, more precise placement, and better purchase in the bone.
  - Positioning rods close to the bone improves stability, as does "double stacking" rods.
- Circular fixators are commonly used for definitive fixation of tibial fractures by enthusiasts of that technique. This option may be chosen in the face of segmental bone loss because it allows use of the frame for bone transport to fill the gap. The patient can frequently bear weight on the frame, allowing early return to function.
- The most common use of external fixation in the tibia is for temporary stabilization, while awaiting another fixation technique. It provides relative stability, preservation of length and alignment, and allows patient mobilization (Figure 19–4). This is used in the face of medical contraindications to surgery or a local soft-tissue injury or swelling that renders early definitive fixation hazardous. Conversion of a temporary external fixator to IM nailing carries a risk of IM osteomyelitis, particularly if there is any history of pin site infection.[8] Because of that risk, such conversions should be done early. One study suggested that use of solid nails rather than cannulated nails in this setting lowers the risk of subsequent infection.[9]

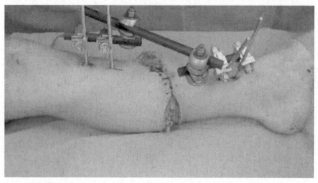

Figure 19–4: **A temporary external fixator for complex soft tissue injury—"traveling traction"**

Internal Fixation: Plates

- Plate fixation of tibial fractures is most commonly done for extreme proximal, extreme distal fractures, or segmental fractures that include a metaphyseal or epiphyseal component.
- Plating tibia fractures must be done carefully. Damage to the soft-tissue envelope from surgical approaches can lead to infection, wound failure, or nonunion. Plate fixation is particularly dangerous in open fractures as a result of the high risk of infection.
- New techniques using minimal incision percutaneous plate placement may reduce the morbidity of tibial plating.
- The plate must be of adequate length (= four plate holes on each side of the fracture is preferable), although not all of the plate holes need to be filled. A screw hole in a plate is an opportunity not an obligation.
- The preferable plate position is on the anteromedial flat surface. Although the plate is more prominent subcutaneously, it interferes less with the tibial blood supply.

Internal Fixation: Intramedullary Nailing

- IM nailing is the most common surgical fixation technique for tibial shaft fractures. The technique provides relative stability, maintaining length and alignment without undue soft-tissue damage at the fracture site.
- Early nail designs were solid, of variable flexibility, and lacked the capacity for interlocking. Examples are Rush rods, Enders nails, and Lottes nails. Modern nail designs incorporate the ability to interlock the nail at both ends and thereby stabilize fractures with comminution or bone loss against shortening and rotation. Interlocking allows for secure fixation of more proximal and distal fractures and fractures in which the isthmus is not intact.
- Smaller diameter, solid section interlocking tibial nails inserted with minimal or no reaming have been successful in both open and closed fracture treatment and have been shown to have a lower reoperation rate than external fixation for open tibial fractures[7,10–13]
- The use of IM reaming for nail insertion allows a larger nail to be inserted, with better bone or nail contact. This improves the stability of fixation but has been postulated to have a negative effect on healing or infection rates resulting from interference with the tibial blood supply.
- However, multiple comparisons in the literature have failed to confirm a detrimental effect of reaming, and indeed show an advantage to reaming, even in open fractures.[11,14–17] Reaming did not delay or impair healing nor promote infection in open fractures.[14] The use of unreamed nails for closed fractures resulted in a trend toward slower healing and the requirement for more secondary procedures in one prospective comparison,[16] a suggestion of more delayed unions in another study,[15] and a significantly longer time to union in a third comparison.[17] All of the studies showed higher rates of screw breakage in unreamed nailings (12% to 52%)

Surgical Technique: Intramedullary Nailing of the Tibia

- As with any fracture operation, the first stage is preoperative planning. Radiographs of the contralateral tibia are useful for predicting the length and diameter of nail necessary. The surgical technique should list the steps of the operation, anticipating potential problems and solutions.
- Preoperative antibiotics are given. A broad-spectrum cephalosporin, such as cefazolin, is a good choice and should be given less than 2 hours but more than 30 minutes before incision. Penicillin-allergic patients can be given clindamycin. Routine vancomycin use should be discouraged.
- The patient is usually positioned supine on a radiolucent fracture table with a bump under the affected hip and knee (Figure 19–5). If assistance is severely limited, the procedure can be done on a fracture table with the hip and knee flexed, and a traction pin through the calcaneus. In that situation, it is important to avoid pressure in the popliteal space from positioning devices.
- The leg is prepped and draped free from mid thigh down, and the foot is covered by wrapping the toes with Coban. If an external fixator is in place, it can be prepped into the field using alcohol followed by Betadine.[18]
- The surgeon stands on the fractured side; the fluoroscopy machine comes in from the opposite side, with the monitor at the foot of the bed.
- Schanz pins are placed from lateral to medial through small stab wounds under fluoroscopic control. The proximal pin is placed posterior to the sagittal midpoint 2 cm or more distal to the plateau and parallel to it. The distal pin is placed in the sagittal midline, parallel to the ankle just above the plafond. In quite distal fractures, this pin can be placed in the talus or calcaneus (Figure 19–6).

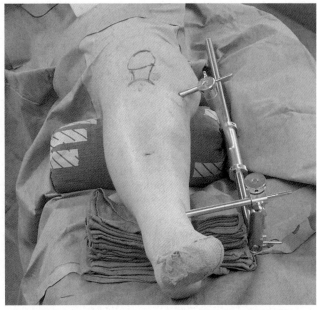

Figure 19–6: **Femoral distractor in place on the medial side.**

- A small bump is placed under the knee to tighten the extensor mechanism. The axis of the tibial shaft is identified using fluoroscopy, and a 1.5- to 2-cm incision is made in this line beginning just at the distal tip of the patella (Figure 19–7). The incision is made deeply through the skin, subcutaneous tissue, tendon, or capsule down to the bone without developing tissue planes. Many surgeons have strong opinions regarding placement of the incision through the tendon or medial to it, but a randomized study has shown no difference.[19] I ignore the position of the tendon and make the incision in line with the shaft axis.

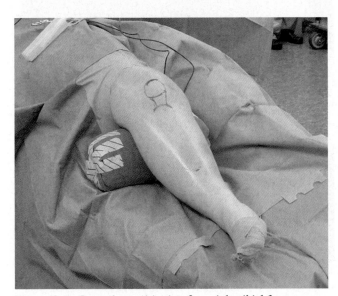

Figure 19–5: **Operative positioning for a right tibial fracture.**

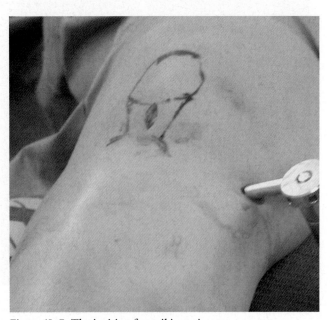

Figure 19–7: **The incision for nail insertion.**

- A proximal starting point is identified by palpation and verified with fluoroscopy. Care should be taken not to make the initial entry into the bone too anterior or too distal. The bone can be opened with an awl, a T-handled reamer, or a drill (Figure 19–8). The opening is enlarged with sequentially larger T-handled reamers. It is important to carefully direct the reamers toward the central canal axis, and it is easy to be fooled and direct the reamer too far medially (Figure 19–9).
- The fracture is reduced manually, and the femoral distractor, if not attached previously, is applied to the Schanz pins to provide improved intraoperative stability. The distractor will control the length and rotation reasonably well. In some cases, angulation is difficult to control with the distractor, or it may be worsened. A tendency to varus resulting from the lateral distractor can be compensated for at the swivel joints or with the use of an assistant's hands. In midshaft fractures, the nail itself will correct the angulation, provided the starting point is correct and reaming has been central in the distal fragment. Oblique or spiral fractures can often be reduced and held anatomically with a percutaneous pointed reduction forceps (Weber clamp). In proximal fractures, blocking screws (as described in the chapter on proximal tibial fractures) may help prevent

deformity and improve reduction. Occasionally, a temporary plate held with clamps or unicortical screws may be useful for reduction while nailing.
- The ball-tipped guidewire (reaming rod) is passed into the bone, across the fracture and into the distal fragment (Figure 19–10). Central position in the distal fragment should be verified in two planes using fluoroscopy (Figure 19–11).
- Sequential reaming is performed over the guidewire using sharp flexible reamers and going up in 0.5-mm increments. Keep the knee and hip flexed. Never use a tourniquet while reaming, to avoid excessive heat generation, which can kill large segments of the bone. Go slowly, frequently clean the flutes of the reamer, and irrigate the canal with saline each time the reamer comes out. Ream at least 0.5 mm (preferably 1 mm) above the planned nail size (Figure 19–12).
- Switch to a smooth-tipped guide wire. Measure the correct nail length using the radio-opaque ruler (Figure 19–13). Before inserting the nail, use fluoroscopy to verify that it is the correct length by holding the nail next to the bone while still in its sterile inner packaging. Insert the nail over the guidewire, and advance with gentle taps of the hammer, with the knee fully flexed.
- Alternatively, the reaming and nail insertion can be performed with the knee only slightly (20 degrees to 40

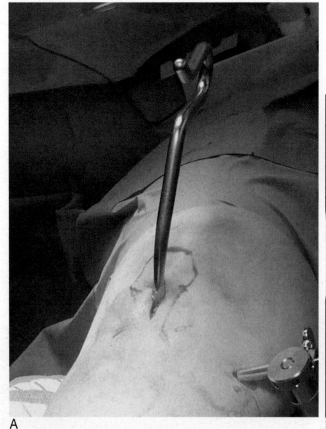

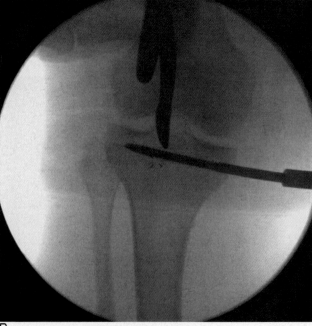

A B

Figure 19–8: **A,** The cortex is opened with a starting awl after palpation of the correct position. **B,** The fluoroscope is used to verify that the starting position is in line with the tibial shaft axis.

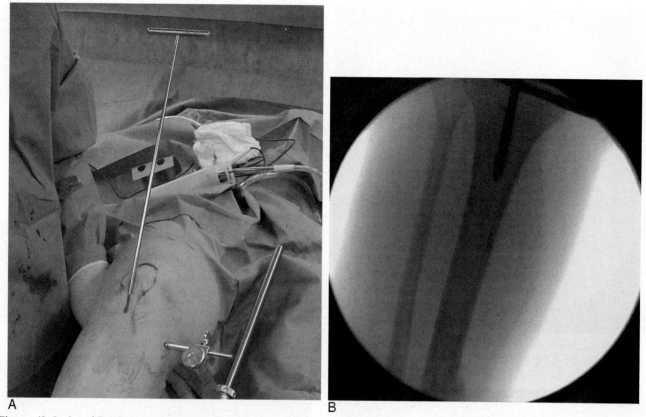

Figures 19–9: **A** and **B,** These images demonstrate the use of the T-handled manual reamers to enlarge the opening in the tibia and direct the path to the intramedullary canal.

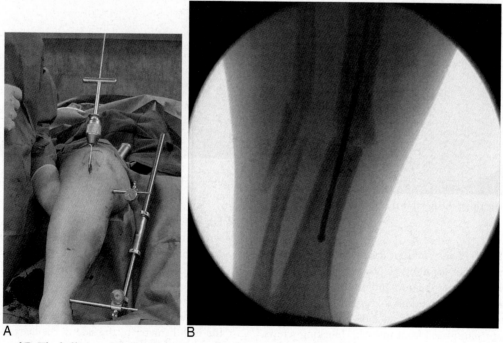

Figure 19–10: **A** and **B,** The ball-tipped guidewire is inserted and directed across the fracture site.

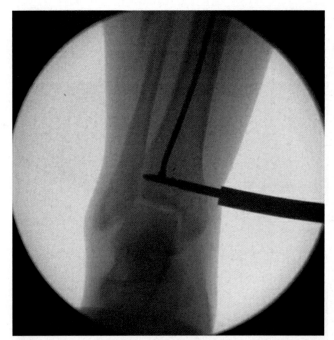

Figure 19–11: **The tip of the guidewire should be centrally positioned in the distal metaphysis.**

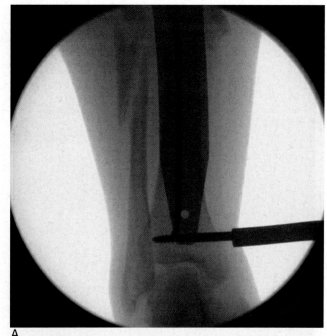

A

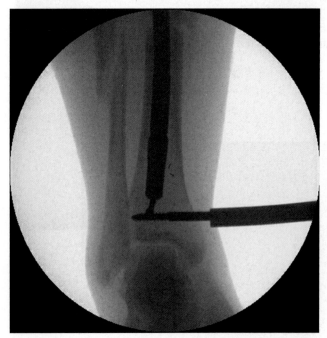

Figure 19–12: **The tip of the flexible reamer in the distal fragment.**

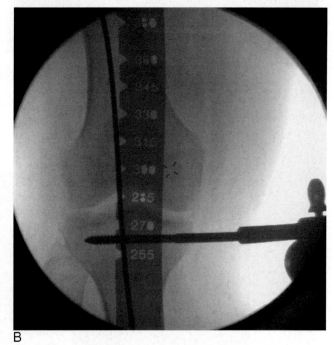

B

Figure 19–13: **A and B,** Measuring the correct length.

degrees) flexed. This position has been advocated to reduce apex anterior deformity in proximal third fractures, but it requires a larger incision and release of the patella for subluxation. Other solutions to the proximal shaft fracture reduction during nailing include percutaneous joy sticks (Schanz pins placed front to back), blocking screws, and temporary plates.

- For fractures of the distal metaphysis, distal blocking screws may be used to maintain a central position of the guidewire, reamer, and nail. This reduces deformities that may occur at this level. As with proximal blocking screws, the screw is placed through the bone in the distal fragment 90 degrees to the plane of the deformity (e.g., front to back for a coronal plane deformity), approximately half the nail diameter to the side of the apex of the deformity (medial for valgus, lateral for varus) (Figure 19–14).

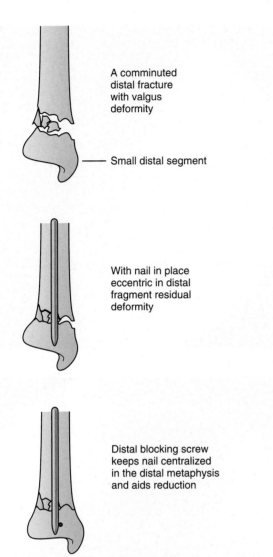

A comminuted distal fracture with valgus deformity

Small distal segment

With nail in place eccentric in distal fragment residual deformity

Distal blocking screw keeps nail centralized in the distal metaphysis and aids reduction

Figure 19–14: **For distal fractures, reduction is hard to control, which can lead to deformity during nailing. Blocking screws placed in the metaphysis on the side of the apex of the deformity will centralize the tip of the nail and help maintain alignment.**

- The nail is seated deeply enough that the proximal end does not extend above the bone.
- Proximal locking is performed with use of the guides attached to the insertion instruments. Distal locking is performed using a free hand technique. The surgeon stands at the foot of the bed, and the C-arm monitor is moved so she can see it. A lateral fluoroscopy shot is obtained that shows perfectly round holes. Distal interlock screws are typically placed medial to lateral to minimize risk of injury to neurovascular structures and to minimize irritation from screws that may be slightly long. A small stab incision is made over the center of the desired hole. A 2-mm cannulated screw guidewire is placed through the incision; the tip is directed to the center of the hole using the C-arm. The wires are drilled across the bone and the position verified. One cortex is drilled over the wire using the

4.5-mm cannulated drill. The drill and wire are removed and the opposite cortex is drilled with the 4-mm drill. Depth gauge is used, and the screw is placed long enough so that at least a couple millimeters of screw tip extend beyond the cortex on the opposite side. This is particularly important with unreamed nailing where the smaller screw diameter leads to a higher incidence of screw breakage (Figure 19–15).

- For midshaft fractures, one interlocking screw on either side is adequate. For proximal or distal third fractures, it is prudent to use two screws in the short fragment for better control (Figure 19–16). Locking the tibia with any gap at the fracture site is a risk factor for nonunion and for reoperation.[20]
- Some systems provide an end cap to prevent in growth of bone into the top of the nail and interfering with extraction.
- The wounds are closed in layers, with heavy absorbable suture in the tendon or capsule. Sterile dressing are applied.
- The drapes and bump are removed, and careful examination of the limb length, rotation, and alignment is performed with the patient still asleep, comparing to the contralateral side. Compartments are palpated. Permanent portable radiographs are obtained in the operating room (OR), including the full length of the tibia, and the patient is not awakened until the radiographs are reviewed.
- The limb is kept elevated, foot pumps are used if possible, and careful periodic evaluation for pain, both at rest and with passive motion, is performed to identify the rare patient who will develop a postoperative compartment syndrome.
- Isometric and active motion exercises can be started as soon as pain allows. In simple fracture patterns with good fixation, partial weight bearing can be begun as soon as tolerated.

Soft-Tissue Management
Open Fracture Wounds

- The tibia is one of the most common sites of open fracture, and open fractures of the tibia have a high incidence of nonunion, malunion, infection, prolonged functional disability, and even ultimate amputation. The general principles of open fracture treatment are covered elsewhere in more detail. This section will review the highlights.
- Early administration of intravenous (IV) antibiotics is vital to prevention of infection. All open tibia fractures should get coverage for gram-positive organisms with a cephalosporin, such as cefazolin, 1 gram every 8 hours. Higher grade or more contaminated fractures should also receive coverage for gram-negative bacteria, and in some situations (e.g., soil contamination) anaerobic coverage is prudent.[21]
- The care of open fracture wounds should be done expeditiously. Delay in wound care increases the incidence of infection, but an absolute threshold of time has not been established. Although most were taught that open fractures

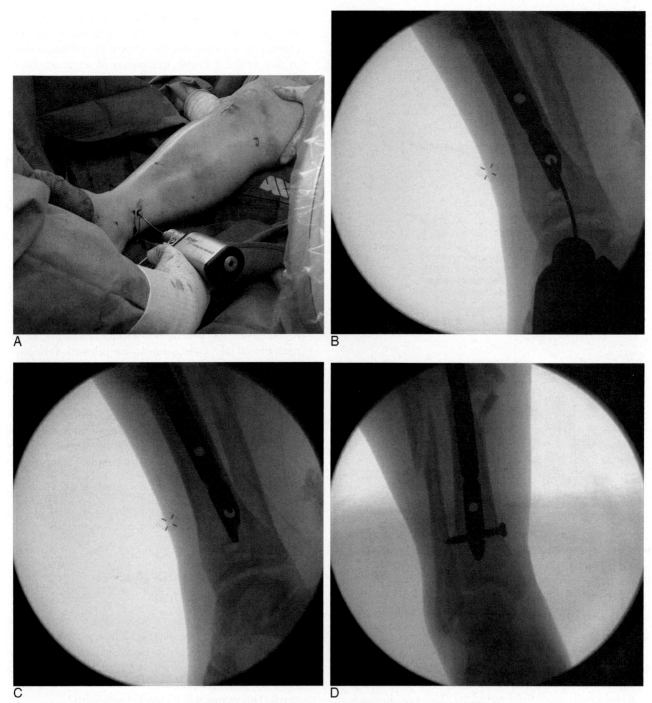

Figure 19–15: **A,** Using a lateral C-arm image, a guidewire is driven across the bone through the distal interlock hole. **B,** The position of the starting tip of the guidewire. Note the close to perfectly round interlock hole on fluoroscopy shows that the X-ray axis is aligned with the interlock hole axis. **C,** The guidewire in place. The fact that the wire shadow does not extend beyond the edges of the nail shadow means the wire must be through the nail and not an airball. **D,** The interlock screw in place. Remember to look at it with the C-arm in both views to verify that the screw passed through the nail.

are an "emergency," in fact some technically open fractures with minor soft-tissue wounds can be managed in similar fashion to closed fractures after evaluation by an experienced trauma surgeon.

- Irrigation and debridement in the OR is usually required and should be performed by an experienced surgeon. The wound is often extended surgically to allow exploration and debridement. The surgical extension of the

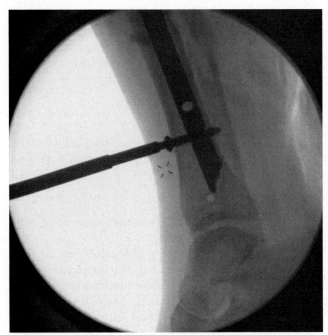

Figure 19–16: **A second anterior to posterior screw was placed for additional stability.**

wound should be longitudinal rather than transverse to avoid problems with closure after skin retraction.

- Debridement should include all clearly devitalized tissue, all foreign material, and debris. Tissues of significant functional importance (nerves, vessels, tendons, or skin in strategic locations), which is marginal in vascularity, may be retained and reevaluated at future procedures within 48 hours; marginal tissues of less importance (fat, fascia, and most muscle) should be debrided at the initial procedure.
- Copious irrigation could be done between debridement of each tissue layer. Although antibiotic additives are widely used, there is no good evidence for efficacy. Liquid castile soap can be used to assist in removal of dirt.[22] Higher pressure irrigation (jet lavage) removes more particulate debris, but the highest pressures have been associated with delayed healing in animal models.
- The size, location, character, and contamination of the soft-tissue wound in addition to the experience and skills of the surgeon will dictate how it is closed or covered. Wound coverage should be done in the first week if possible. Options include:
- Allow healing by secondary intention (granulation). This requires viable tissue in the base of the wound. It may be facilitated with the use of subatmospheric dressings. With this technique, tissues that were formerly believed to require grafts or flaps, such as periosteum, peritenon, or even areas of stripped bone or tendon, can be induced to granulate. Wet-to-dry dressings are an older method that may lead to wound desiccation.
- Delayed primary closure. The use of rubber bands or the vacuum assisted closure (V.A.C) system will help prevent wound retraction and may allow closure at a second procedure.

- Split thickness skin grafting.
- Local fasciocutaneous rotation flaps.
- Local muscle flap with skin grafting.
- Free tissue transfer. Using the technique of microvascular anastomosis, large muscle flaps or composite grafts (including skin, fascia, muscle, or bone) can be autogenously transplanted to fill large defects.

Closed Fracture Wounds

- Even when the skin is not actually broken, the soft tissues of the leg can be damaged significantly, and this can affect fracture healing, functional recovery, and the incidence of complications.
- Crushing injuries and "closed degloving" (separation of the cutaneous and subcutaneous tissue from the underlying fascia) can lead to death of the skin that may be worsened by surgical incisions.
- Signs of soft-tissue injury include abrasion, contusion, swelling, and blistering. These injuries can be classified by use of the Tscherne system as described previously or a more complex system published by the Arbeitsgemeinschaft für Osteosynthesefragen (AO).
- Compartment syndrome results from swelling in the muscles or bleeding into the closed fascial compartments of the leg. Tibial fracture is the most common cause, and the prevalence of compartment syndrome in tibia fracture ranges from 1% to 9%.[23]
  - As discussed previously, compartment syndrome is a clinical diagnosis that begins with a high suspicion based on the history of the injury. Severe or increasing pain, tightness, and subjective sensory changes are common complaints. Physical examination includes palpation for tenseness, evaluation of muscle strength, and elicitation of pain on passive motion of the ankle or toes. Presence of palpable pulses does not rule out a compartment syndrome, in fact, pulses are preserved until late in the disease.
  - Patients at risk for compartment syndrome should be monitored closely with repeated physical examination. Pain complaints and pain medication usage should be followed closely. The leg should not be elevated significantly but should be kept at approximately the level of the heart. No circumferential wrapping for casts, splints, or dressings should be used.
  - A postulated relationship between reamed tibial nailing and development of compartment syndrome has been debunked in several comparative trials that show no difference in the incidence of compartment syndrome between reamed and unreamed nailing.[16,24,25]
  - Transient compartment pressure elevations are seen with fracture reduction, reaming, and nail passage, but these rapidly return to baseline. It is likely that the compartment syndrome seen after tibial nailing is a result of the trauma of the injury rather than to the nailing procedure itself.

- Postoperative compartment syndromes that are identified and treated within the first 6 hours may have no significant sequelae. If treatment is delayed beyond 12 hours, functional outcome is likely to be impaired.

- The use of regional anesthetic technique (spinal or epidural) for nailing of acute tibial fractures may lead to masking of compartment syndrome and delay in diagnosis. The use of patient-controlled analgesia (PCA) has been implicated in delay to diagnosis of compartment syndrome.

- Once compartment syndrome has been diagnosed, the treatment is emergent four-compartment fasciotomy. The author prefers a two-incision approach (Figure 19–17). After the skin is incised, the subcutaneous tissue is divided down to the fascia, which is cleaned off with an elevator. A transverse incision in the fascia is made with the tip of the scalpel, taking care not to cut structures that may lie just below it, such as the superficial peroneal nerve. Once the intermuscular septum is identified, the fascia of the lateral and anterior compartments can be opened longitudinally with scissors under direct vision. The medial incision is 1 to 2 cm medial to the medial border of the tibia. Fascial attachments to the tibia are released with a scalpel and blunt dissection behind the tibia with a finger or elevator releases the posterior compartments. Palpation is used to verify the compartments are all open and loose.

Fasciotomy incisions are left widely open and may be covered with a vacuum assisted closure (V.A.C.) dressing. After swelling subsides, one or both incisions may be closed secondarily, or split thickness skin graft applied.

Complications

In addition to compartment syndrome, other complications of tibial fracture care include infection, nonunion, malunion, and pain.

Infection

- Infection can occur acutely after tibial fracture and is more common after open fractures.

- Prevention of all infections is impossible, but the incidence can probably be reduced with appropriate use of perioperative antibiotics, prompt irrigation and adequate debridement of open fractures, appropriate operative timing and technique for closed fractures, and careful, gentle handling of tissues to preserve vascularity.

- Diagnosis of infection is suggested by a history of worsening or excessive pain, and signs of swelling, erythema, wound drainage or fluctuance, streaks, adenopathy, and fever. The diagnosis may be confirmed by laboratory studies, such as the erythrocyte sedimentation rate (ESR), white blood cell (WBC) count and differential, and

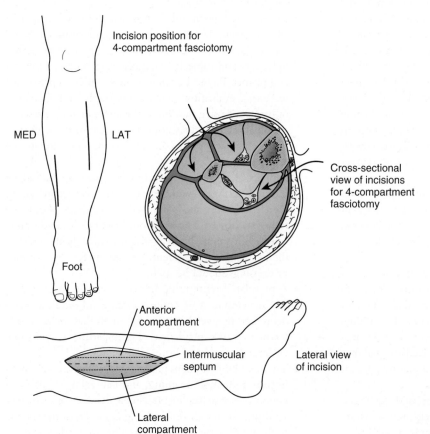

Figure 19–17: Two incision technique of four-compartment fasciotomy. The lateral skin incision is made longitudinally halfway between the tibial crest and the fibula, and the medial incision is made 1 to 2 cm medial to the medial edge of the tibia anteriorly.

C-reactive protein (CRP) level. The CRP is the most sensitive and specific test. Imaging studies include bone scan, radiolabeled leukocyte scan, magnetic resonance imaging (MRI), and positron emission tomography (PET) scanning. PET scanning is the most sensitive and specific modality. Plain films are usually not helpful in diagnosing acute infection.

- The treatment for acute infection with stable hardware is incision and drainage of any purulent collection, irrigation and debridement of wounds, culture, and specific antibiotics delivered systemically or locally with antibiotic beads, dead space management with beads or grafts, and optimized management of any underlying medical problems, such as diabetes, malnutrition, tobacco addiction, or vascular disease.

- The treatment for acute infection with unstable hardware is as above with the addition of hardware removal and stabilization via external fixation.

- Chronic infection is a difficult problem to solve. If the tibia is healed, all hardware is removed, and thorough debridement is performed removing any dysvascular tissues, including reaming the canal. High-dose local antibiotics are delivered with antibiotic beads or rods, and these are changed as necessary, or absorbable local delivery methods are used. Culture-specific IV antibiotics are given, usually for a minimum of 6 weeks. Dead space or soft-tissue defects are covered with healthy vascularized tissue. Hyperbaric oxygen treatments have been used, but the effectiveness is unproven. Medical conditions are treated as noted previously.

Nonunion

- Nonunion after tibia fracture may be obvious or subtle. Open fractures with excessive tibial bone loss may be considered "instant" nonunions; others require that enough time has passed to ascertain that healing has stopped. The designation of a 6-, 9-, or 12-month cutoff is arbitrary. Tibias that have failed to progress in healing clinically or radiographically for 3 consecutive months can be considered nonunions.

- Clinical signs of nonunion include pain that persists or worsens with time, particularly pain on mechanical load like weight bearing. Progressive deformity and gross instability are obvious signs.

- Imaging studies include plain films, which may be hard to interpret as a result of surgical artifact or implants, stress or weight bearing films, and special studies, such as computed tomography (CT), MRI, and, rarely, nuclear scans.

- Nonunions are classified as hypertrophic (vascular) or atrophic (avascular) based on radiographic evidence of callus formation and periosteal reaction to fracture. A synovial pseudarthrosis is a nonunion that has developed a true synovium-lined cavity (false joint) at the nonunion site. Nonunions may also be described as infected or

aseptic and with or without bone loss. All of these distinctions have treatment implications.

- Hypertrophic nonunions have the biological capability to heal but lack the correct mechanical environment. They require provision of stability to heal, most often in the form of internal fixation, although external fixation and functional bracing has also been successful.

- Atrophic nonunions have impaired biology and biomechanics. They need both stability and some sort of stimulation of the healing potential. Often this takes the form of bone grafting, which can be vascularized or cancellous. Growth factors such as bone morphogenetic proteins (BMPs) and electromagnetic or ultrasonic bone stimulators may have a place in treatment as well.

- Treatment of a synovial pseudarthrosis requires excision and grafting of the synovial cavity, along with internal or external fixation.

- Infected nonunions required concurrent treatment of the chronic infection with debridement of avascular tissue, culture specific antibiotics delivered systemically or locally, and coverage with viable vascularized soft tissue.

- Nonunions with significant bone loss need skeletal reconstruction, which can be performed by cancellous grafting, vascularized bone transplant, or distraction osteogenesis.

Management Options

- Detailed discussion of tibial nonunion treatment is beyond the scope of this chapter. A few points can be made.
  - Nonoperative treatments: Optimization of medical conditions, such as diabetes, malnutrition, renal failure, and endocrine disorders, should be part of the management of any nonunion. Tobacco use cessation is believed to be important for bone healing and should be strictly enforced or monitored. The patient should avoid drugs that interfere with bone healing such as antiinflammatory medications, steroids, and biphosphonates, whenever possible. If the patient has been nonweight bearing in a cast for a prolonged period, institution of weight bearing in a functional brace will often stimulate healing. Although many physicians are skeptical about bone stimulators, there is now ample evidence from both animal studies and high-quality human investigations that both electromagnetic and ultrasonic bone stimulators promote bone healing, and in some situations (as in failed surgically treated nonunions) are more effective than surgery. Nonoperative methods can achieve union but cannot correct significant deformity.
  - Surgical treatments: Patients who have failed to heal after closed treatment can usually be healed with internal fixation. IM nailing is commonly used, although the fracture site must sometimes be opened to correct deformity or to open the canal. The femoral distractor can be used to correct alignment. Tension band plating

(dynamic compression plate placed across the apex of the deformity) is another technique with reported success. A nonunion resulting from nailing in slight distraction can sometimes be induced to heal by dynamization or removal of interlocking screws on one side of the nonunion, allowing axial compression at the site during weight bearing. Removal of a smaller diameter nail, reaming of the canal, and placement of a larger diameter nail is known as exchange nailing and can be successful in many cases. If the nonunion is atrophic, refixation should be combined with bone grafting, often with cancellous graft placed along the interosseous membrane through a posterolateral approach. Circular (Ilizarov) wire or ring fixators can be used to treat nonunions, providing stability and compression without a large amount of foreign material at the fracture site. This is a particularly useful technique in the face of infection or bone loss.

Malunion

- The amount of deformity that can be tolerated is somewhat controversial and varies depending on patient expectations and needs.
- The significance of any particular degree of malunion increases the closer the apex it is to the joint.
- The relationship between deformity and arthritis is not clear. The degree of deformity has not been shown to be related to development of arthritis at long-term follow-up.[26]
- Correction of a malunion requires osteotomy.
  - This can sometimes be performed as a single stage procedure, using an oblique cut that allows correction of "multiplanar" deformity and restoration of some length. This is stabilized with a plate and screws. Care should be taken to gently handle soft tissues, cut the bone with sharp osteotomes rather than a power saw to avoid heat necrosis, and plan the closure to avoid excessive skin tension. In a patient above the age of 50 with a longstanding deformity, carefully evaluate the vascular status of the limb because impaired vascular supply (which may be either chronic as a result of peripheral vascular disease (PVD) or acute as a result of correction of deformity) can lead to wound necrosis and infection.
  - Correction can also be performed with a percutaneous corticotomy and gradual correction using an Ilizarov-type external fixator or Taylor Spatial Frame. This technique is gentler on soft tissues and does not require extensive dissection, leading to a lower incidence of incisional infection.
  - With either method, preoperative planning to fully understand the deformity and technique of correction is mandatory. Both methods are technically demanding, have a significant risk for complications, and require an experienced surgeon with special training.

Pain

- Despite the high degree of success of tibial nailing, postoperative pain is a common problem.
- Pain may be related to hardware that is too long or prominent. Fluoroscopic images of interlocking screws may be misleading as a result of the triangular shape of the tibia, especially proximally. These screws should be palpated after insertion to identify prominent tips or heads that can be corrected at the time of surgery. Similarly, the proximal end of the nail may be too prominent and may irritate the patellar tendon or the patella itself. Good lateral images centered at the knee should be obtained at the end of the procedure, and the top of the nail palpated through the insertion incision.
- Anterior knee pain of one of the most common complications after tibial nailing, occurring in more than half of some series.[19,27] When associated with a nail, which is prominent proximally, the cause and solution are obvious, but chronic anterior knee pain can happen even with a well-seated nail.
- Anterior knee pain may affect return to work in up to 10% of patients, interfere with activities of daily living or work in up to a third, affect sports participation in half, and cause difficulty kneeling in 70% of patients treated with tibial nailing.
- Both retrospective and prospective studies have shown no difference in knee pain incidence between transtendinous and paratendinous incision. Other postulated causes are unrecognized injury to the meniscus or to articular cartilage on the tibia or patella, formation of scar tissue, or injury to the infrapatellar nerve.
- Hardware removal has an unpredictable effect on anterior knee pain. Some patients have reduction or elimination of pain, others have no change, and some may have worse pain.[26]

Annotated References

1. Gustilo RB, Anderson JT: Prevention of infection in the treatment of one thousand and twenty-five open fractures of long bones: retrospective and prospective analyses, *J Bone Joint Surg Am* 58:453-458, 1976.

The original description of the open fracture classification system.

2. Tscherne H, Oestern HJ: Pathophysiology and classification of soft tissue injuries associated with fractures, In Tscherne H, Gotzen L editors: *Fractures with soft tissue injuries.* Berlin, 1984 Springer Verlag.

Classic description of soft-tissue injury associated with closed tibial fracture.

3. Sarmiento A: A functional below-the-knee brace for tibial fractures: a report on its use in one hundred thirty-five cases, *J Bone Joint Surg Am* 52:295-311, 1970.

A classic description of the rationale, technique, and outcomes of functional fracture brace treatment for tibial shaft fractures by the foremost authority and advocate.

4. Tibial shaft fractures: intramedullary nailing versus cast immobilization. AO Journal Club/Evidence from the literature, *Orthopaedic Trauma Directions* 2:17-25, 2004.

A review of the literature from 1997 to 2004 turned up three studies comparing intramedullary fixation with casting for tibial shaft fractures. The design and performance of each of the studies are reviewed and quality is discussed. Mean time to union was shorter with nailing, and there were fewer nonunions and delayed unions. Anterior knee pain was more common in the patients who were nailed. Outcome scores including the Iowa Knee scale, Ankle evaluation scale, SF-36, Nottingham Health Profile, and the mean days of sick leave all showed advantage to nailing. The complication rate of both treatments was low.

5. Karladani AH, Granhed H, Edshage B, et al: Displaced tibial shaft fractures, *Acta Orthop Scand* 71:160-167, 2000.

Fifty-three patients with unilateral tibial shaft fractures were randomized to treatment with intramedullary nailing or cast immobilization. However, over half of the cast patients showed early displacement of reduction considered unacceptable and had supplementary cerclage wiring or screw placement. Time to union was longer for cast patients (25 versus 19 weeks, $P < 0.05$). There were twice as many nonunions and three times as many delayed unions in the cast group. The Nottingham Health Profile index scores on physical mobility, social isolation, work ability, and sexual life were significantly better in the nailed tibias. Two compartment syndromes occurred in nail patients.

6. Lindsey RW, Blair SR: Closed tibial shaft fractures: Which ones benefit from surgical treatment? *J Am Assoc Orthop Surg* 4:35-43 1996.

This is a review article that attempts to answer the question of operative indications for closed tibial shaft fractures. The authors note that factors that suggest that surgical treatment will have a better outcome are significant instability, metadiaphyseal location, significant limb edema, and the requirement for repeated manipulations. Patient factors suggesting a benefit to surgical stabilization include obesity, poor compliance, and "health conditions favoring immediate function." Although the authors give "absolute criteria for stabilization" in their abstract (such as "coronal angulation exceeding 5 degrees"), the article actually points out a wide spectrum of opinion in the literature and a paucity of good scientific studies to back those opinions. Nonetheless, it is a useful review of the literature as of mid-1990s.

7. Henley MB, Chapman JR, Agel J, et al: Treatment of type II, IIIA, and IIIB open fractures of the tibial shaft: a prospective comparison of unreamed interlocking intramedullary nails and half-pin external fixators, *J Orthop Trauma* 12:1-7, 1998.

One hundred and seventy four grade II, III-A, or III-B open tibial fractures were prospectively randomized to treatment with unreamed nail or external fixator. Other than method of stabilization the fractures were treated essentially the same. The nail group had fewer instances of malalignment (>5 degrees angulation or >1.5 cm shortening), 8% versus 31%; significantly fewer subsequent procedures, mean 1.7 versus 2.7; fewer infections at the injury site, 13 versus 21%; and at surgical interfaces, 2% versus 50%. There was no difference in haling rates.

8. Maurer DJ, Merkow RL, Gustilo RB: Infection after intramedullary nailing of severe open tibial fractures initially treated with external fixation, *J Bone Joint Surg Am* 71:835-838, 1989.

In this retrospective review of 24 patients who underwent reamed intramedullary nailing of open tibial fractures previously treated with external fixation, the authors found that five of seven patients who had pin tract infections during external fixation subsequently had intramedullary infections around the nail. By comparison, 1 of 17 patients without pin site infections developed nail infections. In the authors' opinion, pin site infection is a contraindication to reamed tibial nailing.

9. Riemer BL, Butterfield SL: Comparison of reamed and nonreamed solid core nailing of the tibial diaphysis after external fixation: a preliminary report, *J Orthop Trauma* 7:279-285, 1993.

In this study of tibial nailing following external fixation, 16 patients treated with unreamed, solid core nails were compared to 16 historical controls that had been treated with reamed, hollow nails. In the hollow nail group, there were seven postnail infections requiring 12 debridement procedures. In the solid nail group, there was only one postnail infection requiring two operations ($P = 0.04$).

10. Schandelmaier P, Krettek C, Rudolf J, et al: Outcome of tibial shaft fractures with severe soft tissue injury treated by unreamed nailing versus external fixation, *J Trauma* 39:707-711, 1995.

This was a retrospective review of 114 fresh tibial fractures, 48 treated with an unreamed nail and 66 treated with external fixation. The unreamed nail group had fewer reoperations, more good outcomes (40% versus 27%), and fewer deformities greater than 5 degrees.

11. Bhandari M, Guyatt GH, Swiontkowski MF, et al: Treatment of open fractures of the shaft of the tibia, *J Bone Joint Surg Br* 83:62-68, 2001.

In this metaanalysis of the nearly 800 citations, the authors found 8 which met all of their stringent inclusion criteria. One study with 56 patients suggested that open tibia fractures treated with external fixation had a lower reoperation rate than those treated with plates. Five studies with nearly 400 patients found that unreamed nails resulted in fewer reoperations, malunions, and superficial infections than external fixators. Two studies compared reamed to unreamed nails and found a lower risk of reoperation with reaming.

12. Gregory P, Sanders R: The treatment of closed, unstable tibial shaft fractures with unreamed interlocking nails, *Clin Orthop* 315:48-55, 1995.

Thirty-eight closed unstable tibial fractures in patients with polytrauma were treated with unreamed intramedullary nailing. Thirty-three (87%) healed within 6 months, two (5%) were delayed unions and three (8%) were nonunions. The authors report that all patients had unlimited ambulation and climbed stairs normally, and those without joint injury regained normal knee, ankle, and subtalar motion. There was one superficial and one deep infection.

13. Sanders R, Jersinovich I, Anglen J, et al: The treatment of open tibial shaft fractures using an interlocked intramedullary nail without reaming, *J Orthop Trauma* 8:504-510, 1994.

One hundred seventeen consecutive open tibia fractures treated with unreamed intramedullary nailing according to protocol were retrospectively reviewed. Average follow up of 2 years was possible in 46 fractures. Mean time to healing increased with increasing grade of fracture: I, 4.8 months; II, 4.7 months; III-A, 8.3 months; and III-B, 9.3 months. Twenty fractures had healing delayed beyond 6 months, including 12 of 15 (80%) of grade III-B fractures.

14. Keating JF, O'Brien PJ, Blachut PA, et al: Locking intramedullary nailing with and without reaming for open fractures of the tibial shaft: a prospective, randomized study, *J Bone Joint Surg Am* 79:334-341, 1997.

This prospective, randomized study of 88 open tibial shaft fractures treated with reamed ($N = 47$) or unreamed ($N = 41$) nailing found no differences between the two groups in technical aspects of the procedure, early complications, healing, infection, pain, range of motion, and return to work or recreation. More screws were broken in unreamed nails, which averaged 9.2 mm in diameter, compared to 11.5 mm in the reamed group. The authors felt there was no risk to reamed nailing in an open tibial shaft fracture.

15. Blachut PA, O'Brien PJ, Meek RN, et al: Interlocking intramedullary nailing with and without reaming for the treatment of closed fractures of the tibial shaft: a prospective, randomized study, *J Bone Joint Surg Am* 79:640-646, 1997.

In this prospective study of 136 closed fractures followed for an average of 12 months, no significant differences were found in healing, infection, requirement for secondary procedures or hardware removal, or malunion. More screws failed in the unreamed group. Nailing without reaming saved an average of 11 minutes of operating time ($P = 0.0013$), but there was no difference in fluoroscopy time or blood loss. There were more delayed unions after unreamed nailing, but the difference was not significant. The authors concluded there was no advantage to nailing without reaming.

16. Finkemeier CG, Schmidt AH, Kyle RF, et al: A prospective, randomized study of intramedullary nails inserted with and without reaming for the treatment of open and closed fractures of the tibial shaft, *J Orthop Trauma* 14:187-193, 2000.

This was a prospective, surgeon randomized study of 94 consecutive patients with unstable tibial shaft fractures treated with reamed or unreamed nailing. Both open and closed fractures were included, but grade III-B and III-C were excluded. There were no differences in infections or compartment syndromes, and for open fractures, no differences in time to healing or number of secondary procedures required. For closed fractures at 4 months there were more healed fractures in the reamed group, but the difference was not present at 6 or 12 months. A insignificant increase in secondary procedures required after unreamed nailing was seen in closed fractures. Broken screws were only seen after unreamed nailing.

17. Larsen LB, Madsen JE, Hoiness PR, et al: Should insertion of intramedullary nails for tibial fractures be with or without reaming? A prospective randomized study with 3.8 years' follow-up, *J Orthop Trauma* 18:144-149, 2004.

After a mean follow up of nearly 4 years in this prospective randomized study of 45 tibial fractures (22 reamed, 23 unreamed),

there was a significantly longer time to union for unreamed nailing, 26 versus 17 weeks. There were more nonunions, malunions, and broken screws in the unreamed group, although these differences were not statistically significant. There were no infections in this series (eight were low-grade open fractures) and equal numbers of compartment syndromes and patients with anterior knee pain.

18. Watson JT, Occhietti MJ, Moed BR, et al: Perioperative external fixator management during secondary surgical procedures, Presented at the OTA annual meeting, Charlotte, NC, October 24, 1999. Abstract available online accessed 8/26/03:www.hwbf.org/ota/am/ota99/otapa/OTA99902.htm

This was a prospective study of 96 patients in external fixators who were taken to the operating room for secondary procedures. The frames were maintained in place and prepped using a protocol of 95% isopropyl alcohol, Betadine scrub for 6 minutes and then Betadine paint. They were then draped into the sterile field. Cultures were obtained of the frame and the incision site. There were four sterile wound complications, two superficial infections, and two deep infections. There was no relation between preoperative cultures and occurrence of complications. The authors concluded that their protocol for maintaining and external fixator intraoperatively was safe and did not lead to an increased risk of postoperative wound infection.

19. Toivanen JA, Vaisto O, Kannus P, et al: Anterior knee pain after intramedullary nailing of fractures of the tibial shaft: a prospective, randomized study comparing two different nail-insertion techniques, *J Bone Joint Surg Am* 84:580-585, 2002.

Forty-two patients who had undergone intramedullary nailing of the tibia were followed for 3 years after surgery. They were randomized to either transtendinous or paratendinous incision for nail insertion. A similar high percentage of both groups had anterior knee pain, 67% for the transtendinous group and 71% for the paratendinous group. Twenty-three of 29 patients with knee pain reported being impaired by the pain. The authors concluded that no difference in knee pain or symptoms resulted from making the incision through or beside the tendon.

20. Bhandari M, Tornetta P, III, Sprague S, et al: Predictors of reoperation following operative management of fractures of the tibial shaft, *J Orthop Trauma* 17:353-361, 2003.

In a retrospective study of 192 patients who underwent tibial nailing at two centers, the authors identified three characteristics that predicted the need for reoperation: open fractures wound (relative risk 4.32, 95% confidence interval [CI] 1.76 to 11.26), lack of cortical continuity—a fracture gap—after fixation (relative risk 8.33, 95% CI 3.03 to 25), and a transverse fracture pattern (relative risk 20, 95% CI 4.34 to 142.86).

21. Olsen SA: Open fractures of the tibial shaft. In Dempsey Springfield, editor: *In* Structional course lectures vol. 46. Rosemont IL, 1997 American Academy of Orthopaedic Surgeons.

This is a comprehensive review of treatment for open tibial shaft fractures from the emergency department to rehabilitation and reconstruction of the nonunions.

22. Anglen JO: A prospective randomized comparison of soap solution and antibiotic solution for irrigation of lower extremity open fracture wounds, *J Bone Joint Surg Am* 87:1415-1422, 2005.

A prospective randomized comparison of antibiotic and soap irrigation for 458 open lower extremity fractures revealed no difference in infection or nonunion rate but did reveal a higher incidence of wound healing problems with antibiotic irrigation.

23. Tornetta P, III, Templeman D: Compartment syndrome associated with tibial fracture, In Springfield Dempsey editor: *In*structional course lectures vol. 46. Rosemont IL, 1997 American Academy of Orthopaedic Surgeons.
A comprehensive review of the topic and the literature.

24. Nassif JM, Gorczyca JT, Cole JK, et al: Effect of acute reamed versus unreamed intramedullary nailing on compartment pressure when treating closed tibial shaft fractures: a randomized prospective study, *J Orthop Trauma* 14:554-558, 2000.
Forty-eight patients with 49 tibia fractures were randomized to reamed and unreamed nailing without traction or a fracture table and compartment pressures were measured intraoperatively. No patient developed compartment syndrome. Transient elevations of pressure were seen during reaming and during unreamed nail passage, but pressures quickly dropped after reduction and fixation. The deep posterior compartment pressures were lower at several postoperative intervals in the reamed group; no differences were seen in the anterior compartment pressure levels between the two treatments.

25. Tornetta P, III, French BG: Compartment pressures during nonreamed tibial nailing without traction, *J Orthop Trauma* 11:24-27, 1997.
Fifty-right tibial fractures were nailed using unreamed technique, no traction, fracture table, leg elevation, or thigh post. Anterior compartment pressures were measured. Transient elevation of the pressure was seen with fracture reduction and nail passage, but it returned to baseline promptly after nail passage. No compartment syndromes were seen.

26. Milner SA, Davis TR, Muir KR, et al: Long-term outcome after tibial shaft fracture: is malunion important? *J Bone Joint Surg Am* 84:971-980, 2002.
One hundred and sixty-four patients with tibial fractures treated closed were evaluated at a minimum of 30 years after injury. Coronal angulation greater than 5 degrees was seen in 47 fractures, and 17 had malalignment of the limb. Although mild osteoarthritis was common (17% with at least moderate disability) and was more common on the ipsilateral side, there was no relationship between malunion and osteoarthritis of knee, ankle, or subtalar joint.

27. Ricci WM: Knee pain, In Ricci WM (ed.). *Complications in orthopaedics: tibial shaft fractures*. Rosemont, IL, 2004 American Academy of Orthopaedic Surgeons.
In this monograph, part of the popular "Complications" series, a thorough discussion of knee pain as well as other complications of tibial shaft fractures is provided, along with literature support.

CHAPTER 20

Pilon Fractures

Joseph Borrelli, Jr., MD

Introduction

- Pilon fractures represent 1% of all fractures and 3% to 9% of all tibia fractures.
- These fractures commonly occur either as the result of direct axial compression to the limb or as a result of a rotational mechanism.
- The axial compression fractures are felt to be of higher energy and commonly occur in falls and motor vehicle crashes, whereas the rotational fractures are more commonly lower energy injuries, which occur in sporting events (i.e., skiing or skateboarding).
- Recognizing the difference between these two types is essential.
- Treatment of these fractures should be individualized and based on objective information and employ proven and accepted methods.
- Unfortunately, despite adequate care of these fractures, limited ankle mobility, pain and long-term disability commonly results, causing patients to modify their activities and change occupations.[1]

Fracture Characteristics

Axial Compression Type Fractures

- Considerable soft-tissue swelling and blistering.
- Open fractures are not uncommon; typically the traumatic wound is either medial or posterior.
- Typically comminuted metaphyseal and articular segments with marked displacement of the fragments and fibula.

Rotational Type Fractures

- Mild to moderate soft-tissue swelling, typically with little blistering.
- Fracture is typically spiral in nature and begins in the distal diaphysis and extends through the metaphysis and into the articular surface.
- Fibula may or may not be fractured.

Diagnostic and Assessment Tools

Physical Examination

- Most of the high-energy tibial plafond fractures can be suspected from a thorough history and physical examination of the distal leg.
- In most cases, swelling, ecchymosis, and deformity are present soon after injury.
- For the rotational type fractures these findings are typically not as obvious, and therefore the diagnosis may need to be confirmed with plain radiographs.

Plain Radiographs

- Anteroposterior (AP), mortice, and lateral radiographs centered on the ankle are generally sufficient to make the diagnosis and properly classify these fractures (Figure 20–1).
- AP and lateral radiographs of the ipsilateral tibia and fibula, including the knee and foot, should also be included to rule out the presence of associated fractures.
- Radiographs of the contralateral foot and ankle and the lumbar spine are warranted in the high-energy axial compression type fractures.

Computed Tomography

- Computed tomography (CT) scans are helpful in the assessment and treatment of pilon fractures and can add information not easily seen on the plain radiographs.[2]
  - Axial CT scans with cuts at the level of the articular surface help to determine the number, size, and position of the articular fracture fragments and the fracture planes (see Figure 20–2A).

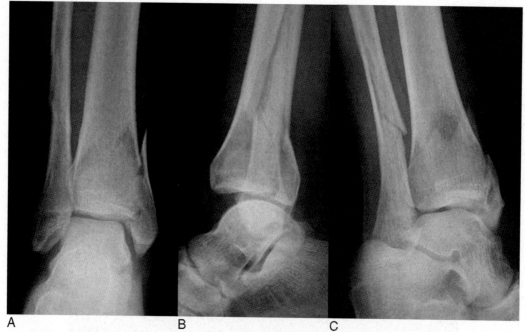

Figure 20–1: **A, B,** and **C,** Anteroposterior, mortice, and lateral radiographs of a type II open axial compression type of pilon fracture.

- Sagittal and coronal reconstructions of the CT scans assist further in the assessment, preoperative planning and ultimately in the treatment of these injuries (see Figure 20–2B and C).
- Investigators are assessing the usefulness of CT scans for determining the amount of energy absorbed at the time of injury, in an effort to correlate energy with injury severity and soft-tissue injury.[3]

Classification

- Traditionally, these fractures have been classified according to the scheme described by Rüedi and Allgöwer[4] (Figure 20–3).
- This simple classification system is somewhat prognostic, although it does not necessarily aid guide treatment.
- Recently the comprehensive classification of long-bone fractures has been published by the AO/Orthopaedic Trauma Association (OTA)[5] (Figure 20–4).
- This classification system is somewhat cumbersome but does allow a more detailed classification of the fracture, aids computer documentation of these fractures, and may be helpful in performing future outcome studies.

General Surgical Indications

- Articular fracture displacement of 2 mm or more and separation between the articular segment and the tibial shaft are generally considered amendable to operative treatment.
- Goals of operative treatment for most surgeons include restoration of articular length, fibular reduction, reestablishment

of limb length, alignment and rotation, stable fixation to allow early mobilization of the limb and of the patient, and occasional bone graft to support fracture healing.

- There are several different operative methods that can be used to achieve these goals. The decision-making process as to which method to employ usually depends on the fracture pattern, condition of the soft tissues, the patients' goals and demands, and the surgeons' ability and training.

Surgical Procedures

- Formal open reduction and internal fixation is commonly performed for most of the low-energy relational-type fractures and many of the axial compression type fractures.
- Limited internal fixation and application of a spanning external fixator is preferentially performed by certain surgeons in an effort to avoid soft tissue complications.
- For severely commuted, periarticular and articular fractures, external fixation plane is often utilized without internal fixation.
- Bone grafting is generally reserved for those fractures with severe comminution or considerable impaction or for those with bone loss (open fractures) on a delayed basis.
- Primary ankle fusions as a treatment for a displaced tibial plafond fracture is rare and is generally reserved for those ankles with advanced osteoarthritis, severe articular comminution, preventing adequate joint reconstruction, and those fractures with associated talar or calcaneal fractures, Also, those fractures in which the soft-tissue injury (open or closed)

precludes safe operative intervention can also be considered for primary ankle arthrodesis once the soft-tissue trauma does eventually resolve.

Surgical Treatment Principles

- Articular fracture fragments should be anatomically reduced and rigidly fixed with interfragmentary lag screws.
- This restores normal weight-bearing forces across the articular surface in an effort to avoid posttraumatic osteoarthritis that may result from residual joint incongruity.
- Once reduced, the articular block should then be reattached to the tibial shaft either with internal or external fixation, with sufficient stability to allow early ankle joint motion.
- Meticulous soft-tissue handling should be carried out throughout the treatment of these fractures in an effort to avoid the potential serious complications associated with wound dehiscence and infection.
- Early mobilization of the ankle joint that aids in cartilage nutrition, minimizes contractures, and potentates the recovery of normal joint motion (Table 20–1).

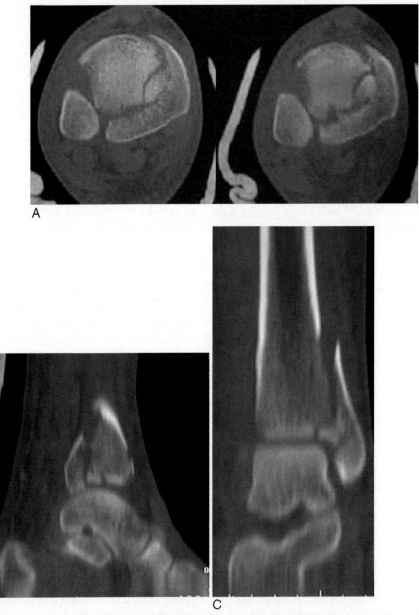

Figure 20–2: **A** and **B,** Anteroposterior and lateral radiograph of a lower energy, rotational type pilon fracture. Plain radiographs underestimate the number of fracture fragments and the extent of their displacement. **C,** Axial computed tomography scan taken through the subchondral bone more clearly demonstrating the articular comminution and fracture displacement.

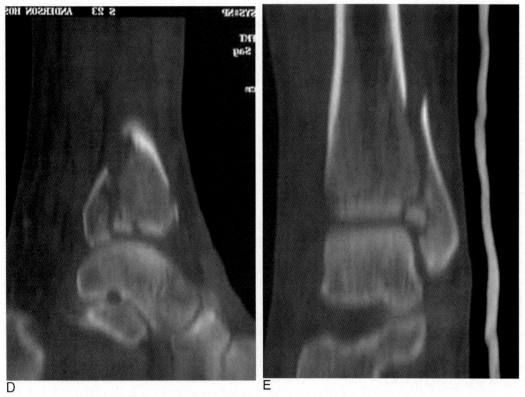

D   E

Figure 20–2, cont'd: **D and E,** Sagittal and coronal plane computed tomography reconstructions of this pilon fracture more clearly demonstrating the articular displacement and the impaction of a portion of the articular surface.

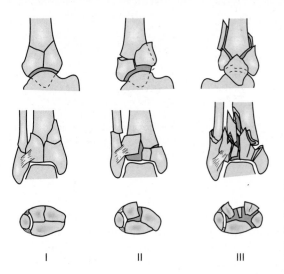

I   II   III

Figure 20–3: Pilon fracture classification as proposed by Ruedi and Allgower. Type I simple cleavage fracture without intraarticular displacement. Type II, displaced intraarticular fracture with little comminution. Type III, displaced intraarticular fracture with articular and metaphyseal comminution. (From Ruedi T, Allgower M: *Injury* 1:92, 1969).

Surgical Techniques
Open Reduction and Internal Fixation

- To decrease the risk of postoperative wound complications informal open reduction and internal fixation (ORIF) of high-energy distal tibial fractures should be treated with a two-stage protocol.[6,7]
- The first stage involves ORIF of the fibula and application of a spanning ankle external fixator.

- This "traveling traction" is designed to reapproximate the displaced fracture fragments through ligamentotaxis and provide enough stability to allow mobilization of the patient and limit further soft-tissue injury.
- Once the spanning external fixator has been applied, patients should maintain the fractured leg elevated and apply ice to the fracture area to help resolve the swelling.
- A CT scan should be obtained at this time and a thorough preoperative plan created.

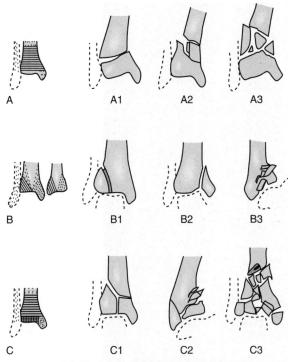

Figure 20–4: AO/Orthopaedic Trauma Association comprehensive classification of long-bone fractures.

with and without locking screw capabilities, are now available and provide fixed-angle fixation that is beneficial for severely comminuted metaphyseal fractures and locking screw technology aids in the treatment of osteoporotic fractures.

- To allow soft-tissue recovery, before the addition of surgical teams ORIF of the distal tibia is generally delayed for 10 to 21 days.[6,7]
- Complications associated with formal ORIF include wound dehiscence, deep infections, metaphyseal nonunions, and painful hardware requiring removal.[8] See Table 20–1.

Limited Internal Fixation and Application of an External Fixator

- Limited internal fixation of the articular fracture fragments can be performed through small incisions the position of which these incisions can be aided by the CT scan.
- Cannulated screws are useful for this type of fixation, including 4- and 4.5-mm screws.
- The articular block can then be reattached to the tibial shaft by the application of a spanning articulated or nonarticulating external fixator or a nonspanning "hybrid" type of external fixator.[9–11] See Figure 20–1.

Table 20–1: Pilon Fracture Techniques		
TECHNIQUE	ADVANTAGES	DISADVANTAGES
Open reduction and internal fixation	Articular reduction, No long-term external fixation Restoration of limb length, alignment, and rotation	Increased risk of wound dehiscence and deep infection
Limited internal fixation and hybrid external fixator	Limited incisions, Indirect reduction and stabilization of the metaphyseal fracture Ankle joint is not spanned	Less than anatomic reduction of articular surface, pin site infections, and metaphyseal nonunions
Limited internal fixation and spanning external fixator	Limited incisions Indirect reduction and stabilization of the metaphysis	Less than anatomic reduction of articular surface, pin site infections, and ankle stiffness

Table 20–2: Pertinent Anatomy of the Ankle Joint
Ankle joint is formed by the relationship between the distal fibula, tibia, and talus.
These bones maintain their normal relationships as a result of a complex array of ligaments and bony contours.
This joint participates in many of the weight-bearing activities of the lower extremity.

- The second stage involves formal ORIF of the distal tibia and removal of the external fixator. Operative stabilization generally employs the use of "small fragment" plates and screws and select "mini-fragment" screws for small articular fragments. Specialty plates, specifically contoured for the distal tibia both

- The spanning frames are generally placed medially and use half pins within the tibial shaft above the fracture and within the talus and calcaneus, below the fracture.[12]
- Hybrid-type frames combine the use of half pins in the shaft of the tibia and thin wires in the articular block. The half pins and the thin wires are connected using a combination of pin to bar clamps and carbon fiber rods and carbon fiber five-eighths rings distally.
- Circular external fixators using all thin wires can also be used to neutralize rotational and axial stresses across the fracture.
- In either case, the external fixator takes the place of the internal plate.

- The external fixators provide enough stability at the level of the metaphyseal fracture while allowing range of motion of the ankle and at least limited weight bearing.
- Complications associated with limited internal fixation and application of an external fixator include pin site infections, superficial nerve injury, deep infections, and metaphyseal nonunions.
- In a recent study reporting the use of a monolateral hinged transarticular external fixator coupled with screw fixation of the articular fragments for high-energy pilon fractures, the results are encouraging. Ankle motion was 62% of the uninjured side whereas subtalar motion averaged 77% of the uninjured side and shortness of the limb averaged approximately 1 cm. In general the patients were satisfied with the results of their treatment and felt that they had improved for a long time after their injury. The Ankle Osteoarthritis Scale showed a dramatic negative effect of this injury on patient function.[13]

Summary

Fractures of the distal tibial plafond are significant injuries that can lead to long-term problems for the patient. These fractures appear to come in two varieties; the high-energy axial compression types and the lower energy rotational types. These fractures typically have their own characteristic fracture patterns and associated soft-tissue injuries. It is important to recognize the two different fracture patterns because it will influence treatment and outcome. Assessment is generally dependent on history and physical examination, plain radiographs, and CT scans. Indications for operative treatment include articular displacement and instability between the articular bloc and the tibial diaphysis. Treatment options include a two-stage protocol with formal ORIF using plates and screws or limited open reduction and internal fixation coupled with either a nonspanning or spanning external fixator. Each treatment modality has its own advantages and disadvantages. These fractures are associated with significant limb-threatening complications and must be treated with the utmost respect and care.

Annotated References

1. Pollack AN, McCarthy ML, Bess RS, et al: Outcomes after treatment of high-energy plafond fractures, *J Bone Joint Surg Am* 85:1893-1900, 2003.

The purpose of this study was to assess midterm health, function, and impairment after pilon fractures and examine injury, and treatment characteristics that influence outcome. Eighty of the originally identified 103 eligible patients either with formal open reduction and internal fixation (ORIF) or with or without internal fixation and application of a spanning external fixator were assessed 3.2 years post-injury. General health (SF-36) was significantly poorer than age and gender-matched norms. Thirty-five percent of the patients reported substantial ankle stiffness; 29% had persistent swelling; and 33% had residual ankle pain. Forty-three percent were not employed at

the time of the follow-up with 68% reporting that the pilon fracture prevented them from working. Multivariate analyses revealed that presence of two or more comorbidities, being married, having an annual personal income of less than $25,000, not having attained a high school diploma, and having been treated with external fixation with or without internal fixation were significantly related to poorer results as reflected by at least two of the five primary outcome measures. The authors concluded that pilon fracture can have persistent and devastating consequences on patients' health and well-being and that certain social demographic and treatment variables seem to contribute to these poor outcomes.

2. Tornetta P III, Gorup J: Axial computed tomography of pilon fractures, *Clin Orthop* 323:273-276, 1996.

The authors investigated the use of computed tomography (CT) scans in the preoperative planning of pilon fractures. The fracture pattern, number of fragments, comminution, impaction, and location of the major fracture lines were recorded. The CT scans revealed an increased number of fragments in 54%, increased articular impaction in 26%, and an increase in the comminution in 50%. As a result the operative plan was changes in 64% of the patients, and additional information was gained in 82% of the patients.

3. Beardsley C, Marsh JL, Brown T: Quantifying comminution as a measurement of severity of articular injury, *Clin Orthop* 423:74-78, 2004.

4. Ruedi TP, Allgower M: The operative treatment of intraarticular fractures of the lower end of the tibia, *Clin Orthop* 136:105-110, 1979.

5. Fracture and dislocation compendium. Orthopaedic Trauma Association Committee for Coding and Classification, *J Orthop Trauma* 10:v-IX, 56-60, 1996.

6. Sirkin M, Sanders R, DiPasquale T, et al: A staged protocol for soft tissue management in the treatment of complex pilon fractures, *J Orthop Trauma* 13:78-84, 1999.

This study also investigated the efficacy of using a two-stage protocol in the treatment of high-energy pilon fractures in an effort to limit surgical wound complications. Fifty AO/Orthopaedic Trauma Association type 43C fractures were included in the study, 34 were closed fractures (group I), and 22 open (group II). Each patient was treated with some part of the following open reduction and internal fixation (ORIF) of the fibula and application of a spanning external fixator initially, and subsequently (average 13 days post-injury) underwent ORIF of the tibia and removal of the external fixator.

7. Patterson MJ, Cole JD: Two-staged delayed open reduction and internal fixation of severe pilon fractures, *J Orthop Trauma* 13:85-91, 1999.

This study evaluated the use of a two-stage protocol involving of a spanning external first and then formal open reduction and internal fixation (ORIF) and removal of the external fixator second. Twenty-one patients, with 22 AO/Orthopaedic Trauma Association C3 pilon fractures were treated by a single surgeon and followed on the average of 22 months after surgery. The definitive fixation was performed on average 24 days after the initial procedure. Twenty-one of the 22 (95%) fractures healed at an average of 4 months. Subjective and objective measures showed 77% good results, 14% fair results, and 9% poor results. There were no infections or soft-tissue complications. The investigators concluded that this protocol was associated with acceptable results and had the advantage over other methods by limiting the degree of soft-tissue complications and improved articular reductions.

8. Sands A, Grujic L, Byck DC, et al: Clinical and functional outcomes of internal fixation of displaced pilon fractures, *Clin Orthop* 347:31-37, 1998.

9. DeCoster TA, Willis MC, Marsh JL, et al: Rank order analysis of tibial plafond fractures: does injury or reduction predict outcome? *Foot Ankle Int* 20:44-49, 1999.

10. Okcu G, Aktuglu K: Intra-articular fractures of the tibial plafond: a comparison of the results using articulated and ring external fixators, *J Bone Joint Surg Br* 86:868-875, 2004.

A retrospective review of 60 pilon fractures treated either with an ankle-sparing diaphyseal-epiphyseal technique ($n = 24$) with an Ilizarov ring fixator or with a monolateral articulated external fixator ($n = 20$). Limited open reduction and internal fixation (ORIF) of the articular fragments was used when deemed necessary. Patients were followed up at an average of 5.5 years and their assessment included clinical and radiographic assessment and assessment of ankle function with the modified Mazur score. Functional outcome scores were similar for both groups, and there was no difference with regard to radiographic score and late complications. However, patients treated with the Ilizarov ring fixator had significantly better ankle and subtalar movement, leading the authors to conclude that although both types of fixators are satisfactory methods of treatment, joint motion is preserved better without bridging the ankle.

11. Wyrsh B, McFerran MA, McAndrew M, et al: Operative treatment of fractures of the tibial plafond: a randomized prospective study, *J Bone Joint Surg Am* 78:1646-1657, 1996.

A randomized, prospective study to compare two methods of treatment for displaced fractures of the tibial plafond. This randomized surgeon designed study had two groups of patients including the first group ($n = 18$) that each underwent open reduction and internal fixation (ORIF) of the tibia and fibula through separate incisions, and the second group ($n = 20$) that were managed with external fixation with or without limited internal fixation. Complications were more common and more severe in the ORIF group as compared to the external fixator group. Average length of followup was 39 months, and the average clinical score was lower for the patients who had had a type II or type III fracture regardless of the type of treatment. Some degree of posttraumatic osteoarthritis was present in each of the ankles with type II or III fractures, and this could not be correlated with the treatment method.

12. Marsh JL, Bonar S, Nepola JV, et al: Use of articulated external fixator for fractures of the tibial plafond, *J Bone Joint Surg Am* 77:1498-1509, 1995.

13. Marsh JL, Weigel DP, Dirschl DR: Tibial plafond fractures. How do these ankles function over time? *J Bone Joint Surg Am* 85:287-295, 2003.

The purpose of this study was to determine the effect of tibial plafond fractures on ankle function, pain, and general health status and to determine which factors predict favorable and unfavorable outcomes. Thirty-one patients, with 35 fractures, were treated with limited open reduction and limited internal fixation and application of a unilateral articulated external fixator. At an average follow-up of 6.5 years, the scores of the SF-36 and the Ankle Osteoarthritis scale demonstrated a long-term negative effect of the injury on the general health and on ankle pain and function when compared with those parameters in age-matched controls. However patients perceived that their conditions had improved for an average of 2.4 years after the injury. Based on this information the investigators warned about recommending early reconstructive procedures to these patients.

Further Reading

14. Anglen JO: Early outcome of hybrid external fixation for fracture of the distal tibia, *J Orthop Trauma* 13:92-97, 1999.

This study was designed to assess the early results of using a hybrid external fixator to treat tibial plafond fractures and compare these results with those of patients treated with formal open reduction and internal fixation (ORIF) of similar fractures. Fracture stabilization was accomplished with the use of a hybrid external fixator ($n = 34$) or with internal fixation ($n = 27$), as determined by preestablished criteria. This study found that patients treated with the hybrid external fixator had lower clinical scores, were slower to return to function, and had a higher rate of complications, including more malunions and nonunions and infections. Based on these data, the authors felt that the hybrid external fixator did not solve the problems associated with treatment of pilon fractures by other means.

CHAPTER 21

Fractures and Dislocations of the Ankle

Keith Heier, MD, and Cory A. Collinge, MD

- Because the ankle is the most commonly injured weight-bearing joint of the body, most orthopaedic surgeons routinely treat ankle injuries.
- The ankle joint may be injured as the result of direct, or more often, indirect trauma (rotational, translational, or axial forces).
- These injuries often result in variable amounts of subluxation or dislocation of the talus from the mortise of the distal tibia and fibula.
- Originally, Ramsey and Hamilton[1] demonstrated that even mild malalignment of the ankle joint leads to abnormal pressure distribution and subsequent arthritis.
- Generally, if a congruent reduction through closed or open means can be obtained and maintained, then the outcome will be positive. However the results are unlikely to be favorable if residual radiographic abnormalities remain after ankle fracture treatment.
- The goals of treatment for an ankle fracture and dislocation are a stable congruent joint that allows for early joint mobility, fracture healing, reduction of complications, and ultimately, arthritis prevention (Box 21–1).
- Soft-tissue problems or wound complications are not uncommon after an ankle injury or subsequent surgery as a result of the thin soft-tissue envelope and the superficial location of the tendons and neurovascular structures; therefore, considerations regarding soft-tissue management in addition to the timing of surgery are critical in minimizing the risks for perioperative complications.
- The decision to use operative or nonoperative treatment of these injuries depends on whether the risks and benefits of open treatment are expected to provide improved results compared to closed treatment.

Box 21–1	Goal of This Chapter: Practical Operative Management of Ankle Fractures

- Surgical indications
- Preoperative management
- Postoperative management
- Clinical pearls to avoid potential complications
- Technical pearls to assist in reductions

Functional and Surgical Anatomy

- The ankle joint consists of the articulation of three bones (tibia, talus, and fibula) that move relative to one another and are restrained by three ligament complexes (Figure 21–1).
- The ankle joint relies on these bony and soft tissues to maintain stability and alignment while allowing the motion necessary for gait.
- Normally, the talus sits in the ankle "mortise" articulating with the weight-bearing tibial plafond and the articular facets of the medial and lateral malleoli. In the neutral position, 90% of the weight borne across the ankle joint passes through the tibial plafond.
- Most of the ankle's motion involves dorsiflexion and plantarflexion of the foot relative to the leg. However when viewed from above, the talus is trapezoidal in shape, thus with ankle dorsiflexion, there is also widening of the mortise and external rotation of the fibula.

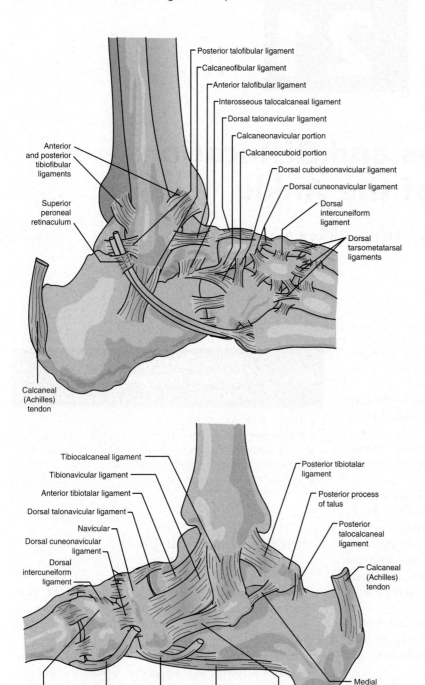

Figure 21–1: The bony and ligamentous anatomy of the ankle.

- The ankle might be regarded most accurately as a complicated hinge.
- An injury to any of the three ligament complexes or bony structures of the ankle can result in an unstable ankle joint.
- Understanding the ankle joint's pathoanatomy is crucial. Typically, a combination of bony and ligamentous injury causes an ankle to become unstable and requires surgical stabilization (Box 21–2).

Injury Classifications

- Optimally, a classification system should guide treatment decisions and provide insight into prognoses.

The distal tibia and fibula are held together by the syndesmosis or inferior distal tibiofibular ligament complex.
1. Anterior inferior tibiofibular ligament
2. Posterior inferior tibiofibular ligament
3. Inferior transverse tibiofibular ligament
4. Interosseous ligament

The lateral ankle ligament complex
1. Anterior talofibular ligament
2. Posterior talofibular ligament
3. Calcaneofibular ligament

The medial ankle ligament complex
1. Superficial deltoid (medial malleolus to calcaneus)
2. Deep deltoid (medial malleolus to talus)

- The two most commonly used classification systems for ankle fractures are the Danis-Weber[2] and Lauge-Hansen[3] systems (Figure 21–2).
- Although orthopaedic surgeons commonly use both systems, neither system is perfect, and their interobserver reliability is unsatisfactory.
- The Danis-Weber system is based on the level of the fibula fracture and is divided into three types:
  1. Type A fibula fractures occur below the level of the tibial plafond.

2. Type B fractures typically rise obliquely from the level of the plafond.
3. Type C fractures are centered well above the plafond and typically have an associated syndesmotic injury.
- The Weber system assumes that the lateral malleolus is the key to stability for an ankle fracture.
- Although the level of the fibular fracture may be used to assess the likelihood of syndesmosis injury,[4] it has been recently emphasized that syndesmosis instability can accompany more distal fractures (Weber type B).[5]
- Although this system is relatively straightforward, it does not provide any guidance regarding treatment of a medial injury, options for fixation (except for the syndesmosis), or prognosis.
- The Lauge-Hansen system is based on the mechanism of injury and is more encompassing than the Danis-Weber system.
- It describes the typical medial injuries and proposes likely reduction maneuvers, which are of prime importance for nonoperative management of ankle fractures.
- Orthopaedic surgeons have criticized the Lauge-Hansen system for having less relevance for the surgical treatment of these injuries.
- The Lauge-Hansen system is based on two terms:
  1. The first describes the position of the foot at the time of injury that dictates which structures are taut and thus, likely to fail at the onset of deformation.

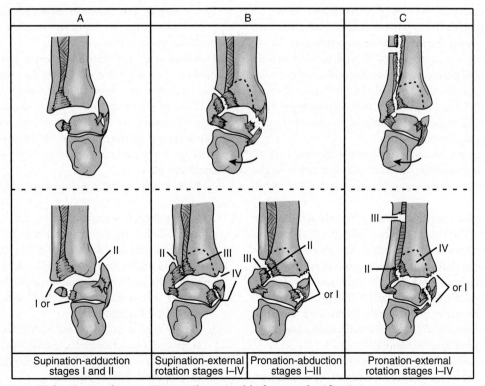

Figure 21–2: The Danis-Weber (top) and Lauge-Hansen (bottom) ankle fracture classifications.

2. The second describes the direction of the force causing the injury.

- The Lauge-Hansen system includes four types of ankle fractures:
  1. Supination-external rotation (S-ER) accounts for up to 85% of all ankle fractures and includes an oblique or spiral fracture of the fibula along with a variable medial injury.
  2. Supination-adduction (S-AD).
  3. Pronation-external rotation (P-ER).
  4. Pronation-abduction (P-AB).
- This chapter will discuss the operative treatment of ankle fractures and dislocations based on anatomic location (medial, lateral, posterior, and syndesmosis), but it also includes and integrates both ankle fracture classification systems into the discussion.
- Isolated ankle dislocations are rarely a purely ligamentous injury; most cases involve a fracture of the ankle mortise. Dislocations of the ankle are typically described by the direction of the dislocated talus.

Fracture Assessment and Decision Making

- The standard radiographic assessment of the ankle includes three views: the anteroposterior (AP), mortise (15 degrees to 20 degrees internal rotation) and lateral views (Figure 21–3).
- With significant injury to the ankle, a consistent pattern of instability occurs: lateral translation and external rotation of the talus relative to the tibial plafond (Figure 21–4).
- Box 21–3 highlights the important radiographic indicators of an unstable ankle fracture that are seen in Figure 21–4.
- Rarely, computed tomography (CT) may be indicated to judge the size and position of a posterior malleolar fragment or involvement of the distal tibiofibular joint (Box 21–3).
- At times, a deltoid ligament injury may accompany a fracture of the lateral malleolus resulting in an unstable injury (bimalleolar equivalent).
- According to recent research, soft-tissue indicators, such as medial pain and swelling, do not reliably predict ankle instability associated with a S-ER fracture of the distal fibula.[6]
- Static radiographic findings may not accurately demonstrate the instability of this injury (Figure 21–5A and B). Dynamic testing or stress views may accomplish the goal of demonstrating radiographically subtle syndesmosis instability.
- A positive stress test shows medial clear space widening relative to the nonstressed radiograph (Figure 21–5C).
- A mortise stress view of the ankle taken with external rotation force may reveal lateral talar subluxation and associated medial joint space widening.[6]
- Michelson and others[7] recommend using a "gravity stress test," which appears less painful for patients yet as effective

as other dynamic tests. When this method is used, the lateral side of the ankle is placed down on the table with the majority of the ankle off the edge of the table (see Figure 21–5B). A cross-table mortise view radiograph is performed.

- Candal-Couto and others[8] demonstrated that disruption of the syndesmosis causes even more displacement in the anteroposterior (sagittal) plane than in the coronal plane, and therefore stress views evaluating anteroposterior displacement of the fibula relative to the tibia may be an even more sensitive indicator of syndesmosis injury.
- The treatment of ankle fractures with special circumstances, including open fractures and those in patients with diabetes mellitus or osteoporosis, will be discussed later in this chapter.

Indications for Surgery

- The goals of treatment for ankle fractures and dislocations, whether treated operatively or nonoperatively, are the maintenance of a stable, congruent joint that allows for early joint mobility, fracture healing, and ultimately the prevention of arthritis.
- Many minor ankle fractures are functionally equivalent to lateral ankle sprains, consisting of a stable, isolated lateral malleolus fracture that will lead to a good outcome if treated nonoperatively.
- Traditionally, joint alignment has been deemed unsatisfactory if radiographs show an increased medial clear space greater than 2 mm or displacement of the medial or lateral malleolus greater than 2 to 3 mm.
- Unfortunately, radiographic criteria can be misleading because they are based on a two-dimensional (2D) static representation of a three-dimensional (3D) dynamic joint. A CT scan may help further define the injury.
- Many fractures are stable and should be considered for nonoperative treatment. Clinical judgment must still be used on every individual fracture when deciding on the treatment plan.
  1. Weber type A fractures not associated with a deltoid injury,
  2. Weber type B fractures not associated with a deltoid injury (S-ER fractures types 1 and 2),
  3. Nondisplaced or distal medial malleolus fractures.
- General guidelines for the surgical treatment of ankle fractures and the authors' recommendations include:
  1. Weber type A fractures associated with a medial injury and S-AD fractures.
  2. Weber type B or S-ER and P-AB fractures that occur as part of a more complex bimalleolar, trimalleolar, or bimalleolar equivalent fracture (fibular fracture with incompetent deltoid ligament).

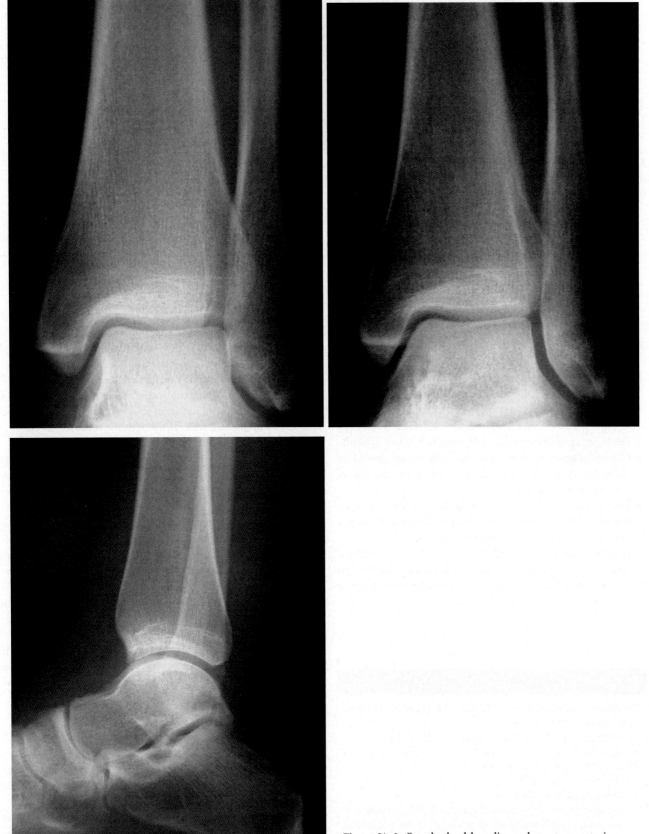

Figure 21–3: Standard ankle radiographs: anteroposterior, 15 degrees to 20 degrees internal rotation mortise, and lateral views.

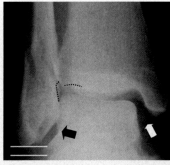 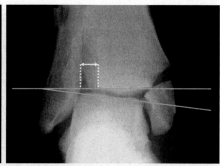

Figure 21–4: **Radiographic signs of significant injury include shortening of the fibula** *(white lines)*, **loss of parallelism of the subchondral lines of lateral malleolus and that of the lateral talus** *(black arrow)*, **loss of normal subchondral lines at incisura** *(hatched black lines)*, **and widened medial joint space** *(white arrow)*.

3. Weber type C and P-ER 2 and P-ER 3 fractures require surgery because of the syndesmosis injury and associated instability.
4. Open ankle fractures.
5. Ankle fracture-dislocations with more extensive bone and soft-tissue injury.

Timing of Surgery

- The timing of surgery is somewhat controversial but ultimately depends on the condition of the soft tissues.
- If possible, surgery is best performed within 6 to 8 hours of injury before significant edema develops. However, the logistics of performing early surgery is often difficult.
- Generally, most experts agree that soft tissues should be quiescent at the time of surgery to minimize the risk of wound complications.
- On the contrary, marked swelling, the presence of acute fracture blisters or other skin changes must delay surgery until the soft tissues have had time to recover.
- If surgery must be delayed, the fracture must be reduced and held in a well-padded splint, a bivalved cast, or even an external fixator, and the limb elevated until swelling subsides.

Box 21–3

Radiographic findings of an unstable ankle fracture (see Figure 21–4)
1. Significant fracture displacement
2. Subluxation or dislocation of the talus under the plafond
3. Widening of the medial joint space
4. Alterations in the talocrural angle
5. Alterations in the talar tilt
6. Widened tibiofibular clear space
7. Loss of alignment of the subchondral plates at the tibiofibular line
8. Shortening of the fibula by loss of parallelism of the subchondral lines of the lateral malleolus and that of the lateral talus

- Most ankle fractures can undergo surgical treatment with no change in technique or complication rates even up to three weeks after the injury.

Implants

- In most cases, we use a small fragment set with a one-third tubular plate laterally, and 4- or 4.5-mm partially threaded cancellous screws (cannulated or solid) medially.
- The one-third tubular plate has been a "work-horse" plate for distal fibula and other ankle fractures because it easily contours to the local anatomy, is low profile, and allows ample mechanical strength for most fractures.
- Specialty implants may be beneficial in particular cases.
  1. "Composite" plates that are one-third tubular distally and 3.5 mm proximally (DePuy, Warsaw, Ind.) may be useful in patients with poor bone quality or in cases with proximal fracture extension.
  2. Locking plate technology may also be useful in some difficult ankle fractures. These plate-screw devices create a fixed angled construct and may be beneficial in patients with poor bone quality and fracture comminution. Care must be taken when using locking plates around the ankle; if they are not placed in a lag fashion like traditional nonlocked plates, they are not useful for aiding in reduction.
  3. Intramedullary (IM) devices may be used for fibular fixation in cases of severe soft-tissue injury. Relative to plate and screw constructs though, nonlocked IM implants poorly control length and rotation.

Examination

- Assessment of the soft tissues and the timing of ankle fracture surgery are among the most important factors in these cases.
- Blisters, considerable swelling, or other signs of soft-tissue trauma should concern the surgeon, and surgery should be delayed until these issues resolve.

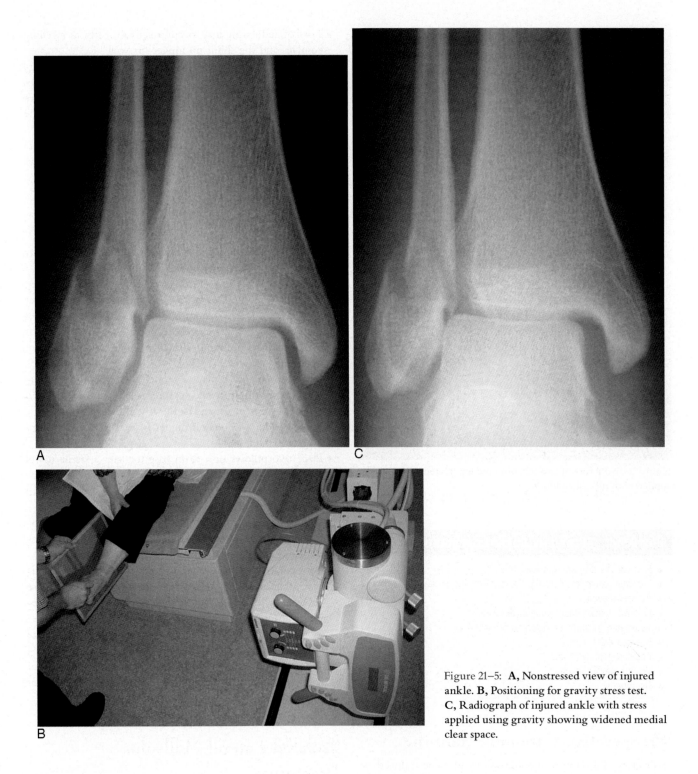

Figure 21–5: **A,** Nonstressed view of injured ankle. **B,** Positioning for gravity stress test. **C,** Radiograph of injured ankle with stress applied using gravity showing widened medial clear space.

- The "wrinkle" sign has been used in other areas of the lower extremity and may be helpful for deciding when the soft tissues are ready for ankle fracture surgery.
- Deformity from an ankle fracture or dislocation may cause pressure necrosis of the skin over the supramalleolar area. For this reason, if surgery is not to be performed immediately, a closed reduction should be performed, and a splint should be applied to maintain reduction of the talus beneath the plafond and decompress the skin "at risk."
- Poorly padded splints or prepackaged fiberglass splints can cause skin injury and blisters if placed incorrectly (Figure 21–6).
- Despite the obvious ankle fracture, a thorough lower extremity examination should be performed (Box 21–4).

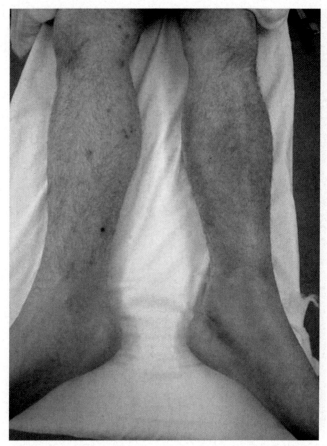

Figure 21–6: **Picture of swollen, blistered leg treated with a splint applied with no cast padding.**

Box 21–4	**Secondary Ankle Examination**

- Skin compromise and previous incisions
- Proximal tenderness over the fibula (Maisonneuve fracture)
- Achilles tendon
- Peroneal tendon subluxation or dislocation
- Associated fractures or dislocations in the foot
- Neurovascular injury
- Compartment syndrome
- Venous stasis changes
- Neuropathy

Preoperative Care and Planning

- Fracture dislocations or subluxations must be reduced as ongoing pressure on the skin may cause further injury or necrosis, especially in patients with preexisting soft-tissue problems.
- The supramalleolar skin over the distal tibia is most often at risk as subluxation of the talus and malleoli, which typically occurs laterally.
- A well-padded posterior and 'U' splint should then be applied to maintain reduction.

- Loss of reduction may occur relatively early as swelling resolves and the splint no longer fits well.
- The importance of preoperative planning cannot be overemphasized. This may be especially true for injuries around the ankle, where multiple surgical incisions are often required and the injuries and soft tissues allow little leeway for surgical errors.
- Forethought as to which injury may need surgical treatment and what approaches should be performed allows for optimal treatment of the patient.

Operative Set Up

- Patients undergoing ankle fracture surgery are typically administered general or spinal anesthesia.
- Local anesthesia and sedation may be used on occasion, although incomplete muscle relaxation will occur that may make fracture reduction difficult.
- For patients being treated for injuries of the medial or lateral ankle, positioning is usually supine on a radiolucent operating table.
- It is often helpful to place a padded bump behind the buttock on the injured side to internally rotate the leg and allow comfortable access to the lateral malleolus.
- A well-padded thigh tourniquet is used to provide a dry surgical field.
- Place two pillows or a foam base (or later a sterile towel roll) under the fractured leg to elevate it above the contralateral leg. This assists in the surgical approaches and in obtaining lateral radiographs.
- A surgical prep of the limb is performed, and a preoperative dose of antibiotic is administered before exsanguination of the leg and insufflation of the tourniquet.
- Postoperatively, wound closure is performed in a multilayer fashion using atraumatic technique because these tissues may have little physiologic reserve and wound problems around the ankle are rarely treated easily.
- Obtaining soft-tissue coverage over the lateral fibular plate with a full-thickness layer of soft tissue is desirable.
- We prefer not to use staples on the skin around the foot or ankle in the setting of acute trauma but instead use 3–0 or 4–0 nylon suture that can be carefully tensioned.

Isolated Lateral Malleolus
Fractures

- The importance of lateral malleolus reduction and its impact on the overall ankle joint congruency and mechanics has been well recognized.[1,9]
- Yablon and others[9] concluded that the lateral malleolus was the key to the anatomic reduction of bimalleolar ankle fractures because the displacement of the talus faithfully followed the displaced distal fibular fragment.

- This concept has recently been challenged by Tornetta,[10] who demonstrated that medial only fixation may be sufficient in many bimalleolar injuries.
- Good results are typically achieved with nonoperative treatment of isolated lateral malleolus fractures without a medial injury.
- These clinical results are supported by cadaveric studies that have shown that isolated displacement of the lateral malleolus does not cause ankle instability.[11]
- The literature supports nonoperative treatment for equal to 2 mm of displacement of the lateral malleolus and a normal medial clear space.[1,11]
- For patients who have a closed, isolated lateral malleolus fracture with minimal displacement, we recommend nonoperative treatment with close follow-up.
- Diagnosis of an associated deltoid ligament injury may be difficult.
- Medial tenderness and swelling may indicate a deltoid ligament injury, but clinical findings of a medial injury are at times quite subtle.
- Initial radiographs must be carefully scrutinized for widening of the medial joint space, which indicates incompetence of the deltoid ligament.
- Other methods of diagnosis include a variety of stress tests (described previously in this chapter) and magnetic resonance imaging (MRI).

Surgical Technique of Fibular Plating

- A direct lateral approach using a longitudinal incision is commonly used for the reduction and plating of fibula fractures (Figure 21–7).
- The fibula is usually palpable beneath the subcutaneous tissues, and its borders can be defined fairly easily.
- At times the skin incision may be moved posteriorly (or anteriorly) depending on the soft tissues, site of plate placement, desire to access the posterolateral and anterolateral tibia, or other reasons.
- It is often beneficial to curve the incision anteriorly near the distal end of the fibula to directly see the syndesmosis anterior inferior tibia fibula ligament (AITFL) and occult fractures off the fibula or tibia.
- The skin incision for the posterior application of an antiglide plate is best placed about 1 cm posterior to the standard lateral incision.
- Additionally, the path of the superficial peroneal nerve is not always consistent, and meticulous dissection is required to assess whether the nerve is crossing through the operative wound, especially as the incision is carried proximally (Figure 21–8).
- Most lateral malleolar fractures that require open reduction and internal fixation (ORIF) are repaired with a prebent one-third tubular plate with or without lag screws.
- The plate can be applied directly laterally or posteriorly (Figure 21–9).
- A laterally applied plate allows for more direct access for plate application and is useful for nearly all fracture patterns but may result in occasional problems with implant prominence.
- A posteriorly applied plate may be more mechanically effective for oblique fibula fractures but has been implicated as a cause of peroneal tendon inflammation.
- The fracture can be "freshened" by removing the organized fracture hematoma from the fracture line that may prevent interdigitation of the fracture's bony interstices.
- Simple fibular fracture patterns, such as the typical oblique or spiral fracture of an SE-4 injury, are relatively easy to reduce with a standard reduction clamp.
- Fracture reduction can be judged by visualizing the proximal fracture spike and checking that it is keyed in at the fracture's apex.

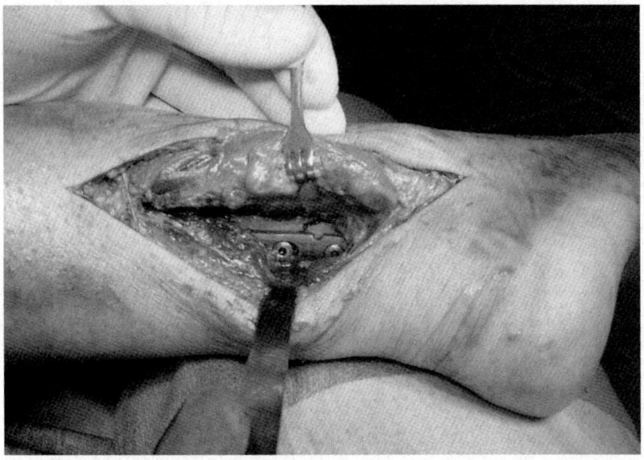

Figure 21–7: **Surgical approach to the distal fibula. The incision can be moved posteriorly to accommodate positioning of the plate on the posterior surface of the fibula or to allow for a posterolateral approach to the posterior malleolus.**

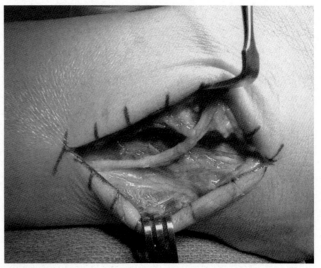

Figure 21–8: **Surgical approach to the fibula showing atypical location of the superficial nerve crossing at a 90-degree angle to the incision.**

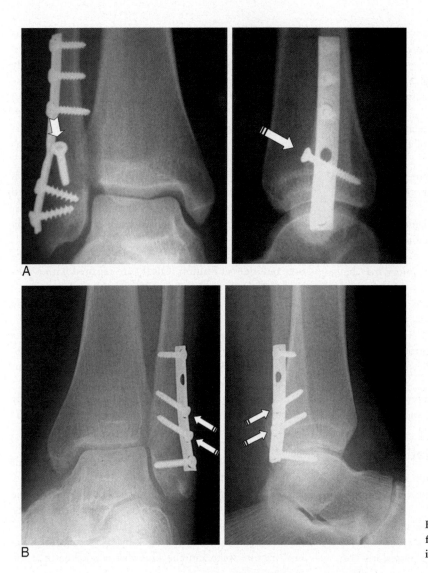

Figure 21–9: **Positioning of plates for the distal fibula. The plate can be positioned on the fibula in a lateral (A) or posterior (B) location.**

- As noted, a one-third tubular plate can be applied laterally or posteriorly for fixation. A lag screw should be applied if possible before plating if a lateral plate is used or through the plate if an antiglide plate is placed posteriorly.
- Comminuted or "crushed" lateral malleolus fractures may be much more difficult to properly reduce and fix. These fractures often involve the syndesmosis.
- Length and rotation of the fibula are restored when the contour of the lateral talus matches that of the medial distal fibula on the mortise view, and the contour of the fibular incisura is restored to the line of the tibial plafond.
- Useful techniques for gaining reduction include indirect reduction methods using the plate as a reduction tool. For example, the plate can be initially applied to one side of the fracture (usually distal) and then length and rotation may be obtained using manual traction or manipulation,

a mini-distractor, or the use of lamina spreaders against a "push-pull" screw.
- The plate is then temporarily secured to the bone proximally with a Verbrugge or other clamp.
- An alternative method is to use a pointed reduction clamp to correct rotation and bring the fibula out to length. One or two small Kirschner wires (K-wires) can then be used to pin the fibula to the talus or distal tibia. A plate can then be secured distally and the K-wires removed.
- The authors typically use a stiffer plate, such as a well contoured 3.5-mm dynamic compression (DC) plate (Synthes USA, Paoli, Penn.) or "composite" plate (DePuy-Ace, Warsaw, Ind.) in cases in which there is considerable fracture shortening, comminution or a more proximal diaphyseal injury (Figure 21–10).
- More rigid plates must be carefully precontoured to include the anatomic rotation of the distal fibular shaft or

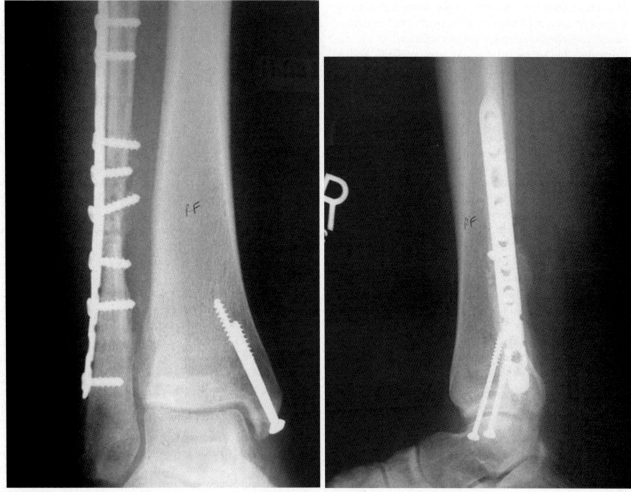

Figure 21–10: Radiographs of open reduction and internal fixation of comminuted lateral malleolus with a composite plate.

they will malreduce the fracture as the bone moves to the plate during screw insertion (Box 21–5).

Medial Malleolus Fractures

- Medial malleolus fractures usually occur in conjunction with lateral malleolus fractures but occasionally occur as an isolated injury in P-ER or P-AB injuries (see Figure 21–2).
- Obtaining radiographs of the entire tibia and fibula is important because an "isolated" medial malleolus may be part of a more complex "Maisonneuve fracture" with a proximal fibula fracture *and* injury to the syndesmosis.
- Medial malleolar fractures may be transverse, oblique, or nearly vertical in orientation.
- Transverse or oblique fractures represent avulsion injuries and may involve the entire medial malleolus or just the anterior colliculus. This distinction is made by careful review of the lateral radiograph. Because the deep deltoid ligament attaches to the posterior colliculus, injury to the

| Box 21–5 | Techniques for Difficult Fibula Fractures |

- Use multiple clamps
- Use the plate as a reduction tool (consider a 3.5-dynamic compression plate or other stiff plate)
- Gain length with manual traction, lamina spreader, or other push and pull tool
- Temporarily pin the distal fibula to the talus to hold length and rotation
- Use direct visualization and fluoroscopy to verify proper reduction
- For osteoporotic fractures, consider modifying plate fixation with supplemental intramedullary pins, locked screws, and placing multiple screws from the fibula to the tibia for increased screw purchase

deep deltoid ligament can coexist with an anterior collicular fracture.
- In this case, repair of the anterior malleolar fragment will not restore competence of the medial ligament, and the ankle may remain potentially unstable.

- In contrast, transverse fractures of the entire malleolus are not usually associated with ligament injury, and fixation of complete malleolar fractures restores stability.[10]
- Currently, long-term studies on outcomes of isolated medial malleolus fractures do not exist.
- We recommend that nondisplaced or minimally displaced fractures be treated with immobilization, but fractures displaced more than 2 mm should be treated with ORIF.
- Plain radiographs provide limited accuracy for imaging the medial malleolus, and even small amounts of residual radiographic displacement of medial malleolus fractures may in reality correlate to much larger amounts of true malreduction.
- One should carefully scrutinize all three radiographic views of the ankle in assessing these injuries, and if the fracture pattern is not clearly visualized, a CT scan should be performed.
- It has been suggested that a sizable malreduced fracture may behave as a deltoid ligament injury and lead to dynamic ankle instability.[7]
- Strong consideration should also be given to open reduction for fractures in which small osseous or osteochondral fragments are in the joint because these can lead to mechanical wear or impingement.
- When the fractured medial malleolus is exposed, the joint should be carefully inspected for free fragments or chondral injuries, which may indicate a more guarded prognosis for the ankle.

Surgical Technique of Medial Malleolar Fixation

- We use a curvilinear incision extending from above the anteromedial aspect of the ankle joint superiorly and curves distally around the tip of the medial malleolus.
- The advantage of this approach is the excellent visualization of the medial ankle joint and fracture reduction proximally and allows for a lag screw to be placed distally.
- Partially threaded lag screws are placed if there is a transverse or oblique fracture.
- The disadvantage of this approach is that the surgeon necessarily encounters the saphenous vein and nerve, which must be carefully preserved.
- Some surgeons prefer a straight longitudinal medial incision extending over the fracture and the tip of the medial malleolus or a curved incision that extends around the posterior aspect of the medial malleolus. A major limitation of these approaches is impaired visualization of the articular reduction and any articular injury.
- Furthermore, making an incision of the skin directly over the bone could lead to potentially catastrophic wound problems that may require a free tissue transfer.
- Reduction of the medial malleolus is typically straight forward, but we have found a few "technical tricks" that are helpful.

- First, a surprisingly large flap of periosteum is often present medially, which may incarcerate in the fracture and prevent accurate reduction or make fracture visualization more difficult.
- This periosteal flap may be amputated as it extends off the bone of the malleolar fragment.
- Second, manipulation of the malleolar fragment may be aided by insertion of K-wires through its tip.
- Once reduction is achieved, these wires may be inserted across the fracture into the distal tibial metaphysis for provisional fixation.
- Maintaining two points of fixation is recommended (provisionally and definitively) to prevent rotational displacement.
- Other potentially useful instruments for this manipulation include the dental pick and the small pointed reduction clamp (a drill hole can be made on the distal tibia's medial cortex proximally).
- Assessment of reduction is accomplished by direct visualization of the extraarticular fracture line medially and anteriorly and at the anteromedial corner of the ankle joint.
- Ideally then, if cannulated screws are to be used, three K-wires should be placed so that when a screw's pilot hole is drilled and that K-wire's stabilizing effect is lost, reduction will be maintained.
- Most medial malleolus fractures are well fixed with two partially threaded cancellous lag screws (Figure 21–11), either cannulated (3.5 to 4.5 mm) or noncannulated (4 mm).
- A technical trick for placing noncannulated screws involves using a cannulated drill and tap over a precisely placed guidewire and then removing the guidewire and placing the solid core screw in the already drilled location.
- Depending on the fracture configuration, smaller fragments may be fixed with a screw and a K-wire (cut short and bent) placed for rotational stability.
- Comminuted fractures may require a tension band construct or even supplemental fixation with minifragment screws.
- S-AD type fractures (see Figure 21–2) or other more vertically oriented fractures that extend further into the tibia should be fixed with an antiglide plate (with or without lag screws) to prevent vertical migration (Figure 21–12).

Bimalleolar Fractures

- Bimalleolar ankle fractures refer to bony injuries typically involving the medial and lateral malleoli, and may include the Weber types A, B, and C and Lauge-Hansen S-AD 2, S-ER 3, S-ER4, P-ER 3, P-ER 4, and P-AB 2 type fractures.
- The vast majority of injuries that involve the medial and lateral malleolus are mechanically unstable and need to be reduced and fixed internally if a good outcome is to be expected.

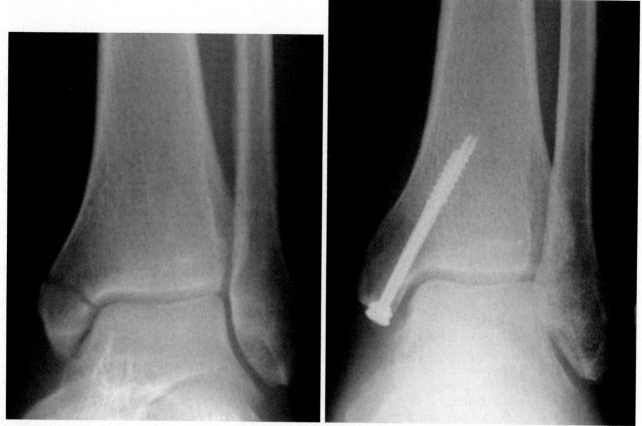

Figure 21–11: Open reduction and internal fixation of medial malleolus fracture using two 4.5-mm cannulated screws.

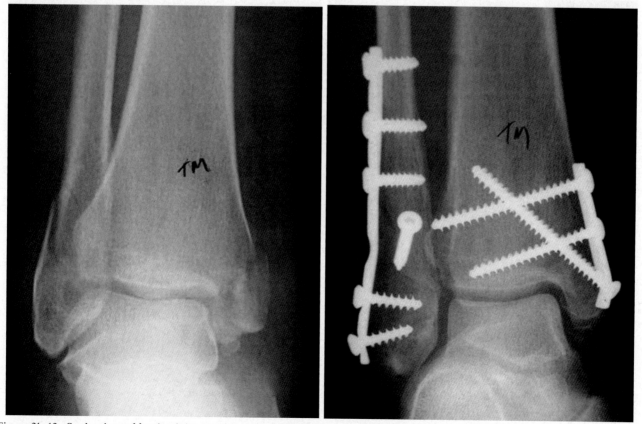

Figure 21–12: Supination-adduction injury to the medial malleolus may be stabilized with an antiglide plate.

- Classically, fixation of both malleoli is recommended, and the methods of fixation for each injured side are discussed individually elsewhere in this chapter.
- The potential for syndesmosis injury must also be considered for almost all of these injuries, but is most common with Weber type C fibular fractures more than 4.5 cm above the plafond.[4,5]
- Recently, Ebraheim and others[5] demonstrated that syndesmosis injury may also be present with more distal fibular fractures that are not typically considered at risk for such injury. We recommended routine intraoperative stress views of the syndesmosis after fixation of all ankle fractures.
- Recent work by Tornetta[10] has demonstrated that many bimalleolar fractures are successfully stabilized by reduction and fixation of the medial malleolus alone.
- This is clinically relevant when fracture blisters, fasciotomy, or other considerations preclude a lateral incision.
- One potential pitfall with medial fixation alone is the isolated fracture of the anterior colliculus.
- Fracture of the anterior colliculus of the medial malleolus may or may not be associated with deep deltoid ligament disruption.
- If one repairs an anterior collicular fracture and is considering medial fixation alone, a stress examination should be done after fixation to determine if medial stability has been restored.
- If the deep deltoid is disrupted, fixation of the anterior colliculus of the medial malleolus does not stabilize the ankle as the associated ligament injury and lateral repair is also necessary.
- We still presently recommend the routine fixation of medial and lateral malleolar fractures in patients with bimalleolar ankle fractures (Figure 21–13).
- The "bimalleolar-equivalent injury" refers to a fibula fracture that is associated with a complete deltoid ligament injury instead of a medial malleolus fracture.
- The deltoid ligament originates on the medial malleolus and inserts on the talus and calcaneus. The superficial portion resists eversion, and the deep component resists external rotation of the talus and is the critical portion that maintains ankle stability.
- The diagnosis of a deltoid injury is often made clinically with swelling and tenderness at or below the medial malleolus.
- Stress views (discussed elsewhere in this chapter) or MRI may be needed to confirm the diagnosis.
- Patients with fibula fractures and an injury to the deltoid ligament rendering the ankle unstable should be treated surgically with an anatomic reduction of the fibula.

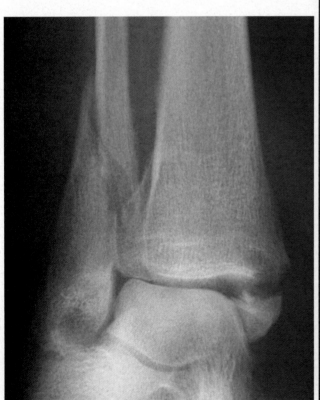 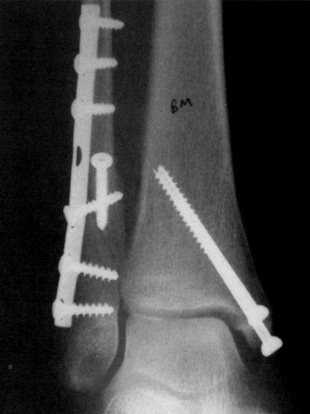

Figure 21–13: **Radiograph of open reduction and internal fixation of bimalleolar ankle fracture.**

- Repairing the deltoid ligament is unnecessary provided an anatomic reduction is obtained of the fibula and the medial clear space has been reduced.
- Even if the medial clear space appears reduced, checking for an associated syndesmosis injury by using intraoperative stress views should be standard.
- These patients should then be treated with immobilization for 6 weeks without early motion to allow the deltoid ligament to heal at its original length.
- Rarely, a portion of the torn deltoid ligament may block complete reduction of the joint and the medial clear space will remain wide; when this occurs, medial exploration is indicated.

Posterior Malleolus Fractures

- Fracture of the ankle's posterior malleolus is caused by external rotation or abduction (Lauge-Hansen P-ER, S-ER 4, and P-AB types) with avulsion of the bone by the posterior inferior tibiofibular ligament (Figure 21–14).
- Most surgeons recommend internal fixation for fractures of the posterior malleolus that comprise greater than 20% to 33% of the distal tibial articular surface if there is posterior instability or greater than a 2-mm step-off.[12]

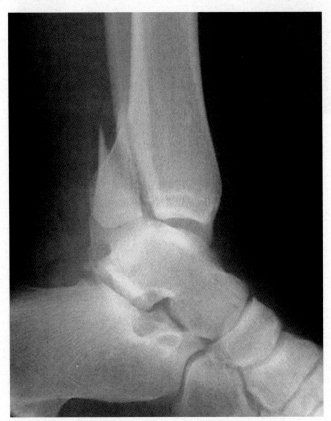

Figure 21–14: **Radiograph of posterior malleolus fracture showing greater than 30% involvement and articular displacement.**

- Stabilization of the fibula can prevent posterior subluxation of the ankle because the fibula and anterior tibiofibular ligament are the primary restraint to posterior instability of the ankle.
- Other studies, however, have shown that patients with posterior malleolar fragments consisting of greater than 25% to 33% of the articular surface had better clinical results with internal fixation.[13]
- One potential pitfall is the assessment of the true size of the posterior malleolar fragment: CT or MRI may be needed to truly assess the proportion of the articular surface that is involved. Additionally, an external rotation view of the ankle can be used intraoperatively to better asses the size of the posterior fragment.
- If the posterior malleolar fracture is not internally fixed, we recommend cast immobilizing the leg for 4 to 6 weeks to minimize the motion at the fracture site (Box 21–6).

Surgical Technique of Posterior Malleolar Fixation

- Displacement of the posterior malleolus frequently reduces indirectly when the fibula is reduced.[13]
- If the fracture is anatomically reduced via indirect methods, the posterior malleolus can be fixed with one or two lag screws placed anterior medial to posterolateral because the posterior malleolar fragment usually involves the lateral portion of the distal posterior tibia (Figure 21–15).
- In this case, lag screws can be inserted percutaneously using cannulated or standard screws.
- Quality fluoroscopic views must be obtained of the fracture reduction and implant position if this method is used.
- If the posterior malleolus fracture is still displaced after the fibula is reduced, it can be reduced and fixed via an open posterolateral approach using the fibular incision (cheated posteriorly) with additional posterior exposure.
- If this open posterolateral approach is anticipated, the patient can be positioned laterally on a bean bag (secured with a seatbelt but without being taped to the table) and can be then gently rolled to a more supine position by deflating the bean bag once the medial side is to be addressed.

Box 21–6	Indications for Internal Fixation of a Posterior Malleolus Fracture

- The fragment is greater than 25% to 33% of the tibial articular surface
- When there is posterior subluxation or dynamic posterior instability of the ankle
- When there is an articular step-off greater than 2 to 3 mm in the posterior tibia, especially if a nonanatomic reduction of the fibula is present (Fig. 21–14).

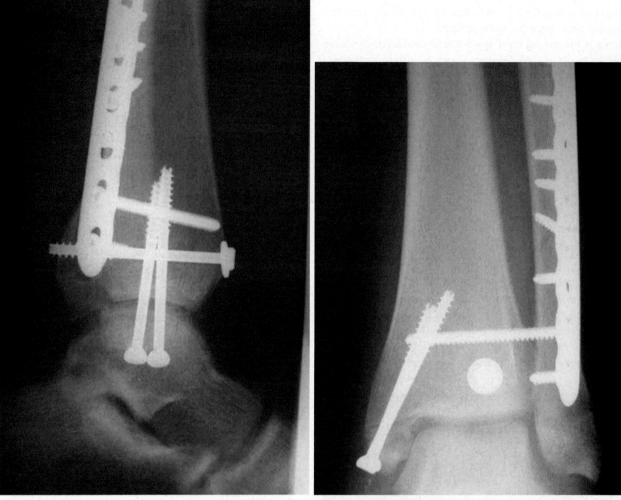

Figure 21–15: Posterior malleolus fixation may be percutaneously applied via anterior-posteriorly placed screws.

- Exposure is gained by opening the superficial interval between the peroneal tendons and the Achilles tendon, then passing lateral to the flexor hallucis longus (FHL).
- The neurovascular bundle of the posteromedial leg is safely protected by the FHL, and wide exposure of the posterior aspect of the distal tibia can be achieved.
- A buttress plate can be placed with lag screws to achieve excellent fixation of the posterior malleolar fragment (Figure 21–16). The fracture is reduced by directly visualizing the tibia cortex posteriorly, which then provides an indirect reduction at the joint level.
- Alternatively, before internally fixing the lateral malleolus, the fractured fibula can be displaced or flipped inferiorly since the syndesmotic ligaments are usually torn.
- By displacing the distal fibula, excellent exposure is now afforded the surgeon and direct visualization is obtained of the distal posterior tibia.
- The posterior fracture can now be reduced and internally fixed, and then the distal fibula can be reduced and fixed in the previously discussed fashion.

Syndesmosis Injury

- The treatment of syndesmosis injuries associated with fractures of the ankle continues to provoke controversy among surgeons.
- Despite multiple anatomic and biomechanical studies addressing the mechanism of injury and diagnosis, surgeons have not reached a consensus regarding specific treatment guidelines, such as the type of fixation needed and postoperative management.
- This chapter addresses only syndesmosis injuries associated with ankle fractures; the article by Wuest[14] is an excellent and comprehensive review article of isolated syndesmosis injuries.
- The syndesmosis is composed of four ligaments: the anterior inferior and posterior inferior tibiofibular ligaments, the inferior transverse tibiofibular ligament, and the interosseous ligament and membrane (see Figure 21–1).
- Syndesmosis injuries may be identified by obvious widening of the distal tibiofibular joint or they may be very subtle.

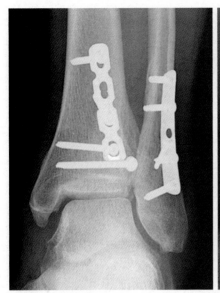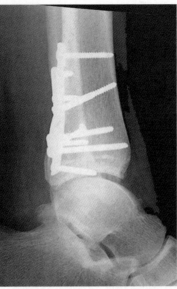

Figure 21–16: Radiograph of posterior malleolus fracture fixed with a posteriorly applied reconstruction plate.

- In the case of a more proximal fibula fracture without a medial fracture, a positive stress test likely shows a deltoid and syndesmosis injury.
- Disruption of the syndesmosis usually occurs as the result of an external rotation force and typically involves "high" distal fibula fractures, (i.e., Weber type C, and Lauge-Hansen P-ER and S-ER 4 fractures).
- The diagnosis is usually made radiographically, although a syndesmosis injury may be obvious or quite subtle and may be revealed only by stress radiographs.
- The medial clear space (the space between the talus and medial malleolus) should be equal to the space superior and lateral to the talus. Figure 21–17 shows the medial widening with stress applied to the ankle.
- Common diagnostic imaging clues include a tibia-fibula clear space of greater than 6 mm on AP and mortise films, and a tibia-fibula overlap less than 6 mm on AP radiographs and less than 1 mm on the mortise view.
- Ebraheim and others[5] report that CT scans comparing the injured to the normal ankle are helpful; signs of syndesmosis injury include tibiofibular diastasis, anterior subluxation of the distal fibula, and a shallow incisura fibularis.
- Sometimes injuries are diagnosed intraoperatively by the Cotton Test, which is performed by pulling the distal fibula with a towel clip in order to determine if it separates from the tibia (Figure 21–18).
- More recently, it has been suggested that AP subluxation may be easier to elicit and may be a more sensitive test of syndesmosis instability.[8]
- The work of Boden and others[4] is commonly quoted during discussions regarding stabilization of the ankle syndesmosis.

- They found that if the deltoid ligament was intact (no medial injury), no amount of syndesmosis disruption altered ankle stability.
- They recommended syndesmosis fixation for patients with fibula fractures occurring greater than 4.5 cm proximal to the mortise (the "critical zone"), provided that they also had a medial injury.
- The degree of ankle instability in patients who had fractures of the fibula from 3 to 4.5 cm proximal to the mortise was not definitive in the study.
- Many surgeons have recommended placing a syndesmosis screw for uncertain injuries because the morbidity of a missed injury may be much greater than that of a syndesmosis screw.
- If in doubt, the surgeon should get intraoperative external rotation or other stress radiographs, such as the Cotton test (see Figure 21–18).
- In many cases, both the fibular fracture and the syndesmosis injury are addressed simultaneously by repair of the fibula with a plate and screw fixation (often through the plate) of the syndesmosis.
- However in some cases, syndesmosis fixation only is appropriate.
- In these cases, the distal fibular fragment is reduced to the talus and one or two syndesmosis screws are placed.
- The rationale for this approach is that the fibula fracture itself is negligible; rather it is the reduction of the distal fibula, restoration of the length of the fibula, and stabilization of the distal tibiofibular joint that are important.
- The previously mentioned Maisonneuve injury combines a proximal fibula fracture with a medial ankle ligamentous injury and includes a syndesmosis injury.

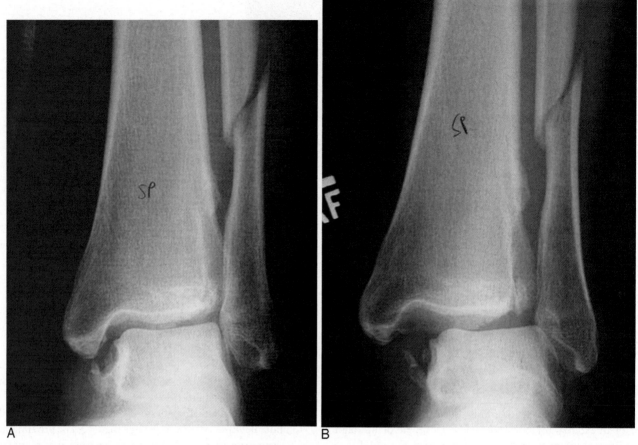

Figure 21–17: **A,** Radiograph of supination-external rotation 4 fracture with proximal fibula fracture but no medial widening. **B,** Stressed radiograph showing medial widening.

- The proximal fibula does not require operative treatment, but the syndesmosis injury should be recognized and addressed.
- To restore normal joint congruity, fibular length and rotation must be restored before placement of the distal syndesmotic screw(s).
- In this case, the authors typically place two syndesmosis screws, sometimes placing them through a two- or three-hole one-third tubular plate to provide a stronger construct (see Figure 21–19).

Surgical Technique of Syndesmosis Screw Fixation

- The lateral or medial fractures should be anatomically reduced and fixed.
- If the medial clear space is still wide (with or without stress test), a large tenaculum or reduction clamp can be placed from the fibula to the distal tibia.
- Intraoperative fluoroscopy allows for assessment of fibular alignment and length and later helps to ensure that the screw is placed parallel to the joint.
- Once the joint is reduced, a syndesmosis screw should be directed parallel to the plafond and aimed slightly anteriorly

from the fibula to the tibia at a level 1.5 to 2 cm proximal to the mortise, above the distal tibia- fibular joint (Figure 21–20).
- It is helpful to tap the pilot hole before screw insertion, even if self-tapping screws are used because the screw may tend to push the tibia away from the fibula when its first few threads engage the tibial cortex.
- A second screw may be added slightly more superiorly, if desired.
- Many surgeons prefer to place syndesmosis screws with the ankle positioned in maximal dorsiflexion "to preserve ankle motion," although Tornetta and others[15] have discredited this thinking.
- A fixation screw (not a lag screw) should be placed to prevent over tightening of the syndesmosis.
- Surgeons typically choose either 3.5- or 4.5-mm screws with three or four cortices of screw purchase, but these points remain controversial.
- No definitive biomechanical or clinical studies demonstrate an advantage of either screw size or number of cortices.
- Hoiness and Stromsoe[16] recently compared one 4.5-mm screw placed through four cortices (removed at 8 weeks)

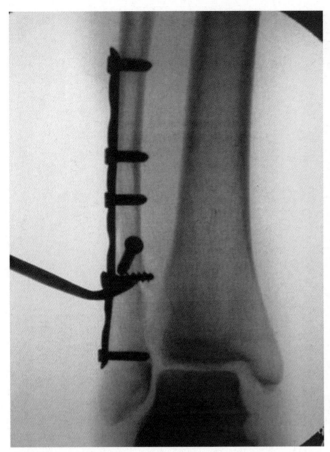

Figure 21–18: Intraoperative radiograph demonstrating a Cotton test and medial joint widening indicative of a syndesmosis injury.

with two 3.5-mm screws which engaged only three cortices (not removed).

- At 1 year, there were no differences between the two groups in pain, functional score, or dorsiflexion.
- Recent articles have demonstrated that good results can also be obtained in the treatment of syndesmosis injuries with 4.5-mm poly-L-lactic acid (PLLA) bioabsorbable screws (Figure 21–21).[17]
- The potential benefit of the absorbable screw is that an additional procedure to remove the screw can be avoided.
- Although this technique is promising, the gold standard for treating the syndesmosis is still metal implants.
- Whether or not to remove the syndesmosis screw before weight bearing may be the most debated of all syndesmosis topics.
- Needleman and others[18] showed that syndesmosis screws cause a decrease in the tibiotalar external rotation.
- Advocates of screw removal point out that leaving the screw in place results in abnormal ankle motion or at least screw breakage (Figure 21–22).
- Advocates of no scheduled removal have shown that patients can be fully weight bearing with the screw in place and that the screws eventually loosen or break with little morbidity.

- Proponents of leaving the screw in place point out that the screws' loosening or breaking allow patients to have near normal ankle motion again.
- The authors typically use a single 3.5-mm cortical screw, placed 1.5 to 2 cm above the mortise, with the ankle positioned in dorsiflexion, and placed through four cortices (see Figure 21–20).
- If the patient is large or obese, or compliance is in question, a second parallel screw may be added.
- The postoperative protocol is as follows:
  1. The patient is kept nonweight bearing for 6 weeks in a cast or boot.
  2. Weight bearing as tolerated in a boot for 6 weeks.
- Screw removal is typically performed between 12 and 14 weeks under local anesthesia with postremoval radiographs obtained to verify a reduced mortise.
- The syndesmosis should absolutely not be removed before 12 weeks because this may lead to an incompletely healed ligament that can result in instability.

Open Fractures

- Open fractures and injuries of the ankle require all of the considerations of closed injuries and additional concerns about the severity of soft-tissue injury and bacterial contamination.
- Open injuries, including ankle fractures, have been shown to be at increased risk for complications and poor outcomes when compared to closed injuries.[19,20,21]
- The treatment of patients who have open ankle fractures begins on arrival to the emergency department (ED) with the administration of intravenous antibiotics and tetanus prophylaxis.
- They should be initially treated as all other open fractures according to the work of Gustillo and others.[21]
- The wound should be examined and then covered with a saline-moistened sterile dressing.
- If the injury is grossly displaced, a reduction maneuver should be performed.
- Antibiotics should be provided according to current recommendations for open fractures.
- Patients who have Gustillo type I and II fractures should receive a cephalosporin (e.g., cefazolin) on admission, continued every 8 hours for at least 24 to 48 hours.
- Patients who have type III fractures should receive the same dose of a cephalosporin plus an aminoglycoside, a broad-spectrum antibiotic (Zosyn), or fluoroquinolone for gram-negative coverage.
- Farm injuries and grossly contaminated wounds should also receive penicillin.
- Timely and thorough wound debridement and lavage is standard.
- An aggressive and organized surgical debridement is performed to remove all foreign material and tissue of questionable viability.

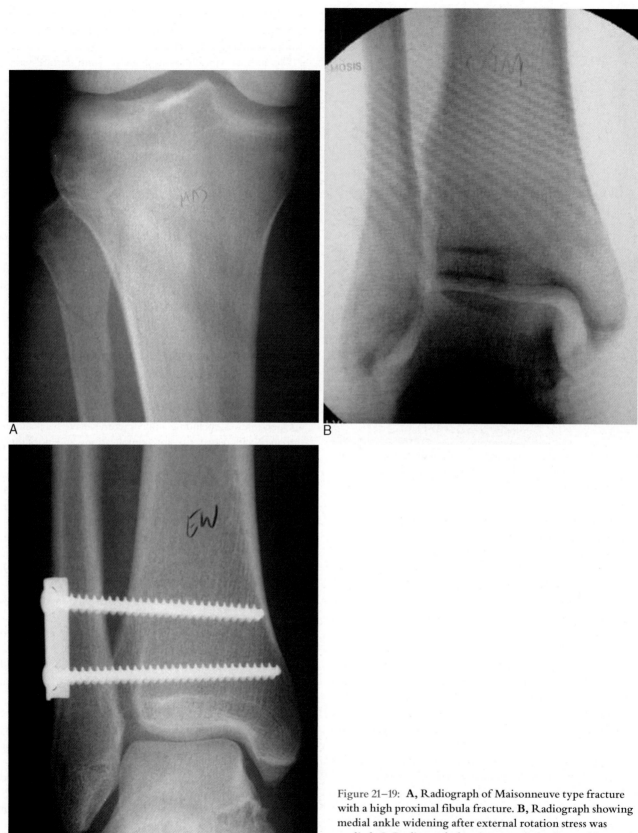

Figure 21–19: **A,** Radiograph of Maisonneuve type fracture with a high proximal fibula fracture. **B,** Radiograph showing medial ankle widening after external rotation stress was applied. **C,** Radiograph showing open reduction and internal fixation of the syndesmosis with two screws and a plate.

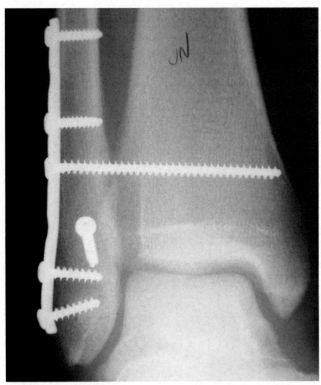

Figure 21–20: **Radiograph showing a fibula fracture reduced with a plate and the concomitant syndesmosis injury treated with non-lag screw fixation.**

- Open types I, II, and III-A fractures can be treated with standard technique using stable internal fixation and wound closure once the wound is clean.
- Bray and others[19] and Franklin and others[20] found that immediate ORIF of open ankle fractures caused no increased incidence of infection compared to those treated with delayed fixation.
- Both groups recommend this approach as the treatment of choice for most open ankle fractures.
- Type III-B fractures may be best stabilized with either minimal internal fixation or an external fixator and delayed definitive fixation.
- Most authors agree that the wound should be re-debrided and irrigated every 48 to 72 hours until the wound is "clean" and then may be safely closed.
- The goal is for wound closure or a wound coverage procedure within 5 to 10 days.

Ankle Fractures in Osteoporotic Bone

- As the nation continues to age, orthopaedic surgeons will continue to be faced with more and more osteoporosis related fractures, including those around the ankle.
- Although treatment goals for the majority of elderly patients are the same as for younger patients, that is restoration of ankle alignment, stability to allow for early motion, and

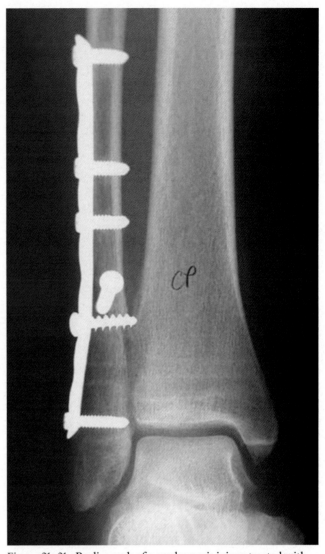

Figure 21–21: **Radiograph of a syndesmosis injury treated with an absorbable screw. The lucent lines parallel to the mortise at the level of the second distal screw hole in the plate mark at the location of the absorbable screw.**

the prevention of posttraumatic arthritis, treatment decisions regarding patients with severe osteoporosis should be made on an individualized basis.

- Unfortunately, nonoperative treatment is usually poorly tolerated in many patients that suffer these injuries, and complication rates are fairly high with nonoperative treatment methods.[22,23]
- With surgery, quality fixation strength may be difficult to achieve in elderly osteoporotic patients and increased complication rates have been seen under these circumstances as well.[22]
- There are several techniques for maximizing fixation strength in patients with osteoporotic ankle fractures:
  1. Plate fixation with all cancellous screws.
  2. Plate and screw fixation supplemented with IM pins (Figure 21–23).

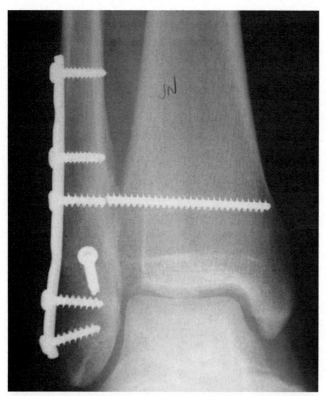

Figure 21–22: **Radiograph of a broken syndesmosis screw.**

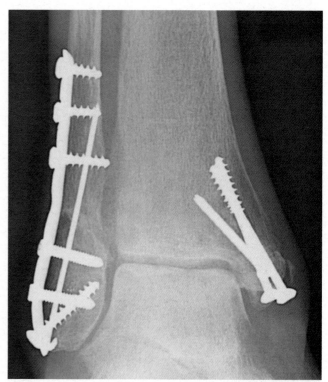

Figure 21–23: **Radiograph of a bimalleolar ankle fracture in an osteoporotic patient. The fibula has a Kirschner wire added for additional fixation.**

3. Use of locked small fragment plates (Figure 21–24).
4. Placing multiple long screws from the fibula into the tibia.
5. Insertion of long overdrilled lag screws for fixation of the medial malleolus (lag screw by technique) that capture the lateral tibial cortex.

- IM fixation of the distal fibula with Rush rods, K-wires, or other similar device may be a consideration for the management of distal fibular fractures in the elderly patient with osteoporosis, although the plate and screw construct should be used in most cases to prevent shortening and rotation.

Ankle Fractures in Diabetic Patients

- The long-term effects of diabetes including peripheral neuropathy, small vessel vascular disease, and skin changes are predictable.
- Ankle fractures in patients with diabetes mellitus are clearly associated with higher complication rates than in those who are unaffected by diabetes.[24]
- Increased rates of surgical infections and wound problems in diabetics are paralleled by increased rates of skin breakdown and other problems in those treated nonoperatively.[25]
- Surgically restoring stability to the unstable ankle in the diabetic with protective sensation, although not without

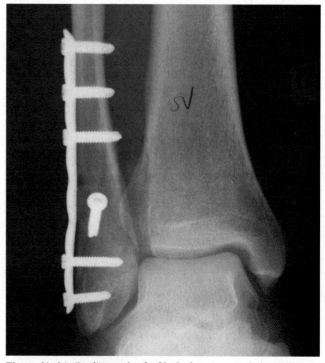

Figure 21–24: **Radiograph of a fibula fracture treated with a locked one-third tubular plate.**

risk, may afford the patient the best chance of a reasonable outcome and minimizes the overall complication rate.

- Careful attention to the soft tissues must be paid both in deciding the timing of surgery and in operative handling of the tissues.
- Initiation of weight bearing should be delayed until radiographic signs of healing are evident as many of these patients may be impaired in their ability to control protected ambulation due to their neuropathy.
- Jani and others[25] achieved relatively good results for severely neuropathic diabetic patients with ankle fractures using a protocol of transarticular pin fixation and an extended period of protected weight bearing.
- The ankle can also be further stabilized with an external fixator for a 3- to 6-week period to enhance the internal fixation stability and minimize the complications of casting in neuropathic patients.
- The unilateral fixator is a better alternative in unstable fractures than Steinmann pins placed across the ankle joint because it does not cause a large cartilage injury in the ankle and also decreases the risk of an intraarticular infection.

Postoperative Management

- Optimizing outcome of ankle fractures requires a balance between obtaining and maintaining a reduction and restoring motion and weight bearing so the patient can return to activities without pain.
- For each type of ankle fracture these guidelines must be modified based on many factors:
  1. The quality of bone and the stability of the fixation
  2. The reliability of the patient
  3. Comorbid conditions
  4. The protection of soft tissues, such as the deltoid ligament and syndesmosis.
  5. The integrity of the deltoid ligament
- Cimini and others[26] assessed early mobilization of ankle fractures after ORIF and showed no loss of fixation with early motion and that early motion results in the same functional outcomes as immobilization.
- In most cases, no difference exists between early weight bearing in a cast and nonweight bearing in a cast so long as adequate stability is attained by surgery.
- The majority of patients continue nonweight bearing or partial weight bearing on the affected limb but are able to safely bear weight by 6 to 8 weeks after surgery.
- However, the surgeon should tailor guidelines for the patients' return to weight bearing according to the stability of the reduction, the quality of the bone, the reliability of the patient, and the health of the patient.
- Weight bearing may be further delayed for elderly and diabetic patients and those with severe osteoporosis, wound problems, and ligament injury (syndesmosis and deltoid).

Complications
Wound Problems and Infection

- After the open treatment of ankle fractures, postoperative complications are similar to those associated with lower extremity articular fractures.
- The most feared complications of operative ankle fracture treatment include postoperative infection (1% to 2%) and wound problems (4% to 5%).
- Many of these may be preventable with a thoughtful, cautious approach to the soft tissues.
- Superficial cellulitis, indicated by periincisional redness and warmth, might be treated with antibiotics and brief observation, but certainly the presence of purulence or other signs of deep infection mandates a more aggressive approach. This aggressive approach typically includes incision, drainage, and intravenous (IV) antibiotic treatment.
- Marginal wound necrosis that results in small areas of dry eschar can usually be observed carefully but does not require immediate action; once the deep tissues granulate beneath the observed areas, these areas can be removed or may fall off spontaneously.
- Larger areas of eschar or frank wound necrosis should prompt a consultation with a plastic surgeon unless the orthopaedic surgeon has experience in complicated soft-tissue problems.
- There is little redundancy to the tissues about the ankle, thus fasciocutaneous or rotation flaps are effective only for small soft-tissue defects in this area.
- Free soft-tissues transfers may be necessary for larger soft-tissue voids.
- Methods to determine if an infection is deep include:
  1. labs (erythrocyte sedimentation rate [ESR], C-reactive protein (CRP), white blood cell count [WBC])
  2. joint or wound aspiration
  3. deep wound culture
  4. WBC labeled indium scan
  5. MRI
- Local wound care with the use of a whirlpool and the "Wound Vac" have been effective techniques for treating infected or complicated wounds.
- In most cases of early deep infection, the wounds can be thoroughly debrided and irrigated, and the implants left in place.
- The infection should be treated with intravenous and then oral antibiotics. Consideration may be given to removing the implants once the fracture has healed (Box 21–7).

Nonunion

- Nonunion of the ankle is not a common problem because most of the bone in the area is metaphyseal and likely to heal.
- Ankle fractures may be prone to nonunion in a few instances, such as cases of medial malleolus fractures and high-energy crush injuries of the lateral malleolus.

Box 21–7	**Reasons for Continued Pain after Open Reduction and Internal Fixation of an Ankle Fracture**

- Malunion of the fracture
- Symptomatic implants
- Osteochondral injury of the ankle
- Arthrofibrosis and Achilles contracture
- Traumatic ankle synovitis
- Neuroma at surgical site
- Subtle infection

- Medial malleolus fractures at the level of the joint may result in residual displacement or interposed soft tissues, which may play a role in healing problems.
- In the authors' experience, these fracture nonunions that occur at the joint level are more prone to be painful than tip avulsion fractures from the medial malleolus that fail to unite.
- Neuropathy is another cause of a nonunion, and an electromyography (EMG) or nerve conduction study should be considered in the workup of a nonunion.
- Infection should always be excluded in the case of a nonunion.
- Surgical treatment of a medial malleolar nonunion typically consists of takedown of the nonunion, reapproximation of the fragments, and fixation with screws or a tension band.
- Both alignment and fixation may be problematic as bony resorption may be significant, and the metaphyseal bone may be quite soft.
- Bone grafting may be necessary if tight interfragmentary compression cannot be achieved; local tibial metaphyseal bone may be used as well.
- Fibula nonunions usually occur in combination with malunions as a result of comminution, loss of length, and an associated syndesmosis injury.
- Treatment of these problems involves restoring fibular length and fixing the syndesmosis (Figure 21–25).
- Fibular length can be restored with a push-pull device to once again align the tip of the fibula with the lateral aspect of the talus.
- A bulk autograft or allograft may often need to be used to maintain the length.

Malunion

- Ankle malunion is now more frequently recognized since the work of Vrahas[27] has shown that malunion significantly alters joint contact stresses, which may lead to arthritis.
- Malunion may involve any portion of the ankle injury.
- Knowledge of the "normal" anatomy and preoperative planning allows the surgeon to minimize this risk.
- Comparison views taken both preoperatively and intraoperatively (usually the unprepped leg can be easily rotated through the draping to allow for C-arm radiography) may

be useful to demonstrate the desired anatomy of the surgical reconstruction.
- Malunion leading to subluxation or incongruity of the joint is likely the most important type because the risks for degeneration of the joint with loss of function can be expected.
- If malunion appears likely to cause these problems, consideration should be given to corrective osteotomy or other operative reconstruction (see Figure 21–25).
- Simply stated, the goal of surgical treatment is to restore normal anatomy and kinematics to the injured ankle.

Arthritis

- Ankle arthritis is usually the result of a malreduction, an osteochondral defect (OCD), or a diffuse cartilage injury at the time of the initial fracture.
- Great effort should be taken to avoid a malreduction, as previously discussed in this chapter.
- For patients who are still having unexpected pain 3 to 6 months after the initial treatment with unremarkable radiographs, an MRI or CT scan may be performed to inspect the joint for an OCD or signs of chondrolysis.
- A complete discussion on the treatment of ankle arthritis is beyond the scope of this chapter, but, options, from mild to severe cases, include:
  1. Activity modification.
  2. Nonsteroidal antiinflammatories.
  3. Corticosteroid injections.
  4. Ankle arthroscopy may be useful as a diagnostic tool and a therapeutic intervention.
  5. Ankle fusion.
  6. Total ankle replacement.
  7. Amputation.

Stiffness

- Stiffness is a commonly discussed complication of ankle fracture and its treatment.
- Joint mobilization and a course of physical therapy may improve motion after the fractures and soft-tissue injuries have healed.
- Stiffness may be caused by ankle synovitis and may be improved with a corticosteroid injection or ankle arthroscopy.
- Most patients will lose some plantarflexion and dorsiflexion relative to the uninvolved leg, but, typically, this does not limit activity.
- Manipulation under anesthesia and formal open releases (gastroc release, tendo-Achilles lengthening, posterior capsulotomy) can be done in recalcitrant cases.

Symptomatic Implants

- Lateral plates with angled distal screws and large medial screws are often symptomatic.

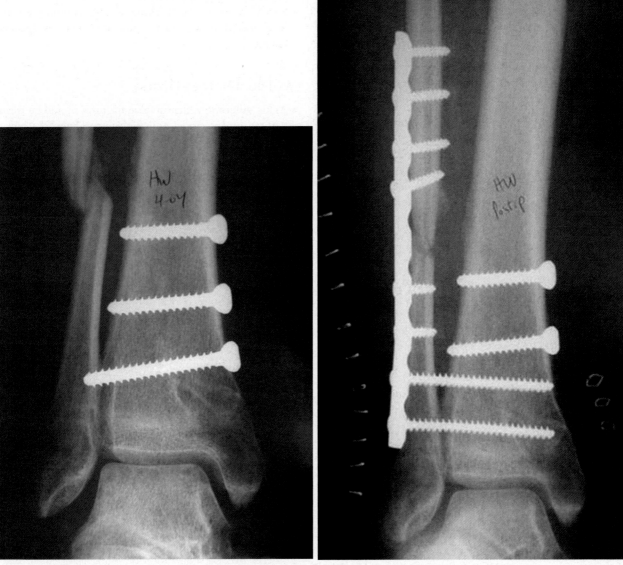

Figure 21–25: Radiographs of a fibula malunion or nonunion. Note the shortening of the fibula and the syndesmosis injury. The fracture was pulled out to length and fixed with a 3.5 dynamic compression plate, and the syndesmosis was secured with two screws.

- Placing the fibular plate posteriorly as an antiglide plate is a useful technique to minimize the risks of symptomatic hardware in patients with a thin soft-tissue envelope.
- Patients with ankle pain resulting from symptomatic implants can have these removed safely after 1 year, but there is no guarantee that their pain will be eliminated at the fracture site.

Neuropraxia or Neuroma

- Neuropraxia is the result of a stretch injury to a nerve at the time of the fracture.

- This most commonly occurs with the laterally based superficial peroneal nerve.
- In this case, sensation will almost always return to normal without intervention.
- In cases of slow improvement of neurologic function, EMG, or a nerve conduction study can be performed between 6 to 12 weeks to document the degree of injury and the likelihood of recovery of the involved nerve.
- A neuroma can develop in a nerve that is compressed or lacerated.

- Nerves that are at risk with open reduction of the ankle are the saphenous nerve medially and the superficial peroneal nerve laterally.
- Both of these nerves are sensory at this level of the ankle, and in cases of refractory pain, these injured nerves can be treated with resection and burying of the free nerve ends deep in muscle or fat.

Osteochondral Fracture

- It appears that chondral and osteochondral injuries occur more commonly with unstable ankle fractures than previously appreciated.
- Loren and Ferkel[28] performed ankle arthroscopy on 48 patients with unstable ankle fractures and found that 30 (63%) had traumatic articular surface lesions greater than 5 mm in the ankle, including 9 of 12 syndesmosis injuries.
- Ono and others[29] performed ankle arthroscopy on 105 patients treated operatively for ankle fractures and found significant cartilage injury in 21 patients (20%), including 8 that had free articular fragments.
- The radiographs should be closely inspected preoperatively and intraoperatively for evidence of a possible OCD.
- A portion of the articular cartilage can be seen during some approaches (e.g., medial malleolus), and if accessible, the joint should be visualized for evidence of an injury.
- Many OCDs are diagnosed during the postoperative period in patients with refractory pain.
- Osteochondral injuries may develop many months after an ankle fracture resulting from an initial injury to the cartilage at the time of the ankle fracture.
- Because these injuries are difficult to detect on plain radiographs, a CT scan should be performed in patients who continue to have persistent pain after having ORIF of their ankle with an apparent anatomic reduction.
- A stable, nondisplaced OCD may heal with a prolonged period of limited weight bearing in a boot that allows range of motion.
- An unstable OCD requires either excision (minimal or no bone on fragment) or ORIF with absorbable or headless screws.

Outcomes

- Most patients with ankle fractures that are operatively treated can expect a return of nearly full function, although as many as one quarter of patients may have a less than satisfactory outcome.[26]
- Recent studies have demonstrated that initial impairment after ankle fracture may show improvement over longer periods of time than previously recognized, even up to 2 years.[26]
- Short form health survey (SF-36) physical function scores remain below population norms even after 2 years.[30]

- Negative predictors for incomplete return to activity may include fracture type (syndesmosis injury, medial malleolus, and posterior malleolus).
- Social factors such as smoking, alcohol consumption, and level of education also affect outcomes after unstable ankle fracture.

Ankle Dislocations

- Ankle dislocations that involve fractures should be treated with an urgent closed reduction to minimize the tension on the soft-tissue envelope.
- Once reduced, the fractures can be treated on a nonurgent basis with formal ORIF.
- Dislocations that do not involve a fracture of the tibia or fibula are relatively uncommon and can usually be treated conservatively with closed reduction and casting.
- The ankle typically dislocates with the foot in plantarflexion resulting from the trapezoidal shape of the talus.
- In the case of a closed dislocation, the ankle should be urgently reduced with conscious sedation or general anesthesia.
- A postreduction CT scan should be considered to verify a congruent reduction and to evaluate for occult fractures.
- Once the ankle is reduced, it should be treated with 3 to 6 weeks of casting in a neutral position depending on the degree of instability on examination.
- Most authors do not recommend primary repair of the ligaments, and long-term follow up has not shown problems with instability.[31]

Annotated References

1. Ramsey PL, Hamilton W: Changes in tibiotalar area of contact caused by lateral talar shift, *J Bone Joint Surg Am* 58:356-357, 1976.
The classic article that used 23 cadaveric tibiotalar articulations to that showed that there is a 42% reduction in the contact area in the ankle with the initial 1 mm of lateral displacement.

2. Weber BG: *Die Verletzungun des oberen sprunggelenkes*, Berlin, 1977, Verlag Hans Huber.
This is the classic description of the Weber classification that divides ankle fractures into the A, B, and C groups based on the level of the fibula fracture relative to the ankle joint. The underlying concept for this system is that the lateral malleolus is the key to stability.

3. Lauge-Hansen N: Fractures of the ankle: analytic historic survey as basis of new experimental roentgenologic and clinical investigations, *Arch Surg* 56:259-317, 1948.
This article is the basis for the Lauge-Hansen ankle fracture classification system.

4. Boden S, Labropoulos PA, Lestini WF, et al: Mechanical considerations for syndesmosis screw, *J Bone Joint Surg Am* 71:1548-1555, 1989.

Classic cadaveric study that demonstrated the need for the placement of a syndesmosis screw in pronation-external rotation (P-ER) type fractures with a fibula fracture 4.5 cm above the mortise.

5. Ebraheim NA, Elgafy H, Padanilam T: Syndesmotic disruption in low fibular fractures associated with deltoid ligament injury, *Clin Orthop* 409:260-267, 2003.

The authors demonstrated that using the level of the fibular fracture as a guideline for application of the syndesmotic screw as suggested by some authors may not be accurate. There are several factors that should be considered including the depth of the incisura fibularis, posterior malleolus fractures, deltoid ligament injury, and subluxation of the fibula. They recommend that the syndesmosis be stressed and evaluated at the time of surgery rather than relying on the plain films alone.

6. McConnell T, Creevy W, Tornetta P: Stress examination of supination external rotation-type fibular fractures, *J Bone Joint Surg Am* 86:2171-2178, 2004.

The authors evaluated a group of 138 patients with supination-external rotation (S-ER) type ankle fractures. Of the 97 patients who presented with an isolated fibular fracture and an intact mortise, 61 had a stable S-ER2 injury and 36 had an unstable stress (+) S-ER4 injury. They showed that stress radiographs allow for the accurate diagnosis of deltoid incompetence in patients with Weber type-B SER fibular fractures and no other osseous injury; however, patients that had medial tenderness, ecchymosis, and swelling were not predictive of deltoid incompetence (instability).

7. Michelson JD, Varner KE, Checcone M: Diagnosing deltoid injury in ankle fractures: the gravity stress view, *Clin Orthop* 387:178-182, 2001.

A cadaveric study that showed that when the deep and superficial deltoid ligaments were cut and the fibular was osteotomized (fractured); the talus always (eight of eight specimens) showed a lateral shift of 2 mm or greater and a valgus tilt of 15 degrees or more. The gravity stress view of the ankle was found to reproducibly document destabilizing deltoid ligament damage.

8. Candal-Couto JJ, Burrow D, Bromage, S, et al: Instability of the tibio-fibular syndesmosis: have we been pulling in the wrong direction? *Injury* 35:814-818, 2004.

A cadaveric study in which the authors sectioned the syndesmotic and deltoid ligaments sequentially and showed that movements were consistently greater in the sagittal plane than in the coronal plane. They concluded that distal tibio-fibular instability should be assessed in the sagittal plane and not in the coronal plane as is done with a hook or Cotton test.

9. Yablon IG, Heller FG, Shouse L: The key role of the lateral malleolus in displaced fractures of the ankle, *J Bone Joint Surg Am* 59:169-173, 1977.

The authors treated 53 patients with bimalleolar fractures by fixing the lateral malleolus with a four-hole plate. There was an anatomic reduction of the talus and medial malleolus in each instance and there were no late cases of degenerative arthritis when these patients were followed for from 6 months to 9 years. They concluded that the lateral malleolus is the key to the anatomic reduction of bimalleolar fractures because the displacement of the talus faithfully followed that of the lateral malleolus.

10. Tornetta P: Competence of the deltoid ligament in bimalleolar ankle fractures after medial malleolar fixation, *J Bone Joint Surg Am* 82:843-848, 2002.

This was a clinical study that revealed that 26% of patients had radiographically evident incompetence of the deltoid ligament after medial malleolar fixation. They concluded that in patients with a bimalleolar fracture, the medial injury may be an osseous avulsion, leaving the deltoid intact on the displaced fragment, or it may be a combination of ligamentous and osseous injury with disruption of the deep portion of the deltoid ligament.

11. Michelson JD, Ahn UM, Helgamo SL: Motion of the ankle in a simulated supination-external rotation fracture model, *J Bone Joint Surg Am* 78:1024-1031, 1996.

This important cadaveric study showed that the primary restraint of the talus to external rotation is the deltoid ligament. Moreover, with an intact deltoid ligament, a complete fibular osteotomy still did not cause abnormal ankle motion. These results give justification for the nonoperative treatment of isolated lateral malleolus fractures and also show that the bimalleolar equivalent ankle fractures need to be immobilized longer to allow the deltoid to heal back to its anatomic length.

12. Hartford JM, Gorczyca JT, McNamara JL, et al: Tibiotalar contact area: contribution of posterior malleolus and deltoid ligament, *Clin Orthop* 320:182-187, 1995.

This was a cadaveric study where the authors created posterior malleolus fractures and measured contact area changes. Displaced posterior malleolus fractures produced a significant decrease in contact area with 33% or greater involvement of the joint and thus should be treated with open reduction and internal fixation. Disruption of the deltoid ligament does not appear to alter contact area further, supporting the concept of repair as optional.

13. Harper MC, Hardin G: Posterior malleolus fractures of the ankle associated with external rotation-abduction injuries, *J Bone Joint Surg Am* 70:1348-1356, 1988.

Study consisted of 38 patients with a posterior malleolus fracture that involved greater than 25% of the articular surface on a lateral X-ray-of which only 13 were fixed. They noted no cases of subluxation of the talus in either group and showed no clinical differences between the group that had open reduction and internal fixation and the group that had no attempt at reduction.

14. Wuest TK: Injuries to the distal lower extremity syndesmosis, *J Am Acad Orthop Surg* 5:172-181, 1997.

Review article on the diagnosis and treatment of syndesmosis injuries of the ankle.

15. Tornetta P, III, Spoo JE, Reynolds FA, et al: Overtightening of the ankle syndesmosis: is it really possible? *J Bone Joint Surg Am* 83:489-492, 2001.

Nineteen cadaveric specimens had syndesmotic compression with a 4.5-mm lag screw with the ankle in plantar flexion. There was no difference between the values for maximal dorsiflexion before and after syndesmotic compression. The authors concluded that maximal dorsiflexion of the ankle during syndesmotic fixation is not required to avoid loss of dorsiflexion and that more attention should be paid to an anatomic reduction of the syndesmosis.

16. Hoiness P, Stromsoe K: Tricortical versus quadricortical syndesmosis fixation in ankle fractures, *J Ortho Trauma* 18:331-337, 2004.

A prospective, randomized study comparing the treatment of syndesmosis injuries: One group had a quadricortical 4.5-mm screw, and the other group had two 3.5-mm screws placed in a tricortical manner. They showed that there was no significant differences between the two groups in functional score, pain, and dorsiflexion at 1 year, and thus concluded that syndesmosis fixation with two tricortical screws is safe and improves early function.

17. Thodarson DB, Samuelson M, Shepherd LE, et al: Bioabsorbable versus stainless steel screw fixation of the syndesmosis in pronation-lateral rotation ankle fractures: a prospective randomized trial, *Foot Ankle Int* 22:335-338, 2001.

A prospective randomized trial with 32 patients with an unstable pronation-external rotation (P-ER) ankle fracture randomized to either a 4.5-mm absorbable poly-L-lactic-acid (PLA) syndesmotic screw or a stainless steel 4.5-mm screw. There were no instances of loss of fixation, osteolysis, or differences between range of motion or complications between the two groups. They concluded that the absorbable screw is safe and effective for syndesmotic fixation.

18. Needleman RL, Skrade DA, Stiehl JB: Effect of syndesmotic screw on ankle motion, *Foot Ankle* 10:17-24, 1989.

A cadaveric study that used eight ankles to determine the loss of motion due to a single 4.5-mm syndesmotic screw. There was a significant loss of ankle external rotation but no less in ankle flexion. Based on their study, the authors recommend removal of the syndesmosis screw before full weight bearing.

19. Bray TJ, Endicott M, Capra SE: Treatment of open ankle fractures, *Clin Orthop* 199:28-37, 1989.

A retrospective review of 31 patients with an open ankle fracture. The authors showed that the patients with immediate open reduction internal fixation of open ankle fractures had a faster recovery with no greater incidence of infection or complications than the conservatively treated group.

20. Franklin JL, Johnson KD, Hansen ST: Immediate internal fixation of open ankle fractures, *J Bone Joint Surg Am* 66:1349-1356, 1984.

A retrospective review of 38 patients with an open ankle fracture that was treated with open reduction and internal fixation and a standard protocol. The protocol included: alignment and splinting of the fracture at the scene of injury if possible, antibiotics administered in the emergency department and continued for 48 hours, surgery as soon as possible, copious irrigation and thorough debridement of the wound, immediate rigid anatomic internal fixation, and delayed primary closure at 5 days. The authors showed good results that were similar to other patients with operatively treated closed ankle fractures.

21. Gustillo RB, Anderson JT: Prevention of infection in the treatment of one thousand and twenty-five open fractures of long bones, *J Bone Joint Surg Am* 60:453-458, 1976.

This is the classic article that establishes the early basis for the standard treatment of open long-bone fractures.

22. Ali MS, McLaren CAN, Rouholamin E, et al: Ankle fractures in the elderly: nonoperative or operative treatment, *J Orthop Trauma* 1:275-280, 1988.

This was a retrospective review of 100 cases of unstable ankle fractures in patients over the age of 60 years. Fifty patients had open reduction and internal fixation, and 50 patients had closed treatment. Worse results were noted in the group with nonoperative care, with a higher proportion of nonunions and malunions.

23. Bauer M, Jonsson K, Nilsson B: Thirty year follow up of ankle fractures, *Acta Orthop Scand* 56:103-106, 1985.

The authors reported on the natural history of the closed treatment of ankle fractures in 143 patients with up to 30-year follow-up. They reported minimal arthritis in most patients despite nonanatomic reductions of the fractures.

24. Blotter RH, Connolly E, Wasan A, et al: Acute complications in the operative treatment of isolated ankle fractures in patients with diabetes mellitus, *Foot Ankle Int* 20:687-694, 1999.

A retrospective review of patients with diabetes and an operatively treated ankle fracture. The relative risk for postoperative complications in the diabetic patients treated with surgical repair of their ankle fracture was 2.76 times greater than the control group's.

25. Jani MM, Ricci WM, Borrelli JJr, et al: A protocol for treatment of unstable ankle fractures using transarticular fixation in patients with diabetes mellitus and loss of protective sensibility, *Foot Ankle Int* 24:838-844, 2003.

Fifteen patients with unstable ankle fractures and diabetes-related neuropathy were treated with open reduction and internal fixation and then an additional large Steinmann pin fired retrograde from the heel to the tibia. There was a 25% complication rate and 13% amputation rate, which are lower than other related series. The authors recommend the use of this approach for this difficult patient group.

26. Cimini J, Schertz D, Limbaugh P: Early mobilization of ankle fractures after open reduction internal fixation, *Clin Orthop* 267:152-156, 1991.

This was a prospective study of 51 patients who underwent open reduction and internal fixation of their ankle and were then treated in a cast or AFO with unrestricted weight bearing. There was no loss of fixation in either group but the patients in the ankle foot orthosis (AFO) group had increased ankle dorsiflexion at the last visit. This study showed that operatively treated patients may be treated with early motion and weight bearing, provided there was stable fixation and normal sensation.

27. Vrahas M, Fu F, Veenis B: Intraarticular contact stresses with simulated ankle malunions, *J Orthop Trauma* 8:159-166, 1994.

Peak contact stresses were evaluated in a human cadaver ankle model of ankle fracture malunion. Their results led them to conclude that other factors besides peak contact stresses were at work in the causation of traumatic arthritis because the lab-created malunions did not significantly raise the peak contact stresses.

28. Loren GJ, Ferkel RD: Arthroscopic assessment of occult intraarticular injury in acute ankle fractures, *Arthroplasty* 18:412-421, 2002.

A prospective study involving 48 patients with unstable ankle fractures who had an ankle arthroscopy before open reduction and internal fixation of their ankle. Sixty-three percent of the patients had a traumatic articular surface lesion (TASL), with 15 of 19 talar lesions in the medial talar dome. The authors note the high incidence of otherwise unknown cartilage injuries associated with ankle fractures and recommend that the patients be scoped at the same time.

29. Ono A, Nishikawa S, Nagao A, et al: Arthroscopically assisted treatment of ankle fractures: arthroscopic findings and surgical outcomes, *Arthroscopy* 20:627-631, 2004.

The authors used a scope to evaluate the joint ankle joint in 105 patients undergoing open reduction and internal fixation (ORIF) of their ankle. They found 21 cartilage lesions and eight syndesmosis injuries. They recommend scoping ankle fractures at the time of ORIF so as not to miss these important injuries.

30. Ponzer S, Nasell H, Bergman B, et al: Functional outcome and quality of life in patients with type B ankle fractures: a two-year follow-up study, *J Orthop Trauma* 13:363-368, 1999.

Forty-one patients with ankle fractures were evaluated 2 years after their injury to assess their functional outcome and quality of life. Only 36% of patients reported a complete recovery from their fracture. The authors suggest that the SF-36 Health Survey may be useful in measuring outcome after an ankle fracture.

31. Rivera F, Bertone C, De Martino M, et al: Pure dislocation of the ankle: three case reports and literature review, *Clin Orthop* 382:179-184, 2001.

This is a case report and literature review of ankle dislocation without a fracture.

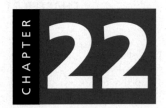

Fractures of the Talus

Eric M. Lindvall, DO

Anatomy

Bone

- Sixty percent cartilage (Figure 22–1)
- Dome, body, neck, and head
- Body with lateral process and posterior process
- Posterior process with medial and posterior tubercles
- Groove for flexor hallucis longus (FHL) between medial and posterior tubercles
- Lateral process articulations: superiorly with fibula, inferomedially is lateral one third of posterior facet articulation
- No muscle or tendon attachments
- Talar dome width: anterior is greater than posterior
- Density of head: lateral is greater than medial

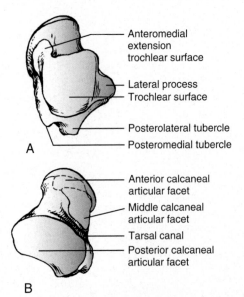

A

- Anteromedial extension trochlear surface
- Lateral process
- Trochlear surface
- Posterolateral tubercle
- Posteromedial tubercle

B

- Anterior calcaneal articular facet
- Middle calcaneal articular facet
- Tarsal canal
- Posterior calcaneal articular facet

Figure 22–1: Superior (*A*) and inferior (*B*) views of the talus (stippling indicates the posterior and lateral processes). (From Coughlin MJ, Mann RA: *Surgery of the foot and ankle,* 7th ed, W. B. Saunders, 1999.)

- Density of body: inferolateral is greater than inferomedial
- Neck angles 15 degrees to 20 degrees medially and is extraarticular

Ligaments

- Posterior talofibular: lateral tubercle of posterior process to fibula
- Posterior deltoid: medial tubercle of posterior process to medial malleolus
- Lateral talocalcaneal: lateral process to posterolateral calcaneus
- Joint capsule provides connection to adjacent structures

Anatomic Regions

- Sinus tarsi: lateral funnel-shaped area inferior to neck, superior to calcaneus, anterior to body, and posterior to head. Funnel narrows medially to connect to tarsal canal.
- Tarsal canal: medial tube-shaped area connecting laterally to sinus tarsi. It contains vascular anastomotic loop.

Blood Supply

- Artery to sinus tarsi: part of anastomotic loop created by perforating artery of peroneal artery and branch of doral pedis artery[1,2] (Figure 22–2).
- Artery of tarsal canal: a branch of posterior tibial artery; gives off deltoid branches to supply medial one third of body
- Artery of sinus tarsi and artery of tarsal canal join inferior to neck providing branches that enter neck and supply neck and head; branches also traverse posterolaterally into body
- Dorsal pedis gives dorsal branches to neck and head
- Peroneal artery gives branches to posterior process or body
- Multiple extracapsular and ligamentous vessels from surrounding joints (tibia, calcaneus, and navicular) add to vascular perfusion

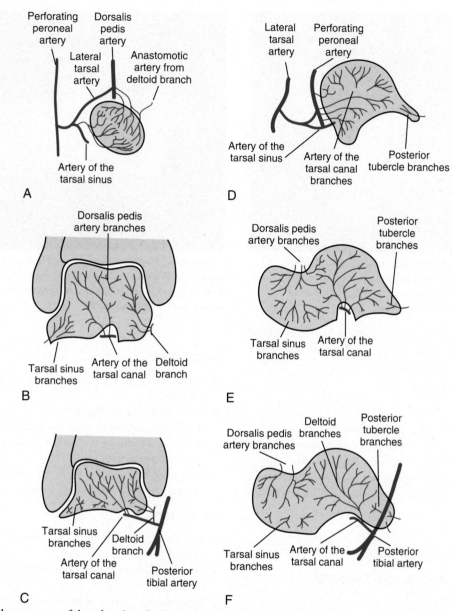

Figure 22–2: Vascular anatomy of the talus. **A** to **C**, Coronal sections. **D** to **F**, Sagittal sections. **A**, Head; **B**, middle third; **C**, posterior third; **D**, lateral third; **E**, middle talus; **F**, medial talus. (From Mulfinger GL, Trueta J: *J Bone Joint Surg Br* 52:160-167, 1970.)

Dislocations
General Information

- Almost half have associated shear fractures
- Pure dislocations better prognosis than those with shear fractures
- Pure dislocations often result of athletic injuries
- Talonavicular and talocalcaneal ligaments weaker than calcaneonavicular ligament allowing for subtalar dislocation
- Most pure dislocations can be reduced closed (>80%)

- Approximately 6 weeks nonweight bearing with immobilization

Subtalar Dislocation

- Also known as peritalar dislocation[3,4] (Figure 22–3).
- Dislocate talo-navicular (TN) and talo-calcaneal (TC) joints as talus remains in ankle mortise.
- Most common direction of foot and calcaneus is medial.
- Talar head commonly dorsolateral to navicular.
- Prognosis good to fair.

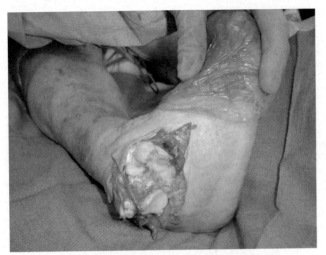

Figure 22–3: Clinical photograph demonstrating an open subtalar dislocation viewed from caudad to cephalad. Note the anterolateral open foot wound with the head of the talus extruded dorsolateral to the navicular.

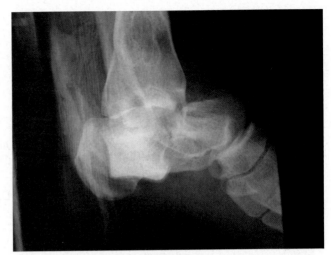

Figure 22–4: Radiograph depicting Hawkins type III fracture (comminution into neck and body) with talar body dislocated from both ankle and subtalar joints. Note talar dome rotated 180 degrees and facing inferiorly.

- Low-energy mechanisms (i.e., sports) reducible by closed methods, whereas high-energy mechanisms fair worse and may require open reduction.[4]

Pantalar Dislocation

- Dislocate TN, TC, and ankle joints
- Less common than peritalar dislocation
- Most are open injuries; controversial to routinely discard talus if extruded without soft-tissue attachments.[5]
- Prognosis worst than peritalar and significant increase in complication rate resulting from infection and avascular necrosis (AVN).

Talar Neck Fractures

Mechanism of Injury and General Information

- Axial load or forced dorsiflexion against resistance: anterior distal tibia impacts talar neck
- Fracture line extraarticular: dorsally between head and neck and plantarly between middle and posterior facets.[6]
- Twenty percent to 28% have associated fractures (malleolar, adjacent bones)
- "Hawkins sign" seen as subchondral lucency in talar dome at 6 to 8 weeks; absence of sign worrisome for AVN.[7]

Classification: Hawkins

- Type I: nondisplaced neck fracture
- Type II: displaced neck fracture with body subluxed or dislocated at subtalar joint
- Type III: displaced neck fracture with body subluxed or dislocated at both subtalar and ankle joints (Figure 22–4)
- Type IV (modified by Canale[8]): same as type III with TN joint dislocation

Diagnosis

- Ankle edema or ecchymosis often just inferior to medial malleolus
- Ankle and foot radiographs: lateral view shows neck in profile and associated joint incongruencies; anteroposterior (AP) and oblique views show ankle and talonavicular joint incongruencies
- Computed tomography (CT) necessary to evaluate subtalar joint; especially following reduction of a dislocation

Treatment

- Any displacement requires open reduction and internal fixation (ORIF).
- Anteromedial approach: from medial malleolus to navicular tuberosity
- Anterolateral approach: lateral to extensor tendons in line with fourth metatarsal; may need dual incisions to correct rotational deformity
- Obtain compression with lag screws if not comminuted; avoid overcompression of medial neck causing varus malreduction
- Must countersink screw heads if anterior to posterior
- Must avoid impingement with posterior to anterior fixation[9] (Figure 22–5)
- Two-incision technique often required when significant displacement or comminution present to avoid rotational malreduction
- Nonweight bearing 10 to 12 weeks

Complications

- Posttraumatic osteoarthritis most common complication and is seen in nearly all displaced fractures with long enough follow-up[10–14] (Figure 22–6)

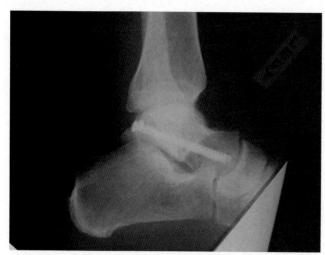

Figure 22–5: Posteriorly inserted screws for Hawkins type II fracture. Screw heads are close to inferior surface of talus because the arc of motion occurs superiorly thus avoiding ankle impingement.

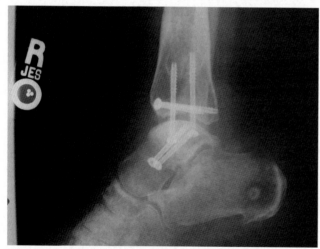

Figure 22–6: Healed fracture/dislocation of talus 9 months after injury in fully ambulatory patient. Although talar dome continues to show increased density and signs of avascular necrosis, no collapse of body has occurred.

- AVN second most common major complication; can be problematic to treat[15,16] (Figure 22–6)
- Pain expected in displaced fractures[12]

Talar Body Fractures

Mechanism of Injury and General Information

- Axial load or forced dorsiflexion against resistance: can shear or comminute body
- Fracture line is into articular surface: superiorly into ankle joint and inferiorly into posterior facet (subtalar joint)[6]

- Osteochondral fractures or lesions[17–19]
  - Acute fractures are result of inversion ankle injury or with axial loading
  - Chronic lesions are often asymptomatic.
  - Classification according to Berndt and Harty[17]
  - Treatment is based on stage of lesion; lower stage lesions should be observed, whereas higher stage lesions require operative intervention.

Classification

- Boyd and Knight[20]
  - Type I: coronal or sagittal shear fracture; subtypes a, nondisplaced; b, displaced only at trochlear articular surface; c, displaced at trochlear articular surface and subtalar dislocation; d, displaced body dislocated from ankle and subtalar joints (Figure 22–7).
  - Type II: horizontal fracture; subtypes a, nondisplaced; b, displaced
- Crush fracture: comminution and loss of body height

Diagnosis

- Ankle edema or ecchymosis distal to malleolli; skin often puckers when dislocated or subluxed.
- Ankle and foot radiographs: mortise and lateral ankle views most helpful
- CT necessary for preoperative planning

Treatment

- Treat like neck fractures; open reduction and internal fixation (ORIF) recommended if any displacement. It may also require medial malleolar osteotomy for adequate exposure.
- Crush fractures: must attempt to maintain body height; severe cases may require fusion.
- Extruded or free bone may be saved; it is the surgeon's preference.

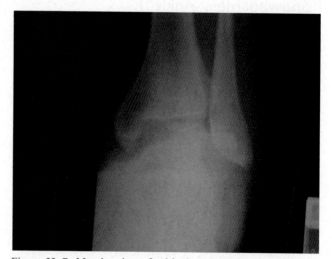

Figure 22–7: Mortise view of ankle demonstrating sagittal fracture/dislocation of talar body. Note bone void medially within mortise and double density seen along lateral talar body and distal fibula representing the extruded talar body fragment.

Complications

- Similar to neck fractures: posttraumatic osteoarthritis is a greater risk than AVN[11,12]
- Chronic pain expected in displaced fractures

Talar Head Fractures

Mechanism of Injury and General Information

- Impaction or crush type fractures result from axial load through metatarsal, navicular, and talus
- Shear fractures result from forefoot adduction and hindfoot inversion
- Isolated head fractures rare
- Often associated with surrounding joint fractures

Classification

- compression[5,21]
- shear[5,21]

Diagnosis

- Foot radiographs usually more helpful than ankle views
- Assess for juxtaarticular fractures

Treatment

- Nondisplaced: 6 weeks nonweight bearing; immobilization[5]
- Displaced: ORIF with small screws, bioabsorbable pins; must countersink screw heads[21]
- Small comminuted fragments can be excised[21]

Talar Process Fractures

Lateral Process Fractures ("Snowboarders' Ankle")

- Usually affects both talofibular and talocalcaneal articulations
- Can involve one third of posterior facet if entire lateral process is involved
- Confused with lateral ankle sprain; also caused by ankle inversion
- Often missed on plain radiographs; CT scan if suspicious
- Mechanism of injury: acute dorsiflexion with eversion and inversion of hindfoot
- Classification: Hawkins[22]
  - Type I: extends from talofibular joint surface down to talocalcaneal joint
  - Type II: comminuted fracture involving both the fibular and posterior calcaneal articular surfaces (the entire lateral process)
  - Type III: chip fracture of anterior inferior portion of posterior articular process of talus; does not extend to talofibular joint
- Nonunion common if fracture is not diagnosed.

- Treatment: size and displacement dictate treatment.
- Early diagnosis allows for potentially better outcome
  - Nondisplaced fractures: nonweight bearing 6 to 8 weeks, immobilization
  - Displaced fractures; larger fractures: ORIF; smaller fractures: excise later if symptomatic

Posterior Process Fractures

- Undersurface is all cartilage and makes up posterior 25% of posterior facet.
- Consists of medial and lateral tubercles; medial tubercle smaller.
- Usually involves pronation of foot in plantarflexion.
- Groove between tubercles houses FHL.
- Medial tubercle less common than lateral tubercle fractures.
- Difficult to recognize on plain radiographs; CT scan if suspicious.
- Lateral tubercle can be seen well on mortise and lateral views.
- Os trigonum is just posterior to lateral tubercle or can fuse to lateral tubercle; bilateral 60% of cases.
- Mechanism of injury is forced plantarflexion (soccer or ballet dancing) or excessive dorsflexion (avulsion) for lateral tubercle.
- Mechanism of injury is avulsion when forced ankle dorsiflexion with pronation for medial tubercle.
- Treatment
  - Lateral tubercle nonsurgical; excise if becomes chronically painful; nonweight bearing, immobilization 6 weeks.[23]
  - Medial tubercle nonsurgical unless large and displaced; excise if becomes chronically painful; nonweight bearing, immobilization 6 weeks.[24]

Annotated References

1. Mulfinger GL, Trueta J: The blood supply of the talus, *J Bone Joint Surg Br* 52:160–167, 1970.

2. Haliburton RA, Sullivan RC, Kelly PJ, et al: The extraosseous and intraosseous blood supply of the talus, *J Bone Joint Surg Am* 40:1115–1120, 1958.

3. Merchan EC: Subtalar dislocations: long-term follow-up of 39 cases, *Injury* 23:97–100, 1992.
Thirty-nine cases of subtalar dislocations (with associated fractures) were reviewed with average follow-up of over 5 years. Closed reduction was performed on most cases and open reduction was used only if unable to be reduced closed. Associated fractures were common and correlated with worse results. Good results correlated with accurate reduction and no associated fractures.

4. Bibbo C, Anderson RB, Davis WH: Injury characteristics and the clinical outcome of subtalar dislocations: a clinical and radiographic analysis of 25 cases, *Foot Ankle Int* 24:158–163, 2003.
Twenty-five cases with mean follow-up of 5 years; 89% of cases showed radiographic subtalar joint changes and 3 out of 4 of those cases also had fractures into the subtalar joint at time of

injury. All closed low energy dislocations were successfully reduced by closed methods. Associated fractures and open injuries carry a worst prognosis.

5. Coltart WD: "Aviator's astragalus", *J Bone Joint Surg Br* 34:546-566, 1952.
Review of 228 talus fractures from World War II. Seventy percent of the more severe injuries were result of flying accidents. Recommended early closed reduction to improve results and noted poor results with talar excision. It remains largest series of talus fractures.

6. Inokuchi S, Ogawa L, Usami N: Classification of fractures of the talus: clear differentiation between neck and body fractures, *Foot Ankle Int* 17:748-750, 1996.
Defined talar neck and body fractures by location of inferior fracture line. Neck fractures exited anterior to posterior facet and were extraarticular, whereas body fractures exited into posterior facet and were intraarticular.

7. Hawkins LG: Fractures of the neck of the talus, *J Bone Joint Surg Am* 52:991-1002, 1970.
Initial classification of neck fractures by Hawkins. Described "Hawkins sign" as subchondral lucency 4 to 6 weeks after injury as a sign of revascularization.

8. Canale ST, Kelly FB: Fractures of the neck of the talus: long term evaluation of seventy-one cases, *J Bone Joint Surg Am* 60:143-156, 1979.
Seventy-one talar neck fractures with average follow-up of greater than 12.5 years. Noted 50% avascular necrosis (AVN) rate in type II fractures and 84% AVN rate in type III fractures. However, only 10 out of 30 type II fractures underwent operative repair, and 11 out of 23 type III fractures had internal fixation.

9. Lemaire RG, Bustin W: Screw Fixation of fractures of the neck of the talus using a posterior approach, *J Trauma* 20:669-673, 1980.

10. Szyszkowitz R, Reschauer R, Seggl W: Eighty-five talus fractures treated by ORIF with five to eight years of follow-up study of 69 patients, *Clin Orthop* 199:97-107, 1985.
Eighty-five talus fractures were reviewed; 36 peripheral or nondisplaced and 49 displaced. Authors reported long-term results of 69 patients with follow-up of 5–8 years: 61% of patients acquired subtalar arthritis and 41% ankle arthritis.

11. Vallier HA, Nork SE, Benirschke SK, et al: Surgical treatment of talar body fractures, *J Bone Joint Surg* 85:1716-1724, 2003.
Twenty-six talar body fractures with at least 1-year follow-up. Authors found 38% incidence of avascular necrosis and 65% incidence of posttraumatic arthritis when all nondisplaced and displaced fractures were included. 100% union rate was achieved.

12. Lindvall E, Haidukewych G, Dipasquale T, et al: Open reduction and stable fixation of isolated, displaced talar neck and body fractures, *J Bone Joint Surg Am* 86:2229-2234, 2004.
Twenty-six displaced, isolated talar neck and body fractures to evaluate incidence of posttraumatic arthritis and avascular necrosis (AVN) without associated juxtaarticular fractures. Minimum follow-up of 4 years. Authors reported AVN rate of 50% and posttraumatic arthritis 100%. Union rate was 88%. No correlation was found between delay in fixation and incidence of AVN.

13. Frawley PA, Hart JA, Young DA: Treatment outcome of major fractures of the talus, *Foot Ankle Int* 16:339-345, 1995.
Sixteen of 28 talus fractures underwent open reduction internal fixation. Twelve cases had casting or closed reduction with casting. Posttraumatic arthritis was the most common complication. Avascular necrosis occurred only in type III and type IV injuries. Overall AVN rate was 4% whereas DJD was 62%.

14. Grob D, Simpson LA, Weber BG, et al: Operative treatment of displaced talus fractures, *Clin Orthop* 199:88-96, 1985.
Twenty-five patients with talar neck or body fractures with average follow-up of 9.8 years. Authors reported avascular necrosis rate of 16% and posttraumatic arthritis rate of 37%. Recommended early anatomic fixation of displaced fractures.

15. Penny JN, Davis LA: Fractures and fracture-dislocations of the neck of the talus, *J Trauma* 20:1029-1037, 1980.
Twenty-seven patients with talar neck fractures and average follow-up of 6.2 years. Reported overall 48% avascular necrosis (AVN) rate: 20% in type II injuries and 100% in type III injuries. Unclear as to exact number of cases that underwent open reduction versus open reduction with internal fixation. Concluded AVN to be the most formidable complication of a talar fracture.

16. Comfort TH, Behrens F, Gaither DW, et al: Long-term results of displaced talar neck fractures, *Clin Orthop* 199:81-87, 1985.
Twenty-eight displaced neck fractures resulted in avascular necrosis in 43%. Authors recommended early open reduction with internal fixation for displaced fractures even if closed reduction may appear accurate.

17. Berndt AL, Harty M: Transchondral fractures (osteochondritis dissecans) of the talus, *J Bone Joint Surg Am* 41:988-1020, 1959.

18. Canale ST, Belding RH: Osteochondral lesions of the talus, *J Bone Joint Surg Am* 62:97-102, 1980.

19. Anderson IF, Crichton KJ, Grattan-Smith T, et al: Osteochondral fractures of the dome of the talus, *J Bone Joint Surg Am* 71:1143-1152, 1989.

20. Boyd HB, Knight RA: Fractures of the astragalus, *South Med J* 35:160-167, 1942.
The classification system for talar body fractures that has been referenced comes from this article and is based on the fracture plane. The classification subtypes are related to the degree of displacement.

21. Pennal GF: Fractures of the talus, *Clin Orthop* 30:53-63, 1963.

22. Hawkins LG: Fractures of the lateral process of the talus, *J Bone Joint Surg Am* 47:1170-1175, 1965.

23. Paulos LE, Johnson CL, Noyes FR: Posterior compartment fractures of the ankle: a commonly missed athletic injury, *Am J Sports Med* 11:439-443, 1983.

24. Cedell CA: Rupture of the posterior talotibial ligament with the avulsion of a bone fragment from the talus, *Acta Orthop Scand* 45:454-461, 1974.
This fracture of the medial tubercle of the posterior process had been coined the "Cedell fracture" from this report. Closed treatment unless large fragment; if chronically painful then recommend excision.

Fractures of the Calcaneus

Michael P. Clare, MD

Introduction

- Calcaneal fractures were first described in 1843[1] and account for approximately 2% of all fractures.
- Sixty percent to 75% of all calcaneal fractures are displaced, intraarticular fractures.
- Historically, closed manipulation or nonoperative treatment of these fractures were advocated, often necessitating delayed reconstruction of the malunited fracture.
- Operative treatment was first advocated by Bohler in 1931,[1] and early open reduction and internal fixation (ORIF) techniques were first reported by Palmer[10] in 1948 and Essex-Lopresti in 1952.[2]
- Nonoperative treatment was still considered the treatment of choice well into the 1970s. Technologic advances in the ensuing 20 years led to renewed interest in surgical management.
- Despite ongoing controversy in the literature, ORIF has become the treatment of choice for the majority of displaced, intraarticular fractures of the calcaneus.

Anatomy and Biomechanics
Osteology and Anatomic Relationships

- The posterior third of the calcaneus consists of the calcaneal tuberosity, which provides the broad insertion of the strong gastrocnemius-soleus complex at the posterior-inferior margin.
- The middle third includes the articular surface of the posterior facet, which has a substantial anterior down slope in addition to a distinct plantar down slope medially.
  - On the lateral wall, the peroneal tubercle provides an anchor point for the inferior peroneal retinaculum, through which run the peroneus longus and brevis. The

origin of the calcaneofibular ligament lies directly posterior to the peroneal tubercle.
  - Medially, the sustentaculum angles anteriorly and plantarly and contains a groove along its inferior surface for the flexor hallucis longus tendon. The flexor digitorum longus tendon courses over the sustentaculum. The sustentaculum anchors the calcaneotibial portion of the superficial deltoid ligament, which provides stability to this fragment in a displaced intraarticular fracture, the medial talocalcaneal ligament, and other supporting ligaments.
  - Along the medial wall superficial to these supporting ligaments also run the posterior tibial artery and vein and the posterior tibial nerve.
- The anterior third consists of the middle and anterior facets and the saddle-shaped articulation with the cuboid.
  - The posterior facet is separated from the middle and anterior facets by the calcaneal sulcus, which runs obliquely and forms the floor of the tarsal canal and into which the talocalcaneal ligament inserts.
  - The tarsal canal expands anteriorly to form the sinus tarsi, which provides insertion for multiple supporting subtalar joint ligaments.
  - The adjacent crucial angle of Gissane is formed by the dense cortical bone underlying the posterior, middle, and anterior facets and supports the lateral process of the talus.
- The sural nerve is located midway between the peroneal tendons and Achilles tendon at the level of the ankle joint and course just posterior to the peroneal tendons over the lateral wall of the calcaneus. The nerve crosses the peroneal tendons superficially just distal to the inferior peroneal retinaculum.
- The soft tissues overlying the lateral portion of the calcaneus receive blood supply from a confluence of three arterial branches: the lateral calcaneal artery, the lateral malleolar artery, and the lateral tarsal artery. The lateral calcaneal artery arises most commonly as a branch of the

peroneal artery and supplies most of the full-thickness flap created with an extensile lateral approach.[3]

- The heel pad is composed of highly specialized, condensed adipose tissue contained by fibrous septa. These septa are oriented in a spiral pattern to resist torsional forces during gait and form chambers that are supported by transversely arranged elastic fibers. This unique arrangement is crucial to shock absorption with gait and may become compromised in the event of a calcaneal fracture, often leading to scar tissue formation and becoming a source of chronic pain.[4]

Radiographic Anatomy

- Two important angles are seen on the lateral view of the hindfoot: Böhler's angle and the crucial angle of Gissane.
  - Böhler's angle[1] is formed by a line drawn from the highest point of the posterior facet to the highest point of the anterior process and a line tangential to the superior edge of the tuberosity. The angle normally ranges between 20 degrees and 40 degrees; a decreased angle is indicative of collapse of the posterior facet, with shifting of the body weight anteriorly (Figure 23–1).
  - The crucial angle of Gissane[2] is found directly beneath the lateral process of the talus. The angle is formed by the dense cortical struts of bone beneath the lateral margin of the posterior facet and extending anterior to the beak of the calcaneus, respectively, which form an obtuse angle (see Figure 23–1).

Biomechanics of the Calcaneus

- The calcaneus plays an integral role in ankle and hindfoot function in providing a lever arm for the gastrocnemius-

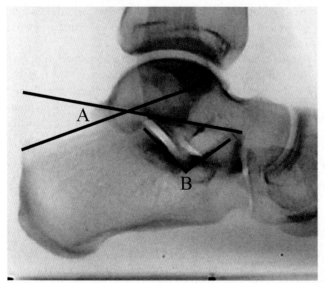

Figure 23–1: **Normal lateral radiograph of the foot demonstrating Böhler's angle** *(A)* **and the crucial angle of Gissane** *(B).*

soleus complex, supporting body weight, and maintaining length of the lateral column of the foot to protect the posterior-medial arch.

- The vertical plane orientation of the calcaneus determines the orientation of the talus, and thus indirectly affects ankle dorsiflexion.

Mechanism of Injury and Pathoanatomy
Intraarticular Fractures

- Displaced intraarticular calcaneal fractures are typically the result of high-energy trauma, such as a motor vehicle accident or a fall from a height. The pathoanatomy of the fracture (pattern of fracture lines, comminution, etc.) depends on the position of the foot at the time of impact, the force involved, and the quality of the patient's bone at impact.
- Essex-Lopresti[2] described two major fracture patterns: joint depression-type and tongue-type fractures. He postulated that at the time of impact, the subtalar joint was forced into eversion, causing the lateral process of the talus to impact the crucial angle of Gissane, thereby dividing the lateral wall and the body of the calcaneus and producing the primary fracture line. The remainder of the energy was dissipated medially toward the sustentaculum. With continued force, the fracture line exited either in the anterior process of the calcaneus or the calcaneocuboid joint, thus producing an anterolateral fragment. A secondary fracture line resulted from increased force: If the force extended posteriorly, the fracture line exited both into and posterior to the posterior facet, resulting in a joint depression-type fracture pattern; if the force extended inferiorly, the fracture line exited posterior to the posterior facet, resulting in a tongue-type fracture pattern (Figure 23–2).
- Carr,[5] in a cadaveric study of experimentally produced fractures, identified two primary fracture lines: one fracture line dividing the calcaneus into medial and lateral fragments, with the fracture line exiting in the anterior facet or the calcaneocuboid joint; and the second fracture line dividing the calcaneus into anterior and posterior fragments, starting laterally at the crucial angle of Gissane and extending medially toward the sustentaculum. Similarly, these primary fracture lines resulted in a variety of fracture patterns, including both joint depression-type and tongue-type fractures, in addition to anterolateral and superomedial fragments (see Figure 23–2; Box 23–1).

Dislocations of the Calcaneus

- Dislocations of the calcaneus typically occur as a high-energy, combination fracture-dislocation variant, with a significant intraarticular fracture component. The mechanism of injury, although poorly understood, is believed to

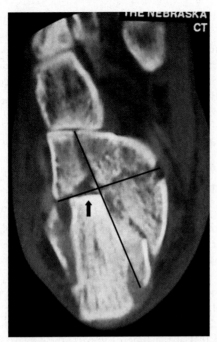

Figure 23–2: Axial computed tomography scan of a displaced intraarticular (tongue type) calcaneal fracture showing primary fracture lines *(bold lines)*. Note extension of the vertical line into the calcaneocuboid joint, forward displacement of the posterior facet *(arrow)*, and the adjacent lateral wall expansion.

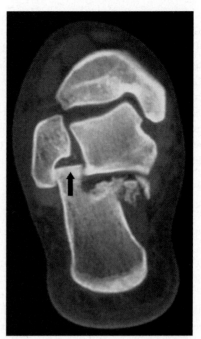

Figure 23–3: Semicoronal computed tomography scan of a fracture-dislocation of the calcaneus. Note the superolateral portion of the posterior facet *(arrow)* wedged within the talofibular joint, as well as the asymmetry of the talus within the ankle mortise, indicating disruption of the lateral ligaments of the ankle.

Box 23–1	**Common Sequelae of Displaced Intraarticular Calcaneal Fractures**

- Displacement of the posterior facet articular surface with variable impaction into the body of the calcaneus.
- Expansion of the lateral wall with relative widening of the calcaneal body.
- Loss of height through the posterior facet in the vertical plane.
- Shortening of the calcaneus in the axial plane, with varus angulation of the calcaneal tuberosity.
- Superior displacement of the anterior process (anterolateral fragment) with variable extension into the calcaneocuboid joint.

include axial load with forceful inversion of the hindfoot, which leads to disruption of the lateral ankle ligaments and causes the superolateral fragment of the posterior facet to be wedged within the talofibular joint as the limb recoils (Figure 23–3). The calcaneal body may also fully displace, whereby the medial wall of the calcaneal body may become locked against the lateral portion of the posterior facet, which can cause the flexor hallucis longus tendon or the medial neurovascular bundle to become entrapped within the fracture site, thus blocking fracture reduction.

Extraarticular Fractures

- Extraarticular fractures result from a variety of different injury mechanisms but are typically lower energy injuries than intraarticular fractures.

- Anterior process fractures occur from a forced inversion-plantarflexion injury, producing an avulsion injury from tension on the bifurcate ligament. The fracture line exits in the calcaneocuboid joint and usually involves only a minimal amount of articular surface (Figure 23–4).
- Anterior process fractures may also result from a forced abduction injury, producing an impaction fracture of the calcaneocuboid articular surface. In this case, the fracture fragment is typically larger with more articular surface involvement.
- Sustentaculum fractures occur from a combination of axial load and forced inversion, and are rare.
- Tuberosity fractures result from a forced dorsiflexion injury, whereby the strong pull of the gastrocnemius-soleus complex produces an avulsion fracture of variable size (Figure 23–5).

Clinical Evaluation

Intraarticular Fractures

Injury to the Soft-Tissue Envelope

- Fracture displacement and the extent of soft-tissue disruption are proportional to the amount of energy involved in the injury: lower energy injuries may result in only mild swelling and ecchymosis, whereas high-energy injuries typically result in severe disruption of the soft-tissue envelope, which may include an open fracture.

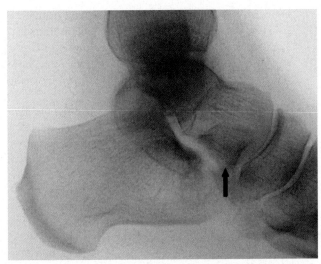

Figure 23–4: Lateral radiograph demonstrating a displaced fracture of the anterior process of the calcaneus *(arrow)*. Note the extent of involvement of the calcaneocuboid articulation.

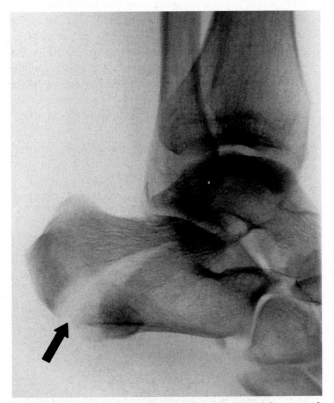

Figure 23–5: Lateral radiograph showing a displaced fracture of the calcaneal tuberosity *(arrow)*. Note the possible extension of the fracture into the posterior facet articular surface.

- Patients with open fractures may present with a small puncture wound, typically medially from a prominent spike of bone from the medial wall of the calcaneus or may present with a larger wound with significant soft-tissue disruption, which typically occurs laterally.

- Patients are usually unable to bear weight and experience severe pain at the fracture site resulting from fracture hematoma developing in the tight fascial compartments of the hindfoot. The ensuing soft-tissue swelling usually eliminates creases in the skin overlying the fracture.

- If soft-tissue swelling is severe, fracture blisters can develop. These result from cleavage at the dermal-epidermal junction. The fluid within the blister is considered a sterile transudate and may contain either clear fluid, indicative of the presence of epidermal cells within the dermis, or blood, in which case the dermis is devoid of epidermal cells.

- Severe soft-tissue swelling may also lead to the development of a compartment syndrome of the foot, which occurs as a result of severely increased pressure within a closed fascial space. When this increased pressure affects pulse pressure, arterial flow is affected, and the localized ischemia produces pain out of proportion to the injury. The surgeon may encounter difficulty in distinguishing the pain of a compartment syndrome from the pain of a calcaneus fracture.

  - There are four compartments in the foot: medial, lateral, central, and interosseous compartments. The central compartment consists of the superficial and deep, or calcaneal, compartments.

  - The calcaneal compartment contains the quadratus plantae muscle and the lateral plantar nerve and has direct communication with the deep posterior compartment of the leg.

  - An unrecognized compartment syndrome of the foot may result in clawtoe deformities, weakness, contractures, and sensory abnormalities.

Associated Injuries

- A high index of suspicion must be maintained for associated injuries, including lumbar spine fractures or other lower extremity fractures, which can occur in up to 50% of patients with calcaneus fractures.

- An estimated 10% of patients with calcaneus fractures will also have fractures of the lumbar spine, whereas 25% will have other fractures in the lower extremity.

- A thorough clinical evaluation is thus of paramount importance, with appropriate radiographic evaluation when necessary.

Extraarticular Fractures

- Patients with anterior process fractures usually present with pain, swelling, and ecchymosis in the anterolateral ankle and hindfoot area, which may mimic that of a simple ankle sprain. Direct palpation of the anterior process fragment will elicit tenderness. A high index of suspicion must be maintained for this particular fracture because there may not be an obvious foot deformity.

- Patients with sustentaculum fractures typically present with pain and swelling in the medial hindfoot, anterior and distal to the medial malleolus. Tenderness may be elicited with passive motion of the adjacent flexor hallucis longus tendon.
- Patients with calcaneal tuberosity fractures present with pain and swelling in the posterior hindfoot and may exhibit weakness with resisted ankle plantarflexion, as a result of the shortened gastrocnemius-soleus complex. Displacement of the fragment may lead to necrosis of the overlying skin because the surrounding soft-tissue envelope is indeed limited. Therefore assessment of the overlying soft tissue is of paramount importance, and expeditious care of the fracture may be required to avoid skin slough.

Diagnostic Tools
Plain Radiography

- Initial radiographic assessment of the patient with a suspected calcaneal fracture includes a lateral view of the ankle and hindfoot, an anterior-posterior view of the foot, and a Harris axial view of the calcaneus. Routine lumbar spine radiographs may also be indicated because of the association with lumbar spine fractures.
- The lateral view of the hindfoot usually confirms the presence of an intraarticular calcaneal fracture, whether the fracture is a joint depression type or tongue type, according to the Essex-Lopresti classification[2] and also reveals a loss of height in the posterior facet (Figure 23–6).
  - If the entire posterior facet is separated from the sustentaculum and depressed, a decreased Böhler's angle and an increased crucial angle of Gissane will result. If only a portion (typically lateral) of the posterior facet is

involved, the displaced articular surface will manifest as a double density, and Böhler's angle remains normal.
- The displaced articular fragment of the posterior facet is visualized within the body of the calcaneus, typically rotated up to 90 degrees forward relative to the remaining intact posterior facet.
- The lateral view of the hindfoot also identifies the presence of an extraarticular calcaneal fracture, including fractures of the anterior process and calcaneal tuberosity.
- The anterior-posterior view of the foot demonstrates extension of intraarticular fracture lines into the calcaneocuboid joint and isolated anterior process fractures.
- The Harris axial view of the calcaneus provides visualization of the articular surface and increased width, varus angulation, and loss of height of the tuberosity fragment. Isolated sustentaculum fractures are also seen in this view.
- Additionally, a Brodén's view may be used to further visualize the posterior facet articular surface. The view is obtained much like that of a mortise view of the ankle, with the leg internally rotated 30 degrees to 40 degrees. The X-ray beam is centered over the lateral ankle, and four total views are obtained with the X-ray tube angled at 10 degrees, 20 degrees, 30 degrees, and 40 degrees, respectively, toward the head of the patient. The 10-degree view shows the posterior-most portion, and the 40-degree view shows the anterior-most portion, of the posterior facet. These views may be reproduced intraoperatively to verify reduction of the posterior facet articular surface (Figure 23–7).
- If plain radiographs demonstrate intraarticular involvement of the fracture, computed tomography (CT) scanning is indicated. Additionally, CT scans are useful in delineating fracture patterns and extent of involvement in extraarticular fractures.

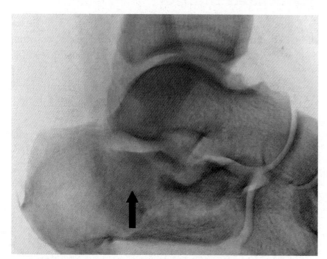

Figure 23–6: **Lateral radiograph of a displaced intraarticular (joint depression-type) calcaneal fracture. Note the impaction of the superior-lateral fragment (arrow), thereby disrupting the crucial angle of Gissane. Note also the loss of calcaneal height as indicated by the decreased Böhler's angle.**

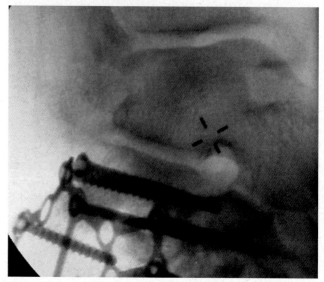

Figure 23–7: **Intraoperative Brodén's view of a displaced intraarticular calcaneal fracture confirming anatomic restoration of the posterior facet articular surface.**

Computed Tomography Scanning

- CT scanning is invaluable in further defining the pathoanatomy of the fracture, the number and location of the various specific fracture fragments, and in assisting with preoperative planning. Standard images for a calcaneal fracture include views in the axial (transverse), 30-degree semicoronal, and sagittal planes.
- The axial (transverse) views provide information as to primary fracture lines extending into the calcaneocuboid joint, anterior-inferior base of the posterior facet (crucial angle of Gissane), and sustentaculum and the extent of varus angulation of the tuberosity fragment (see Figure 23–2).
  - The axial views also define the extent of involvement of the calcaneocuboid joint in anterior process fractures and the fracture line in tuberosity fractures.
- The 30-degree semicoronal views reveal the extent of involvement of the posterior facet articular surface, impaction of the superior-lateral fragment of the posterior facet in the talofibular joint, such as in a fracture-dislocation variant pattern, expansion of the lateral wall, shortening and widening of the calcaneal body, varus angulation of the tuberosity, and the position of the peroneal and flexor hallucis longus tendons (Figure 23–8).
  - Particular attention is paid to the number, location, and displacement of the articular fracture fragments because these factors are of prognostic importance.
  - These views are also beneficial with sustentaculum fractures in defining the size and displacement of the fragment and in identifying any intraarticular extension of the fracture line.
- The sagittal reconstruction views identify the fracture as either a joint depression-type or tongue-type fracture and reveal the forward rotational displacement of the superior-lateral fragment of the posterior facet and displacement of the tuberosity fragment. Additionally, the extent of involvement of the anterior process region is further delineated, including superior displacement of the anterior-lateral fragment (Figure 23–9).

Fracture Classification

- Classification systems are used to facilitate communication among surgeons and to aid in decision making and management strategies. Thus, they are useful only if they are reproducible with adequate interobserver and intraobserver reliability.
- Essex-Lopresti[2] described two distinct fracture patterns based on plain radiography in 1952: tongue-type fractures and joint depression fractures. His work was an extension of a previous classification system described by Palmer in 1948; however, it provided limited prognostic information.

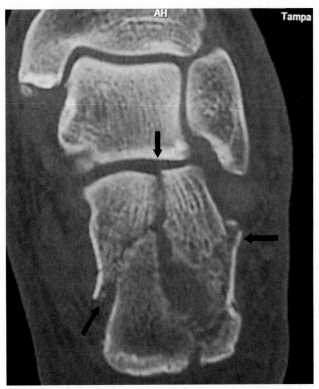

Figure 23–8: Semicoronal computed tomography scan of a displaced intraarticular calcaneal fracture. Note the displacement of the superior-lateral fragment of the posterior facet articular surface (*vertical arrow*), lateral wall expansion (*horizontal arrow*), and varus angulation of the tuberosity fragment with axial shortening (*oblique arrow*).

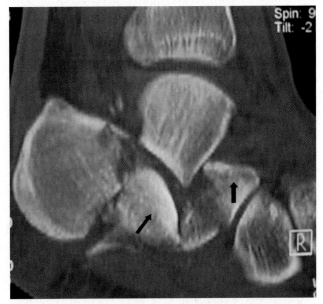

Figure 23–9: Sagittal reconstruction computed tomography scan of a displaced intraarticular (joint depression-type) calcaneal fracture. Note the marked impaction and forward displacement of the superior-lateral fragment (*oblique arrow*) and superior displacement of the anterior process fragment (anterior-lateral fragment, *vertical arrow*).

- Multiple classification schemes have been developed based on CT scanning.
  - That described by Zwipp and others[6] was the first to apply the CT scan findings into a rational understanding of fracture pathoanatomy.
  - The Crosby-Fitzgibbons[7] classification was the first to correlate fracture patterns on CT scan with clinical outcome.
  - The Sanders[8] classification is currently the most commonly used classification system based on CT evaluation. The system is based on the 30-degree semi-coronal section with the widest undersurface of the posterior facet of the talus, which is divided into three equal columns thereby producing three potential fracture fragments: lateral, central, and medial. These fragments, in addition to the sustentaculum, result in four potential articular fragments in the posterior facet of the calcaneus. The classification is thus based on the number and location of the articular fragments, and does have prognostic implications.

Management Options
Nonoperative Treatment

- Specific indications for nonoperative management include:
  - Nondisplaced extraarticular (Sanders type I) fractures.
  - Anterior process fractures with less than 25% involvement of the calcaneocuboid articulation.
  - Sustentaculum fractures with no intraarticular involvement or minimal displacement.
  - Fractures in patients with severe peripheral vascular disease, insulin dependent diabetes, or other medical comorbidities prohibiting surgery.
- Nonoperative treatment may also be necessary in certain situations in which the severity of the injury precludes early surgical intervention:
- Severe open fractures, particularly those in which the traumatic laceration is lateral (where an extensile lateral approach would normally be completed).
- Fractures associated with severe soft-tissue compromise, such as blistering and massive prolonged edema, which excessively delays surgery.
- Fractures in patients with life-threatening injuries.
- A standard protocol for nonoperative treatment includes:
  - Use of a bulky, supportive splint to allow resolution of the acute fracture hematoma in the initial 2 weeks following injury.
  - Conversion thereafter to a prefabricated fracture boot locked in neutral dorsiflexion-plantarflexion to counteract the pull of the Achilles tendon and an elastic compression stocking allow dissipation of residual limb edema. Early

subtalar and ankle joint range-of-motion exercises are also instituted at this time.
  - Nonweight-bearing restrictions are continued for approximately 10 to 12 weeks, until radiographic union is confirmed.
  - Nonoperative treatment of a displaced intraarticular fracture in an appropriate surgical candidate will result in a calcaneal malunion, in that the articular surface remains residually displaced, the heel remains shortened and widened, the residual loss of calcaneal height causes the talus to remain relatively dorsiflexed in the ankle mortise, and the persistent lateral wall expansion leads to impingement of the peroneal tendons.[9] These factors thereby provide the patient limited opportunity to return to normal function.

Operative Treatment

- Indications for operative management include:
  - Displaced intraarticular fractures involving the posterior facet (Box 23–2).
  - Anterior process fractures with greater than 25% involvement of the calcaneocuboid articulation.
  - Displaced sustentaculum fractures, particularly those with intraarticular extension.
  - Displaced tuberosity fractures.
- Ideally, surgery is performed within 3 weeks of the injury before early consolidation of the fracture. Beyond this time, the fracture fragments become increasingly difficult to separate in obtaining an adequate reduction, and the articular surface may delaminate away from the underlying subchondral bone.
- Surgery must, however, be delayed until the soft-tissue swelling in the foot and ankle has adequately resolved, as evidenced by a positive wrinkle test.
  - The wrinkle test is performed by gentle palpation of the skin overlying the lateral calcaneus as the foot is positioned in slight dorsiflexion and eversion. The presence of skin wrinkles indicates a positive test and that surgery may then be safely performed.

Box 23–2 | **Goals of Surgery with Displaced Intraarticular Calcaneal Fractures**

- Restore congruity of the posterior facet articular surface.
- Reestablish calcaneal height, thereby restoring the normal orientation of the talus.
- Recreate the normal narrow shape of the calcaneal body by addressing the lateral wall expansion, thus lessening the potential of peroneal tendon and subfibular impingement.
- Restore alignment of the anterior process to facilitate subtalar range of motion.

- Several different methods may be employed to reduce soft-tissue swelling in the fractured extremity, from simple elevation and immobilization in a bulky compressive splint to commercially available pneumatic compression foot pumps, cyclical cold therapy devices, or a venous compression stocking used in combination with a prefabricated fracture boot.

Open Reduction and Internal Fixation with Extensile Lateral Approach

- Several approaches have been previously described for surgical management of a displaced intraarticular calcaneal fracture, including various lateral approaches, medial approaches, and combined medial and lateral approaches. The extensile lateral approach is currently favored by most fracture surgeons, and is generally considered the gold standard.[10]

Positioning

- The patient is positioned in the lateral decubitus position on a beanbag, with the lower extremities in a scissor-like configuration, such that the operative limb angles toward the distal, posterior corner of the operating table, and the nonoperative limb lies away from the surgical field (Figure 23–10).
- An operating "platform" is created beneath the operative limb with foam padding and blankets, and the nonoperative limb is secured to the operating table.

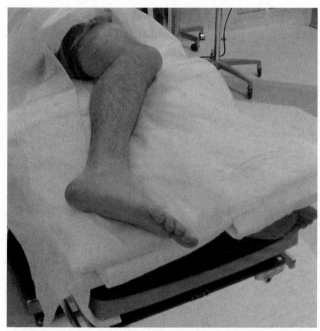

Figure 23–10: **Intraoperative photograph demonstrating the lateral decubitus position for an extensile lateral approach to the calcaneus. Note the scissor configuration of the limbs and multiple blankets forming the "operating platform."**

Incision and Approach

- An extensile lateral right-angled approach is used, with the vertical limb of the incision placed just anterior to the Achilles tendon to avoid injury to the sural nerve and the lateral calcaneal artery, a branch of the peroneal artery, which supplies the majority of the full-thickness flap. The horizontal limb of the incision is placed at the junction of lateral and plantar skin and is continued distally to the level of the calcaneocuboid joint while avoiding injury to the peroneal tendons.
- Using meticulous "no-touch" technique, a full-thickness, subperiosteal flap is elevated, including the calcaneofibular ligament and peroneal tendons. Dissection continues to the sinus tarsi and subtalar joint anteriorly and to the superior-most portion of the calcaneal tuberosity posteriorly to allow "window" visualization of the posterior facet and distally to the calcaneocuboid joint.
- Three 1.6-mm Kirschner wires (K-wires) are placed in the distal fibula, talar neck, and cuboid, respectively, for retraction of the full-thickness flap.

Essential Steps to Fracture Reduction

- Excision and preservation of lateral wall expansion fragments.
- Disimpaction of the superolateral fragment of the posterior facet from the calcaneal body. The fragment may be either rotated posteriorly or fully excised and preserved in saline on the back table.

Restoration of Calcaneal Height

- A periosteal elevator is used to disimpact the sustentaculum from the tuberosity and calcaneal body, and the tuberosity is subsequently repositioned beneath the sustentaculum.
- This maneuver includes a combination of longitudinal traction, medial translation, and valgus angulation and may be facilitated with use of a 4.5-mm Schanz pin.[11]
- Reduction of the anterolateral fragment and other anterior process fragments.
  - Dental picks are used to mobilize the fragments inferiorly, thereby restoring the distal portion of the crucial angle of Gissane. The fragments are provisionally held with 1.6-mm K-wires.

Reduction of the Superolateral Posterior Facet Fragment(s)

- Using "window visualization," the articular surface fragments are reduced anatomically and provisionally stabilized with multiple 1.6-mm K-wires.
- If the superolateral fragment includes two or more pieces, small bioresorbable pins may be used systematically reduce the articular surface from medial to lateral.[10]
- An accurate reduction allows restoration of articular surface congruity to the posterior facet and in combination with proper repositioning of the anterior process, complete

reestablishment of the crucial angle of Gissane, which is critical for subtalar joint motion.
  ● Intraoperative lateral, Brodén's, and axial fluoroscopic views are obtained to verify fracture reduction and alignment.

Fracture Stabilization

● Definitive fixation commences at the posterior facet where 3.5-mm cortical lag screws are placed just beneath the articular surface, aiming slightly plantarly and distally toward the sustentaculum to avoid violation of the articular surface.
● A low-profile neutralization plate is applied and initially secured distally at the anterior process. The tuberosity is then secured with several screws while simultaneously applying a lateral-to-medial force on the plate and a laterally directed valgus force on the medial undersurface of the tuberosity to avoid varus angulation and reshortening of the tuberosity.
● The final reduction is verified and fluoroscopic images are obtained.

Closure

● A deep drain is placed exiting above the proximal extent of vertical limb of the incision, and the full-thickness flap is closed in layered fashion.
● Deep absorbable sutures are passed, beginning at the proximal and distal ends of the incision and progressing toward the apex. The sutures are temporarily clamped until all sutures have been placed and are passed such that the full-thickness flap is progressively advanced toward the apex of the incision. The sutures are then hand-tied in similar fashion, working from opposite ends of the incision toward the apex.
● The skin layer is closed in similar fashion with 3–0 nylon suture using the modified Allgöwer-Donati[11] technique, followed by application of a bulky splint.

Postoperative Protocol

● The limb is immobilized for 2 to 3 weeks postoperatively, followed by conversion to a compression stocking and fracture boot locked in neutral position and initiation of early subtalar joint range-of-motion exercises. The sutures are typically maintained for 3 to 6 weeks until the incision is fully sealed and dry.
● The fracture boot is used throughout the day and night so as to neutralize the Achilles tendon and prevent contracture.
● Weightbearing is not permitted until 10 to 12 weeks postoperatively. The patient is then transitioned into regular shoe wear thereafter.
● Most patients are able to return to moderate activities by 4 to 5 months postoperatively.

Prognosis

● Although controversy continues to surround the management of these injuries, several studies have indicated that surgical treatment of displaced intraarticular calcaneal fractures, when properly executed, is superior to nonsurgical treatment.[8,12,13]
● An anatomic articular reduction is needed to obtain a good or excellent result but does not necessarily ensure a good or excellent result, likely as a result of articular cartilage injury at the moment of impact.[8]
● An anatomic reduction becomes increasingly difficult to achieve as the number of articular fragments increases. Thus the more comminuted the articular surface, the worse the prognosis. Indeed, those patients with Sanders type IV fractures have a poor prognosis with attempted ORIF.[8]
● There is a definite learning curve associated with surgical management of these injuries, and up to 50 cases may be necessary before consistent, reproducible results are obtained.[8]

Percutaneous Fixation Techniques

● Manipulative fracture reduction and percutaneous fixation, known as the Essex-Lopresti technique, is indicated for Sanders type 2-C fractures, particularly tongue-type fractures.[2,14]

Technique

● The patient is placed in either the lateral decubitus or prone position. With fluoroscopic assistance, two large terminally threaded guide pins are placed in parallel fashion into the tongue fragment from the superior edge of the tuberosity fragment parallel to the fracture line in the axial plane.
● The guide pins are levered plantarward while simultaneously plantarflexing the foot. As reduction of the tongue fragment is confirmed fluoroscopically and the foot is held in plantarflexion, the guide pins are advanced distally just beneath the crucial angle of Gissane into the plantar portion of the anterior process region.
● A Brodén's view is obtained to confirm reduction of the articular surface, and placement of the guide pins in confirmed with lateral, axial, and anteroposterior fluoroscopic views.
● Definitive fixation is obtained with two large cannulated screws (6.5, 7.3, or 8 mm); alternatively, multiple 3.5-mm cortical screws may be used (Figure 23–11). Additional screws may be placed transversely just beneath the posterior facet articular surface for supplemental fixation.
● If a satisfactory reduction cannot be obtained, the guide pins are removed and a formal ORIF through an extensile lateral approach is performed.

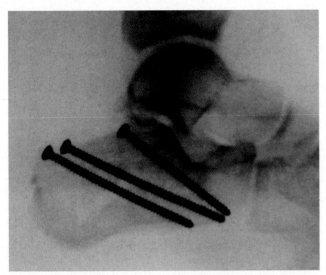

Figure 23–11: Intraoperative lateral radiograph demonstrating percutaneous fixation of a displaced tongue-type calcaneal fracture following reduction using the Essex-Lopresti technique.

- The identical postoperative protocol is used as described previously.
  - Several other percutaneous, minimally invasive, or arthroscopic-assisted techniques have been recently described and are best reserved for patients with specific fracture patterns and performed by experienced fracture surgeons.

Bilateral Fractures

- Bilateral calcaneal fractures may be surgically addressed with the patient placed either in the prone position, which eliminates the need for repositioning, or in the lateral position for each fracture. Each fracture is then managed using the techniques as described previously.
- Although there are few studies in the literature specifically assessing treatment of bilateral injuries, the general consensus is that patients with bilateral calcaneal fractures have a worse prognosis that those with unilateral injuries.

Open Reduction and Internal Fixation with Primary Subtalar Arthrodesis

- ORIF with primary subtalar arthrodesis is indicated for Sanders type IV highly comminuted intraarticular fractures, whereby the articular surface is unsalvageable.[8,15] By restoring calcaneal morphology and the so-called talocalcaneal relationship, both ankle range of motion and complex hindfoot motion in the transverse tarsal joints are optimized.[15]

Technique

- The identical technique as for a displaced intraarticular calcaneal fracture is used.
- Once the provisional reduction has been obtained as described previously, including restoration of calcaneal height and length, the posterior facet articular surface is then assessed.
- If the posterior facet is confirmed to be unsalvageable, the remaining articular surface is removed while preserving the underlying subchondral bone. The subchondral surface is drilled with a 2.5-mm drill bit for vascular ingrowth and supplemental allograft material is placed.
- A low-profile neutralization plate and associated screws are then placed as described previously. Fixation of the arthrodesis is completed with two 6.5- to 8-mm cannulated screws from posterior to anterior in diverging fashion into the talar dome and neck. The screws are placed perpendicular to the plane of the posterior facet, and care is taken to avoid violation of the talofibular joint. One or more of the 3.5-mm screws may need to be removed or redirected to facilitate placement of the larger screws.
- The patient is kept nonweightbearing in serial short leg casts for 12 weeks, until healing of the fracture and arthrodesis is confirmed radiographically.

Open Fractures

- Despite limited studies in the literature specifically addressing these fractures, the general consensus is that open calcaneal fractures are distinct injuries requiring different treatment and are associated with higher complication rates relative to closed injuries, including deep infection, osteomyelitis, and possible need for amputation.[16]
  - The wound complication rate with open fractures is up to three times higher than that associated with closed fractures.[17,18]
  - The severity of the soft-tissue injury appears to be the most important variable in predicting outcome because the incidence of major complications increases with increasing severity of the traumatic wound.[16]

Principles of Management

- Initial management of an open calcaneal fracture includes immediate intravenous (IV) antibiotics and tetanus prophylaxis, emergent aggressive surgical debridement of the wound, and temporary limb stabilization.
- Serial debridements are performed until the wound bed is clean, followed by definitive soft-tissue coverage where necessary.
- All open type I fractures and those open type II fractures with a medial wound can be treated by standard techniques once the soft-tissue swelling has adequately dissipated.[16]
- External fixation or limited percutaneous techniques are used for open type II fractures with a nonmedial (lateral,

posterior, or plantar) wound and for all open type III-A fractures.[16]

- Late reconstruction is performed for all open type III-B fractures or for those fractures resulting from penetrating trauma.[16]

Delayed Reconstruction of the Malunited Fracture

- Delayed reconstruction of the malunited fracture is necessary in certain clinical situations in which appropriate treatment of the acute fracture is not possible, including:
  - Patients with severe open fractures.
  - Patients with life-threatening injuries.
  - Patients with severe soft-tissue compromise, such as marked, prolonged edema or fracture blisters.
  - Patients for whom initial evaluation is delayed beyond 3 to 4 weeks from the date of injury or patients initially treated nonoperatively.
- In these instances, early consolidation of the fracture has occurred, and attempted manipulation of the articular fragments will typically result in delamination of the articular surface (Box 23–3).
- Historically, various techniques have been described in managing the malunited calcaneus. Currently, the preferred techniques focus on relieving subfibular impingement and peroneal tendon irritation and restoring calcaneal height and alignment, in combination with arthrodesis of the subtalar joint where necessary.
- A CT scan is obtained and the calcaneal malunion can be assessed according to the Stephens-Sanders classification[19]:
  - Type I: lateral wall exostosis with or without far lateral subtalar arthrosis.
  - Type II: lateral wall exostosis with subtalar arthrosis.
  - Type III: lateral wall exostosis with subtalar arthrosis and residual hindfoot malalignment (typically varus).

Technique

- The identical positioning and extensile lateral approach as for a displaced intraarticular calcaneal fracture is used.

Box 23–3   Pathoanatomy of the Malunited Calcaneus

- Residual incongruity of the posterior facet articular surface leading to posttraumatic subtalar arthritis.
- Persistent widening of the lateral calcaneal wall resulting in subfibular impingement and peroneal tendon irritation.
- Loss of calcaneal height resulting in relative dorsiflexion of the talus in the ankle mortise, causing anterior ankle impingement and loss of ankle dorsiflexion.
- Residual hindfoot malalignment (typically varus) leading to an altered gait pattern.

- A lateral wall exostectomy is performed for all three malunion types so as to provide decompression of the subfibular impingement.[9]
  - Starting posteriorly, the large saw blade is angled slightly medially relative to the longitudinal axis of the calcaneus, preserving more bone plantarly.
  - Care is taken to avoid violation of the talofibular joint.
  - The exostectomy is continued to the level of the calcaneocuboid joint and completed with an osteotome, thus removing the fragment en bloc.
- The peroneal tendon sheath in incised along the undersurface of the subperiosteal flap and a tenolysis is completed.[9]
- In those patients with a type II or III malunion, the articular surface of the subtalar joint is debrided and drilled as described previously. The previously excised lateral wall fragment is placed within the subtalar joint as an autograft bone block, with care taken to avoid varus malalignment of the hindfoot. The bone block restores calcaneal height and thus the more vertical orientation of the talus.[9]
- Definitive stabilization is achieved with two 6.5- to 8-mm cannulated screws placed from posterior to anterior in diverging fashion as described previously. A third screw may be added in the anterior process region extending into the talar neck while avoiding violation of the talonavicular joint (Figure 23–12).
- In patients with a type III malunion, correction of hindfoot malalignment within the calcaneal tuberosity is completed prior to implant placement. A Dwyer-type closing wedge osteotomy is used for varus malalignment, whereas

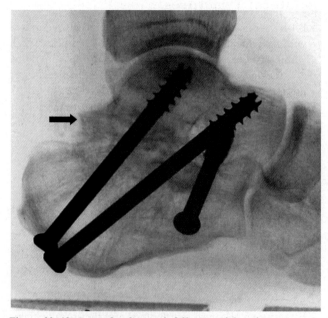

Figure 23–12: Lateral radiograph following delayed reconstruction of a Stephens-Sanders type II calcaneal malunion. Note the excised lateral wall fragment used as an autograft bone block (*arrow*) with restoration of calcaneal height.

a medial displacement osteotomy is used for valgus malalignment.

- Layered closure over a deep drain is completed as described previously. Weight-bearing and range-of-motion exercises are initiated in type I malunions once the incision has healed, whereas those with type II and III malunions are kept nonweight bearing for 12 weeks postoperatively, until radiographic union is confirmed.
  - Alternatively, a subtalar distraction bone block arthrodesis with iliac crest autograft[20] may be used; however, this technique offers limited access to the lateral wall exostosis and peroneal tendons. Additionally, overdistraction of the subtalar joint may result in varus malalignment as a result of tethering of the deltoid ligament medially.

Technique

- With the patient placed prone, a Gallie-type vertical incision is made just lateral to the Achilles tendon.[20]
- A lamina spreader is used to distract the subtalar joint, and the articular surface is prepared and drilled. Iliac crest tricortical autograft is harvested according to the amount of distraction obtained by the lamina spreader and wedged within the subtalar joint. Care is taken to avoid overdistraction of the subtalar joint, resulting in varus malalignment.
- Definitive fixation is obtained as described previously and the identical postoperative protocol as for a type II or III malunion is utilized.

Open Reduction and Internal Fixation of Anterior Process Fractures

- Surgical management of anterior process fractures is indicated for those fractures involving greater than 25% of the calcaneocuboid articulation on CT evaluation.

Technique

- The patient is placed supine, and a modified Ollier's approach is performed. The origin of the extensor digitorum brevis muscle is reflected distally in subperiosteal fashion.
- The calcaneocuboid joint is exposed, and the fracture is reduced and provisionally stabilized with 1.2- to 1.6-mm K-wires. The reduction is confirmed fluoroscopically on oblique and lateral views of the foot.
- Definitive fixation is obtained with small or minifragment screws.
- Excessively small, comminuted articular fragments may require primary excision; however, emphasis is placed on preserving as much articular surface as possible.
- Layered closure is performed over a drain, and a bulky splint is applied. The patient is converted to an elastic stocking and fracture boot at 2 weeks postoperatively, and early range-of-motion exercises are initiated. Weightbearing is not permitted for 10 to 12 weeks postoperatively.

Open Reduction and Internal Fixation of Sustentaculum Fractures

- Although most sustentaculum fractures can be treated nonoperatively, ORIF of fractures of the sustentaculum tali is indicated for larger fragments that are displaced greater than 2 mm or when the fragment extends into the posterior facet articular surface.

Technique

- With the patient supine, the fracture is exposed through an incision centered over the sustentaculum, which is found directly inferior to the medial malleolus.
- Dissection continues along the plantar margin of the posterior tibial tendon through the tendon sheath of the flexor digitorum longus tendon. The tendon is retracted and the floor of the tendon sheath is incised and elevated in subperiosteal fashion both dorsally and plantarly. Extreme care is taken to protect the adjacent neurovascular bundle.
- The fracture site is identified and provisional reduction is obtained with multiple 1.2- to 1.6-mm K-wires. The reduction is verified fluoroscopically, particularly through the lateral, Brodén's, and axial views. Definitive fixation is obtained with small or minifragment screws, depending on the size of the fragment.
- The floor of the tendon sheath is approximated with 2-0 permanent suture, and the tendon sheath is closed in similar fashion. A deep drain is placed and the tourniquet is deflated, evaluating for vascular compromise. Routine layered closure is performed and a bulky splint is applied.
- The patient is converted to an elastic stocking and fracture boot at 2 weeks postoperatively, and early range-of-motion exercises are initiated. Weightbearing is not permitted for 10 to 12 weeks postoperatively.

Open Reduction and Internal Fixation of Calcaneal Tuberosity Fractures

- ORIF of calcaneal tuberosity fractures is indicated for displaced fractures, resulting from the strong pull of the gastrocnemius-soleus mechanism, which typically makes maintenance of a closed reduction difficult.

Technique

- With the patient prone, a sterile bump is placed against the dorsal foot, which plantarflexes the ankle and relaxes the pull of the gastrocnemius-soleus mechanism.
- Because of the limited surrounding soft-tissue envelope, a percutaneous approach is preferred; meticulous handling of the soft tissues must be observed.

- With the ankle plantarflexed, the tuberosity fragment is reduced with large pelvic reduction forceps under fluoroscopy and held with multiple 1.6-mm K-wires. The reduction is verified using both lateral and axial views.
- A variety of options exist for definitive fracture fixation.
  - In younger patients with good bone quality, multiple small fragment screws may be placed in lag fashion perpendicular to the fracture line starting at the superior portion of the tuberosity angling just beneath the subchondral bone of the posterior facet, and exiting in the plantar cortex distally. Additional screws are then sequentially placed working distally toward the Achilles tendon insertion.
  - In an older patient with poor bone quality, two large 6.5- to 8-mm cannulated screws may be placed in similar fashion and supplemented with 16- or 18-gauge tension band wire through small stab incisions medially, laterally, and posteriorly. The wires are passed through the cannulated portion of the screws, as in fractures of the patella, and tensioned with the ankle in plantarflexion. Care is taken to pass the wire proximal to the Achilles tendon insertion posteriorly and deep to the plantar fascia plantarly.
- The stab incisions are closed, and bulky splint is applied with the ankle in plantarflexion, so as to relax the pull of the gastrocnemius-soleus mechanism.
- The patient is converted to an elastic stocking and fracture boot with a layered, tear away heel lift, and gentle early range-of-motion exercises are initiated at 2 weeks postoperatively. Weightbearing is not permitted for 10 to 12 weeks postoperatively, at which point the heel lift is gradually eliminated, and the patient is transitioned into regular shoe wear.

Complications
Wound Dehiscence

- The most common complication following operative treatment of a calcaneal fracture is wound dehiscence, which may occur in up to 25% of cases.[17,18,21]
- The incision will typically close relatively easily at the time of surgery; however, the wound later dehisces, most commonly at the apex of the incision.
- Risk factors for wound dehiscence and wound complications include smoking, diabetes, open fractures, high body mass index, and a single-layered incision.[17]

Management Technique

- All range-of-motion exercises are stopped so as to prevent further dehiscence.[10]
- The wound is managed with a combination of whirlpool treatments, damp-to-dry dressing changes or other granulation-promoting wound agents, and oral antibiotics.

- The majority of wounds will eventually heal, so long as the wound includes only partial thickness of the skin flap. Once the wound is sealed and dry, range-of-motion exercises are restarted.

Deep Infection and Calcaneal Osteomyelitis

- Deep infection or osteomyelitis will develop in approximately 1% to 4% of closed displaced intraarticular fractures and in up to 19% of open fractures.[8,15–18,21]
- Clinical evaluation includes a thorough assessment of the wound and surrounding soft tissues, and for systemic signs of infection (fevers, chills, malaise, etc.), and laboratory evaluation, including a complete blood cell count (CBC), erythrocyte sedimentation rate (ESR), and C-reactive protein (CRP).
- Radiographic evaluation includes repeat plain X-rays for assessment of fracture healing and the integrity of existing implants. CT scanning may also be beneficial if plain radiographs are inconclusive.

Management Technique

- Preoperative prophylactic antibiotics are held until deep cultures are obtained.
- The previous extensile lateral incision is used and full-thickness flap is developed.
- Deep cultures are obtained, and the wound is thoroughly debrided, removing all nonviable tissue. If fracture consolidation has been confirmed preoperatively, the indwelling implants may then be removed. The wound is irrigated with 6 to 9 L of sterile saline via pulsed lavage.
- If gross purulence is encountered, however, serial surgical debridements must be performed, typically at 48-hour intervals. In most cases, diffuse osteomyelitis is not encountered but rather superficial osteomyelitis as a result of direct extension from an adjacent source.
- In the event of diffuse osteomyelitis, all fixation implants are removed, and all necrotic and infected bone is aggressively and serially debrided until only healthy viable bone remains. Limb salvage may be attempted or amputation may be required, depending on the remaining calcaneal bone stock.
- Once the wound bed is deemed clean, wound closure is obtained through a free tissue transfer or other soft-tissue flap procedure. Alternatively, a negative-pressure device may be used (Vacuum-Assisted Closure, KCI, Inc., San Antonio, Tex.) for wound healing.
- Culture-specific IV antibiotics are typically used for 6 weeks, with continued monitoring of laboratory infection parameters.

Posttraumatic Subtalar Arthritis

- Posttraumatic subtalar arthritis requiring arthrodesis develops in approximately 3% of calcaneal fractures treated operatively and in up to 16% of fractures treated nonoperatively.[21]
- Arthritis may develop from an inadequate articular reduction, prominent hardware protruding into the joint, or from significant articular damage at the time of original injury, even if a truly anatomic reduction has been obtained.[4,8]
- Factors predictive of the need for a late subtalar arthrodesis include a work-related injury, Sanders type IV fractures, fractures with an initial Böhler's angle less than 0 degrees, and initial nonoperative treatment of a displaced intraarticular fracture.[22]
- Patients with posttraumatic subtalar arthritis will experience pain with weight bearing, particularly when ambulating on uneven surfaces. Tenderness is typically exhibited with palpation in the sinus tarsi. Weight-bearing radiographs will exhibit joint space narrowing, osteophyte formation, and even subchondral cyst formation. CT scanning may be beneficial to better assess the subtalar joint.
- The subtalar joint should, however, be verified as the true source of pain. This may be confirmed by either differential anesthetic injections or by a short period of immobilization in a fracture boot or cast.
- Nonoperative management includes: shoe modifications; a University of California Berkeley Laboratory (UCBL) orthosis, lace-up ankle brace or other insert; ambulatory aids, such as a cane or walker; and nonsteroidal antiinflammatory medication.
- If nonoperative measures fail, then removal of the indwelling hardware and an in-situ subtalar arthrodesis is indicated.[10]

Technique

- The patient is placed in the lateral decubitus position, and the previous extensile lateral approach is used, developing a full-thickness flap as previously described.
- The existing implants are removed, and the subtalar joint is debrided of residual articular cartilage with a periosteal elevator and pituitary rongeur, while preserving the subchondral bone. The subchondral bone is then perforated with a 2.5-mm drill bit, and supplemental bone graft material is placed within the joint.
- With the hindfoot held in neutral position, definitive fixation is obtained with two large (6.5- to 8-mm) cannulated screws placed from posterior to anterior in diverging fashion into the talar dome and neck. Care is taken to avoid violation of the talofibular joint.
- The incision is closed in layered fashion over a drain as previously described, and the patient is maintained in serial nonweight-bearing casts. Weightbearing is initiated at 10 to 12 weeks postoperatively, once radiographic union is confirmed.

Peroneal Tendinitis and Stenosis

- Peroneal tendon problems, such as tendonitis and stenosis, are most commonly the result of lateral subfibular impingement following nonoperative management. In this instance, the displaced, residually expanded lateral wall subluxes the peroneal tendons against the distal tip of the fibula. Management of these problems focuses on decompression of the subfibular area through excision of the prominent lateral wall as described previously in the calcaneal malunion section.
- In some cases, frank dislocation of the tendons may occur, requiring reconstruction of the superior peroneal retinaculum following subfibular decompression.
- Tendon adhesions, scarring, or tenosynovitis may also develop following operative treatment and is typically the result of either the extent of the surgical dissection itself or prominent hardware. Physical therapy modalities and tendon mobilization and strengthening exercises may provide relief. If these measures fail, a peroneal tenolysis or removal of symptomatic hardware may be necessary.

Ankle Pain

- Lateral ankle pain may result following a calcaneal fracture and is usually the result of residual stiffness in the subtalar joint.[9]
- In these cases, coronal plane inversion and eversion motion is borne by the ankle joint, resulting from the coupled nature of the ankle and subtalar joint complex. Because the ankle joint is not intended to bear these stresses, the patient will experience chronic, sprain-like pain in the lateral ankle.
- These symptoms will usually respond to nonoperative measures, including nonsteroidal antiinflammatory medication, temporary immobilization, and use of a lace-up ankle brace.

Heel Pad Pain and Exostoses

- Patients may develop chronic pain in the plantar heel pad following a calcaneal fracture, resulting from either disruption of the unique septa in the heel pad[4] or less commonly from a prominent exostosis.
- Nonoperative management includes a visco gel heel cushion or other similar pad; few other management options exist, however, in the absence of a bony exostosis.
- Painful plantar exostoses may be surgically removed through a lateral approach because a plantar incision should be avoided.

Conclusions

- Calcaneal fractures remain a therapeutic challenge for the orthopaedic surgeon.

- The calcaneus plays a critical role in ankle and hindfoot function and a normal gait pattern.
- Despite continued controversy, surgical management is the treatment of choice for the majority of displaced, intraarticular calcaneal fractures and certain extraarticular fractures.
- Some fractures, despite an anatomic reduction, may result in posttraumatic subtalar arthritis resulting from damage to the articular surface at the time of injury.
- Future developments in percutaneous and arthroscopic techniques may allow similar restoration of the articular surface and bony architecture of the calcaneus while limiting wound complications and deep infection.

Annotated References

1. Böhler L: Diagnosis, pathology and treatment of fractures of the os calcis, *J Bone Joint Surg* 13:75-89, 1931.

This classic paper demonstrates the pathoanatomy of the displaced intraarticular calcaneal fracture and the biomechanical implications of the untreated fracture on gait and foot function. The author also describes the tuber joint angle, now known as "Böhler's angle," and the closed traction and manipulation technique that also bears his name.

2. Essex-Lopresti P: The mechanism, reduction technique, and results in fractures of the os calcis, *Br J Surg* 39:395-419, 1952.

This classic paper discusses the mechanism of injury and radiographic features of the fractured calcaneus, and correlates the radiographic findings into the two major fracture types, tongue-type and joint depression-type. The author also describes management techniques using the Gissane spike, including: percutaneous manipulation for tongue-type fractures still used today and open reduction and percutaneous manipulation for joint depression-type fractures.

3. Borelli J Jr, Lashgari C: Vascularity of the lateral calcaneal flap: a cadaveric injection study, *J Orthop Trauma* 13:73-77, 1999.

This cadaveric study demonstrates the vascular supply to the full-thickness flap of an extensile lateral approach. The apex of the flap is supplied primarily by the lateral calcaneal artery, a branch of the peroneal artery. The lateral malleolar and lateral tarsal arteries also contribute.

4. Paley D, Hall H: Intra-articular fractures of the calcaneus: a critical analysis of results and prognostic factors, *J Bone Joint Surg Am* 75:342-354, 1993.

This study was a retrospective review of 52 displaced intraarticular fractures in 44 patients managed surgically through a medial approach. Those patients with tongue-type fractures had superior results relative to those with joint depression-type fractures; those patients with comminuted fractures had the poorest results. Prognostic variables associated with an unsatisfactory result included age greater than 50 years, increased residual heel width, residual loss of calcaneal height and lateral subfibular impingement, and residual subtalar joint incongruity. Those patients with an unsatisfactory outcome experienced pain most commonly in the plantar heel pad.

5. Carr JB, Hamilton JJ, Bear LS: Experimental intra-articular calcaneal fractures: anatomic basis for a new classification, *Foot Ankle* 10:81-87, 1989.

This was a cadaveric study involving experimentally produced calcaneal fractures. Two primary fracture lines were consistently observed, which were similar to those described by Essex-Lopresti, and resulted in a variety of fracture patterns. The authors also proposed a classification scheme based on a two-column theory for the calcaneus.

6. Zwipp H, Tscherne H, Thermann H, et al: Osteosynthesis of displaced intraarticular fractures of the calcaneus: results in 123 cases, *Clin Orthop* 290:76-86, 1993.

This was a retrospective review of 123 displaced intraarticular calcaneal fractures managed by a variety of surgical approaches based on the fracture pattern as determined on computed tomography scan. The authors also describe a detailed classification system, applying their scheme to the pathoanatomy of the fracture in determining the optimal surgical approach and internal fixation construct for each fracture type.

7. Crosby LA, Fitzgibbons TC: Computerized tomography scanning of acute intra-articular fractures of the calcaneus, *J Bone Joint Surg Am* 72:852-859, 1990.

This study was a retrospective review of 30 displaced intraarticular calcaneal fractures in 27 patients managed by a variety of methods, including simple immobilization, closed manipulation and casting, and closed manipulation and percutaneous pinning. They also devised a classification scheme based on computed tomography scan, which was used to determine prognosis of closed treatment: patients with nondisplaced fractures had better outcomes than those with displaced fractures, whereas those with comminuted fractures had the poorest outcome.

8. Sanders R, Fortin P, Dipasquale T, et al: Operative treatment in 120 displaced intraarticular calcaneal fractures: Results using a prognostic computed tomography scan classification, *Clin Orthop* 290:87-95, 1993.

This study was a retrospective review of 120 displaced intraarticular calcaneal fractures surgically managed through an extensile lateral approach with lag screw fixation for the articular fragments and a lateral neutralization plate. The authors also devised a classification system based on computed tomography (CT) scan which was prognostic of outcome, and remains the most commonly used classification system today. Patient outcomes were correlated with postoperative CT scans: clinical results were found to deteriorate as the number of articular fragments increased, indicating that an anatomic reduction was necessary for an excellent result. They also presented legitimate evidence of a true learning curve with these fractures.

9. Clare MP, Lee WE III, Sanders RW: Intermediate to long-term results of a treatment protocol for calcaneal fracture malunions, *J Bone Joint Surg Am* 87:963-973, 2005.

This was a retrospective review of 45 calcaneal fracture malunions in 42 patients managed according to a standard treatment protocol based on the Stephens-Sanders classification. The authors also include a detailed description of the pathoanatomy of the malunited calcaneus, the biomechanical rationale for their treatment protocol, and their surgical technique.

10. Sanders R: Current concepts review: displaced intra-articular fractures of the calcaneus, *J Bone Joint Surg Am* 82:225-250, 2000.

This is a comprehensive review of the clinical evaluation, pathoanatomy, and treatment rationale for displaced intraarticular calcaneal fractures; the author incorporates the historical evolution in the management of these fractures, from closed manipulation to modern internal fixation constructs. Thorough descriptions of surgical technique and treatment of complications are also included.

11. Sangeorzan BJ, Benirschke SK, Carr JB: Surgical management of fractures of the os calcis, *Instr Course Lect* 44:359-370, 1995.

This is another excellent review paper detailing fracture reduction and internal fixation techniques for displaced intraarticular calcaneal fractures. A highlight of the paper includes a description of reducing of the calcaneal tuberosity through the primary fracture line with use of a Schanz pin in restoring calcaneal length and height. The authors' postoperative protocol is also included.

12. Thordarson DB, Krieger LE: Operative vs. nonoperative treatment of intra-articular fractures of the calcaneus: a prospective randomized trial, *Foot Ankle Int* 17:2-9, 1996.

This study was the first randomized, prospective trial comparing operative treatment through an extensile lateral approach with nonoperative treatment of displaced intraarticular calcaneal fractures. Those patients managed surgically had significantly higher outcome scores and superior clinical and radiographic results.

13. Buckley R, Tough S, McCormack R, et al: Operative compared with non-operative treatment of displaced intraarticular calcaneal fractures, *J Bone Joint Surg Am* 84:1733-1744, 2002.

This study was a large multicenter, randomized, prospective trial comparing operative with nonoperative treatment of displaced intraarticular calcaneal fractures. Those patients treated operatively were managed with a variety of surgical approaches and fixation techniques. Although the overall functional results of the two groups were not significantly different, the authors reported certain factors to be associated with superior clinical outcome in patients undergoing operative treatment, including: an anatomic or near-anatomic articular reduction, younger patient age, and a moderately lower Böhler's angle (indicative of a less severe initial injury). Additionally, patients treated nonoperatively were 5.5 times more likely to require a subtalar arthrodesis for posttraumatic arthritis than those patients treated operatively.

14. Tornetta PI II: The Essex-Lopresti reduction for calcaneal fractures revisited, *J Orthop Trauma* 12:469-473, 1998.

This was a prospective study of 26 consecutive tongue-type calcaneal fractures managed by percutaneous reduction and fixation using the Essex-Lopresti technique. The reduction was satisfactory in all but three fractures using this technique. A detailed description of the reduction technique and fracture fixation is also included.

15. Clare MP, Sanders RW: Open reduction and internal fixation with primary subtalar arthrodesis for Sanders type IV calcaneal fractures, *Tech Foot Ankle Surg* 3:250-257, 2004.

This is a review paper of the surgical technique for managing highly comminuted intraarticular calcaneal fractures, emphasizing restoration of calcaneal morphology before arthrodesis fixation. A detailed explanation of patient positioning, surgical approach, fracture reduction and fixation techniques, and postoperative protocol is included.

16. Heier KA, Infante AF, Walling AK, et al: Open fractures of the calcaneus: Soft-tissue injury determines outcome, *J Bone Joint Surg Am* 85:2276-2282, 2003.

This was a retrospective review of 43 open calcaneal fractures in 42 patients managed by a standard protocol. There was a 37% infection rate and a 19% osteomyelitis rate overall; those patients with type III open wounds had a significantly higher infection and osteomyelitis rate. The authors developed a treatment algorithm based on wound location and severity, and concluded that severity of the soft-tissue injury was the most important factor in patient outcome.

17. Folk JW, Starr AJ, Early JS: Early wound complications of operative treatment of calcaneus fractures: analysis of 190 fractures, *J Orthop Trauma* 13:369-372, 1999.

This study was a retrospective review of wound complications following surgical management of 190 displaced intraarticular calcaneal fractures through an extensile lateral approach. Overall, 25% of patients in their series developed some type of wound problem following surgery. The authors identified certain risk factors associated with wound complications, including: diabetes mellitus, smoking, and open fractures. The presence of more than one risk factor further increased the relative risk.

18. Benirschke SK, Kramer PA: Wound healing complications in closed and open calcaneal fractures, *J Orthop Trauma* 18:1-6, 2004.

This was a retrospective review of wound complications following surgical treatment of 341 closed displaced intraarticular calcaneal fractures and 39 open calcaneal fractures, all managed through an extensile lateral approach. There was a 1.8% infection rate with closed fractures and a 7.7% infection rate in open fractures; a difference of over fourfold. The authors concluded that patient noncompliance was the most important factor in the development of wound complications following surgery.

19. Stephens HM, Sanders R: Calcaneal malunions: results of a prognostic computed tomography classification system, *Foot Ankle Int* 17:395-401, 1996.

This was a prospective study of 26 consecutive calcaneal fracture malunions managed according to a standard treatment protocol. The authors developed a classification scheme and treatment protocol based on computed tomography scan, and their classification was prognostic of patient outcome.

20. Carr JB, Hansen ST, Benirschke SK: Subtalar distraction bone block fusion for late complications of os calcis fractures, *Foot Ankle* 9:81-86, 1988.

This study was a retrospective review of 16 calcaneal fracture malunions treated according to a standard technique developed by the authors. They describe in detail the pathoanatomy of the malunited calcaneus and their surgical technique.

21. Howard JL, Buckley R, Tough S, et al: Complications following management of displaced intra-articular calcaneal fractures: a prospective randomized trial comparing open reduction internal fixation with non-operative management, *J Orthop Trauma* 17:241-249, 2003.

This study analyzed complications following both operative and nonoperative management of displaced intraarticular calcaneal fractures. Although the overall major complication rate was significantly higher for those undergoing operative treatment, the incidence of posttraumatic subtalar arthritis requiring arthrodesis was over fivefold higher among those patients undergoing nonoperative treatment.

22. Csizy M, Buckley R, Tough S, et al: Displaced intraarticular calcaneal fractures: variables predicting late subtalar fusion, *J Orthop Trauma* 17:106-112, 2003.

This study analyzed variables associated with the need for late subtalar arthrodesis following a displaced intraarticular calcaneal fracture; the authors identified several factors, including: the amount of initial injury (Böhler's angle < 0 degrees, Sanders type IV fractures), a work-related injury, and initial nonoperative treatment. The authors concluded initial operative treatment of a displaced fracture minimized the likelihood that a subtalar arthrodesis would be required.

CHAPTER 24

Midfoot and Forefoot Fractures

A. Samuel Flemister, Jr., MD

Introduction

- Midfoot and forefoot fractures involve the bones distal to the talus and calcaneus.
- Injuries to these structures occur through a variety of mechanisms (Box 24–1).
- As a result of the diverse nature of these fractures multiple treatment modalities are required.
- Although many of these injuries will heal adequately with little treatment, others require an absolute anatomic reduction to restore full function.
- If neglected, midfoot and forefoot injuries often lead to long-term functional disabilities.

Clinical and Radiographic Evaluation

- Patients with fractures of the midfoot and forefoot present with diffuse swelling and tenderness. In cases of high-energy trauma or crush injuries the associated soft-tissue damage may be severe. Compartment syndrome, although rare, should be considered. Surgery for any closed foot fracture should not be preformed until soft-tissue swelling has subsided and skin wrinkles have returned; usually 10 to 14 days post-injury.
- Anteroposterior (AP), lateral, and oblique radiographs of the foot should be obtained for all foot injuries. Computed tomography (CT) scans are often required to completely evaluate fracture patterns.

Box 24–1 Common Mechanisms for Midfoot and Forefoot Fractures

- Crush injuries
- Motor vehicle accidents
- Falls from height
- Athletic injuries

Navicular Fractures

- The navicular functions as the main support to the medial longitudinal arch of the foot. It has strong ligamentous attachments with the cuneiforms distally and the talus proximally. Medially it is further strengthened by the insertion of the posterior tibial tendon.
- There is minimal motion between the navicular and the cuneiforms as a result of their relatively flat articulations. However the proximal concave articulation with the talus accounts for about 80% of hindfoot motion.
- An accessory navicular bone located medial to the tuberosity is present in about 10% to 14% of normal feet.
- The blood supply to the navicular enters dorsal from the dorsalis pedis artery and plantar from the medial plantar artery. The central third is poorly vascularized leaving this area of the bone vulnerable to stress fractures, nonunions, and avascular necrosis (AVN).
- Navicular fractures are grouped into four major categories: dorsal lip avulsion, tuberosity, body, and stress.[1]
- Dorsal lip avulsion fractures are the most common navicular fractures and are the result of a forced plantar flexion injury (Figure 24–1). Most of these avulsion fractures are small, and the overall injury can be treated as a sprain with a 2- to 4-week course of protected weight bearing. Non-united fragments, which remain symptomatic, can be treated with excision.
- Tuberosity fractures are also avulsion-type fractures that occur with forced eversion of the foot against a contracting posterior tibial tendon. Resulting from the multiple attachments of the posterior tibial tendon significant displacement is uncommon.
- Fractures of anterior process of the calcaneus, mid tarsal subluxation, and cuboid fractures may occur with tuberosity fractures (Figure 24–2).
- Nondisplaced or minimally displaced tuberosity fractures are treated for 4 to 6 weeks in a short-leg weight-bearing

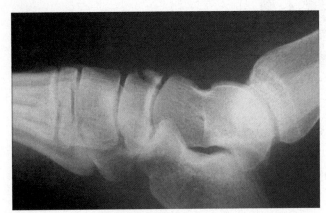

Figure 24–1: **Navicular dorsal lip avulsion fracture.**

cast. Small fragments (<1 cm), which are displaced greater than 5 mm can be excised, followed by reattachment of the posterior tibial tendon (see Figure 24–2). Larger fragments should be treated with open reduction and internal fixation (ORIF).

- Avulsion injuries of the accessory navicular are rare and occur through the synchondrosis. Treatment is similar to tuberosity avulsions, with smaller fragments being excised and larger fragment being fused to the navicular tuberosity.

- Navicular body fractures are uncommon and usually the result of crushing injuries or high-energy trauma with axial loading. They are classified into three types (Box 24–2). Nondisplaced fractures are treated with a short leg nonweight-bearing cast for 6 to 8 weeks. Fractures with greater than 2 mm of displacement should be treated with ORIF. In general, navicular body fractures are approached surgically through an anteromedial incision made just distal to the medial malleolus between the anterior and posterior tibialis tendons. The prognosis for each type of fractures is based on the likelihood of achieving an anatomic reduction with type 1 fractures having the best prognosis and type 3 fractures having the worst.

- Complications associated with the operative and nonoperative treatment of navicular body fractures include hindfoot stiffness, AVN, varus deformity, arthrosis, nonunion, and persistent pain.

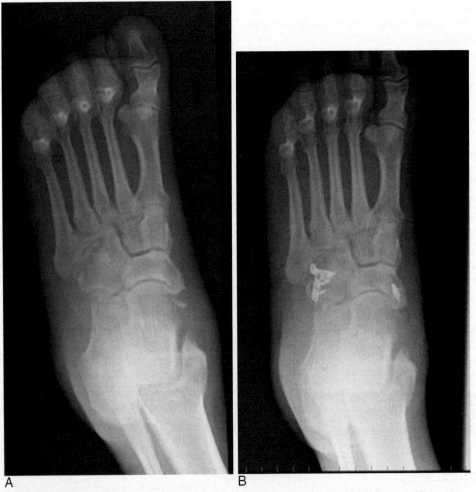

A   B

Figure 24–2: **A,** Preoperative radiograph of navicular tuberosity avulsion associated with cuboid fracture. **B,** Radiograph after excision of fragment and reattachment of posterior tibial tendon and open reduction and internal fixation of cuboid.

Box 24–2	Mechanism and Classification of Navicular Body Fractures

- Type 1: Caused by a force applied to the central axis of the foot. A transverse fracture is produced with dorsal and plantar fragments but minimal comminution (Figure 24–3)
- Type 2: The most common type. They are produced by axial compression exerted on the forefoot. The primary fracture line is directed from dorsolateral to plantar medial. The medial fragment is the largest and often displaced medially (Figure 24–4). The talonavicular joint is subluxed or dislocated and the foot appears adducted.
- Type 3: A comminuted and displaced fracture of the central body involving impaction of the lateral portion of the navicular. The forefoot appears abducted. Laterally directed forces applied to the forefoot cause these fractures.

- Navicular stress fractures usually occur in athletes, such as basketball players, sprinters, and gymnasts, involved in explosive push-off maneuvers. These fractures are rare and present with poorly localized midfoot pain and swelling. Plain radiographs are often negative, and a delay in diagnosis is common. Bone scans, CT scans, and magnetic resonance imaging (MRI) are all helpful in making an accurate diagnosis (Figure 24–5).
- Nondisplaced navicular stress fractures are treated in a short leg nonweight-bearing cast for 6 weeks. Return to activity should not be considered until there is a complete absence of tenderness.[2] Displaced fractures and nonunions should be evaluated with a CT scan to delineate the fracture pattern and then treated with ORIF.

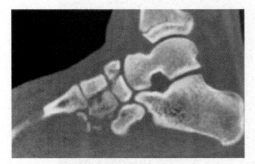

Figure 24–3: **Type 1 navicular body fracture.**

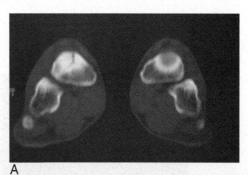

A

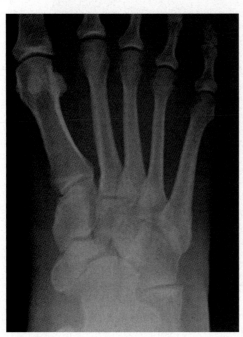

Figure 24–4: **Type 2 navicular body fracture.**

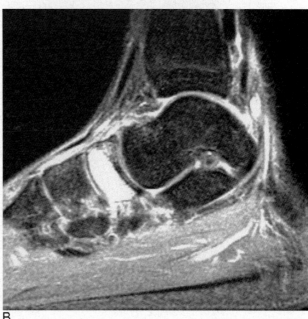

B

Figure 24–5: **A,** Computed tomography scan of navicular stress fracture. **B,** Navicular stress fracture seen on magnetic resonance imaging scan. Note marked edema within the navicular.

Cuneiform and Cuboid Fractures

- Isolated fractures of the cuneiforms are extremely rare. The majority of these injuries are associated with tarsometatarsal fracture-dislocations.[3]
- Isolated fractures of the cuboid are also uncommon with the majority of these fractures being small avulsions along the lateral aspect of the calcaneocuboid joint. These avulsion fractures are treated in weight-bearing cast or fracture boot until they become asymptomatic, usually in 4 to 6 weeks.
- The most significant cuboid fracture is a compression or "nutcracker fracture" that occurs as a result of an abduction force applied to the forefoot. This injury is another variant of tarsometatarsal fracture-dislocations and occurs as the cuboid is impacted between the lateral metatarsals and the calcaneus. If neglected, these fractures result in shortening of the lateral column with subsequent abduction deformity and arthrosis of the metatarsal-cuboid and calcaneocuboid articulations. Therefore these fractures require operative treatment to restore cuboid length with bone grafting, internal or external fixation[4] (Figure 24–6).

Tarsometatarsal Fracture-Dislocations

- Fracture-dislocations of the tarsometatarsal joints are commonly referred to as Lisfranc fractures. These injuries may involve the intertarsal articulations and tarsometatarsal articulations. To adequately treat these injuries one must have a through understanding of the complex anatomy of these joints (Box 24–3).

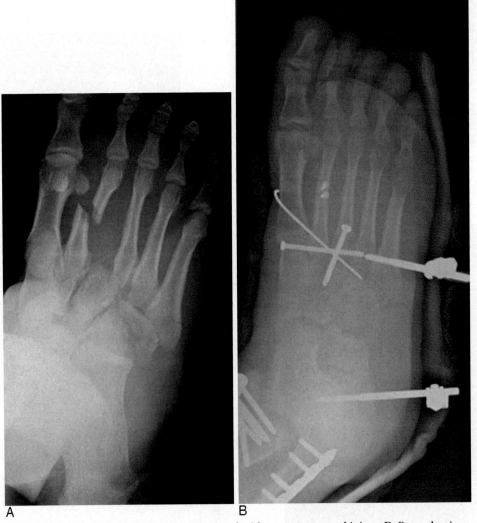

A   B

Figure 24–6: **A,** Radiograph showing cuboid crush injury associated with a tarsometatarsal injury. **B,** Postreduction radiograph following bone grafting and external fixation of the cuboid and open reduction and internal fixation of this Lisfranc variant.

- Lisfranc injuries may result from high-energy or low-energy trauma.[5] These injuries occur by both direct and indirect forces. Indirect injuries are much more common than direct (crushing) injuries. The majority of indirect mechanisms involve forces applied to a plantarflexed foot. In low-energy trauma, such as athletic injuries, an axial load is applied to the heel with the ankle plantarflexed. This load forces the metatarsals into further plantarflexion resulting in disruption of the relatively weak dorsal tarsometatarsal ligaments. In higher energy trauma, most commonly motor vehicle accidents, a plantarflexed foot is loaded against the floorboard of the vehicle resulting in disruption of the dorsal ligaments.

- Lisfranc injuries can also be caused by abduction forces applied to the forefoot with the hindfoot in a fixed position. This type of indirect mechanism results in lateral displacement of the metatarsals often with a fracture of the base of the second metatarsal as it is forced out of its recessed position.

- Lisfranc injuries are classified by the direction the metatarsals displace relative to each other and by the degree of joint incongruity (Box 24–4).

- Clinically, patients with Lisfranc injuries present with various degrees of midfoot pain, swelling, and inability to ambulate. In patients with multiple trauma, these injuries are often missed or neglected. In lower energy trauma, spontaneous reduction of the dislocation may occur and initial radiographs may appear normal. Therefore a high

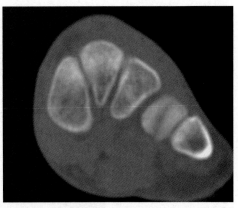

Figure 24–7: Computed tomography scan thru base of the metatarsals demonstrates wedge shape of second and third metatarsal bases and arch configuration.

Box 24–4 | Classification of Lisfranc Injuries

- Type A: All five metatarsals are involved (total incongruity) and displaced in the same direction (homolateral): usually dorsolateral (Figure 24–8a)
- Type B: One or more but less than five metatarsals are displaced (partial incongruity) and in the same direction (homolateral; Figure 24–8b)
- Type C: Medial and lateral metatarsals are displaced in opposite directions (divergent) and may be total or partial congruity (Figure 24–8c)

---

index of suspicion for these injuries is required in all patients with midfoot pain and swelling.

- Radiographic evaluation of tarsometatarsal injuries starts with AP, oblique, and lateral views of the foot. On the AP view the first metatarsal cuneiform joint should be congruent and the medial border of the second metatarsal should form a continuous line with the medial border of the middle cuneiform (Figure 24–9). On the oblique view the medial aspect of the fourth metatarsal forms a continuous line with the medial border of the cuboid (see Figure 24–9). On the lateral radiographs there should be no dorsal or plantar displacement of the metatarsals relative to tarsal bones (Figure 24–10). Any abnormality of these relationships is indicative of a midfoot injury. Other radiographic findings suggestive of Lisfranc injuries include a small avulsion fracture (fleck sign) between the bases of the first and second metatarsals (Figure 24–11) and any fracture of the second metatarsal base, cuneiforms, or cuboid.

- Suspected Lisfranc injuries with normal radiographs should be further evaluated with comparison standing AP and lateral radiographs of both feet. If the patient is unable to stand, stress radiographs in adduction and abduction are performed under ankle block or general anesthetic. CT scans are helpful in defining the extent of the

---

Box 24–3 | Anatomy of the Tarsometatarsal (Lisfranc) Joints

- The midfoot is divided into three columns. The medial column consists of the first metatarsal, medial cuneiform, and the medial navicular facet. The middle column consists of the second and third metatarsals, middle cuneiform, and their navicular facets. The lateral column is made up of the fourth and fifth metatarsals and their articulations with the cuboid.
- The tarsometatarsal articulations form an arch in the coronal plane.
- The second and third metatarsals are wedge shaped. This wedge-shaped anatomy adds greater stability to the tarsometatarsal arch (Figure 24–7).
- The second metatarsal is the longest and is recessed between the medial and lateral cuneiforms. This recessed articulation is the keystone to the tarsometatarsal joints accounting for the majority of their stability.
- Ligamentous attachments exist between each metatarsal and its corresponding tarsal bone. The intermetatarsal ligaments connect the second thru fifth metatarsals. The first metatarsal is not connected to the second. The second metatarsal is attached to the medial cuneiform by the oblique Lisfranc ligaments.
- In general, the plantar ligaments are significantly stronger than the dorsal ligaments.

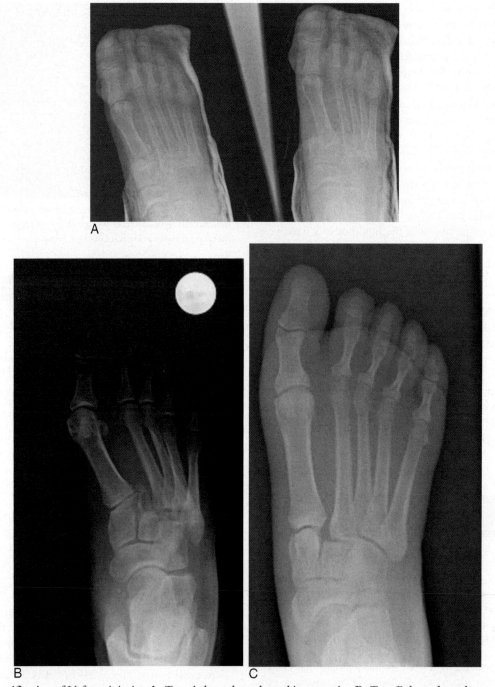

Figure 24–8: Classification of Lisfranc injuries. **A,** Type A, homolateral, total incongruity. **B,** Type B, homolateral partial incongruity. **C,** Type C, divergent with partial incongruity.

injury and in preoperative planning but are rarely helpful in making the diagnosis of the Lisfranc injury.

- Anatomic alignment following any Lisfranc injury is essential for a good outcome. Purely ligamentous injuries that demonstrate no instability on standing radiographs or stress radiographs can be treated as a midfoot sprain. These sprains require 2 to 4 weeks of immobilization in a short-leg nonweight-bearing cast, followed by protected weight bearing in a fracture boot for another 2 to 4

weeks. Patients often continue to have some degree of midfoot pain and swelling for up to 6 months. Nondisplaced purely bony Lisfranc fractures are rare and may be treated in a short-leg nonweight-bearing cast for 6 weeks.

- Closed reduction followed by casting has led to overall poor outcomes following displaced Lisfranc fracture-dislocations. Therefore operative treatment should be considered for Lisfranc injuries that demonstrate any degree of displacement or instability.

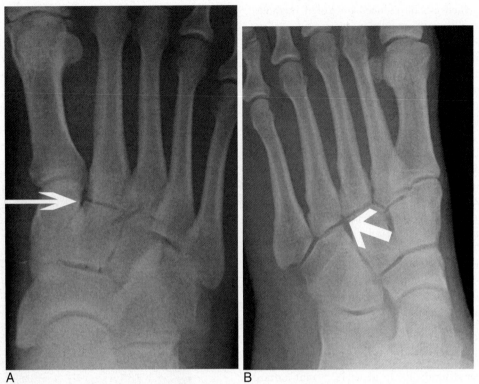

Figure 24–9: **A,** The arrow points out the congruent nature of the second metatarsocuneiform joint seen on anteroposterior view in a normal foot. **B,** The arrow points out the congruent nature of the fourth metatarsal cuboid joint seen on an oblique view in a normal foot.

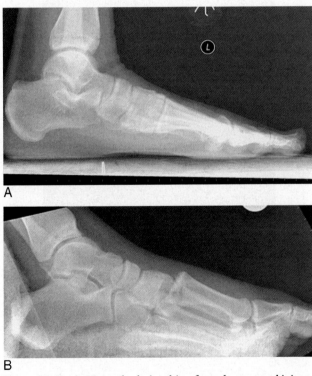

Figure 24–10: **A,** Normal relationship of tarsal metatarsal joints on lateral radiograph. **B,** Dorsally subluxed metatarsals seen with Lisfranc injury.

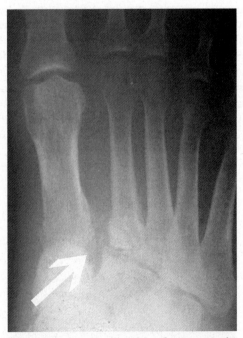

Figure 24–11: Fleck sign: Small avulsion fracture seen between first and second metatarsal.

- Dislocations, which can be reduced by closed methods, are amenable to percutaneous fixation. However, an absolute anatomic reduction must be ensured. Both screw and Kirschner wire (K-wire) fixation have been described. K-wire fixation has been associated with infection requiring early pin removal, pin migration, and loss of reduction following pin removal. Because of these disadvantages screw fixation is preferred.

- The majority of Lisfranc injuries are treated with ORIF.[6] Surgery is delayed until soft-tissue swelling has resolved, and skin wrinkles have returned, usually in 10 to 14 days. Two dorsal longitudinal incisions are routinely required (Figure 24–12). A medial incision is made in line with the first intermetatarsal web space centered over the bases of the first and second metatarsal. This incision allows access to the first, second, and medial third metatarsal base. A second lateral incision is made over the fourth metatarsal base. This incision allows access to the third, fourth, and fifth metatarsal bases.

- The first metatarsocuneiform joint is stabilized first, followed by the second metatarsocuneiform joint. Once the second joint is reduced the third metatarsocuneiform will often also reduce as a result of the connections of the intermetatarsal ligaments. In general 3.5-mm cortical screws, placed in a variety of configurations, are used to treat Lisfranc injuries. Whether screws should be placed in a lag or noncompression fashion is controversial and likely inconsequential. Screws used to stabilize the first metarsocuneiform joint may be started distal in the metatarsal or proximal in the medial cuneiform. Screws used to secure the second and third metarsocuneiform joints are started distally in the metatarsals (Figure 24–13). Alternatively, the second metatarsal may be secured using a lag screw inserted from the medial aspect of the medial cuneiform obliquely into the base of the second metatarsal. This so called "Lisfranc screw" is designed to recreate the force of the natural Lisfranc ligament (see Figure 24–13C).

- Most surgeons advocate stabilizing the fourth and fifth metatarsocuboid joints with smooth K-wires versus screws (Figure 24–14). These lateral two joints are significantly more mobile than the medial three and prone to stiffness

with prolonged screw fixation. K-wires are easily removed after 6 weeks decreasing the risk of stiffness. Late displacement of the fourth and fifth metatarsals is usually not an issue as a result of their connections to the second and third metatarsals, which remain stabilized with screws.

- In cases of severe comminution at the metatarsal bases screw fixation may not be possible therefore requiring the use of K-wires or spanning plates. More recently,

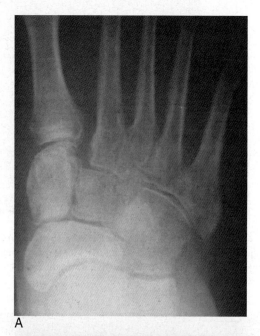

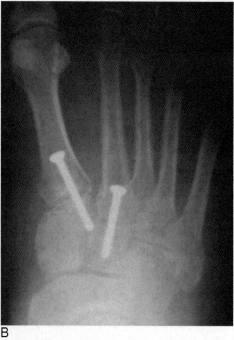

Figure 24–13: **A,** Radiographs showing first and second metatarsocuneiform joint incongruity. **B,** Postoperative radiograph showing screw placement.

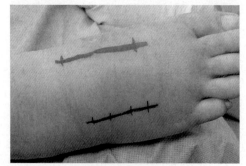

Figure 24–12: **Dorsal incisions for Lisfranc injuries.**

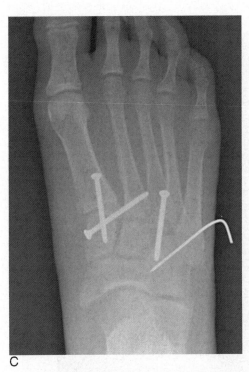

C

Figure 24–13, cont'd: **C,** Oblique "Lisfranc screw."

primary arthrodesis has been advocated for these severely comminuted injuries[7] (Figure 24–15).

- If a "nutcracker fracture" of the cuboid is also present and the lateral column of the foot is markedly shortened, reduction of the medial dislocated joints may not be possible as a result of the valgus pull of the fourth and fifth metatarsals. In this case the cuboid will require ORIF or open reduction with external fixation and bone grafting before medial column stabilization (see Figure 24–6).

- Various postoperative protocols have been used following Lisfranc injuries. Patients are routinely splinted for about 2 weeks and then placed in a short-leg nonweight-bearing cast. Some surgeons allow range-of-motion exercises after as little as 4 weeks, others prefer casting for up to 12 weeks. Most agree weight bearing should not begin for 10 to 12 weeks.

- The need for screw removal is debatable. Screws should be left in place for a minimum of 4 months. During this time frame, weight bearing is protected. If the screws are not removed, patients should be informed about the possibility of breakage. Currently, bioabsorbable screws are being investigated as an alternative to metal implants.[8]

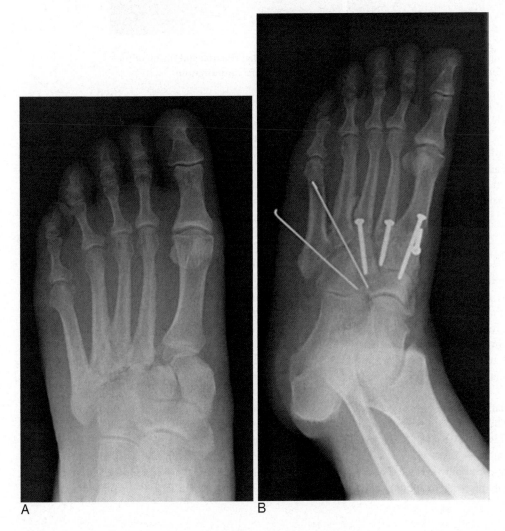

A   B

Figure 24–14: **A,** Comminuted Lisfranc fracture dislocation. **B,** Fixation with screws medially and Kirschner wires laterally.

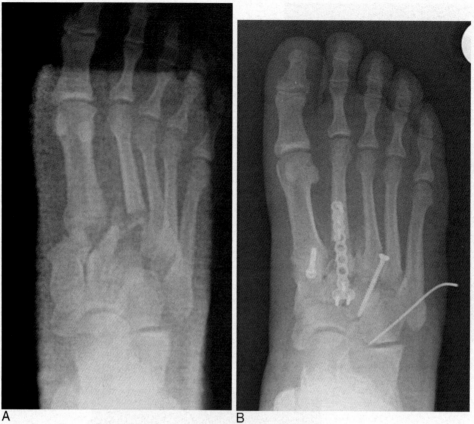

A   B

Figure 24–15: **A,** Type A Lisfranc injury. **B,** Treatment with open reduction and internal fixation and fusion of the second and third tarsometatarsal joints. A spanning plate was required because of severe comminution.

- Residual disability is common following Lisfranc injuries, and outcomes following purely ligamentous injury appear to be worse than bony injuries.[9] Anatomic reductions give the best outcomes. Posttraumatic arthrosis is the most common complication after Lisfranc injuries following both operative and nonoperative treatment.[10] Neglected tarsometatarsal injuries develop painful pes planus and abduction deformities.[11]

Metatarsal Fractures

- Metatarsal fractures most commonly occur as a result of a direct blow, inversion injury, or overuse. Fractures may involve the metatarsal neck, shaft, or base.
- Nondisplaced fractures of the metatarsal neck and shaft are treated with protected weight bearing in fracture boot or postoperative shoe for 4 to 6 weeks. Regular shoe wear is then allowed as tolerated and activity gradually progressed.
- In cases of nondisplaced metatarsal base fractures, a Lisfranc injury must be considered. These injuries are treated in a short-leg nonweight-bearing cast for 4 weeks and then with protected weight-bearing for another 2 to 4 weeks.
- Metatarsal stress fractures most commonly involve the second and third metatarsals. Patients seek treatment when

they have a painful, swollen foot but no history of acute trauma. When asked, the patient will usually report a recent increase in the level of activity. Initial radiographs appear normal; however, given this clinical scenario one must have a high index of suspicion for a stress fracture. By about 2 to 3 weeks the fracture site becomes evident on radiographs and early callus can be seen (Figure 24–16). Patients with suspected stress fractures should be treated in a postoperative shoe or fracture boot for about 4 weeks.

- Dorsally displaced or angulated metatarsal fractures lead to increased weight bearing on the more lateral metatarsal heads causing intractable plantar keratotic lesions. Plantar displacement or angulation causes increased plantar pressure beneath the metatarsal head, also leading to an intractable plantar keratotic lesion. First metatarsal fractures with varus angulation can lead to a hallux valgus deformity, and those with valgus angulation lead to a hallux varus deformity.
- Fractures with 3 to 4 mm of displacement or greater than 10 degrees of angulation require operative treatment. Intramedullary (IM) pins, screws, and low-profile plates have used to treat these fractures.[12]
- Fractures from the midshaft to the metatarsal neck are fixed with IM K-wires. If closed reduction of the fracture is possible K-wires are inserted percutaneous distal to

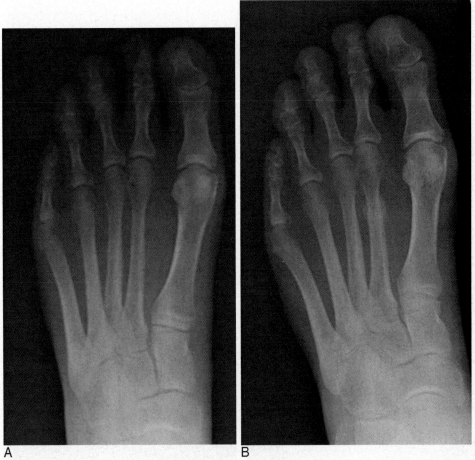

Figure 24–16: **A,** Radiograph of a 65-year-old female 3 days after the onset of forefoot pain and swelling. **B,** Patient's radiographs 3 weeks later. Note callus at second metatarsal.

proximal from the metatarsal head across the fracture site. The toes are held in a dorsiflexed position while the K-wires are inserted. If open reduction is required, a dorsal incision is made over the fracture site or in the web space between two fractured metatarsals. K-wires are then inserted from the fracture site distally through the metatarsal head with the toes held dorsiflexed (Figure 24–17). The wires are then passed proximally across the fracture site. The most common complication from this type of fixation is metatarsophalangeal joint stiffness.

- Fractures from the midshaft to the metatarsal base are treated with screw or plate fixation. If significant bone loss is present, as is the case with many gunshot wounds or open fractures, a small external fixator may be used to maintain length before subsequent bone grafting.
- The majority of fifth metatarsal fractures are the result of inversion injuries. Most commonly these fractures involve the tuberosity or the proximal metaphyseal-diaphyseal junction.
- The peroneus brevis inserts into the tuberosity of the fifth metatarsal. An inversion mechanism against this powerful everter produces an avulsion fracture of the

tuberosity. Because the peroneus brevis has a broad insertion these fractures are usually nondisplaced (Figure 24–18A).
- Nondisplaced tuberosity fractures are treated in a short-leg weight-bearing cast or fracture boot for 4 to 6 weeks. Fractures with significant displacement or joint incongruity require ORIF (see Figure 24–18B and C).
- Owing to the excellent blood supply in this area of the metatarsal these tuberosity fractures heal uneventfully. In rare cases of nonunion small avulsions can be excised. Larger fragments require ORIF with bone grafting.
- The metaphyseal-diaphyseal junction of the fifth metatarsal is a watershed area to its blood supply. This tenuous blood supply makes this area prone to stress fractures and nonunions.
- Proximal fifth metatarsal fractures involving the metaphyseal-diaphyseal junction are commonly called Jones' fractures. Jones' fractures are divided into acute and stress fractures.
- Acute fractures result from a combination of adduction and inversion forces. These fractures should be treated in a short-leg nonweight-bearing cast for at least 6 weeks.

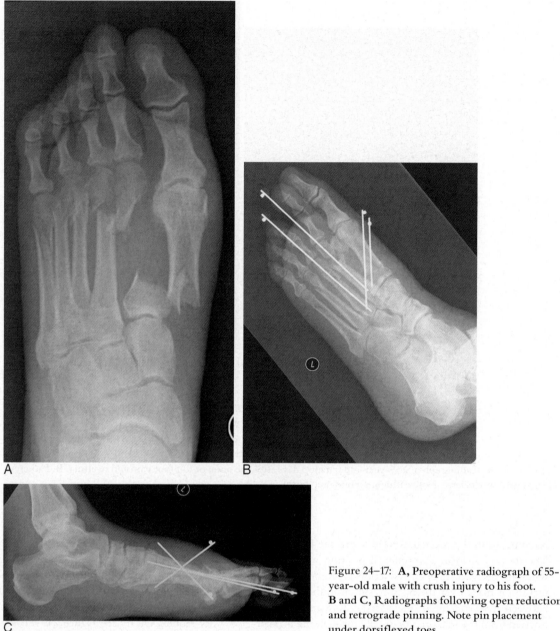

Figure 24–17: **A,** Preoperative radiograph of 55-year-old male with crush injury to his foot. **B** and **C,** Radiographs following open reduction and retrograde pinning. Note pin placement under dorsiflexed toes.

As a result of the relatively higher incidence of nonunion, some surgeons advocate internal fixation in athletes.[13]

- Internal fixation is accomplished using IM screw fixation. Screws ranging from 4-mm cannulated screws to 6.5-mm cancellous screws have been recommended.[14] In general the largest screw the canal will safely accommodate should be used (Figure 24–19). Adequate healing and return to full activity is between 7 and 8 weeks. Failure of the procedure is associated with return to sports before complete bony healing.[15]

- Stress fractures occur due to repetitive forces and may be associated with a cavovarus foot.

- Patients with fifth metatarsal metaphyseal-diaphyseal stress fractures present with prodromal symptoms of vague lateral foot pain. Radiographs show sclerosis at the fracture site and narrowing of the IM canal (Figure 24–20). Non-weight bearing in a short-leg cast for 6 to 8 weeks is the recommended initial treatment. However, the poor blood supply to this area makes these fractures especially prone to delayed union and nonunion. Therefore some authors have recommended IM fixation and local bone grafting as initial treatment. Patients with cavovarus feet require correction of their deformity at the time of fracture fixation.

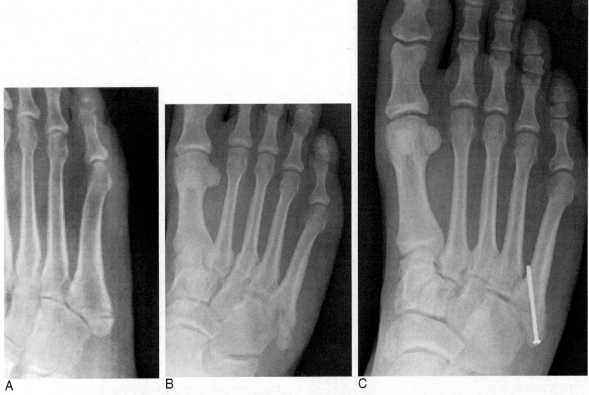

Figure 24–18: **A,** Nondisplaced fifth metatarsal tuberosity fracture. **B,** Displaced fifth metatarsal tuberosity fracture in active duty Marine. **C,** Tuberosity fracture stabilized with 3-mm cannulated screw.

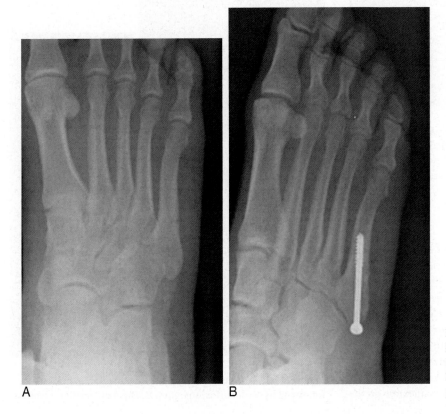

Figure 24–19: **A,** Acute Jones' fracture in 20-year-old basketball player. **B,** Fracture treated with 4-mm cannulated screw. Patient returned to full activity at 7 weeks postoperatively.

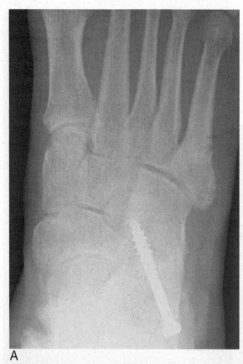

A

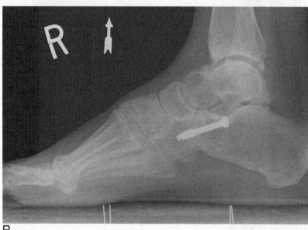

B

Figure 24–20: **A,** Anteroposterior view of Jones' stress fracture. The canal is narrowed and sclerotic. Patient had an unrelated previous calcaneocuboid fusion. **B,** Lateral view of same patient showing cavovarus foot and Jones' stress fracture.

Sesamoid Fractures

● The medial and lateral sesamoids articulate with the plantar aspect of the first metatarsal head. These bones are contained within the tendons of the flexor hallucis brevis tendons and are connected by the intersesamoidal ligament. The sesamoids function to absorb weight-bearing forces and to provide a mechanical advantage for the flexor hallucis brevis. The sesamoids may be multipartite with bipartite medial sesamoids occurring in 10% to 30% of the population.

● Sesamoid fractures most commonly occur as a result of one of three mechanisms: (1) forced dorsiflexion of the great toe resulting in an avulsion fracture, (2) direct trauma by a fall from a height, or (3) repetitive trauma resulting in a stress fracture.

● It may be difficult to differentiate a sesamoid fracture from an inflamed bipartite sesamoid. Each of these conditions may have tenderness over the sesamoid and pain with dorsiflexion of the great toe. To evaluate the sesamoids standard foot radiographs should be obtained and include a tangential sesamoid view. Acute fractures will demonstrate an irregular lucent line, whereas the bipartite sesamoids usually are larger with smooth sclerotic borders (Figure 24–21). If there is doubt, a bone scan is usually helpful.

● Acute sesamoid fractures are treated in a short-leg nonweight-bearing cast with an extended toe box for 6 weeks. Patients are then progressed into a shoe with a metatarsal pad. Many patients will continue to experience discomfort for several months.

● Sesamoid nonunions have been treated in a variety of ways. Whereas some authors have recommended complete or partial excision of the sesamoid, others have recommended bone grafting if the articular surface remains intact.[16]

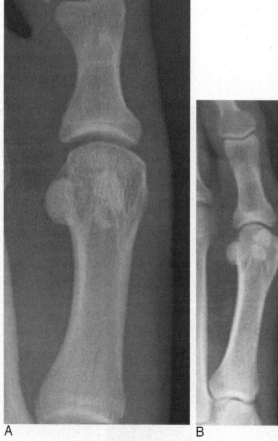

A   B

Figure 24–21: **A,** Avulsion fracture of the medial sesamoid following hyperdorsiflexion injury. **B,** Bipartite medial sesamoid.

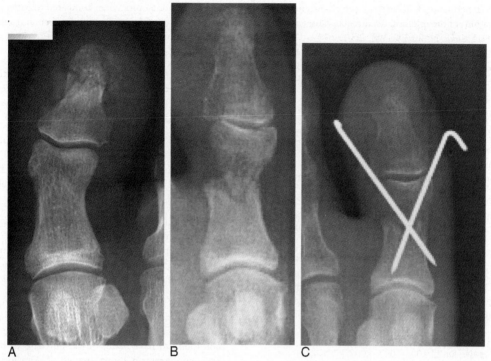

Figure 24–22:   **A,** Tuff fracture of great toe distal phalanx. **B,** Displaced and angulated great toe proximal phalanx fracture. **C,** Closed reduction and percutaneous pinning of proximal phalanx fracture.

Lesser Toe Phalanx Fractures

- The majority of lesser toe phalanx fractures occur by kicking a heavy object. Patients present with a painful swollen toe. These fractures are usually minimally displaced, and the diagnosis is easily confirmed with plain radiographs. Treatment consists of buddy taping to the adjacent toe and ambulation in a postoperative shoe. Regular shoe wear is generally tolerated within 1 to 2 weeks but discomfort may persist for several weeks. Surgery is indicated only for severely angulated fractures that cannot be reduced by closed methods.

Great Toe Phalanx Fractures

- Fractures of the great toe phalanges most commonly result from kicking a heavy object or having a heavy object dropped on the toe.
- Distal tuff fractures frequently involve a nail bed injury (Figure 24–22A). In these cases the nail should be preserved as it functions as a biologic dressing and splint. The patients are treated with a short course of oral antibiotics and allowed weight bearing as tolerated in a postoperative shoe for 3 to 4 weeks
- Nondisplaced fractures of either the distal or proximal phalanx are treated in postoperative shoe for 3 to 4 weeks.
- Because of the functional demands of the great toe displaced or angulated fractures must be reduced and then pinned with K-wires if unstable (see Figure 24–22B and C).

Significant intraarticular incongruity is also an indication for open reduction and pinning.[16]

Annotated Reference

1. Digiovanni CW: Fractures of the navicular, *Foot Ankle Clin* 1:25-71, 2004.

This is comprehensive review of navicular fracture anatomy, classification, and treatment. An emphasis is placed on the complicated nature of these fractures, and a detailed description of state-of-the-art operative techniques is presented.

2. Lee S, Anderson RB: Stress fractures of the tarsal navicular, *Foot Ankle Clin* 1:85-104, 2004.

This is a comprehensive review of the anatomy, pathophysiology, presentation, evaluation, and treatment of navicular stress fractures.

3. Klaue K: Chopart fractures, *Injury* 35:SB64-SB70, 2004.

This is a detailed review of fracture-dislocations about the talonavicular and calcaneo-cuboid joints. Principles of operative treatment are discussed at length and the need for anatomic reduction is stressed.

4. Weber M, Locher S: Reconstruction of the cuboid in compression fractures: short to midterm results in 12 patients, *Foot Ankle Int* 23:1008-1013, 2002.

Patients with cuboid crush injuries were treated with iliac crest bone grafting and internal fixation. Good restoration of length and intraarticular congruity were achieved. Residual symptoms were frequently related to associated midfoot injuries.

5. Richter M, Wippermann B, Krettek C, et al: Fractures and fracture dislocations of the midfoot: occurrence, causes and long term results, *Foot Ankle Int* 22:392-398, 2001.

The etiology and outcome of 155 patients with midfoot fractures occurring over a 25-year period were analyzed. The majority of these injuries (72.2%) were the result of traffic accidents. Patients treated with early open reduction and internal fixation had the least long-term impairment.

6. Thordarson DB: Fractures of the midfoot and forefoot, In Myerson MS editor, *Foot and ankle disorders*. Philadelphia, 2000, WB Saunders.

A through discussion of all aspects of midfoot and forefoot injuries is presented.

7. Mulier T, Reynders P, Dereymacker G, et al: Severe Lisfranc injuries: Primary arthrodesis or ORIF? *Foot Ankle Int* 23:902-905, 2002.

Three groups of patients with severe Lisfranc dislocations were compared at a follow-up of 30 months. Patients undergoing open reduction and internal fixation or arthrodesis of the medial three tarsometatarsal joints had less pain than those undergoing arthrodesis of all five tarsometatarsal joints.

8. Thordarson DB, Hurvitz G: PLA screw fixation of Lisfranc injuries, *Foot Ankle Int* 23:1003-1007, 2002.

Polylactic acid bioabsorbable screws were used to treat 14 patients with Lisfranc fracture-dislocations. At an average follow-up of 20 months, there were no adverse soft-tissue reactions, osteolysis, or loss of reduction.

9. Teng AL, Pinzur MS, Lomasney L, et al: Functional outcome following anatomic restoration of tarsal-metatarsal fracture dislocation, *Foot Ankle Int* 23:922-926, 2002.

Gait analysis revealed that 11 patients with anatomic surgical reductions following Lisfranc fracture-dislocations were found to have a return of normal walking parameters. Clinical outcomes, however, were less than satisfactory.

10. Kuo RS, Tejwani NC, DiGiovanni CW, et al: Outcome after open reduction and internal fixation of Lisfranc joint injuries, *J Bone Joint Surg Am* 82:1609-1618, 2000.

Forty-eight Lisfranc injuries were retrospectively evaluated at an average of 52 months. Patients with purely ligamentous injuries had poorer outcomes when compared to patients with combined ligamentous and bony injuries. Best clinical results were associated with an anatomical reduction. Posttraumatic arthrosis was the most common complication.

11. Philbin T, Rosenberg G, Sferra JJ: Complications of missed or untreated Lisfranc injuries, *Foot Ankle Clin* 8:61-71, 2003.

This is a review details treatment options for the late sequelae of untreated Lisfranc injuries.

12. Rammelt S, Heineck J, Zwipp H: Metatarsal fractures, *Injury* 35:SB 77-SB 86, 2004.

This is a comprehensive review of metatarsal fractures. Patient evaluation, operative indications, and surgical techniques are discussed.

13. Portland G, Kelikian A, Kodros S: Acute surgical management of Jones' fractures, *Foot Ankle Int* 24:829-833, 2003.

Twenty-two patients with acute Jones' fractures or proximal diaphyseal stress fractures were treated intramedullary screw fixation. There was a 100% union rate at about 6 to 8 weeks.

14. Kelly IP, Glisson RR, Fink C, et al: Intramedullary screw fixation of Jones fractures, *Foot Ankle Int* 22:585-589, 2001.

In this cadaver study, 6.5-mm screws were compared to 5-mm screws and found to have better thread purchase within the medullary canal and greater pull out strength. The majority of the cadaver fifth metatarsals were able to accommodate the 6.5-mm screw.

15. Larson CM, Almekinders LC, Taft TN, et al: Intramedullary screw fixation of Jones fractures: analysis of failure, *Am J Sports* 30:55-60, 2002.

In 15 patients treated with cannulated screw fixation for acute Jones' fractures, failure of the procedure was noted to be higher in elite athletes. Return to full activity before complete radiographic union was also associated with nonunion.

16. Mittlmeier T, Haar P: Sesamoid and toe fractures, *Injury* 35: SB 87-SB 97, 2004.

Review of sesamoid, great toe, and lesser toe phalanx fractures. Clinical evaluation, nonoperative, and operative treatment are highlighted.

The Role of Electricity and Ultrasound in Fracture Healing

Steven D. Steinlauf, MD

Introduction

- The common goal of fracture treatment is to obtain fracture union in the shortest period of time possible.
- Approximately 5% to 10% of the fractures occurring annually in the United States will show some signs of impaired healing.
- In a nonunion, healing has stopped and will not proceed without some type of intervention. This failure of the healing process must be documented by two sets of radiographs separated by 90 days.
- Operative treatment to obtain stability and bone grafting to stimulate healing comprise the traditional treatment for nonunion.
- To decrease the need for further, often complex operative procedures or alternative forms of treatment to stimulate the healing process have been developed. These include bone growth stimulation with physical modalities.
- The various modalities include low-intensity ultrasound (US), pulsed electromagnetic fields (PEMFs), combined magnetic fields (CMFs), capacitive coupling stimulation, and direct electrical stimulation (Table 25–1).
- In the past, arguments against the use of these devices have included the limited knowledge of the mechanism of action and the significant cost.
- However, there exists a rapidly expanding scientific basis that supports the reported benefits of this adjunct modality.
- It is essential to better define the patients and conditions that would realize the greatest benefit from the application of this technology.
- Although the basic mechanisms of action are not completely understood, it is known that bone cells are sensitive to the physical forces that they encounter.
- The cells respond to their environment, according to Wolf's law, leading to remodeling of bone.

- Bone growth stimulators are devices that impart a physical force on the skeleton or deliver an electrical current to alter the process of bone healing.
- They were originally designed with the intent of stimulating healing in cases of nonunion. As research has advanced, new indications have evolved. These include the use of stimulators to speed the healing of certain fresh fractures, the use of stimulators to accelerate the rate of fusions, and various other applications.
- Numerous devices have been developed to achieve these goals. They employ a number of different technologies, all of which seem to arrive at a common pathway of turning on or speeding up the process of osseous healing (Figure 25–1).
- The purpose of this review is to better educate the orthopaedic surgeon about the current technology available and the indications for the use of this valuable adjunctive modality.

History

- Investigators initiated the study of electrical and US stimulation of bone starting in the 1950s.
- Interest in elucidating the effects of electrical stimulation on bone developed after Fakuda and Yasuda[1] noted that mechanical stress on bone leads to the generation of "piezoelectric potentials," which are not dependent on cell viability.
- In a separate area of research around the same period, Corradi and Cozzolino[2] used US for the first time to stimulate fracture healing.
- During the 1960s, Brighton and others[3] began studying the electrical properties of nonstressed living bone. Their observations led to numerous studies that demonstrated that the application of small electrical currents to bone stimulates osteogenesis. The amount of new bone formed was greatest at 20 microamps.

Table 25–1	Bone Growth Stimulators	
MODALITY	**AVAILABLE DEVICE**	**INDICATIONS**
Low-intensity ultrasound	Exogen (Smith and Nephew)	Nonunions, certain fresh fractures*
Capacitive coupling	Biomet, EBI, Orthopak	Nonunions, spinal fusion
Direct current	EBI's implantable device	Nonunions, spinal fusion
Pulsed electromagnetic fields	EBI, Orthofix	Nonunions, spinal fusion
Combined magnetic fields	Don Joy OL1000 (DJ Orthopaedics)	Nonunions, spinal fusion

*Fresh closed or grade 1 open tibia fractures treated nonoperatively;fresh closed, dorsally displaced distal radius fractures treated nonoperatively

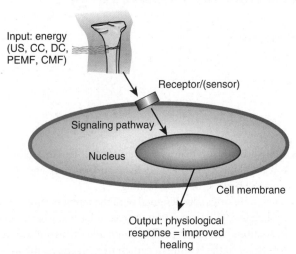

Input: energy
(US, CC, DC, PEMF, CMF)

Receptor/(sensor)

Signaling pathway

Nucleus

Cell membrane

Output: physiological response = improved healing

Figure 25–1: The bone growth stimulators use either mechanical force or electricity to "turn on"cells. The exact mechanism by which this is accomplished is unknown. However it likely involves an affect on the cell surface receptor that leads to the stimulation of the cellular processes leading to the production of certain proteins. These proteins in turn lead to the physiologic response of improved osseous healing.

- The clinical use of electricity and electromagnetic fields for fracture healing began in the 1970s.
- In 1971, Friedenberg and others[4] reported the first successful treatment of an established nonunion with electrical stimulation. The case involved a nonunion of the medial malleolus treated for 9 weeks with an implantable stimulator.
- In 1979, the Food and Drug Administration (FDA) approved the use of direct current for the treatment of established nonunions.
- Over the ensuing years additional technologies have been developed to stimulate bone healing. These modalities include PEMF, which induces electrical fields in bone similar in magnitude and time course to endogenous electric fields produced in response to strain. The PEMF device was approved by the FDA in 1979 for the treatment of nonunions.
- Furthermore, animal research, such as that by Pilla and others[5] in the 1980 and 1990s, supported the use of low-intensity US to enhance osseous healing. Over the

ensuing years US has been used to successfully stimulate the healing of nonunions and to accelerate the rate of healing of certain fresh fractures.
- In addition to the use of stimulators in the treatment of nonunions and fresh fractures, bone growth stimulation has been investigated in high-risk arthrodesis, the treatment of avascular necrosis (AVN), osteotomies, and distraction osteogenesis.

Direct Current Stimulation

- Using the knowledge gained through basic science studies, Brighton and others[3] developed a bone growth stimulation system and began clinical trials in 1970.
- Direct current stimulation of osteogenesis is accomplished with an implantable device, which produces a localized electric current between electrodes inserted at the fracture site.
- The cathode consists of fine wires wrapped throughout the site of the nonunion and is the site where stimulation occurs. No contact can occur between the wires and metallic implants.
- The battery based anode is inserted into the subcutaneous tissues close to the site of treatment. The subcutaneous nature of the battery may lead to irritation of the overlying tissues necessitating removal after fracture healing.
- A constant direct current of 20 microamps and 0.83 V is established between electrodes placed at the fracture site.
- No problem with patient compliance occurs because of the implantable nature of the device.

Basic Science

- Although the understanding of the mechanism of action of direct electrical stimulation is not complete. Brighton and others[3] noted that the local oxygen tension is lowered, and the pH is raised at the cathode. This leads to cellular changes that result in osteogenesis.
- In addition, increased proteoglycan and collagen synthesis is noted, and preliminary data indicate that direct current stimulation leads to up-regulation of important growth factors.

Clinical Studies

- Clinical studies have demonstrated the effectiveness of direct current stimulation in the treatment of established nonunions.

- In the 1970s, Brighton and others[3] evaluated constant direct current in the treatment of established, posttraumatic nonunions. A nonunion was defined as a fracture that demonstrated no interval healing on serial radiographs made over a 3-month period. The average duration of nonunion was 2.7 years from the time of fracture; 72% of the patients had undergone previous surgery. The treatment period was 12 weeks. However 29 of the patients required more than one treatment period. One hundred forty-nine of 178 nonunions (83.7%) healed. A significant number of patients (74.4%) with previous osteomyelitis also healed. There was an apparent decrease in the rate of healing in nonunions present for greater than 40 months.
- In a similar report, Patterson and others[6] reported a rate of successful healing of 86% in 84 patients with delayed union and nonunion of long bones. The majority of fractures involved the tibia, and many patients had failed previous surgical treatment of the nonunion. The treatment involved an implantable stimulator and casting.

Ultrasound

- The use of low-intensity US to stimulate osteogenesis has been studied extensively.
- US is a form of mechanical energy that can be transmitted into the body as high-frequency acoustical pressure waves at 30 mW/cm^2.
- In the clinical setting the transducer must be placed in direct contact with the skin over the site to be treated and is used for one 20-minute treatment session daily.

Basic Science

- The exact mechanism of action is unknown. However a rapidly expanding knowledge of the basic science has demonstrated that US leads to:
  - Increased activity of certain enzymes.
  - Up-regulation of signaling pathways in osteoblasts.
  - Release of growth factors.
  - Increased expression of certain genes.
- This is demonstrated in the study by Wang and others.[7] They showed that US stimulation leads to increased nitric oxide production, which leads to increased vascular endothelial growth factor-A (VEGF-A) production by osteoblasts. This in turn leads to angiogenesis and chondrocyte and osteoblast differentiation.
- Kortstjens and others[8] also demonstrated that US also leads to increased bone cell differentiation and calcified matrix production.
- US may have an effect on all stages of fracture healing.
- Animal studies have also been used to study the effects of US on osseous healing.

- In 1990, Pilla and others[5] used a rabbit fibular osteotomy model and demonstrated that the osteotomies exposed to US showed biomechanical healing accelerated by a factor of 1.7 compared to controls.

Clinical Studies

Fresh Fractures

- Clinical studies have demonstrated the positive effects of low-intensity US stimulation on the fracture healing process in certain well-controlled settings.
- Heckman and others[9] performed a prospective, randomized, double-blind, placebo controlled study of 67 closed or grade I open fractures of the tibial shaft treated with a cast and either US or a sham device. There was a significant decrease in the time to clinical healing for the actively treated group, 86 days versus 114 days. There were no complications related to the device, and there was good compliance. Smokers also showed a faster rate of healing in the active treatment group.
- Kristiansen and others[10] performed a similar study in patients with dorsally angulated distal radius fractures treated with a short arm cast and US for 20 minutes per day for 10 weeks or a sham device. In the US-treated group, there was a statistically smaller loss of reduction, a decrease in the mean time until loss of reduction ceased, and more rapid healing, 61 days versus 98 days.
- In 2004, Leung and others[11] performed a randomized, double-blind study on a small group of patients with high-energy tibial shaft fractures treated operatively with or without the addition of ultrasound. Although some benefits were noted in the US group, only one delayed union was present in each group.
- Other studies have failed to demonstrate a beneficial effect of adjunctive US treatment in the fresh fracture setting.
- Emami and others[12] performed a prospective, randomized, double-blind, placebo controlled study of acute closed or grade I open tibial fractures treated with a reamed, locked intramedullary (IM) nail and either US or a sham device. In this study US did not shorten the healing time. Possible reasons for this include the fact that reaming and early weight bearing may stimulate fracture healing enough to negate any additional benefit from US.
- From the few studies on the use of adjunctive US in the setting of fresh fractures some benefit has been demonstrated. However, US should not be used in the vast majority of acute fracture settings for which there is no supporting literature.
- More studies will be performed in the future and may give orthopaedic surgeons better insight into which fractures would benefit from the addition of early US treatment.

Nonunions

- All studies of nonunions (Figure 25–2) are retrospective and some are based on registry data. However the studies

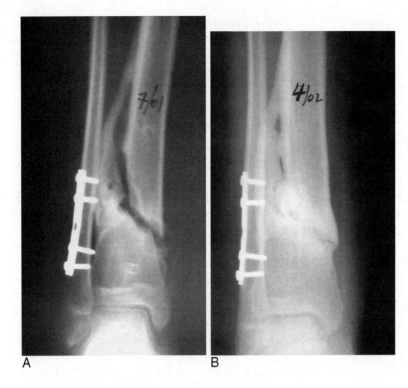

A   B

Figure 25–2: These are the radiographs of a 16-year-old boy who sustained a closed fracture of the distal tibia and fibula after being hit by a car. He was originally treated with external fixation of the tibia and plating of the fibula and then referred for further management 4 months after the original surgery. **A,** Demonstrates no significant healing of the tibia. Surgical intervention was proposed but the family refused. Thus low-intensity pulsed ultrasound was initiated for 20 minutes per day. The patient was maintained at full weight bearing in a short leg cast. **B,** Illustrates that at 9 months after initiation of treatment the fracture had healed. The patient was pain free and had resumed all activities.

are consistent in design and demonstrate similar outcomes. The patients typically have not undergone any type of surgery for the nonunion in the past year before US is started, and the fractures have typically demonstrated no healing for at least 3 months. In the studies ultrasound is the only new treatment that is initiated.

- Nonunions of long bones and non-long bones show similar rates of successful healing.
- In a review of the registry by fracture age Rubin and others[13] demonstrated that 83% of 1546 nonunions healed. The average time to healing was 172 days. Sixty-nine percent of humeral nonunions, 84 % of tibial nonunions, and 82% of femoral nonunions healed with ultrasound.

Distraction Osteogenesis

- The goal of using US during distraction osteogenesis is to speed healing of the regenerate. This would then allow for earlier removal of the external fixator, decreasing the associated risks, and allowing the patient to regain function more rapidly.
- Numerous animal studies have been performed to evaluate the effects of US on osteogenesis. Some have demonstrated a beneficial effect of supplemental US. However, others have shown either no benefit or poorer healing.
- In a clinical study El-Mowafi and Mohsen[14] evaluated 20 patients who underwent bone lengthening. After the completion of distraction, 10 patients received US stimulation, and 10 patients continued with the external fixation alone. The healing index in the patients treated with US was significantly shorter than in the patients

who did not receive the adjunct therapy (30 days/cm versus 48 days/cm).

Pulsed Electromagnetic Fields

- PEMF was developed to induce electrical fields in bone similar in magnitude and time course to the endogenous electrical fields produced in response to strain.
- The indications for the utilization of PEMF include nonunions, failed fusions, and congenital pseudoarthrosis in the appendicular skeleton
- Contraindications to the use of PEMF include a fracture gap greater than 10 mm and synovial pseudoarthrosis.

Basic Science

- PEMFs have multiple effects on cell function and promote angiogenesis.
- Aaron and Ciombor[15] in 1996 developed a hypothesis that PEMFs exert their effect on receptor mediated transmembrane signaling mechanisms of cytokines pertinent to cell differentiation. This in turn alters the signal transduction process influencing the regulation of transcriptional and synthetic activities. The results include:
  - Up-regulation of TGF-B mRNA.
  - Enhanced differentiation of mesenchymal stem cells.
  - Increase in extracellular matrix synthesis.
  - Stimulation of endochondral ossification.
- Bodamyali and others[16] in 1998 helped to elucidate the mechanism by which PEMF stimulates osteogenesis. They demonstrated that PEMF leads to an increase in the levels

of bone morphogenetic protein-2 (BMP-2) and BMP-4 mRNA and an increase in the number and size of bone nodules in a mammalian cell culture model.

- In an animal study, Cane and others,[17] using transcortical drill holes in the metacarpals of horses, demonstrated that the amount of bone formed and the mineral apposition rate were significantly greater in the group treated with PEMF for 30 days compared to a sham device on the opposite side.

Clinical Studies

- Bassett and others[18] used for 10 hours per day to treat patients with long-standing nonunions of the tibial diaphysis. The average period from the time of fracture to the initiation of treatment with PEMF was 28 months, and the patients had an average of 2.4 previous surgeries. They achieved an 87% rate of healing in 127 nonunions of the tibial diaphysis. The median healing time was 5.2 months.
- Heckman and others[19] used for 12 hours per day to treat patients with nonunions of various bones. They achieved a 64% success rate overall in 149 nonunions. For lower extremity nonunions, cast immobilization and nonweight bearing were used. The average period from the time of fracture to the initiation of treatment with PEMF was 30.2 months. Twenty-six nonunions were actively infected. At 11.1 months posttreatment 96 of 149 (64%) were healed. Seventy-one percent of tibias, 52% of femurs, and 44% of humeral nonunions had healed.
- Sharrard[20] reported the results of a placebo controlled, double-blind, randomized trial using PEMF for 12 hours per day for 12 weeks for tibial shaft fractures, which showed poor healing. Fifty-one patients were treated with long leg casting, no weight bearing and either an active or a sham device. Nine out of 20 (45%) with active devices healed, only 3 out of 22 with placebo devices healed (14%). These results show significantly improved healing with the active device. The author attributes the low overall rate of healing to the severity of the fractures.
- In 1991 Garland and others[21] evaluated 139 nonunions treated with PEMF. They showed that when the PEMF device was used for less than 3 hours per day only 5 of 14 (35.7%) nonunions healed. When the PEMF device was used for greater than 3 hours per day 108 of 135 (80%) healed. They noted no significant difference in success rate for long- and short-bone fractures, open and closed fractures, all durations of nonunion, recalcitrant and first-time treatment, infected and noninfected nonunions, fracture gaps up to 1 cm, patient age, and for weight bearing versus no weight bearing treatment. Long-term healing was maintained, and no long-term complications of PEMF treatment were noted.

Combined Magnetic Fields

- The CMF device used an external pair of coils that produce two parallel low-energy magnetic fields, an alternating magnetic field combined with a static magnetic field.
- The device is used for a single daily 30-minute treatment session. This treatment time was chosen based on growth factor release studies and animal studies that demonstrated that 30 minutes was as effective as longer treatment periods.
- The indications for CMF include nonunions (Figure 25–3) and adjunctive treatment in spinal fusion.
- CMF induces an electric field that is in the low range of the endogenous potentials associated with mechanical loading.
- Control of the direct current, or static, magnetic field is believed to increase the sensitivity of cells to the low-energy alternating current or time varying magnetic field.

Basic Science

- The basic science research on combined magnetic fields has focused on identifying the mechanism that links external stimuli, such as CMF, with the process of bone growth and repair. The studies to date have evaluated the effects of CMF on insulin-like growth factor II (ILGF-II). This is a predominant growth factor in human bone. It is responsible for the regulation of chemotaxis, proliferation, and differentiation of normal human osteoblasts.
- In 1995, Fitzsimmons and others[22] demonstrated that short-term CMF exposure, 10 minutes, stimulates the production and release of ILGF-II from human TE-85 osteosarcoma cells. They theorize that this in turn leads to an increase in cell proliferation.

Clinical Studies

- In both published and unpublished studies, and in review of the manufacturing company's registry data, CMF has been shown to successfully heal recalcitrant nonunions.
- In 2000, Longo[23] reported the results of a retrospective evaluation of 20 patients with 23 nonunions treated with CMF. The immobilization techniques that had been employed before the addition of CMF were continued throughout the course of treatment with CMF. The average time from the original injury to the initiation of CMF was 389 days. The average number of surgeries before CMF was 2.1. The duration of treatment was 6 months. Greater than 90% compliance was noted. All patients healed.

Capacitive Coupling

- The modality of capacitive coupling was developed by Brighton and Pollack.
- Two surface electrodes are coupled to the skin, producing an electric field at the fracture site. The internal electric field is from 0.1 to 20 mV/cm and has a current density of 300 microamps/cm^2.

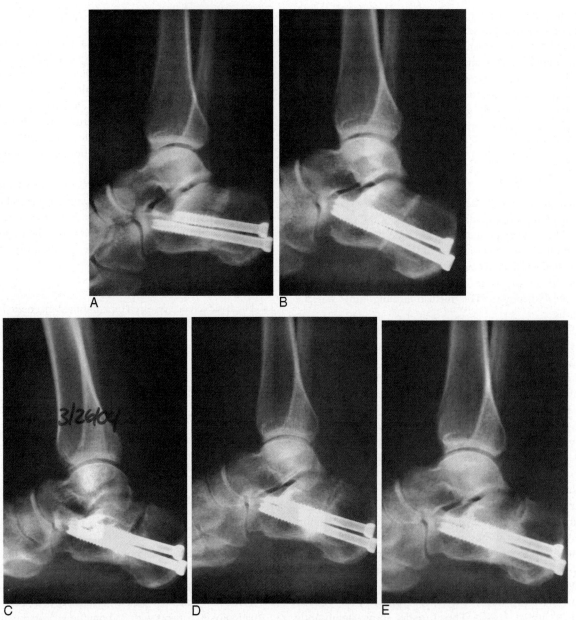

Figure 25–3: These are the radiographs of a 55-year-old woman with painful adult-acquired flat foot deformity. Reconstructive surgery, including a medial calcaneal slide, was performed. The threads of the top screw did not cross the osteotomy in this immediate postoperative X-ray **(A)**. X-ray taken at 5 weeks postoperatively **(B)**. This resulted in a painful nonunion with obvious resorption noted on X-ray taken 4.5 months postoperatively**(C)**. Revision surgery was offered, but the patient refused. Thus a combined magnetic field device was begun and used for 30 minutes each day. The patient was allowed to remain weight bearing in a fixed walker boot. Approximately 2.5 months after the combined magnetic field stimulator was started the patient's pain had started to decrease, and healing is noted on X-ray **(D)**. Four months after the combined magnetic field stimulator was started the patient was pain free, had resumed all activities, and the X-rays demonstrate a healed osteotomy **(E)**.

- The recommended treatment time is 24 hours per day.
- The indications for capacitive coupling include nonunions of long bones and of the scaphoid, and an adjunct to spine fusion.

Basic Science

- Using cell cultures Zhuang and others[24] demonstrated that capacitively coupled electric fields increase TGF-B1 mRNA and lead to increases in the proliferation of osteoblastic cells.

Clinical Studies

- Scott and King[25] published the results of their experience with capacitive coupling in the treatment of nonunions. This was a double-blind study. The device was used for 24 hours per day for 6 months for 23 nonunions of long bones. Sixty percent of the patients using the active device healed in a mean of 21 weeks. None of the 11 patients with the placebo device healed. In the crossover group of six patients, two healed, two showed progress, and two did not heal.

Summary

- Basic science studies, including cell culture and animal studies, have demonstrated that all of the devices discussed can stimulate a healing response in bone. The mechanism of action of the various modalities has been studied to a great extent as well. Although the exact mechanisms of action are not yet clear, the fundamentals are known.
- It appears that all of the various modalities lead to a common pathway.
- Pilla[26] compared electromagnetic field (EMF) stimulation, US, and strain-generated potentials (SGP) in a rabbit fibular osteotomy model. A time-varying electrical field E(t) is associated with each type of stimulus. This is directly induced by EMF and indirectly induced by the streaming potentials generated by the mechanical movement of ionic fluids within bone caniculi or past cell surfaces from US and SGP signals. It was demonstrated that both EMF and the mechanical stimuli accelerate mechanical strength to the same degree.

- The majority of clinical studies evaluating the treatment of nonunions are not randomized, placebo, controlled studies. However, the patients often act as their own controls. In other words, they have often failed multiple previous surgeries and have shown no progression toward healing for an extended period of time. The bone growth stimulator is the only new treatment added. If the nonunion then heals, the successful result can be attributed to the stimulator.
- It should be noted that atrophic nonunions are more resistant to healing than hypertrophic nonunions.
- The literature supports the use of bone growth stimulators for the treatment of nonunions as an adjunct treatment for spinal arthrodeses and in the treatment of certain fresh fractures. More randomized prospective studies are needed to prove that the stimulators are not only efficacious but also cost effective in clinical settings, such as complex arthrodeses (Figure 25–4), distraction osteogenesis, AVN, osteotomies, and complex fractures at risk of nonunion.
- Future research must also focus on the results of combining bone growth stimulation with other treatment modalities, such as bone grafting, and revision fixation in the treatment of nonunion, and how bone growth stimulators will interact with the other biologic agents now used to stimulate healing.
- These noninvasive modalities for the treatment of nonunions offer a viable alternative to traditional operative techniques.

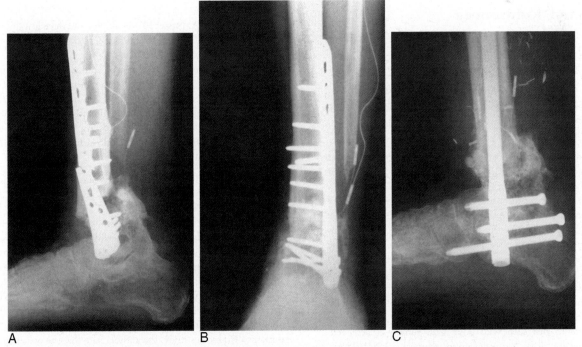

A   B   C

Figure 25–4: Sixty-year-old man who sustained a grade III-A open tibial pilon fracture originally treated with open treatment and internal fixation but developed a nonunion. Revision surgery was performed including an ankle arthrodeses, which also resulted in a nonunion (**A and B**). The patient was then referred for evaluation. The patient was treated with a retrograde nail, autograft bone graft, and an implantable direct current stimulator (**C and D**).

(Continued)

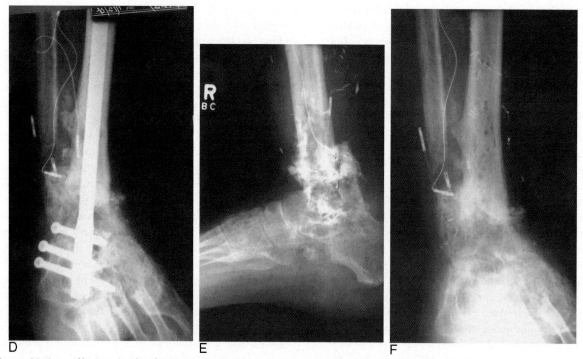

Figure 25–4, cont'd: Despite developing a wound dehiscence and a deep infection, which necessitated flap coverage, long-term antibiotics, and hardware removal, the patient healed both the soft tissues and the bone and has resumed activities with much less pain than preoperatively **(E and F)**.

Annotated References

1. Fakuda E, Yasuda I: On the piezoelectric effect of bone, *J Physiol Soc Jap* 12:1158, 1957.
Historical reference.

2. Corradi C, Cozzolino A: The action of ultrasound on the evolution of an experimental fracture in rabbits, *Minerva Ortop* 55:44-45, 1952.
Historical reference.

3. Brighton CT, Black J, Friedenberg ZB, et al: A multicenter study of the treatment of nonunion with constant direct current, *J Bone Joint Surg Am* 63:2-13, 1981.
In this article the investigators present a concise history of the study of direct current stimulation of bone. In addition, they present the results of a retrospective study of constant direct current in the treatment of acquired nonunions secondary to trauma. The authors report that in the University of Pennsylvania series 149 out of 178 nonunions (83.7%) united. When the study was expanded to an outside group of orthopaedists, 58 out of 80 nonunions (72.5%) united. The results indicate that with constant direct current and prolonged cast immobilization a rate of union comparable to that seen with bone graft surgery is achieved. Inadequate electricity, active infection, synovial pseudoarthrosis, and dislodgement of electrodes are causes for failure.

4. Friedenberg ZR, Harlow MD, Brighton CT: Healing of nonunion of the medial malleolus by means of direct current, *J Trauma* 11:883-885, 1971.

5. Pilla AA, Mont MA, Nasser PR, et al: Non-invasive low-intensity pulsed ultrasound accelerates bone healing in the rabbit, *J Orthop Trauma* 4:246-253, 1990.
The investigators studied the effects of a 20-minute daily ultrasound (US) treatment on a midshaft fibular osteotomy. One limb of each rabbit served as a control while the other received the ultrasound treatment. The limb treated with the US showed more rapid biomechanical healing, attaining the strength of an intact bone earlier than that of the control limb. At day 28 no difference in ultimate strength was noted.

6. Paterson DC, Lewis GN, Cass CA: Treatment of delayed union and nonunion with an implanted direct current stimulator, *Clin Orthop* 148:117-128, 1980.
Eighty-four patients were included in the study. Forty-seven patients were classified as delayed unions, no healing within 6 months and 37 as nonunions, no healing within 12 months. Seventy-two fractures involved the tibia. Over 30 surgeons were involved in the study. The implanted stimulator and cast immobilization were used. Seventy-two of 84 fractures (86%) healed. The average time to achieve union was 16 weeks. Many of the patients had failed previous surgical attempts to achieve union. In contrast to Brighton's study, the authors state that the presence of infection is not a contraindication to direct current stimulation. One important finding should be noted. By today's standards many of these fractures were recalcitrant nonunions that healed after electrical stimulation and casting alone, demonstrating the great potential of implantable stimulators.

7. Wang FS, Kuo YR, Wang CJ, et al: Nitric oxide mediates ultrasound-induced hypoxia-inducible factor-1 alpha activation and vascular endothelial growth factor: a expression in human osteoblasts, *Bone* 35:114-123, 2004.

In this study human osteoblasts were treated with or without low intensity ultrasound (US) stimulation for 20 minutes. The researchers demonstrated that osteoblasts respond to US by increasing nitric oxide mediated vascular endothelial growth factor-A (VEGF-A) induction. VEGF-A is important in the regulation of osteochodrogenesis and angiogenesis during fracture healing. They showed that nitric oxide acted as a critical mediator to communicate US stimuli into intracellular responses. They suggest that hypoxia-inducible factor-1 alpfa (HIF-1alpha), an angiogenic transcription factor, is likely a target of the US stimulus leading to the angiogenesis promoting activities.

8. Kortstjens CM, Nolte PA, Burger EH, et al: Stimulation of bone cell differentiation by low-intensity ultrasound: a histomorphometric in vitro study, *J Orthop Res* 22:495-500, 2004.

This is a basic science study investigating the effects of low-intensity ultrasound (US) on metatarsal bone rudiments of fetal mice. One group was exposed to the US treatment for 20 minutes per day. The researchers concluded that low-intensity US likely stimulates endochondral ossification by stimulating bone cell differentiation and calcified matrix production.

9. Heckman JD, Ryaby JP, McCabe J, et al: Acceleration of tibial fracture-healing by non-invasive, low-intensity pulsed ultrasound, *J Bone Joint Surg Am* 76:26-34, 1994.

This article describes the effects of a single, daily 20-minute treatment with low-intensity ultrasound (US) on fresh, low-energy, tibial shaft fractures in a homogenous population. The fractures were either closed or grade I open and were treated with long leg casting. The patients in the treatment group received an active US unit, whereas those in the control group received a sham device. Numerous exclusion criteria existed. The studies strong points include its randomized, prospective, placebo-controlled design. However, there were a large number of patients either lost to follow-up or removed from the study secondary to protocol "deviations." The study demonstrated a statistically significant increase in the healing rate in the treatment group.

10. Kristiansen TK, Ryaby JP, McCabe J, et al: Accelerated healing of distal radial fractures with the use of specific, low-intensity ultrasound, *J Bone Joint Surg Am* 79:961-973, 1997.

The authors have made a good effort to demonstrate the effectiveness of ultrasound (US) in the treatment of acute fractures of the distal radius, a cancellous bone model. The study's strong points include the double-blinded, randomized, prospective nature. The authors demonstrated a more rapid cessation of and smaller loss of reduction in the treatment group. However, the acceleration in healing that was noted may not have practical benefit. Furthermore, patient satisfaction and return of function were not evaluated. In addition, no cost analysis was performed to see if a cost benefit was produced by the use of the US device.

11. Leung KS, Lee WS, Tsui HF, et al: Complex tibial fracture outcomes following treatment with low-intensity pulsed ultrasound, *Ultrasound in Med Biol* 30:389-395, 2004.

The investigators do a good job of studying the effects of low-intensity ultrasound (US) on 30 high-energy tibia fractures. The fractures were either comminuted closed fractures or open fractures. All closed and Gustilo grade II or II open diaphyseal fractures were treated with reamed, locked nails. All grade III-A and metaphyseal fractures were treated with an external fixator. The treatment group received ultrasound treatment for 20 minutes per day for 90 days. The treatment group demonstrated earlier callus formation, earlier full weight bearing, earlier external fixator removal, higher bone specific alkaline phosphatase levels, and higher bone mineral content levels. However, all fractures in both groups healed with one delayed union in each group. Thus, further investigation is needed to demonstrate that the improved healing indices reported in this study actually translate into an improved functional outcome and improved patient satisfaction. In addition a cost analysis would be beneficial to determine if US leads to a cost savings by accelerating the healing process.

12. Emami A, Petren-Mallmin M, Larsson S: No effect of low-intensity ultrasound on healing time of intramedullary fixed tibial fractures, *J Orthop Trauma* 13:252-257, 1999.

This is a randomized, prospective, double blind study investigating the effects of low-intensity ultrasound (US) on the healing of closed or grade I open tibial shaft fractures treated with reamed, statically locked nails. No acceleration of healing was noted in the treatment group versus the control group. The effects of reaming, early weight bearing and increased stability of intramedullary (IM) nailing may make addition of US unnecessary. However, the patient selection criteria excluded high-energy fractures, and many factors that may predispose a patient to delayed or nonunion. Thus the data cannot be extrapolated to all tibial fractures treated with IM nails.

13. Rubin C, Bolander M, Ryaby JP, et al: The use of low-intensity ultrasound to accelerate the healing of fractures, *J Bone Joint Surg Am* 83:259-270, 2001.

This is a well-written current concepts review on low-intensity ultrasound. The article cites the authors' own review of the nonunion prescription-use registry as of June 2000. Nonunions were defined as fractures that had not healed by 255 days after injury. The average fracture age of the nonunions was more than 1.9 years. The healing rate ranged from 69% for humeral nonunions to 89% for metatarsal nonunions.

14. El-Mowafi H, Mohsen M: The effect of low-intensity pulsed ultrasound on callus maturation in tibial distraction osteogenesis, *Int Orthop* 29:121-124, 2005.

In this study the authors evaluated the effect of ultrasound (US) started during the consolidation phase of distraction osteogenesis. Twenty patients were included in the study. Eighteen patients sustained traumatic bone loss, whereas two presented with congenital deformities. The mean length of the defects was 6.1 cm. A monofocal osteotomy was used, and distraction was performed at 1 mm/day in four increments. After distraction the patients were randomized to either adjunct treatment with the US device for one 20-minute treatment daily or an inactive device while external fixation was maintained. The authors demonstrated that the addition of ultrasound after the completion of lengthening leads to a significantly shorter healing index, allowing for earlier removal of the external fixator.

15. Aaron RK, Ciombor D: Acceleration of experimental endochondral ossification by biophysical stimulation of the progenitor cell pool, *J Ortho Res* 14:582-589, 1996.

The authors implanted decalcified bone matrix subcutaneously into rats. Previous pulsed electromagnetic fields (PEMF) dose response studies from the same lab demonstrated a maximal effect on endochondral ossification at 8 hours per day. Thus the animals were subjected to 8 hours per day of electromagnetic stimulation at different time periods after implantation (during the mesenchymal, chondrogenic, or calcific phases). They were able to demonstrate that stimulation during the mesenchymal stage of endochondral bone formation leads to increased extracellular matrix synthesis and bone formation presumably through enhanced differentiation of mesenchymal stem cells. They hypothesize that the electromagnetic stimulation has an effect on the transmembrane signaling mechanisms, altering the signal transduction processes and influencing regulation of transcriptional and synthetic activity of cells.

16. Bodamyali T, Bhatt B, Hughes FJ, et al: Pulsed electromagnetic fields simultaneously induce osteogenesis and upregulate transcription of bone morphogenic proteins 2 and 4 in rat osteoblasts in vitro, *Biochem Biophys Res Comm* 250:458-461, 1998.

It is known that bone morphogenic proteins exert influence over many stages of endochondral bone formation. In this basic science study the authors studied the effects of pulsed electromagnetic fields (PEMF) on bone nodule formation and on bone morphogenetic protein-2 (BMP-2) and four mRNA in murine calvarial osteoblast cultures. Six hours of PEMF exposure, characteristics designed to mimic those produced in the clinical setting, increased both the number and size of bone nodules formed compared to unexposed controls. In addition PEMF induced a significant increase in the levels of BMP-2 and 4 compared to controls. The effect on the BMPs was directly related to the duration of PEMF exposure. This study along with others provides strong insight into the mechanisms by which bone growth stimulators "turn on" the healing process in fracture nonunions.

17. Cane V, Botti P, Soana S: Pulsed magnetic fields improve osteoblast activity during the repair of an experimental osseous defect, *J Orthop Res* 11:664-670, 1993.

The authors studied the effects of continuous exposure to pulsed electromagnetic fields (PEMFs) for 30 days on transcortical drill holes in the metacarpal bones of horses. The left side was treated with an active device and the right side with a sham device. Analysis showed that the amount of bone formed was significantly greater between treatment and sham groups. Tetracycline labeling demonstrated that the mineral apposition rate during a 10-day period was also significantly greater. The mineral apposition rate was used as a direct correlate of bone appositional growth rate, the osteogenic phase of healing.

18. Bassett CAL, Mitchell SN, Gaston SR: Treatment of ununited tibial diaphyseal fractures with pulsing electromagnetic fields, *J Bone Joint Surg Am* 63:511-523, 1981.

The authors review their results of treatment of 127 tibial diaphyseal nonunions in 125 patients. The treatment protocol included the use of pulsed electromagnetic fields (PEMFs) for 10 hours per day. The nonunions were stabilized in a long leg cast for an average of 4 months, followed by a short leg cast with axial loading for an average of 1.5 months. The average number of previous surgeries was 2.4 per patient, and the average period of disability was 28 months. Patients had to demonstrate 4 months of no changes clinically or radiographically before beginning treatment. The average treatment duration was 5.2 months. The overall success rate of healing was 87%. The subpopulation of 19 actively infected individuals showed a healing rate of 79% with concomitant resolution of the infection. The authors concluded that ununited fractures that have not progressed to synovial pseudoarthrosis often can be healed with PEMFs. Contraindications to the use of PEMFs include soft-tissue interposition and gaps greater than 1 cm. The authors noted that the healing process begins when gap tissues progressively calcify and are invaded by vessels from the bone margins, similar to endochondral ossification. The calcified cartilage is then replaced by bone. The success rate was not affected by the age or sex of the patient, the length of prior disability, the number of previous failed surgeries, or the presence of metal fixation.

19. Heckman JD, Ingram AJ, Loyd RD, et al: Nonunion treatment with pulsed electromagnetic fields, *Clin Orthop* 161:58-66, 1981.

This is a retrospective review of all of the nonunions treated by the authors over a 5-year period. The authors evaluated two groups of patients. Patients who were considered to have nonunions based on clinical findings and serial radiographs that showed no signs of healing for 2 months. The second group of patients consisted of those in whom fracture healing was so slow that the internal fixation devices were at risk for failure. Eighty-seven percent of the patients had no surgery within 3 months of the initiation of the pulsed electromagnetic field (PEMF) device. The treatment protocol included 12 hours of treatment with the PEMF device, cast immobilization, and no weight bearing for lower extremity nonunions. The authors noted that at 3 months after the treatment is started, if there are early signs of healing, then the patients have a good chance of going on to union. If there is no sign of healing at 3 months, then the fractures have a high likelihood of not uniting. Twenty-five patients did not complete treatment. One hundred forty-nine patients (153 nonunions) completed treatment. The overall success rate was 64.4%. The tibial nonunions had a higher success rate than did the femoral and humeral nonunions. The authors speculated that this was secondary to better immobilization for tibial nonunions. Infection, either quiescent or active, did not seem to influence the results. The authors noted that PEMF is more effective when started within 2 years of the injury.

20. Sharrard WJW: A double-blind trial of pulsed electromagnetic fields for delayed union of tibial fractures, *J Bone Joint Surg Br* 72:347-355, 1990.

This multicenter study analyzed the results of pulsed electromagnetic field (PEMF) treatment for fractures of the tibial shaft that showed poor healing between 16 and 32 weeks after the initial trauma. The author only included fractures with predisposing factors for poor healing. The fractures were all treated nonoperatively from the onset with a long leg cast and no weight bearing. In the active treatment group PEMF was utilized for 12 hours per day for 12 weeks. The results of healing were determined radiographically by both a blinded radiologist and a blinded orthopaedic surgeon. In an attempt to maintain homogeneous populations multiple exclusion criteria were utilized. The two groups were similar with the exception of an increased age in the control group and greater comminution in the control group. However, the author states that these factors did not influence the results to a sufficient enough extent to account for the difference noted in healing. The study shows a significant improvement in the rate of healing when PEMF is used for fractures with delayed union.

21. Garland DE, Moses B, Salyer W: Long-term follow-up of fracture nonunions treated with PEMFs, *Contemp Ortho* 22: 295-302, 1991.

The authors evaluated the effects of pulsed electromagnetic field (PEMF) treatment on a core group of 139 established nonunions. They determined that a minimum of 3 hours per day of treatment is necessary to achieve union. In addition, they evaluated multiple variables, noting no significant affect on healing by nonunion duration, patient age, open or closed fracture status, recalcitrant versus first time treatment, infection, fracture gaps up to 1 cm, or weight-bearing status. Although 131 investigators were involved in the study and there was a large loss to follow-up, the study has a number of strong points. The nonunions were of long duration, average 2.6 years. Eight-one percent of the fractures underwent an average of two previous surgeries that had failed. Fractures of long and short bones and failed arthrodesis were evaluated. At long-term follow-up a healed status was noted in 92% of the fractures with no long-term sequelae noted from the use of PEMF.

22. Fitzsimmons RJ, Ryaby JT, Mohan S, et al: Combined magnetic fields increase insulin-like growth factor-II in TE-85 human osteosarcoma bone cell cultures, *Endocrinology* 136:3100-3106, 1995.

This is a well-done basic science study comparing the effects of a combined magnetic field (CMF) device versus a sham device on cell cultures of TE-85 human osteosarcoma cells. The researchers demonstrated that 10 minutes of CMF exposure leads to increased release of insulin-like growth factor-II (IGF-II; a major regulatory growth factor in bone) and that the increased release of IGF-II leads to increased deoxyribonucleic acid (DNA) synthesis and cell proliferation. Exposure times greater than 10 minutes demonstrated a varying stimulatory effect. Overall, the authors feel that these data support the hypothesis that local growth factors may link biophysical stimuli such as CMF with physiologic responses.

23. Longo JA: Successful treatment of recalcitrant nonunions with combined magnetic field stimulation, *Surg Tech Int* VI:397-403, 2000.

The author evaluated 23 nonunions from multiple sites. Fractures that had not healed at least 6 months after the initial injury and showed no progression of healing within 3 months of beginning the CMF device were classified as nonunions. No other treatment parameters were changed when the CMF device was started. The average time from injury to treatment was 389 days. Good compliance was noted, and all nonunions healed after and average treatment time of 6 months.

24. Zhuang H, Wei W, Seldes RM, et al: Electrical stimulation induces the level of TGF-B1 mRNA in osteoblastic cells by a mechanism involving calcium/calmodulin pathway, *Biochem Biophys Res Comm* 237:225-229, 1997.

This basic science study evaluated the effect of capacitively coupled electrical stimulation on osteoblast cell cultures. The authors found that the stimulation leads to an increase in transforming growth factor B1, TGF-B1, mRNA, and subsequently an increase in TGF-B1 activity. Increased cell proliferation was also noted. Using various techniques it was discovered that the cytosolic calcium-activated calmodulin-axis plays a major role in the signal transduction of an electrical signal into increased osteoblast proliferation through a calmodulin-dependent pathway. Although the increase in TGF-B1 was noted, the authors are still not sure what effect this has on the osseous repair process and further research is needed to elucidate the mechanisms by which external stimuli enhance healing.

25. Scott G, King JB: A prospective, double-blind trial of electrical capacitive coupling in the treatment of non-union of long bones, *J Bone Joint Surg Am* 76:820-826, 1994.

This is a well-done prospective, blinded study that demonstrates the effectiveness of external electrical stimulation in the treatment of long-standing nonunions of long bones. Nonunions were defined as fractures that had not healed at least 9 months after injury and that showed no signs of healing for at least 3 months before beginning treatment. Exclusion criteria included synovial pseudoarthrosis and gaps greater than 50% of the width of the bone at the location of the fracture. The same immobilization and weight-bearing status were continued after the electrical stimulation was initiated. The two groups were comparable. The mean duration of nonunion was 31 months for the active group and 26 months for the placebo group. In the active group 6 of 10 healed and in the placebo group 0 of 11 healed.

26. Pilla AA: Low-intensity electromagnetic and mechanical modulation of bone growth and repair: are they equivalent? *J Orthop Sci* 7:420-428, 2002.

The author compared electromagnetic stimulation, ultrasound (US), and strain-generated potentials (SGP) in a rabbit fibular osteotomy model. The study shows that the primary messenger affecting cellular activity is the time varying electric field produced by these external stimuli. The different methods of electrical bone growth stimulation include capacitive coupling, direct current, pulsed electromagnetic fields (PEMF), and combined magnetic fields (CMF). The study demonstrates that the electrically and mechanically (US and SGP) induced electric fields have common waveform characteristics at the treatment site and deliver similar doses of electrical stimulation. Thus the different types of bone growth stimulators all share a common pathway to enhance osseous healing.

Index

Page numbers followed by *f* denotes figures; *b* denotes boxes; and *t* denotes tables.